Third Edition

Essentials of Nursing

a medical-surgical text for practical nurses

CLAIRE BRACKMAN KEANE, R.N., B.S.

Formerly Director, Athens General Hospital School
of Practical Nursing, and Clinical Instructor, Athens
School of Practical Nursing, Athens, Georgia; Formerly
Director of Nursing Education and Instructor in Medical-Surgical
Nursing, Grady Memorial Hospital School of Nursing, Atlanta, Georgia

W. B. SAUNDERS COMPANY · Philadelphia · London · Toronto

W. B. Saunders Company: West Washington Square
Philadelphia, PA 19105

12 Dyott Street
London, WC1A 1DB

833 Oxford Street
Toronto, Ontario M8Z 5T9, Canada

Essentials of Nursing   ISBN   0-7216-5312-X

Last digit is the print number: 9   8   7   6   5   4   3   2

Love your patient,
not for what you can help him to be,
but for what he is.
With mutual respect and trust
you can both become something better.

PREFACE

PREFACE

The decade that has passed since the first edition of this text was written has reminded all of us that nothing is so constant as change. Every segment of our society has felt in some way the impact of the social and cultural revolution that has been the hallmark of the sixties and seventies. Nursing, as part of the health care delivery system, has been forced to take a new look at its values, attitudes and knowledge and to appraise them in terms of relevancy and immediacy. It is hoped that the revisions that have been made and the material included in this third edition will not disappoint those who expect to find in its pages information that is relevant and useful.

It is a healthy sign of growth and maturity in the field of nursing that we are looking to the patient, the consumer if you will, for assistance in defining the role of the nurse and determining the direction nursing should take to serve the health needs of our communities. For this reason, Chapter 1 has been revised to include the expectations patients have of nurses and the needs they feel should be met by nursing. This chapter also considers the health-illness continuum and its meaning to nursing and the community. Chapters 2, 3, 4, 5 and 6 are intended to give the reader an orientation to and an overview of the causes, symptoms and diagnosis of medical-surgical disorders and their implications for nursing. Chapters 7 and 8, which were originally one chapter, have been rewritten to include all aspects of the continued and coordinated care of the aged and chronically ill. An attempt was made to develop in the reader empathy with the aged and the disabled and an understanding of the problems one must face when one is old or chronically disabled.

The remaining chapters deal with more specific conditions of illness and the patient needs created by these conditions. The preventive aspects of health care and patient teaching are woven throughout the text. An effort was made to update the written text, illustrations and suggested student reading lists. The rapidly increasing amount of information available and required as reading for student and graduate nurses demands familiarity with a variety of resource materials and references for more in-depth study. Hopefully their exposure to additional information will develop in them the habit of continued reading and study throughout their nursing careers. It is to this end that the suggested reading lists are included in the text. Many instructors and students have expressed satisfaction with the clinical case problems and outlines at the end of each chapter, so these have remained as part of the third edition.

The author is indebted to the many instructors, students and interested persons who have taken the time to offer comments, criticisms and suggestions for improvement of the text. Decisions that must be made regarding deletions and additions during revision are never lightly made, but with the help of others, the task is always easier.

CLAIRE B. KEANE

CONTENTS

Breast exam 444

1

Introduction To Nursing Conditions Of Illness

VOCABULARY

Anxiety
Assess
Bizarre
Continuum
Criterion
Fantasies
Reciprocity

THE NURSE AND HER PATIENT

Of all the principles and practices that a student nurse must learn as she begins her career in nursing, and all that she continues to learn throughout her life, the most important are those that relate to the personal relationship that exists between a nurse and her patient. Each patient can teach her something new about herself and strengthen her commitment to the service of others. But how does one go about building a satisfactory relationship between the helper and the helped so that together they will grow and develop into something better? What does the nurse know and do that sets her apart from others and makes her relationship with a patient different from other experiences in her life and the patient's?

Virginia Henderson, a noted leader and educator in nursing, has written: "The unique function of the nurse is to assist the individual, sick or well, in the performance of those activities contributing to health or its recovery (or to peaceful death) that he would perform unaided if he had the necessary strength, will or knowledge. And to do this in such a way as to help him gain independence as rapidly as possible."[4]

The nurse therefore does for another person those things he cannot do for himself to prevent illness and, if illness occurs, to help him regain his independence insofar as it is possible for him to do so. She has something unique to give because she gives her *self,* her own individuality. Margaret Colliton asks, "What is the use of self in clinical practice but being willing to accept the risks, face the uncertainties, take the good with the bad, and stick with the patient until he is on his own?"[2] And there are risks and uncertainties in nursing just as there are in any other experience of life. There are, however, some things we can learn about nursing that will help us become more effective helpers and will relieve

1

some of the uncertainties involved in the nurse-patient relationship.

We can find some answers to our questions about satisfying a patient's needs by asking the patients themselves what they want from nursing. The findings of surveys and studies indicate that patients can be very definite and clear about what they want. First, *the patient wants to be treated as an individual*. This means that he wants to be called by name, not by room number or diagnosis. He wants to be a person, not a case study or a locality. He resents having someone talk *about* him rather than *to* him in his presence, as if he were another piece of furniture or machinery in his room. To talk about a person rather than to him is dehumanizing and renders him a nonperson.

Second, *he wants to be given an explanation of his care*. He wants to know what is going to be done to him, why it is being done and what he is expected to do before, during and after the procedure. He also wants the explanation given to him in language he can understand. Imagine, if you will, a formerly healthy and active person's reaction to being placed in a situation in which everyone is busily working, using words and initials that might as well be in a foreign tongue and showing precious little interest in him beyond their dedication to administering medications and performing treatments. He is stripped of his usual attire and given a hospital gown to wear. Someone walks into his room (she hasn't told him *her* name), removes his water pitcher and glass and places a sign over his bed. The sign reads N.P.O., and when he asks the meaning of the letters, he is told, "You're having a G.I. series in the morning." Now, few of us would settle comfortably in our beds and have a good night's sleep after this experience. We surely could not feel secure in the knowledge that we were in the hands of people sincerely interested in us as human beings with our own personal fears and anxieties.

There will be times when the nurse will not know the answers to all of her patient's questions. She cannot speak for the physician or other members of the health team. Unfortunately, we must still live with the fact that various health professionals and paramedicals involved in the care of a patient frequently do not communicate with one another as often or as effectively as they should. Many times the patient suffers because the right hand has not been told exactly what the left hand is doing. This places a limit on the information a nurse may be able to communicate to her patient. It is not, however, an excuse for ignoring his anxiety. He has a right to know what diagnostic and therapeutic procedures are planned for him. The nurse may be limited in the information she can give him, but she is never limited in the interest and compassion that she can show.

A third wish of patients is closely related to the first and second; that is, *the patient would like to be considered a partner in his care*. He doesn't want people doing things *for* him and *to* him without consulting him on the matter or considering the fact that whatever is being done is extremely important to him and his future. We often ask a patient to cooperate without understanding the true meaning of that word. "Cooperate" means "working with." It means giving the patient an opportunity to have some control over the things that are happening to him.

Fourth, but no less important, is *the patient's desire to have his behavior accepted as part of his illness* and not necessarily typical of the way he might react under more normal circumstances. This requires kindness, understanding and quite often firmness on the part of the nurse. People often become childlike and fearful when they become ill, and they appreciate having someone with them who can guide them through their ordeal in a gentle and kind manner. If there appears to be some correlation between nursing and "mothering" here, that is because there is a similarity and patients recognize it. Just as a child wants his mother to be near when he is ill and frightened, patients want to know that a nurse will be there' when needed. Beland tells us of a group of patients who requested that a nurse not be transferred from night duty because they could depend on her being there when they needed her.[1] We leave it to the reader to decide how well that nurse fulfilled her role and lived up to the expectation of her patients.

Up to this point we have emphasized attitudes and skills related to feeling and doing. Of course there is more to nursing than this. Patients also have expectations about what the nurse knows and how she uses that knowledge to help them. They want a nurse to know what she is doing and to act like she knows what to do. They expect her to have the necessary equipment at hand before she begins a procedure, to know how to use it and to perform repeated procedures in the same way as far as possible under the circumstances.

Finally, and perhaps most important to a patient's feeling of security and confidence in the nurse, is her ability to assess a situation quickly, make a decision and promptly set about doing something to solve the problem. This ability implies a thorough knowledge of the patient as a person, an understanding of his illness and how it is affecting him, the plan of treatment set up for him by his physician and the results expected from the plan. These are the essentials of nursing, the knowledge that is basic to all aspects of nursing care.

NEEDS CREATED BY ILLNESS

Concepts of Health and Illness

All of us react to events in our lives in our own special ways. Illness is an event that can have a severe and permanent effect—even to the point of death—or it can be a relatively minor occurrence that interferes only slightly with the activities of daily life. Between these two extremes are varying degrees of well-being (see Fig. 1–1). It is important for the nurse to realize that

THE HEALTH CONTINUUM

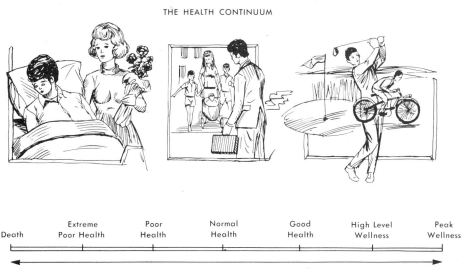

| Death | Extreme Poor Health | Poor Health | Normal Health | Good Health | High Level Wellness | Peak Wellness |

Figure 1–1. Health may be viewed as a continuum that ranges from extreme states of ill health to peak wellness. (From Du Gas: *Kozier-Du Gas' Introduction to Patient Care,* 2nd Ed., W. B. Saunders Co., Philadelphia.)

many factors enter into the health-illness continuum. It is never a static situation and depends on whether a person sees himself as ill or well, how society views health versus sickness and the age of the person involved.

A person's judgment about whether he is sick or well can directly affect the way in which he avoids illness or accepts and responds to treatment and nursing care when he does become ill. His attitudes toward his state of health can also influence how well he maintains his health and utilizes community resources to avoid illness. People generally judge their position on the health-illness scale on the basis of three criteria: (1) The presence or absence of symptoms. Pain, bleeding or breathing difficulties are examples of the kinds of things a person feels or sees about himself that tell him he is not well. (2) The way in which he feels in general. He may have some vague impression that he is not well and that for some reason he feels "sickly." (3) His ability to continue his day-to-day life at home and at work. Of course, attitudes toward work and home life can affect his ability to do this. One person may not feel well enough to go to work but he may feel able to mow the lawn or do the family laundry. On the other hand, another person's home situation may be so unpleasant that he leaves home to go to work and then checks into the employee health clinic for a rest or lounges around on the job all day.[3]

We can see, therefore, that many situations in the patient's environment as well as his internal physical and emotional make-up can affect his attitudes toward his physical well-being. These factors are important to an understanding of the ways in which illness can affect an individual and the needs that can be brought about by his illness (see Fig. 1–2).

Physiologic Needs. The physical needs of the person who is ill are essentially the same as those of the well person. The difference lies in the ill person's physical and mental ability to meet those needs. Everyone has a need for adequate exchange of oxygen and carbon dioxide, good nutrition, proper elimination, adequate physical activity and the host of other general functions performed by the systems of the body.

The nurse who wishes to meet the physiologic needs of her patient will first evaluate his condition and determine which of these needs can be met by the patient alone, which he can maintain only with her assistance and which will require attention beyond the scope of nursing. A patient who is having difficulty breathing may need only a change of his position to meet his needs for respiration. He may require administration of additional oxygen to insure adequate oxygenation of

PERSONAL FACTORS

Age
Personality
Emotional stability
Religious and spiritual
  values
Role in the family
Standing in the community
General state of health
  prior to present illness
Concept of health and
  illness

♦ PATIENT ♦

ENVIRONMENTAL FACTORS

Cultural background
Past experiences with
  illness in others close
  to him
Knowledge of modern medicine
  and methods of treatment
Community in which he lives
Available sources of health
  care
Physical environment at
  home and at work

Figure 1–2. Factors affecting a person's attitudes toward his physical and mental well-being and his reactions to illness.

his blood to meet the needs of the tissues for oxygen. If he has a respiratory tract obstruction that cannot be removed by nursing measures, it may be necessary for the surgeon to perform a tracheostomy and to insert a tube attached to a respirator to maintain adequate respiration for the patient. Between these two extremes the nurse will find that her patients depend on her to varying degrees.

If the plan of medical treatment for a patient is successful, and if nursing care provides for his physical needs as they arise, the goal of restoring the patient to a state of independence in which he can meet his own physical needs has been reached.

Psychosocial Needs. In the introductory section of this chapter we reviewed some of the things patients expect and want to receive from nurses. Almost all these expectations center upon the patient's feelings and attitudes toward his nurse and her personal relationship with him. These feelings and attitudes are directly related to meeting a person's psychologic and social needs when he is ill. All people have in common some basic emotional and social needs that affect every aspect of their lives. The words we use to express these needs and the ways in which they are satisfied are words that convey feelings of love, security, trust, confidence, respect and acceptance. Everyone needs to feel good about himself, to know that others understand him and his feelings and that they respect him as someone who is worthwhile.

When a person becomes ill, he often has difficulty controlling his emotions, and he becomes more sensitive to the words and actions of others. He is placed in a position of dependence that is often difficult to accept. He loses control over many of the things that are happening to him, and he becomes fearful, anxious about himself, depressed and sometimes hostile and bitter about his situation.

Nurses are frequently told that they must give "emotional support" to their patients and that they must "reassure" them that there is no need for worry and anxiety. These vague directions may be useful to the nurse as long as she knows how to determine whether a patient is suffering from anxiety and, if the patient does feel threatened by a situation, how she can relieve his anxiety.

We have all been fearful about a new and different or unknown situation in our lives. Our hands begin to perspire and we feel our pulses throbbing, our hearts pounding. Perhaps we talk faster, louder or in a higher pitch than normal, or we stutter and cannot think clearly. Among us are the floor-pacers, the nail-biters and the tabletop-drummers. If the reader will consider what she might do when she is anxious or if she will look at herself and her classmates just before and during an important written examination, the morning of the first day on duty or even the first day in class together, she will have a good picture of the signs and symptoms of anxiety.

What are some things a nurse can do to relieve a patient's anxiety? Du Gas suggests that, although the particular needs of the patient will be met on an individual basis, there are some guiding principles that may be helpful.[3]

First, _it is easier to relieve anxiety when we know what is causing it._ This means that the patient should be given an opportunity to talk about what is worrying him or what he is afraid of. It does not mean that the nurse pries into his personal life or practices amateur psychotherapy. She simply listens when the patient wants to talk and lets him know that she is interested in helping him.

Second, _people feel less anxious when they know what is going to happen to them and that whatever happens they are in good hands._ This is simply another way of looking at the previously discussed expectations that patients have of nurses. They want to be told what is going to happen to them, and if they are told in a manner that they can understand, much of their anxiety and fear can be eliminated. The success of this second point, however, depends on the nurse's honesty and the patient's trust in her honesty.

Third, *loneliness and loss of control of the situation aggravate a patient's anxiety* and give him the impression that things are much worse than they really are. Why else would everyone ignore him and avoid his questions, if not because they are afraid to tell him the awful truth? Why can he not have some voice in when he eats and bathes and whether he stays in bed or walks down the hall, if not because he is much sicker than anyone dares to admit to him? If these seem to be ridiculous fantasies that are not very likely to cross an average patient's mind, just ask a friend or relative who has been hospitalized for a period of time about the thoughts that went through his mind when he was alone and was not sure exactly what was happening around him and to him.

In meeting the psychosocial needs of the patient, we listen to what patients tell us they want from nurses and we continue to listen to each patient in order to be better able to give him emotional support that is meaningful and helpful to him as an individual.

Gertrude Ujhely, an expert psychiatric nurse, writes that nurses on a medical-surgical service in a general hospital can and must provide some emotional support to their patients. She tells us that "usually, as the nurse listens, the patient will develop in front of her eyes three kinds of themes: the content theme (the "what" of his story), the mood theme (how he tells his story), and the interaction theme (the way he relates to the nurse and, by reciprocity, sets up how he would like her to relate to him."[8]

Nurses who have not had opportunities to practice the techniques of giving encouragement and emotional support should not be discouraged. Even the most experienced nurse may encounter a situation that is unlike any she has ever experienced before. The most important point to remember is that no two patients are alike and that the more a nurse knows about her patient, and the more she listens to what he has to say, the easier it will be to give him the individualized emotional support that he needs.

We cannot ignore the fact that nurses themselves are human and that they will experience emotional reactions and feelings toward their patients. Some may not be pleasant reactions. The nurse is entitled to have feelings toward a patient, regardless of their nature. But she is not entitled to express those feelings openly in his presence.[8] She cannot use her position as a weapon to remind the patient who is in charge or who is the stronger of the two. Remember, he has enough problems trying to salvage some kind of control over his life, and he needs to be accepted as he is, without fear of reprimand or ridicule.

EFFECTS OF ILLNESS ON THE FAMILY

No normal, emotionally stable person wants to be ill. It is a great inconvenience to him and also affects those who know and love him. The family, friends and other social groups can, in turn, have a deep and lasting effect on the success of medical treatment and the restoration of the patient to his former status, or at least to an acceptable way of life.

The inconveniences and hardships imposed on the family by an illness will depend to some extent on the patient's place in the household. If it is the father and family wage-earner who is ill, or the mother on whom the family depends for making the house into a home, everyone in the family group will be greatly inconvenienced. The person who is ill may worry and become upset because he can no longer assume responsibilities for the family and arrangements must be made for someone else to take over his former duties. This may be a temporary or a permanent arrangement, depending on the type of illness and whether or not the patient will be able to resume his former activities. Whatever the case, definite and practical plans must be made to keep the family together. Juvenile delinquency, overdependence on welfare agencies and other socioeconomic problems can grow out of a disturbance in the family life.

Illness within the family will usually make the ties stronger or weaker. A family that is closely knit will most likely draw still closer together and work together for the good of all. A family group that has always been at odds with one another and unable to work together will probably drift even farther apart under the pressures of misfortune. There are exceptions, of course, but the general rule is that additional problems most often aggravate a situation rather than minimize the problems already existing.

Illness and disability create needs for the family members just as they do for the patient. Family members often feel guilt because the patient has been hospitalized, viewing the transfer of care from the home to the hospital as a sign of their failure to give adequate care to the patient. Others may feel a great sense of relief that they have placed the patient in the hands of others who are more competent than they in the care of the patient. Some family members may be resentful of the inconvenience the patient's illness has caused. The family, whatever their feelings, need an opportunity to express their feelings and to obtain advice and assistance in coping with the problems brought about by illness.

In the past nurses have too often considered relatives of the patient a nuisance and an unnecessary complicating factor in patient care. Visiting hours were severely limited (and in some cases still are) and when the family was allowed into the hospital they came only as observers. Today we recognize the need to include family members as participants in the care of the patient, particularly in cases of long-term illness in which the goal is the patient's eventual return to his home, where much of his care will be the responsibility of the family. The recognition of this goal means that we are beginning to see the family and community as an extension of the patient and his needs. We must determine the needs of the patient and his family in the light of what they should know and be able to do to participate effectively in the rehabilitation of the patient. (See Chapter 8 for further discussion of rehabilitation.)

HEALTH CARE IN THE COMMUNITY

Since the 1940's there has been general dissatisfaction with the traditional health care delivery system in this country and increasing pressure from individuals and groups to improve the system. We have become more aware of the fact that in the past good health care has not been available to everyone who needed it, and although we have provided "crisis" care in the treatment of disease and injury, we have to a large extent ignored disease prevention and health maintenance.

The 1960's and 1970's have seen a revolution in our health care programs. The traditional way is no longer satisfactory to the general public. There is a new way of looking at persons needing health care; they are now called *consumers* and *clients,* which implies that they have some voice in the kind of services provided for them. Health professionals are responding to the consumer demands in a number of ways. They are realizing that one of the best ways to provide health care is to go to the people needing their services. Large medical centers that have tried to be all things to all people are now giving way to small centers in the community. There are growing numbers of neighborhood health centers, community clinics and some home health services that go beyond the care provided by public health departments.

The nurse who wishes to help meet all the needs of the patient must begin to think of health care that extends beyond the walls of our traditional institutions. She needs to be aware of the many individuals and agencies that are available sources of help for the patient, and she must prepare herself to help patients utilize the community resources.

Each community is different and the kind of services provided today will not necessarily be the same tomorrow. We are living in a time of rapid change that affects every aspect of our lives. The nurse who wishes to give effective and coordinated care to her patients will recognize the need to keep abreast of these changes and to grow and develop within the new system of health care delivery.

CLINICAL CASE PROBLEMS

1. Miss Thomas is a practical nursing student who is assigned to the care of three patients from 7:00 A.M. to 11:00 A.M. She has been a student for three months and works under the direct supervision of her clinical instructor. When she receives her morning report at 7:00 A.M., Miss Thomas learns the following about her patients:

Mr. Allman, aged 35, sustained multiple and deep lacerations of the arms when he fell through a pane of glass while working at a construction site. He has been in the hospital for three days. He is very despondent because he cannot use his arms to care for himself and has been told that he will need extensive physical therapy before he regains full use of them.

Mrs. Smith, age 50, is scheduled for surgery at 8:00 A.M. She has been pre-

pared for surgery and has received all of the preoperative medications.

Mrs. Johnson, age 26, has undergone an appendectomy, is in her third postoperative day and is to be dismissed from the hospital today.

Identify the individual nursing needs of each of Miss Thomas's three patients.

How will Mr. Allman's injury affect his family, which consists of his wife, three small children and his mother, who lives with them?

Where might Mrs. Johnson find herself on the health-illness continuum if she has no other illnesses and considered herself healthy before surgery?

2. Mr. Muzak is a university professor who is admitted for diagnostic studies. His illness might possibly be quite serious, involving the nervous system and producing a variety of bizarre symptoms. He is very demanding and sarcastic to the nursing staff and frequently refuses medication and other forms of treatment, stating, "No one around here knows what she is doing, and I refuse to allow you to practice on me."

Can you think of some possible reasons for Mr. Muzak's behavior?

What might be done to relieve some of Mr. Muzak's anxiety?

REFERENCES

1. Beland, I. L.: *Clinical Nursing: Pathophysiological and Psychosocial Approaches,* 2nd edition. New York, The Macmillan Co., 1970.
2. Colliton, M. A.: "Foreword: Symposium on the Use of Self in Clinical Practice." *Nurs. Clin. N. Amer.,* Vol. 6, No. 4., 1971, p. 691.
3. Du Gas, B. W.: *Kozier-Du Gas' Introduction to Patient Care,* 2nd edition. Philadelphia, W. B. Saunders Co., 1972.
4. Henderson, V.: "The Nature of Nursing." Am. Journ. Nurs., Aug., 1964, p. 62.
5. Popiel, E. S.: "We're Headed for Hospitals Without Walls." Nursing '72, April, p. 4.

6. Shafer, K. N., et al.: *Medical-Surgical Nursing,* 5th edition. St. Louis, The C. V. Mosby Co., 1971.
7. Sorenson, G. S.: "Dependency — A Factor in Nursing Care." Am. Journ. Nurs., Aug., 1966, p. 1761.
8. Ujhely, G.: "What Is Realistic Emotional Support?" Am. Journ. Nurs., April, 1968, p. 758.

SUGGESTED STUDENT READING

1. Babcock, C. G.: "Stress and Illness." Journ. Pract. Nurs., May, 1962, p. 16, and June, 1962, p. 18.
2. Boulette, T. R.: "Anxiety and the Nurse." Journ. Pract. Nurs., Aug., 1967, p. 28.
3. Dennis, R. J.: "Ways of Caring." Am. Journ. Nurs., Feb., 1964, p. 107.
4. Drummond, E. E.: "Impact of a Father's Illness." Am. Journ. Nurs., Aug., 1964, p. 89.
5. Francis, G.: "How Do I Feel About Myself?" Am. Journ. Nurs., June, 1967, p. 1244.
6. Robinson, A. M.: "Anxiety, Apprehension, and Fear." Journ. Pract. Nurs., June, 1971, p. 20.
7. Robinson, A. M.: "Anger." Journ. Pract. Nurs., July, 1971, p. 14.

OUTLINE FOR CHAPTER 1

I. The Nurse and Her Patient

A. The nurse does for her patient those things he cannot do for himself to prevent illness, and if illness occurs, to help him recover.

B. Patients have definite ideas about what they want from nursing. Patients want:

    1. to know what is happening.
    2. to be treated as individuals and as partners in their own care.
    3. to be accepted.
    4. to be cared for by a nurse who knows what she is doing and acts like she knows.

II. Needs Created by Illness

A. Concepts of health and illness—a continuum.

    1. One judges himself to be ill or well by the presence or absence of symptoms, how he feels in general and his ability to continue daily activities of life.
    2. One's attitudes toward his state of health can influence his well-being.

B. Physiologic Needs—essentially the same as for well person. Difference lies in patient's ability to meet his physical needs.

    1. Dependence of patient varies according to his individual situation.
    2. Goal is met when patient is restored to a state of independence.

C. Psychosocial Needs—illness poses a situation in which the patient loses some control over what is happening to him.

    1. Anxiety frequently accompanies illness.
    2. Symptoms of anxiety familiar to all of us.
    3. Needs should be met according to cause of anxiety.
    4. Nurse can give realistic emotional support.
    5. Family needs also must be considered.

III. Health Care in the Community

A. Health care system in this country is rapidly changing.

B. "Clients" or "consumers" will have a voice in the kinds of care they will receive.

2.

Causes of Disease and the Body's Response to Injury

INTRODUCTION

The human body is a very complex organism that must work constantly to maintain the delicate balance needed for normal function of the millions of cells of which it is composed. Each of these cells is itself in a constant state of change, absorbing nutrients, excreting wastes and adapting chemically and physically to the many stresses that are present in the cell's ever-changing environment. The human body must also continually adapt to its external environment and to the changes taking place internally.

The pathologist views disease on a cellular level; that is, he recognizes disease or illness as being a condition in which some of the body cells are seriously injured. These injured cells must adapt to the changes brought about by the injury or they will eventu-

ally die. If the cells can recover, then the patient recovers, but if the cells die and there are so many of them destroyed that one or more of the essential organs in the body cannot function, the patient succumbs.

There are many possible causes of cell injury and death. Some causes may be very obvious, as, for example, a severe chemical burn in which the cells of external organs or perhaps internal digestive organs are severely damaged. Other causes of cellular injury such as those that involve hormonal imbalance or deficiency may not be as obvious and may cause subtle changes in cells for a period of time before the patient begins to exhibit outward symptoms of a disease.

It is possible to categorize the causes of disease and injury in a number of different ways, but since we are concerned with disease prevention and health maintenance as well as treatment of illness and injury, it might be well to consider the factors that can interfere with normal *cellular* function. In this way we are able to gain an understanding of how disease occurs and how it might be prevented, or, if prevention is not possible, how disease can be recognized in its earliest stages before it causes irreversible damage or death.

Generally the factors that can interfere with normal cellular function include (1) inadequate oxygen supply (*anoxia*), (2) physical injury, (3) chemical injury, (4) genetic defects, (5) nutritional imbalance, (6) aging, (7) neoplasms, (8) disorders of immunity and (9) biologic agents.[6] Another factor that is less clearly understood but nonetheless important is that of emotions and their physical effects on the body.

OXYGEN DEFICIENCY

An adequate oxygen supply is essential to the normal functioning of all cells. Some tissues of the body are more sensitive to anoxia than others. Brain cells, for example, cannot survive more than four to six minutes without oxygen; after that period of time they are damaged beyond repair. Cells of other types of tissues can survive without oxygen for slightly longer periods of time, but eventually these cells also will be irreversibly damaged.

All cells receive their oxygen supply via the blood. It follows that disorders which interfere with the flow of blood will result in cellular anoxia. These disorders include blood clots within the arteries or veins which slow down or completely stop the flow of blood through the vessels, and arteriosclerosis and atherosclerosis, which narrow the lumen of the arteries and interfere with the flow of blood. A heart attack (coronary occlusion) or a stroke (cerebrovascular accident) are examples of disorders in which the interruption of the flow of blood results in

cellular anoxia. In a heart attack, the blood supply to the heart muscle is obstructed. In the case of stroke, the brain cells are denied an adequate oxygen supply because of damage to one or more of the cerebral blood vessels.

We know the red blood cells carry oxygen to the various cells of the body. If, as in anemia, there are insufficient numbers of red blood cells, or if they are unable to perform their normal functions, the body tissues will suffer from a deficiency of oxygen.

Another possible cause of cellular anoxia is inadequate intake of oxygen into the lungs. If there is obstruction of the air passages or damage to the cells of the lung where oxygen passes from the exhaled air into the red blood cells, the cells will not have oxygen available to be transported to the body cells.

Cells, and eventually tissues, that are deprived of sufficient oxygen will undergo two kinds of changes. The cells will first begin to swell as they fill with water, and their membranes will be damaged. If this swelling continues, the substance of the cell body will undergo chemical changes that eventually completely destroy the cell.

PHYSICAL INJURIES

Physical injury such as that caused by a severe blow to or penetration of the body tissues is called physical *trauma*. Traumatic injury can also occur as a result of extremes of heat and cold, as in frostbite or thermal burns. Another type of physical injury is caused by electrical energy which produces burns and also profound shock. Radiation injury can result from ultraviolet rays from the sun, x-rays from high voltage x-ray machines and emissions from radioactive products. (For further discussion of radiation, see Chapter 10.)

CHEMICAL INJURIES

We are all familiar with at least a few of the many chemicals around our homes or at work that can seriously damage cells and tissues. Many of the chemical agents in our kitchens and laundry rooms have killed or injured far too many children who have accidentally swallowed them. We must also realize, however, that such apparently harmless substances as salt and glucose can cause severe injury or death to the cells if used improperly in highly concentrated solutions. Several years ago infants in a newborn nursery died as a result of an accident in which the nurse preparing the infants' formulas used salt instead of granulated sugar. In the April edition of *Nursing '72*, we are warned of the danger of using more than the prescribed amount of soap when preparing a soapsuds enema.

There is still much to be learned about the ways in which chemicals affect the body cells. We still do not know exactly how specific chemical agents act and we cannot assume that those that we use every day are completely harmless. Nurses, who use a wide variety of chemicals in carrying out routine nursing procedures, must be alert to possible dangers. We cannot allow familiarity with the use of chemicals to lull us into carelessness in measuring proper amounts and reading labels when preparing solutions.

Drugs present a relatively new hazard to health and are a rapidly growing cause of illness. We are not referring to drug abuse, which in itself is a serious health problem in this country, but to drug reactions and interactions. Modern research in pharmacology has provided an abundance of new drugs for combating illness. These discoveries are a mixed blessing, however. It is estimated that 3 to 5 per cent of all patients admitted to hospitals are suffering primarily from a drug reaction and that 30 per cent of these patients experience a second reaction during their hospital stay.

A disorder that is produced inadvertently as a result of treatment for some other disorder is called an *iatro-genic* disorder. Drug reactions can be classified as iatrogenic disorders. We must remember that drugs are toxic agents; the same drug that causes no difficulty in one patient may trigger a serious reaction in another. A drug may also cause side effects that may be relatively minor in one patient and extremely serious in another. The steroids, so valuable in the treatment of many types of inflammatory diseases, can cause serious loss of sodium and potassium. Sulfonamide administration can result in an extremely low blood sugar level. These are only a few examples of drug reactions. Of course the nurse does not prescribe medications, but she should be aware of the fact that drugs are toxic and can cause injury to the cells. She should also be alert for signs of allergic idiosyncratic reactions to drugs, and to report signs and symptoms of these conditions as soon as they are observed in a patient.

GENETIC DISORDERS

Genetic disorders are physical and mental defects that are transmitted through the genes. Genes are units of heredity; they transmit the physical, biochemical and physiological traits that children inherit from their parents. Genetic disorders may or may not be apparent at the time of birth, and they need not be present in the parents of the child who has inherited the disorder. Diseases that are a result of genetic disorders include *sickle cell anemia, thalassemia* and other blood dyscrasias resulting from abnormalities in hemoglobin.

Some genetic disorders are inborn errors of metabolism in which there may be faulty or incomplete metabolism of carbohydrates, proteins or fats. Metabolism is the sum of all the physical and chemical processes taking place in the body, and there are many individual steps involved in these processes. The absence of a necessary enzyme can lead to a metabolic "block" which then results in the accumulation of products formed part of the way through the metabolic process; or there may be a deficiency of a product that is normally found in the series of metabolic reactions. *Galactosemia* and *phenylketonuria* (**PKU**) are examples of inborn errors of metabolism. In galactosemia there is a lack of the enzyme necessary for proper metabolism of galactose (a sugar). This enzyme would normally change galactose, which cannot be utilized by the body, into glucose, which can be used. Since the galactose cannot be metabolized, it accumulates in the blood. In **PKU** there is a disturbance in the metabolism of an amino acid (phenylalanine). This results in the lack of a substance necessary for producing the hormones adrenalin and thyroxin. A deficiency of these hormones leads to severe mental retardation unless the condition is detected early in the infant's life and corrected.

In some genetic disorders there is an imbalance of genetic material; for example, there may be too many or too few chromosomes. Such imbalances can lead to severe mental and physical defects. *Down's syndrome* (mongolism) is an example of this type of genetic disorder. The infant with Down's syndrome has 47 chromosomes instead of the normal 46.

Research into genetic disorders and an increasing awareness of the importance of early diagnosis and treatment have greatly improved the prognosis and reduced the danger of permanent disability from such defects.

Congenital defects are sometimes confused with genetic disorders. The two terms are not synonymous. The word *congenital* simply means that the defect is one that has resulted from an abnormal development during fetal life and is apparent at birth or immediately after. Not all congenital disorders are hereditary. They may be acquired during fetal life, as in the case of congenital syphilis, which the fetus ac-

quires from its mother. In maternal measles, the development of the fetus is affected by the measles virus that has infected the mother. Rubella (German measles) during the first three months of pregnancy can cause a defect in the structure of the infant's heart and a variety of other defects, including deafness. In either case the congenital disorder is not in any way related to the genetic make-up of the infant.

NUTRITIONAL IMBALANCE

The disorders of this type include the vitamin deficiency diseases and severe protein-calorie deficiencies. In many parts of the world where hunger is a part of everyday life, these disorders are still major health problems, but in the developed countries of the world, we are now faced with cellular injury resulting from excessive intake of food. Obesity, for example, is a disorder that, aside from the emotional and social problems it presents, also can lead to heart disease, aggravate arthritis and impede circulation.

Other types of disorders that fall into the category of nutritional imbalance are those that result from improper storage of nutrients or inadequate utilization of these food elements. For example, glycogen storage can be hampered by disorders of the liver, and iron cannot be utilized in pernicious anemia.

AGING

Although we consider cell deterioration a natural consequence of growing old, there are many unknown factors involved in these physiologic changes. We accept these changes as a "normal abnormality," but we cannot explain exactly why they take place and why some individuals age more rapidly than others. We do not know why some races and ethnic groups have a longer life span than others. Today there is increasing interest in the study of the aging process. Some experts predict that by the end of this century we will be able to forestall some of the deterioration that we now consider the inevitable consequence of growing older. The aging process and nursing implications are discussed in more detail in Chapter 7.

NEOPLASMS

A neoplasm is literally a *new growth.* Frequently the word "tumor" is used to describe a neoplasm, even though it is not a true description. "Tumor" simply means "a swelling." It does not necessarily mean the development of new cells. The new cells in a neoplasm do not behave as normal cells do; they serve no purpose and become troublesome when they interfere with the functions of normal tissues. A neoplasm may be benign or malignant. *Benign neoplasms,* as the name implies, do not wreak as much havoc as malignant ones, but they should never be thought of as completely harmless. They may develop into malignant growths or grow so large that they cause damage to nearby tissues and organs.

Malignant growths are referred to as *cancerous.* The cells of a malignant growth interfere with and sometimes destroy the cells of normal tissue; they use up essential nutrients intended for the normal cells and usually multiply and spread rapidly. This spreading of the malignant cells to other parts of the body from their original site is called *metastasis.*

Neoplasms may also be classified according to their origin. Those which include new growth of bone, fat, blood vessels or lymphatic tissue are said to be of *mesenchymal* origin and are called *sarcomas.* Epithelial neoplasms arise from the coverings of the internal and external surfaces of the body, such as the skin and mucous membranes. The term *carcinoma* refers to malig-

nant tumors of this type. Neoplasms that contain more than one type of tissue are called *teratomas.* These are mixed tumors that represent all three germ layers of the body tissues and often show attempts at organ formation. Malignancy is discussed in more detail in Chapter 10.

DISORDERS OF IMMUNITY

The immune system of the body is essential to the body's defenses against invasion by foreign agents such as bacteria and other proteins. The system functions as a defense mechanism whereby lymphoid tissues and reticuloendothelial cells react to foreign substances entering the body by producing antibodies specifically designed to destroy the foreign agents. An understanding of the immune system, especially the antigen-antibody reaction, is preliminary to a discussion of disorders of immunity.

Antigen-Antibody Reaction

The term *antigen* refers to any substance that can generate or stimulate the production of antibodies. *Antibodies* are specific proteins which act against the antigens, causing their neutralization. When we say that the antibodies are specific, we mean that those which are produced to destroy a particular type of antigen will affect only that type of antigen and no other. It is for this reason that immunity toward measles, for example, will not provide immunity for chickenpox or any other type of viral infection.

Antigens that are important to the health of man are usually proteins. For example, bacteria and viruses are mainly protein, as are the toxins they produce. Other antigens that can stimulate the production of antibodies include all the proteins and some of the polysaccharides (sugars) in nature, all of which can be interpreted by the body as foreign agents to be rejected. It is apparent, therefore, that the antigen-antibody reaction is very beneficial when one is exposed to bacteria and other harmful substances. But when the body interprets a useful protein such as milk or even a transplanted organ as a harmful foreign agent and reacts by setting up a mechanism to reject the protein, the antigen-antibody reaction can create problems.

The immune system is an automatic response, but where do the antibodies come from and how do they destroy or neutralize the antigens? Almost all antibodies are formed in the lymph nodes, spleen, bone marrow and lymphoid tissue of the gastrointestinal tract. As soon as the antigens enter the body, the plasma cells of these tissues and organs begin to multiply very rapidly, thus increasing the production of antibodies. This is an *immediate response* in which the antibodies that react with the invading antigens are released in the plasma. Another type, called the *delayed response,* involves an apparent involvement of the cells from the lymphoid tissues; that is, the lymph cells themselves also react with the antigens and destroy them.

The antibodies that are produced in the immediate response act in a number of ways to neutralize the antigens. If the antigen is a toxin, or poisonous substance from bacteria, the antibody produced is an *antitoxin* that is capable of chemically neutralizing the toxin. Other antibodies combine with their specific antigens, causing their precipitation and rendering them ineffective. These antibodies are called *precipitins.* Some antibodies (called *agglutinins*) attach themselves to the surface of the antigens, causing them to clump together (agglutinate) and assume a heavy, nonaggressive aggregate form, thereby rendering them harmless. We know that red blood cells will agglutinate when exposed to other red blood cells of a different blood type. This is the basis of a blood transfusion reaction and is the result of antibodies present on the surface of the red blood cells of the person receiving the transfusion.

Another means by which antibodies destroy antigens is by causing *cellular lysis.* In this situation the antibodies (called *lysins*), with the help of a substance in the plasma that is called *complement,* react with the membrane of the antigen cell and cause the cell to rupture. *Opsonins* are antibodies which affect the membrane of the antigen cell so that it can be more easily engulfed and ingested by the *phagocytes* (to be discussed later).

Immunity

The term *immunity* refers to security or insurance against a particular disease-producing organism or antigen. It is because of the antigen-antibody reaction that the human body is able to develop immunity for specific diseases. For reasons not yet fully understood, some diseases confer a lasting immunity while others, such as influenza and the common cold, do not. It is also true that certain body cells are immune to particular types of organisms, but if those organisms find their way to other parts of the body they will cause disease in those cells. There are some bacteria in the intestinal tract, for instance, which do no harm and are actually helpful in digestion. Yet they can cause serious infections if they get into the urinary tract.

Immunity is only a relative term. It may guarantee complete avoidance of a disease or it may simply lessen the severity of the disease when it occurs. It also varies with each individual because some of us are more proficient in our ability to manufacture antibodies than others.

Types of Immunity. There are three types of immunity: (1) natural, (2) active and (3) passive. They may be obtained in various ways and will offer varying degrees of safety from disease.

NATURAL IMMUNITY. This is an innate resistance to disease which some

TABLE 2–1. TYPES OF IMMUNITY

Natural	Species Race Sex Cell and tissue resistance Individual ability to manufacture immune bodies	
Active	1. An attack of the specific disease	
	2. Artificial means	a. Vaccines—weakened or harmless living organisms b. Bacterins—dead organisms c. Toxoids—modified toxins
Passive	1. To fetus from mother	
	2. Artificial means	a. Immune serum—contains ready-made antibodies: some also contain antitoxins b. Gamma globulin—contains antibodies

are fortunate enough to have simply because they are of a certain species, race, sex and constitution. The fact that we are human protects us from some diseases common to lower animals. Race, sex and our general state of physical and mental health also help us resist attacks from certain diseases.

ACTIVE IMMUNITY. Before vaccination and inoculation became commonplace, it was believed that the only way an individual could acquire immunity was to suffer an attack of the disease and through a strong constitution and good fortune manage to survive. Once he had survived this "trial by fire," he was immune and no longer needed to fear that particular disease.

Establishment of immunity artificially by vaccination became widely accepted through the efforts of an English country doctor, Edward Jenner. He had heard a milkmaid remark, "I cannot take the smallpox for I have already had the cowpox." Dr. Jenner knew that this was a common belief among his patients of that district and in 1796 he set about to prove the theory. He performed the first crude form of vaccination on an 8-year-old boy by scratching the surface of the boy's skin and rubbing in some purulent material from the sore of the hand of a milkmaid infected with cowpox. Six weeks later a potentially fatal amount of the deadly smallpox exudate was introduced into the boy's arm. The young man was immune! He did not develop smallpox, and Dr. Jenner was hailed as the father of preventive medicine. The same method, with some refinements and safety control of dosage and strength of cowpox organisms, is used in smallpox vaccinations today.

To provide for active immunity to other diseases by artificial means, the actual pathogenic microorganisms are grown and cultured in the laboratory (see Fig. 2–1). They are divided into single doses under rigid controls and made into vaccines. These specially treated microorganisms are so weakened that they will stimulate the production of antibodies but will not cause the disease itself. Vaccines from cowpox viruses, tetanus and tubercle bacilli and most recently the polio vaccine are all examples of agents used to produce an active immunity in humans.

This method of stimulating the production of immunizing substances in the body is quite successful in situations in which there is time to wait for the person to build up his own defenses. But what can be done if a person has no immunity and contracts the disease? Obviously there is no point in adding insult to injury by injecting more antigens into his body.

PASSIVE IMMUNITY. As the name implies, passive immunity is acquired

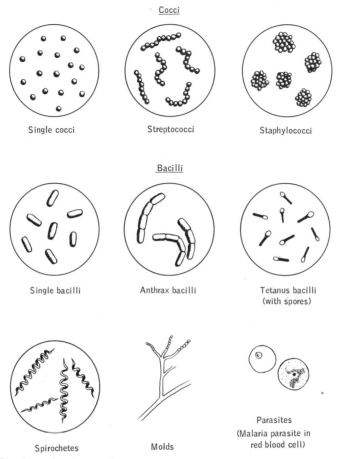

Figure 2-1. Drawings of various pathogenic microorganisms as they appear under the microscope. Their shape and groupings determine their classification.

through the efforts of someone else. Usually the "someone else" is a horse or rabbit. The serum from the blood of one of these animals contains ready-made antibodies and antitoxins. The serum is produced in the laboratory by giving increasingly stronger injections of specific antigens to the animals over a period of time so that they build up the necessary antibodies and antitoxins. The most common diseases in which passive immunity is an effective means of treatment to bolster the patient's defenses are diphtheria and tetanus. Immune serum is also useful in treating victims of bites from venomous snakes. It must be remembered, however, that these injections for pas-

sive immunity should be given in the earliest stages of the disease, since they can only help prevent damage to tissues; they cannot repair damage already done.

Sometimes passive immunity is established before the disease is contracted. In instances of contact with a disease such as measles, when the exposed person is considered too weak to withstand the rigors of a full-blown disease, gamma globulin is given to prepare the body in advance and lessen the severity of the disease should the person exposed contract it.

The fetus in the uterus can *passively* receive some natural immunity from its mother. Most antibodies in the mother's blood stream can pass through the placenta and become mixed with the blood of the fetus, so that they are present in the infant's blood at birth. Thus an expectant mother who has a high level of immunity to diphtheria, tetanus and whooping cough can be assured that her newborn baby will have some immunity to these diseases. This is only a temporary arrangement, however, and the child must be immunized again when it has reached the age of two or three months.

passive

Actually, all passive immunity is useful only as a temporary safety measure and cannot be expected to guarantee a permanent safeguard against attacks from specific disease. In fact, for some diseases the antibody content may drop to a very low level over a period of years, even with active immunity. It is then necessary that the body be reminded of the need to produce more antibodies. To achieve this, single doses of antigens are given. These are so-called "booster doses."

Disorders of the Immune System

The disorders of the immune system fall into four broad categories: (1) deficiencies of the immune system in which the necessary antibodies are not produced, (2) autoimmune diseases, (3) abnormal growth of the cells of the immune system and (4) abnormal reaction (hypersensitivity) to antigens.

Deficiency States. Many, but not all, of these disorders are genetic syndromes; that is, the individual inherits the trait of deficient antibody production. He may produce too few antibodies of a certain type and he may have lymphoid cells that are incapable of functioning normally, which means that both the immediate and delayed responses to antigens are defective and his resistance to infection is dangerously low or nonexistent.

Acquired forms of immunologic deficiencies can occur as a result of leukemia or some other type of malignant disease involving the lymphatic system. The most outstanding manifestation of these types of immunologic deficiencies is an absence or extremely low level of gamma globulins in the blood (*agammaglobulinemia* and *hypogammaglobulinemia,* respectively).

Autoimmune Disease. Normally the body is able to recognize the difference between its own protein substances and those that are exogenous or foreign to it. Usually antibodies are formed only in the presence of exogenous proteins, but in autoimmune disease the individual forms antibodies against his own cells. In these cases the antigen is called an *autoantigen* and the antibodies are called *autoantibodies.* The reason for autoimmunity is not yet clearly understood; however, it is believed to be related to the production of abnormal proteins during infectious disease.[4]

Diseases that usually are classified as autoimmune disorders include systemic lupus erythematosus, myasthenia gravis, certain forms of glomerulonephritis and rheumatoid arthritis. The autoimmune diseases are also referred to in medical literature as "collagen diseases."

Neoplastic Diseases. These disorders have in common the development of *neoplasia* or new growth of plasma cells. As a result of this new growth and increased number of plasma cells, there are increased amounts of the gamma globulins (*hypergammaglobulinemia*). The gamma globulin molecules form almost all the antibodies produced by the immune system. There is still little known about the exact cause of these neoplastic diseases, and they are only recently being recognized as disease entities. The disorders, which include multiple myeloma and plasma cell leukemia, usually affect older persons and are twice as common in men as in women.

Hypersensitivity. In this type of disorder, the individual's immune system simply over-reacts to the antigens with which the individual comes in contact. Examples of this type of disorder include hay fever, food and drug allergies, asthma and anaphylactic shock. Of these, the least dangerous, but nonetheless annoying, is a mild allergic reaction to food or other substances in the environment. The most serious is anaphylaxis, which is characterized by circulatory collapse and can be fatal in a matter of minutes if not properly treated.

When the allergic reaction occurs, the cells begin to swell. Some of them rupture, releasing substances such as histamine, heparin and choline into the body fluids. Some of these substances are toxic. Histamine, or a histamine-like substance, is believed to be responsible for many of the serious reactions in allergy. Drugs called antihistamines are frequently used to relieve the symptoms of an allergic reaction.

Factors influencing the type of reaction are (1) the kind of antigen, (2) concentrations of antigens and antibodies, (3) the kind of antibody and (4) the location and kind of tissue cells involved.

Since allergic reactions are antigen-antibody responses, an allergy will not develop until an individual has become "sensitized." This means that on first contact with an *allergen* (antigen that causes allergic reactions) there will be no specific antibodies present in his body; therefore, no antigen-antibody reactions can occur. Upon the second exposure to the antigen, however, the antibodies are available and the reaction takes place. Many allergens are proteins such as those present in animal products and plants.

TREATMENT OF ALLERGY. It is thought that allergies occur only when a person is mildly sensitized to an allergen. For example, an infant may be temporarily allergic to a substance such as egg albumin or meat extracts, but as he becomes more exposed to the allergen he develops greater immunity and eventually the allergy disappears. The *desensitization* of patients suffering from an allergy is based on this principle. Under the supervision of an allergist the allergen is given in small but progressively larger doses over a period of time until the patient builds up a strong immunity to the allergen.[5]

Antihistamine drugs work as blocking agents to the histamine released during an antigen-antibody reaction. These drugs are especially useful in preventing the effects of histamine in hay fever, urticaria (hives) and anaphylaxis.

Epinephrine acts as a neutralizing agent and is used to counteract the effects of histamine in an allergic reaction. The drug causes constriction of the blood vessels, which is the reverse of the histamine effect. It also produces dilatation of the bronchi, which is helpful in the relief of asthma and other respiratory difficulties due to allergy.

Cortisone and hydrocortisone, which are hormones of the adrenal cortex, are sometimes used in the treatment of allergy. These hormones are anti-inflammatory agents that reduce the effects of the allergic reaction. In large doses they also act to depress the formation of antibodies.

Nursing care of a patient with an allergy will depend on the way in which the allergy is manifested. Skin disorders resulting from an allergic reaction are discussed in Chapter 13; respiratory disorders are discussed in Chapter 16. Whatever the type of allergic disorder, it should be remembered that the emotional state of the patient will greatly affect the progress of the disease and the effectiveness of the treatment. His environment should be as quiet and nonstimulating as possible. Situations that produce anxiety, fear and anger should be avoided, and the nurse should do whatever she can to help the patient achieve serenity and peace of mind.

PREVENTION OF SERIOUS ALLERGIC REACTION. Everyone concerned with the administration of medications should be aware of the dangers of giving drugs to patients who are highly sensitive. One should always ask the patient about specific allergies before administering any antibiotic or immunizing agent such as vaccines. It should also be remembered that predisposition to other allergies makes the individual a good candidate for anaphylaxis. Although the nurse cannot always foresee the development of a serious allergic reaction, she must be prepared for such an eventuality. Epinephrine (Adrenalin) should always be readily at hand when allergy-producing drugs are administered. The symptoms of an allergic reaction should be familiar to the nurse, and if they appear she should notify the physician at once. These symptoms include apprehension, generalized rash or hives, choking sensation, wheezing, cough, incontinence, shock, fever, loss of consciousness and convulsions. In anaphylaxis the patient often has severe dyspnea, and death may occur in five to ten minutes.

BIOLOGIC AGENTS

Introduction

The invasion of the body by biologic agents refers to an infection by living organisms such as bacteria, fungi or viruses. Inflammation is a characteristic of infection and will be discussed in detail later, but it is mentioned here to emphasize that the terms infection and inflammation are not synonymous. Inflammation is actually the body's response to some irritating agent, its attempt to defend itself. A sunburn is an example of an inflammation in which there are no bacteria and no infection

present. If the burn is very deep, however, and the wound is not kept sterile, bacteria will invade the tissues and an infection will result.

Types of Bacteria. Organisms capable of producing disease in humans are called pathogenic. Not all bacteria, yeasts and molds are pathogenic, however, and many serve useful functions in the body as aids to digestion and absorption of food. Those which are usually not harmful to cells and tissues are called nonpathogenic.

Bacteria belong to the plant family, as do viruses, yeasts and molds, and they are classified according to their characteristics. There is no need for the practical nurse to learn and know all the many varieties under these classifications. Since bacteria are the most common causative agents in infections, however, and because the practical nurse will hear the terms "strep throat" and "staphylococcal infection," she may wish to understand something about these terms and what they mean.

Generally, bacteria are divided into three main groups according to their shapes (see Fig. 2-1): (1) cocci (round), (2) bacilli (rod-shaped) and (3) spirochetes (spiral or corkscrew).

Since bacteria in their natural state are seen through the microscope as tiny, colorless organisms, they must be stained with a dye. This dye is usually methylene blue. The procedure is called the Gram stain after the scientist who first used this method of classifying bacteria. Those bacteria which "take" the dye are called gram-positive. Those which will not retain the color are called gram-negative. All streptococci and all staphylococci are gram-positive. The bacillus which causes tuberculosis is gram-negative.

Bacteria may be grown in the laboratory in a specially prepared broth or jelly. They become visible to the naked eye as a large group or colony of specific types, all members of the colony having grown from one microscopic cell. The manner in which these bacteria arrange themselves as a group is also a means of classifying them. Some grow in pairs (diplococci), some in chains (streptococci) and some in clusters (staphylococci).

Thus we see that "strep throat" (short for streptococcal infection of the throat) is an infection caused by round organisms which grow in chains. A "staph" infection is an abbreviated way of saying that there is an infection present caused by round organisms which grow in clusters.

Viruses. Viruses are extremely small living pathogenic organisms that are increasingly causing disease and death. They are known to be responsible for at least 50 diseases in humans, among them the common cold, poliomyelitis, most childhood diseases and a variety of respiratory disorders. Investigations are under way to determine whether viruses are a contributing factor in the development of cancer.

The study of viruses is difficult because they are so small; they cannot be seen without an electron microscope. The process of growing colonies of viruses similar to cultures of bacteria is difficult because viruses propagate only within living cells. Another difficulty in research on viruses as a cause

of disease in man is the problem of growing human viruses in experimental animals. Before their effects on animals can be determined, the viruses often change their characteristics and in effect evolve into different viruses. This characteristic of adaptability in the virus means that scientists who start out working with the same virus in different laboratories may, after some time, find themselves working with different viruses. Because of this adaptability and changing of characteristics, the diagnosis and treatment of viral diseases can be very difficult. In addition, establishing immunity against certain viruses may be almost impossible, primarily because immunity is specific, and immunity against one virus will not guarantee immunity against another type. This does not mean that there is no immunity for any viral disease. We already have an immune vaccine for smallpox, measles and mumps, all of which are viral diseases.

Biologists and biochemists are interested in viruses because they are excellent subjects for the study of the fundamental processes of cell growth and multiplication.

Classification of viruses can be based on a variety of characteristics including size, nucleic acid composition and

TABLE 2–2. CLASSIFICATION OF VIRUSES*

Nucleic Acid	Virus Group	Size, Mμ	Types Pathogenic to Man
RNA	Picorna	17-30	Poliovirus; Coxsackie viruses A and B; echovirus; rhinovirus (common cold)
	Reovirus	74	Types 1, 2, 3
	Arbovirus	20-100	Encephalitis (many varieties)
	Myxovirus	80-200	Influenza; mumps; parainfluenza; measles; respiratory syncytial
DNA	Papovavirus	40-55	Papilloma (wart)
	Adenovirus	68-85	Common cold (28 types)
	Herpesvirus	120-180	Herpes simplex; herpes zoster; cytomegalovirus
	Poxvirus	150-300	Variola (smallpox) Varicella (chickenpox)

*From French: The Nurse's Guide to Diagnostic Procedures. 3rd edition. Copyright McGraw-Hill, Inc., 1971. Used by permission of McGraw-Hill Book Company.

affinity for certain types of tissues in the human body.

Fungi. A fungus is any member of a class of vegetable organisms of a low order of development, including molds and yeasts (see Fig. 2-2). They thrive in warm, moist places and are easily spread. A fungal infection of the skin, hair and nails is called a *dermatomycosis.* Examples of this type of fungal infection include athlete's foot and ringworm. Systemic fungal infections *(systemic mycoses)* are usually acquired by inhaling the spores of the fungus. The primary site of infection is the lung. From there the infection may spread throughout the body by the lymph vessels or blood stream. Histoplasmosis, blastomycosis and actinomycosis are examples of systemic mycoses. The recent discovery of specific antifungal drugs, such as griseofulvin and amphotericin B, has greatly changed the prognosis for fungal infections with the result that long-standing cases that have resisted other forms of treatment can now be completely cured.

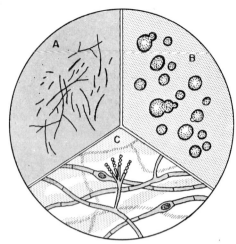

Figure 2–2. Fungal types. *A*, Actinomycete. *B*, Yeast. *C*, Mold. (From Brooks: *Basic Facts of Medical Microbiology*, 2nd Ed., W. B. Saunders Co., Philadelphia.)

Nursing Implications

We must realize that bacteria, viruses and fungi are always present in our environment. They are likely to be present in much greater numbers in a hospital, where infections of all kinds are constantly being treated. A proportionately large number of people within the hospital walls are quite likely to serve as carriers and sources of infectious agents.

From the beginning of her experiences as a practical nurse, the student is admonished to wash her hands before and after every nursing procedure. Though this may seem a simple and sometimes annoying task, its importance can never be overstated. The principles of cleanliness and good personal hygiene taught at the beginning of and throughout the course of practical nursing are of vital importance in the prevention of cross-infection and self-contamination. In all nursing procedures we are taught to clean and dry equipment after it is used, and we must never underestimate the importance of plain soap, water and "elbow grease." In Chapter 9 of this text are presented the special procedures necessary for isolation and care of patients with specific infectious diseases, but the underlying principles of cleanliness are the same in all nursing procedures. Unfortunately we cannot see infectious agents without special microscopes, but we must be aware that they are always with us. By applying your knowledge of infectious agents to all aspects of nursing care, you will do much to protect your patients, yourself and your family from needless sickness and misery.

INFLAMMATION AND REPAIR

Introduction

Inflammation and repair are two closely related responses to injury of the cells and tissues. The human body's cells respond to a physical or chemical injury in the same manner that a normal individual will react to anything that he sees as a threat to his well-being. He will take measures to defend himself against attack and then engage in active battle if necessary to rid himself of the enemy and repair the damage that has been done.

Although a distinction should be made between infection and inflammation, it is important to note that bacteria, viruses and fungi are among the most important causes of inflammation.

The inflammatory and reparative processes are influenced by a variety of factors. These include (1) the intensity of the agent causing the injury and the number of cells damaged—for instance, a widespread and acute inflammation that can occur in hypersensitivity to allergens can be extremely serious and possibly fatal; (2) the patient's state of nutrition and general state of well-being—persons with diabetes mellitus, for example, have great difficulty in the repair of cell injury; (3) the presence of foreign bodies which can impede repair—for instance, sutures can facilitate invasion by pathogenic organisms; and (4) the adequacy of blood supply to the injured cells and a normal functioning of blood cells.

The Process of Inflammation

Inflammation involves changes in the injured cells and also in the blood, blood vessels and connective tissues. The outward signs of these internal changes are *redness, heat, swelling, pain* and *loss of function*. These are the classic signs of inflammation, and although the internal changes presented below can account for the redness, heat and swelling, we are still not sure exactly why pain and loss of function occur.

Vascular Changes. As soon as cell injury occurs, whether by infectious agents, heat or cold, chemicals or phys-

ical trauma, a substance called *necrosin* is liberated by the damaged cells. It enters the surrounding tissue fluids and affects the adjacent capillaries so that there is an increased flow of fluid and protein to the area. The blood vessels enlarge and the blood flow becomes slow and sluggish. This reduced blood flow to and from the inflamed area delays the spread of infectious agents or other toxic substances. The redness and heat are external signs of these vascular changes.

Leukocytosis. The inflamed tissues also liberate a substance known as *leukocytosis promoting factor*. As the name implies, this substance causes increased production of leukocytes (or white blood cells) from the bone marrow. The leukocytes gather in large numbers at the site of the inflammation. There a group of leukocytes called *phagocytes* engulf and ingest bacterial cells and dispose of them. Other white cells (*lymphocytes*) carry enzymes which dissolve or digest bacteria.

Transudation and Exudation. The term *transudation* refers to the passage of fluid from the blood plasma into the tissue fluid. Mild injuries bring about the release of this type of serous and watery fluid. An example is the fluid in a blister that has been produced by a second degree burn. Exudation is more often associated with infection and the presence of large numbers of leukocytes and bacterial cells. The exudate is then known as pus and is composed of plasma and debris from the site of the inflammation. It is helpful in the removal of dead bacteria, tissue cells and blood cells. It also brings immune bodies into the area as well as necessary enzymes, all of which are helpful in removing the debris. It is necessary that this exudate have an outlet so that the body can repair the damaged tissues. That is why a surgical procedure called "incision and drainage" is sometimes needed for abscesses and other localized inflammations when drainage cannot be achieved any other way. In some cases a strip of rubber or a piece of tubing is placed in the wound to facilitate drainage.

Reparative Process

The process of repairing the damage done to cells and tissues begins almost immediately after the inflammatory process begins. There are three possible outcomes of an injury to cells. First, if the cells are not damaged beyond recovery, they will restore themselves, leaving no permanent evidence of injury. If an infection is present and localized, the exudate is removed and the tissues return to normal. This process is called *localization and resolution.*

A second possibility is that some of the cells may be damaged so severely that they die (*necrosis*). The affected area must then heal by *regeneration,* which means that new cells similar in structure and function to the dead ones are produced as replacements. Regeneration is not possible in all types of tissues. The epithelial, fibrous, bone and lymphoid tissues regenerate well, but the nervous, muscular and elastic tissues do not.

The third possible outcome in the reparative process involves replacing the damaged tissue with fibrous scar tissue (*scarring*). The exudate mentioned earlier in the inflammatory process contains fibrin, which forms a network of strands upon which granulation tissue forms. As the debris from the inflammatory site is removed by the leukocytes, capillaries and immature fiber cells begin to move into the space left. These small blood vessels and fiber cells give the granulation tissue a soft, reddish appearance. Sometimes there is too much granulation tissue formed and the epithelial cells and fiber cells do not have a proper network upon which to build new tissue. This excessive granulation tissue is sometimes called "proud flesh" and occurs when wound infection or prolonged wet dressings overstimulate the production of granulation tissues. This "proud flesh" must be removed by cautery or surgical debridement before the wound can heal properly.

Scarring. This is a natural result of the repairing process. The capillaries and connective tissue cells in the wound shrink and become taut, first appearing as hard reddish tissue, then gradually becoming white and glossy, forming the typical scar tissue with which we are all familiar. Internally the formation of scar tissue may create some difficulties. Adhesions may form and become troublesome when these tough fibrous tissues interfere with the normal functions of the internal organs around which they are formed. If the scar tissue is very large, it may disable the tissues of an organ, as, for example, a large area of scar tissue in the myocardium after recovery from a coronary occlusion (heart attack).

Wound Healing

There are two general types of wound healing: (1) by primary union ("first intention") and (2) by secondary union ("second intention"). In the first type, the two edges of the wound are close together. A crust forms between them to seal the wound, resulting in a thin scar. In healing by second intention, the edges of the wound are far apart and cannot be brought together. There is usually a loss of a large amount of tissue because of necrosis or physical trauma. The ulcerated area in the middle fills with granulation tissue so that the wound heals from the edges inward. A healing decubitus ulcer is an example of a wound healing by second intention.

Factors that speed up or delay healing are of interest to the nurse caring for a patient with any type of wound, whether it be a surgical wound, a result of physical trauma or a decubitus ulcer.

Age. Older persons heal more slowly than children and young adults. The exact reason for this is not known; however, elderly persons often have circulatory disturbances and nutritional deficiencies.

Blood Supply. The blood vessels and blood cells transport many elements essential to the inflammatory process and the repair of damaged cells. Therefore, it is obvious that a good blood supply and healthy blood cells will enhance the healing of a wound. Edema, tight bandages or arterial damage will delay healing.

Nutrition. New tissues are built of amino acids, the building blocks of proteins, so an inadequate intake of protein foods will hamper wound healing.

Another nutritional element, vitamin C, is necessary for the repair of tissue.

Mechanical Injury. Friction, pressure, blows to the wound or foreign objects in the wound will delay healing. Physical injury destroys granulation tissue, which is the framework upon which new cells grow and mature to form a covering for the wound. Infection, a form of mechanical and chemical injury, also delays healing.

Hormones. The steroids (hormones from the cortex of the adrenal gland) significantly hamper repair and healing. Since prolonged stress results in an increase of these hormones, it is believed that anxiety and physical stress can delay repair.

TABLE 2–3.

Factors Affecting Wound Healing	Nursing Implications
1. Blood supply	Avoid tight bandages or other sources of pressure against blood vessels in the vicinity of the wound. Relieve edema by proper positioning of the affected part. Apply, as ordered, cold compresses for relief of edema or warm packs for improvement of circulation to wounded area.
2. Nutrition	Encourage patient to eat high-protein diet. Give citrus fruits and juices and other sources of vitamin C.
3. Mechanical injury	Protect wound from friction and direct blows. Devise protective bandages using foam rubber, plastic cups, tongue blades or other supplies (see Fig. 2–3). Handle affected part gently. Use great care in applying and removing dressings and bandages.
4. Infection	Observe patient for early signs of infection and report immediately any elevated temperature, redness, swelling or pain beyond the norm. Wash hands thoroughly before and after each contact with patient. Use strict aseptic technique during dressing changes and wound cleansing.
5. Hormones	Provide rest, relieve anxiety as much as possible.

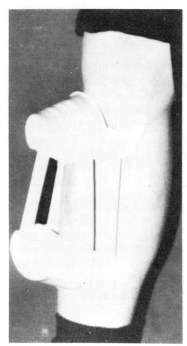

Figure 2–3. Protective device for wound, improvised from plastic cups and tongue blades. (From Auld, Craven, and West: Nursing, October, 1972.)

REFERENCES

1. Auld, M., Craven, R., and West, Jr.: "Wound Healing." Nursing '72, Oct. 1972, p. 36.
2. Beland, I.: *Clinical Nursing: Pathophysical and Psychosocial Approaches,* 2nd edition. New York, The Macmillan Co., 1970.
3. Du Gas, B. W.: *Kozier-Du Gas' Introduction to Patient Care,* 2nd edition. Philadelphia, W. B. Saunders Co., 1972.
4. Frobisher, M., and Fuerst, R.: *Microbiology in Health and Disease,* 13th edition. Philadelphia, W. B. Saunders Co., 1973.
5. Guyton, A. C.: *Basic Human Physiology: Normal Function and Mechanisms of Disease.* Philadelphia, W. B. Saunders Co., 1971.
6. Robbins, S. L., and Angell, M.: *Basic Pathology.* Philadelphia, W. B. Saunders Co., 1971.
7. Watson, J. E.: *Medical-Surgical Nursing and Related Physiology.* Philadelphia, W. B. Saunders Co., 1972.

SUGGESTED STUDENT READING

1. Craven, R. F.: "Anaphylactic Shock." Am. Journ. Nurs., April, 1972, p. 718.
2. Johnson, K. J.: "Allergen Injections." Am. Journ. Nurs., July, 1965, p. 121.
3. Rodman, M. J.: "Drugs for Allergic Disorders." RN, July, 1971, p. 53.

OUTLINE FOR CHAPTER 2

I. Introduction

A. Human body works constantly to maintain delicate balance needed for normal cellular function.

B. Cells must continually adapt to changing environment.

C. Pathologist views disease on a cellular level.

D. Many causes of cell injury and death.

II. Oxygen Deficiency—Anoxia

A. One of the most common causes of cell injury.

B. May be result of circulatory disturbance, blood disorders or respiratory disease.

III. Physical Injuries—Trauma.

A. May be result of violent blow or other physical force.

B. Other kinds of injury involve heat, cold, electrical energy and radiant energy.

IV. Chemical Injuries

A. Can be caused by any of the strong chemicals in our environment.

B. Can be relatively harmless chemicals if they are used improperly and in high concentration.

C. Drugs must also be included. *Iatrogenic* disorders are often chemically induced.

V. Genetic Disorders—Transmitted by Genes

A. May or may not be present at birth.

B. Not all congenital disorders are genetic; for example, congenital syphilis and heart defects.

C. Sickle cell anemia, thalassemia, Down's syndrome are examples of genetic disorders.

VI. Nutritional Imbalance—Possible Causes

A. Inadequate or excessive intake.

B. Faulty storage and utilization of food elements.

VII. Aging

A. Deterioration of cells currently accepted as consequence of growing old.

B. Research may show that deterioration not always inevitable.

VIII. Neoplasms—New Growths, Benign or Malignant

IX. Disorders of Immunity

A. Antigen-antibody reaction essential to body's defense against invasion by foreign bodies.
   1. Immediate response—antibodies react with antigens.
   2. Delayed response—apparent involvement of cells from lymphoid tissues.
B. Immunity—security against a particular disease-producing organism or antigen.
C. Types of Immunity:
   1. Natural.
   2. Active.
   3. Passive.
D. Disorders of immune system include:
   1. Deficiency states of immunologic agents.
   2. Autoimmune diseases.
   3. Abnormal growth of the cells of the immune system.
   4. Hypersensitivity:
     a. Ranges from hay fever to anaphylaxis.
     b. Treatment of allergy—antihistamines and desensitization.
     c. Prevention of serious allergic reaction—use caution in giving antibiotics and immunizing agents such as vaccines to patients with known allergies.

X. Biologic Agents—Infection by Living Organisms Such as Bacteria, Fungi or Viruses

A. Types of bacteria—belong to plant family. Classified according to characteristics such as shape, growth formation and resistance to dyes.
B. Viruses—responsible for at least 50 diseases in humans.
C. Fungi—thrive in warm, moist places.
D. Nursing implications—good handwashing technique and basic sanitation important to prevent infection and spread of disease.

XI. Inflammation and Repair—Closely Related Processes

A. Influencing factors:
   1. Number of cells damaged.
   2. Patient's state of nutrition and well-being.
   3. Presence of foreign bodies.
   4. Adequacy of blood supply and normal blood cells.
B. Process of inflammation—involves changes in the injured cells, the blood and blood vessels and the connective tissues.
   1. Outward signs include heat, redness, swelling, pain, loss of function.
   2. Internal changes include vascular changes, leukocytosis, transudation and exudation.
C. Reparative process begins almost immediately after start of inflammatory process—possible outcomes:
   1. Localization and resolution.
   2. Regeneration.
   3. Scarring.
D. Wound Healing.
   1. Two general types: primary and secondary union.
   2. Factors affecting wound healing include age, nutrition, blood supply, mechanical injury, infection and hormone level.

3

Symptoms
of Illness

VOCABULARY

Analgesic
Aspiration
Capillary
Catalyst
Contraction
Delusion
Dilatation
Disoriented
Enzyme
Flatus
Hallucination
Intermittent
Indices
Noxious
Placebo
Reaction
Toxic
Vascular
Vital

INTRODUCTION

The diagnosis of disease from the symptoms presented by the patient and the prescription of treatment for illness lie within the realm of the physician. But when continued treatment and personal care are required, it is the nurse who spends the longest periods of time with the patient. During his absence from the bedside, the physician must rely on the nursing staff for intelligent observation and accurate reporting of the patient's progress and the symptoms his illness produces. Of all the duties involved in nursing care, observation is probably the most vital. Florence Nightingale, in describing the role of the nurse, said, "Without the habit of ready and correct observation,

we [nurses] shall be useless for all our devotion."[5]

This talent for "ready and correct observation" is not easily achieved and can only be developed with experience and a full understanding of what intelligent observation really means. It requires much more than merely watching. First, there must be a sincere interest in the patient, a willingness to listen to his complaints and an understanding of his individual personality and personal reactions to his illness. Secondly, the observer must have a sound knowledge of the usual course of the patient's particular condition or illness so that she can recognize deviations from that course. Third, the observer must make a critical judgment between the usual and the unusual, and finally, she must make a decision of action based on her observations.

An example of this is a situation in which the practical/vocational nurse observes a patient having slight respiratory distress. She changes his position to facilitate breathing, but the dyspnea does not improve and the patient becomes restless. The nurse knows that this patient has had gastric surgery and she realizes that dyspnea is not usually associated with this condition. She recognizes it as an unusual occurrence and decides to report the patient's dyspnea to the nurse in charge. This nurse has made an intelligent observation and has chosen a wise course of action on the basis of her observations.

Much can be learned about a patient by observing his general appearance. With experience, one realizes that facial expressions, posture in bed, bodily movements and ability to cooperate are all significant clues to the physical and mental condition of a patient.

There are also specific signs which nurses must learn to look for while caring for patients. These signs of the presence of illness, or a change in the progress of an illness, are called *symptoms*. They are the warning signals that something is amiss. These symptoms may be *subjective* or *objective*. Subjective symptoms are those the patient must tell us about; for example, itching, pain, nausea and fatigue are subjective symptoms. Objective symptoms are those which can be determined with instruments and laboratory tests, or those which we can see for ourselves. Pallor, high blood pressure, increased blood sugar or skin rash are examples of objective symptoms.

The observant nurse uses all her senses to detect signs and symptoms of illness. With her sense of touch she distinguishes between normal, healthy skin and that which is coarse, dry, dehydrated, edematous or cold and clammy. She feels the extremities and other body parts to determine whether they are cold because of poor circula-

tion or hot because of a localized inflammation. She listens for normal breathing and distinguishes between a cough that is dry and hacking or one that is moist and "bubbly." She hears the wheezing of an asthmatic patient or the crowing sound produced by an obstruction of the air passages. These are but a few of the ways in which the nurse uses her hearing to evaluate a patient's condition.

In some instances specific odors can be of help in diagnosing certain disorders. For example, the sweetish, fruity odor of acetone can indicate diabetic acidosis; the smell of new-mown clover may accompany hepatic coma. The odor of alcohol is usually detected rather easily in acute alcoholism unless the patient has been drinking vodka, which is relatively odorless. A patient who is suffering from acute alcoholism may also smell of liquid Sterno, lighter fluid, after-shave lotion or other sources of alcohol.

Mouth odors that are fetid or metallic usually indicate poor oral hygiene and periodontal disease (disease of the tissues around the teeth). A nasal odor may be due to chronic sinusitis with postnasal drip or an obstruction in the nasal passages. In children one might suspect a foreign object such as a bean or pea in the nose when there is a distinctly fetid nasal odor. The patient who wears excessive amounts of perfume or cologne may be hiding a serious body odor problem that is symptomatic of anemia, endocrine dysfunction or an abnormality of the central nervous system. The nurse who suspects that the patient is trying to hide an embarrassing odor should seek to gain the patient's confidence and trust so that he can talk freely about his problem and receive help in coping with it.

Since the nurse is not called upon to diagnose an illness, she is not expected to be familiar with all of the symptoms of specific diseases. She should, however, be aware of the more common symptoms of illness and what these symptoms mean to the patient in terms of discomfort and danger. Later in this text, symptoms of specific diseases will be discussed, but there are many symptoms which are common to a variety of diseases.

VITAL SIGNS

The vital signs, or signs of life, are perhaps the most familiar and frequently used "yardsticks" for measuring a patient's state of health or degree of illness. They include the body temperature, rate and character of pulse and respiration, and blood pressure.

The Patient With an Abnormal Body Temperature

Fever. When a person has a body temperature one or more degrees above his normal range, he is said to have a fever. An elevated body temperature is part of the body's response to tissue injury and therefore is not a disease but a symptom of some disturbance within the body. It is believed that fever occurs as a result of certain *pyrogenic* (fever-producing) substances released by white blood cells or other cells during the inflammatory process.[1]

Fever is accompanied by an increase in the metabolic rate, which produces increased sweating, elevated pulse and respiratory rate, flushed skin and weight loss. In addition to these outward signs of fever, the patient feels exhausted, he has a headache and generalized aching all over his body, and his eyes are sensitive to light.

NURSING IMPLICATIONS. The nurse caring for the patient with a fever can use some simple but very effective nursing measures to relieve his discomfort and avoid complications of fever. An ice cap to the head or cool compresses to the forehead will help relieve the headache. Rest can conserve strength and reduce fatigue, and a quiet environment can promote rest.

The patient's eyes should be protected from bright lights. If the fever is prolonged or extremely high, it will be necessary to increase carbohydrate and protein intake to combat weight loss and repair tissue damage. Extra fluids are needed to replace those lost through excessive perspiration. The mucous membranes of the nose and mouth will require special attention to prevent cracking and drying. Adequate intake of fluids, whether by mouth or intravenously, is helpful in avoiding sores (fever blisters), highly concentrated urine and other general effects of dehydration.

When the fever becomes excessively high, there is some danger of damage to tissue cells, and the physician will then order specific measures to reduce the body temperature. These methods will vary, but usually include sponging the patient with a solution of alcohol and water to cool the surface of the body by evaporation. Ice bags applied to the head, axillae and groin, a cool-water enema and antipyretic drugs such as aspirin will also reduce the body temperature. Caution should be taken that the body temperature is not lowered too suddenly. The nurse should check the temperature of a feverish patient 30 minutes after temperature measures have been taken and at least every two hours thereafter unless otherwise ordered.

Chills, with violent shivering, often accompany or immediately precede high temperatures. These uncontrollable muscular activities are the body's attempt to raise the temperature (as a defense against infection) by increased muscular activity. The patient suffering from a chill will need extra warmth in the form of blankets and hot water bottles. When the chill subsides, the patient's linens may be wet with perspiration, and extreme care should be taken that he is not exposed to drafts. The linen should be changed with as little fanning of the covers as possible.

Hypothermia. An abnormally low

body temperature occurs much less frequently than fever. The deliberate lowering of body temperature (induced hypothermia) is a therapeutic measure used during surgery of the heart, large blood vessels and brain. Its purpose is to reduce the activity of the cells so that they will require less oxygen during the surgical procedure. This type of hypothermia is discussed more fully in Chapter 6.

Some causes of hypothermia other than that which is artificially induced include prolonged exposure to cold, particularly if the person's clothes are wet or if he is inebriated from too much alcohol. The wet clothes increase heat loss through evaporation, and the alcohol causes vasodilation. Oversedation by barbiturates or other nervous system depressants can also lead to hypothermia.

NURSING IMPLICATIONS. When a patient's temperature is 96.4°F. (35.8°C.) or lower, he is considered hypothermic. His body is slowly rewarmed—usually at the rate of one to two degrees Fahrenheit per hour—to avoid shock. External heat, if applied at all, must be used cautiously to avoid local damage to the tissues, which are especially susceptible to burning when the body temperature is well below normal. It is recommended that the patient be rewarmed at room temperature, using light blankets for cover to conserve body heat and allow a gradual return to normal body temperature.

Because there is danger of shock and cardiac arrest during the rewarming process, the patient's pulse and blood pressure should be checked regularly along with his temperature. An irregularity of the pulse, drop in blood pressure or rapid rise in body temperature should be reported immediately.

Pulse Rate And Rhythm

Pulse is the expansion of an artery that occurs with each heart beat. As the ventricle contracts, it sends a wave of blood through the aorta and into the arteries, where increased pressure from the wave causes them to expand. As the arteries stretch, a small amount of blood moves through; then the arterial walls return to their normal size, or recoil. With each expansion and recoil, blood is moved along the arteries and into the capillaries. Determinations of pulse rate, rhythm, volume and tension or thickness of the arterial wall are all important sources of information about the status of the heart and blood vessels.

Abnormalities in the rhythm or pattern of the pulse beat are called arrhythmias. There are three general types of arrhythmia: (1) a changing rate in which no regular rhythm can be detected, (2) a normal beat quickly followed by a small beat that is followed by a normal rhythm and (3) an irregular rhythm and beats of varying strength. The most common site for palpating the pulse is the wrist, where the radial pulse can be felt. Other sites include the neck (carotid), the groin (femoral), the temple (temporal) and the top of the foot (dorsalis pedis). The apical pulse is determined by placing a stethoscope over the apex of the heart. This can be located just below the left nipple, or about 2 to 3 inches to the left of the sternum.

Sometimes the physician will request an apical-radial pulse reading to determine whether a patient with cardiovascular disease has a pulse deficit. The apical pulse is determined by one nurse using a stethoscope, while at the same time another nurse counts the radial pulse. The difference between the apical pulse and the radial pulse is called the pulse deficit. Thus, if a patient in congestive heart failure has a radial pulse rate of 110 and an apical pulse rate of 150, his pulse deficit is 40.

An increase in the rate of the pulse to over 130 beats per minute is considered to be an indication that the heart contractions are not behaving normally. This increase in the rate of the heart beat is called tachycardia and is usually an indication of an increase in the basal metabolism resulting from a need for a greater supply of blood somewhere in the body. It may be present in persons who are merely excited, of course, and this is a normal reaction, but a fast pulse also frequently accompanies fever, hyperthyroidism, congestive heart failure and hemorrhage.

A slowing of the heart rate to below 60 per minute is called bradycardia. This is considered normal for some persons (for example, young male adults and athletes), but it may also be an indication of a disease. Wherever there is a possibility of brain damage from head injury, the slowing of the pulse is a very alarming sign and should be reported at once. Bradycardia in some cardiac patients might also be considered dangerous. Some drugs, such as digitalis, slow the heart beat and should not be given if the pulse rate is below 60 per minute.

Blood Pressure

The degree of pressure exerted by the blood against the arterial walls is called blood pressure. The normal range varies with individuals, and a person's blood pressure can vary from one time of day to another. The average blood pressure is considered to be about 120 mm. of mercury for the systolic pressure and about 80 mm. of mercury for the diastolic pressure. The difference between the systolic and the diastolic pressures is called the pulse pressure. Hypertension (high blood pressure) becomes dangerous when it places such a strain on the arterial walls that they may rupture, resulting in damage to the surrounding tissues. The most likely place for this to occur is within the cranial cavity, where there is less room for expansion of the blood vessels. This is what sometimes happens at the time of a cerebrovascular accident or "stroke."

There are various theories about the exact cause of hypertension, but we do know that it often accompanies circulatory diseases, such as arteriosclerosis, and kidney diseases. Generally, the treatment for high blood pressure consists of rest and quiet, a dietary regimen aimed at preventing obesity and administration of drugs which dilate the blood vessels. Hypertension and hypertensive heart disease are discussed in more detail in Chapter 14 of this text.

Hypotension is in itself not dangerous unless it becomes extreme, as in shock and hemorrhage. (See Chapter 6, Preoperative and Postoperative Care.) Anemia is sometimes accompanied by hypotension, but as one authority has said, "Therapeutically the patient with low blood pressure may be congratulated." It is the marked deviation from what is normal for the patient that is cause for alarm. The blood pressure must be checked carefully in patients with head injuries and any marked change in the readings reported immediately, since it may indicate changes in the pressure within the cranial cavity and resultant brain damage.

A condition known as postural hypotension can occur in a number of instances. It is related to the person's posture or body position and frequently occurs when a patient who has been on bed rest for a period of time gets up into a sitting or standing position too quickly. There are certain drugs that can produce postural hypotension in persons who are relatively active but who, after lying down for a while, suddenly stand up and experience dizziness or fainting from a sudden drop in blood pressure. Another phenomenon that has recently been noted is that of postural hypotension in late pregnancy or during the early stages of labor, when the pregnant uterus presses against the inferior vena cava, thereby interrupting the blood flow to the upper part of the body and producing a sudden drop in blood pressure. This situation occurs when the mother is lying on her back and can be remedied very quickly and simply by turning her on her side.

The nurse should always be aware of the possible causes of postural hypotension, and when a patient experiences symptoms of extreme hypotension after suddenly rising or assuming a certain position, the incident should be brought to the attention of the physician and noted on the patient's chart.

RESPIRATION

Normal respiration depends on a variety of factors, each one being essential to breathing and having a direct influence on the adequate exchange of oxygen and carbon dioxide in both external and internal respiration. These factors include (1) adequate supply of oxygen in the air, (2) an open airway, (3) sufficient and healthy lung tissue, (4) nervous and chemical control, (5) an intact rib cage and diaphragm, (6) sufficient hemoglobin in an ample volume of blood and (7) a healthy heart to pump blood through an intact circulation.

Each patient with a respiratory difficulty will have individual needs, depending on which of the preceding factors are involved in his particular illness. The nurse will most often be concerned with the first two, however, and it is her responsibility to assure proper positioning of the patient, maintenance of an open airway and an oxygen supply as prescribed by the physician. It is obvious, however, that oxygen therapy and other heroic measures to maintain respiration may be all but useless if there is little or no air flowing into the patient's lungs. Many times the value of simple nursing measures is overlooked in a frenzied concern over the proper functioning of complicated machinery and bedside equipment. This is not to say that such equipment is unimportant, but one should not lose sight of its purpose and the ways in which it is expected to meet the needs of the patient.

The Patient With Respiratory Difficulty

Respiratory problems can accompany many kinds of disease or injury to the cells and tissues. Environmental factors such as availability of adequate oxygen in the air or the presence of noxious fumes or poisonous gases must also be considered as possible causes of dyspnea. Infections and chronic inflammation of the respiratory tract can obstruct the air passages or prevent normal functioning of the respiratory organs. Circulatory diseases often bring about respiratory difficulties because they interfere with the transportation of oxygen to the cells and the elimination of carbon dioxide.

NURSING IMPLICATIONS. We have all probably experienced at some time in our lives the near panic one feels when he cannot breathe properly. It is understandable that the patient who struggles for breath or feels that he is smothering is truly suffering from mental anxiety as well as physical distress. Unfortunately his mental state of fear and anxiety can only aggravate his physical condition and increase his distress. The nurse who knows what to do for him and does so promptly and efficiently relieves both his physical and emotional discomfort. Her actions are directed toward providing an adequate supply of oxygen to the body cells and assuring the patient that everything possible is being done to bring relief. (The effects of anoxia on the cells are discussed more fully in Chapter 2.)

Proper Positioning. We know the advantages of proper posture while walking, standing and sitting; these principles of good posture are equally important to the patient with dyspnea. A position sometimes referred to as the "coffin" position can be especially hazardous to adequate expansion of the lungs and maintenance of an open airway. In this position the individual is lying on his back, pillow under the head, chin resting on the chest and one or both arms lying across the abdomen.

The reasons for avoiding this position in a patient with respiratory difficulty become quite clear when we consider the ways such a position hampers normal functioning of the organs of respiration. First, the tracheal opening is narrowed considerably when the head is bent forward. Second, a person in the supine position, even without a pillow under his head, is in danger of aspirating mucus, vomitus or other accumulations in the mouth. In addition, the tongue may fall to the back of the throat, thereby obstructing the flow of air. Third, the weight of one or both arms on the chest can interfere with complete expansion of the thoracic cavity.

A good position to insure optimum breathing when lying flat in bed is on the side with the neck extended and the head and chin supported by a small pillow. The uppermost leg is flexed and the uppermost arm is also bent and supported by a pillow. There will be times when a patient's particular condition of illness prevents positioning him in this manner. In this case the nurse should consult with the head nurse or the physician and determine proper positioning for the patient.

Some patients cannot breathe comfortably in any lying position and must sit up or stand to breathe adequately. These patients are said to have orthopnea. Proper positioning of the orthopneic patient will require some special arrangement of the bed, pillows and supportive structure for adequate rest. These patients often rest more comfortably and perhaps are able to sleep if an overbed table is raised to the height of the patient's chest and covered with pillows. The patient's arms are then placed across the pillow and his head is allowed to rest between his arms (see Fig. 3–1). The author recalls a patient with an acute asthmatic attack who was admitted to the hospital with severe dyspnea and fatigue. A student nurse placed the patient in the orthopneic position, and, speaking softly to her, assured her that she would be very close at hand should the patient need her. The patient promptly fell asleep. When she awoke several hours later, she praised the student nurse and said, "That is the first time I have slept in

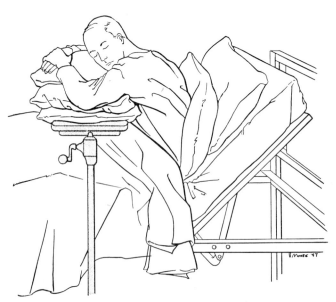

Figure 3–1. Orthopneic position, used when the patient has difficulty breathing and is more comfortable in a sitting position. Pillows are used to support back. Other pillows are placed on overbed table to support weight of arms, shoulders and head. (From Montag and Swenson: *Fundamentals in Nursing Care,* 3rd Ed., W. B. Saunders Co., Philadelphia.)

three days and three long nights. I can't tell you how good it was to finally get some sleep."

Many patients can obtain relief from dyspnea when placed in the simple Fowler's position with the back well supported and the neck straight or slightly extended. This position improves respiration because it allows for better expansion of the diaphragm owing to a downward gravitational pull of the abdominal contents.

Another factor to consider in caring for the dyspneic patient is that of pressure from organs below or near the lungs and diaphragm. A full stomach aggravates breathing difficulty, and for this reason, small frequent feedings are preferable to three large meals a day. Abdominal distention due to a collection of flatus and fecal material in the intestines can also make breathing more difficult. If the nurse queries her patient and observes that the abdomen is distended, she should report her findings and request a mild laxative, suppository or enema for relief of the distention.

The patient with a respiratory disorder needs adequate sleep and rest for recuperation and for reduction of his need for oxygen. The less active and restless he is, the less his body cells will suffer from hypoxia. His nursing care and treatments should be planned so that there are a minimum of interruptions during the day, allowing the patient some periods of time when he can take short naps.

Observations. There are several observations that are important in assessing the needs of the patient with difficult breathing. These observations can be valuable to the physician in his diagnosis of dyspnea. The patient's skin color is a good indicator of sufficient oxygen supply or adequate circulation. Is his skin bluish (cyanotic)? red and flushed? In observing his general appearance, the nurse looks for signs of labored breathing such as flaring nostrils, distended neck muscles

and prominent eyes. She listens for sounds produced as the patient inhales and exhales. Is he wheezing? Are there moist bubbling sounds (rales) on exhalation, or is there a coarse, high-pitched sound on inhalation? Does he inhale with relative ease but seem to "push" the air out when he exhales? Does he use his abdominal muscles when breathing? Do his cheeks puff outward each time he exhales?

The nurse also takes note of the patient's apparent mental status: whether he is alert, or drowsy and somewhat confused. She recognizes dizziness, mental sluggishness and sleepiness as signs of anoxia. She checks for coughing, its frequency, whether it is dry and nonproductive or wet and productive of sputum. If it is a productive cough, she observes the amount and character of the sputum and any unusual odors that may indicate infection or stagnation of sputum in the respiratory tract.

Each of the many observations made by the nurse in her assessment of the patient should be clearly and concisely written on the patient's chart.

Oral and Nasal Suctioning. Patients who are extremely weak or semiconscious often need assistance in removing secretions from the air passages. In these cases a suction apparatus is used to remove thick mucus and other tenacious material. The following rules should be observed when suctioning the mouth, throat and nose:

1. The bottle used for collecting wastes suctioned from the air passages is never filled above the line designated on the bottle.

2. The catheter is pinched off or suction is otherwise withheld until the tube has been inserted into the throat. This measure prevents damage to the mucous membranes. After the catheter is in the throat, suction is applied and the catheter is moved gently up and down the throat in order to clear mucus from all areas.

3. During the suctioning procedure, the catheter may become plugged with

thick mucus. It must then be removed from the throat and placed in a glass of water or saline to rinse and clear the catheter.

4. Remember that the suctioning procedure removes air as well as liquid, which can increase a patient's air hunger. Allow for periods of rest and do not continuously suction the throat for more than 20 to 30 seconds at one time.

5. The catheter and tubing are rinsed clean after each suctioning by placing the catheter in a glass of water or saline while the motor is still on.

6. There are times when the physician may place a tube or "airway" made of rubber, metal or plastic into the throat of a patient to facilitate breathing. When an airway is in place, the catheter is inserted through the opening of the airway and mucus is thus removed from the throat.

7. When the nasal passages require suctioning, it is recommended that two catheters be used, one for the nose and the other for the throat. This is especially important when a surgical incision in the area is likely to become infected.

Oxygen therapy is discussed in detail in Chapter 16 of this text.

CONVULSIONS

A convulsion or seizure is an attack of uncontrollable muscular contractions. Generally, there are three types of convulsion: (1) tonic, in which there is continued contraction of all muscles; (2) clonic, in which there is alternate contraction and relaxation of the muscles, giving the body a jerking motion; and (3) jacksonian seizures, in which the muscular twitching begins in one area and spreads to other parts of the body.

These attacks of uncontrollable muscular contractions may appear in many diseases. The most common ones are epilepsy, infectious diseases in which there are extremely high temperatures,

tetanus, uremia and brain injuries.

It is very important that the practical nurse be aware of the possibility that the patient may hurt himself during a convulsion. She must remain with the patient during the convulsion in order to observe him and to help protect him from injury. The bed should be fitted with side rails and the head of the bed well padded with a pillow or folded bath blanket. A tongue depressor padded with gauze should be at the bedside. This is placed between the patient's teeth to prevent biting the tongue or the inside of the mouth when the strong jaw muscles contract. No effort should be made to pry open the mouth, since this may loosen the patient's teeth. If the patient having the convulsion was not in his bed, but was up and had fallen to the floor during the seizure, no attempts should be made to move him during the seizure. The only choice then is to protect the patient from injury as much as possible, making sure that his head is placed on a pillow or blanket so that he does not injure the skull during the convulsion. No restraint should be used.

The following observations should be made during the convulsion and reported in detail on the patient's chart or directly to the nurse or doctor in charge.

1. When convulsion began and length of time it lasted.

2. Type of convulsion, whether tonic, clonic or jacksonian.

3. Area of the body in which the convulsion began and whether it was restricted to one particular part or was generalized over the entire body.

4. If the patient lost consciousness or was incontinent of urine or feces.

5. Effect of convulsion on the pulse and respiration of the patient.

6. Changes in skin color and whether or not there was profuse perspiration.

7. Any complaints the patient may have had before or after the convulsion.

DELIRIUM

The delirious patient is confused and disoriented as to place and time. Because of disturbances in the nerve cells of the brain, he may suffer from delusions and hallucination, and he cannot act rationally until the delirium subsides. Fortunately, delirium is usually only temporary and can be relieved when the underlying cause is eliminated. Conditions that can produce delirium include infectious diseases which are accompanied by high fevers, alcoholism (delirium tremens) and drug addiction.

The nursing care of the delirious patient is primarily concerned with protecting the patient from harm and avoiding circumstances in his environment which may stimulate the brain and excite him. While delirium is present, someone should remain with the patient to prevent him from injuring himself. Restraints should be used only when absolutely necessary, since they may disturb the patient and increase his restlessness. One must be careful about windows and doors which the patient may try to use as a means of escape during his confusion.

Bright lights, noises and sudden movements of persons around the patient can serve as stimuli which aggravate the delirium and give rise to delusions. Conversation in the patient's presence should be kept at a minimum because of the possibility of his misinterpreting what he hears, but the nurse should always explain in a calm voice what she is going to do for the patient and why it is being done. One must avoid arguing with a delirious person. It is often helpful to remind him where he is and who is caring for him, thus assisting him in orienting himself. Finally, an attitude of sympathy and understanding on the part of the nurse can help relieve the patient's anxiety. He cannot control his behavior, and no amount of reprimanding or so-called disciplinary measures will relieve his unhappy situation. In fact, such practices will only further confuse and upset him.

INCONTINENCE

The patient who is unable to control his functions of elimination presents many physical and emotional problems for himself as well as for those who must care for him. We do not mean to imply that improvement of the situation is impossible, though at times it may appear so. If there is to be any progress made, it is necessary that the nurse begin with a positive attitude and discourage feelings of hopelessness on the part of the patient and his family. Once the nurse has convinced herself and the patient that something can be done, she has already begun to do something about the problem. Since there are many different causes of incontinence, the next step is to try to determine why the patient cannot control the passage of feces and/or urine. If the incontinence is a result of trauma to the nerve pathways or muscular deficiencies in which there is no possibility of removing the cause or remedying the original condition, some type of permanent appliance or receptacle should be used. The use of these in specific diseases and surgical procedures will be discussed more fully later in the text.

All nursing measures will be aimed at keeping the patient clean, odorless and dry. A bit of imagination and use of available waterproof materials can help in improving ways of protecting the patient's clothing and bed linens. A regularity in routine of eating and elimination can also prevent episodes of embarrassment to the patient. It is rare that the first thing tried will work well and those easily discouraged will soon sink into despair. If, however, the nurse can imagine herself in the patient's place and try to appreciate how the family must feel, she will persist until her patient is at least more comfortable and socially acceptable.

JAUNDICE

Jaundice is a symptom, *not* a disease, and is the result of increased accumulation of bile pigments in the blood. To say that a patient has jaundice is similar to saying that he has nausea or dyspnea. Jaundice may be due to an obstruction of the flow of bile from the liver through the ducts to the gallbladder and intestines, to inability of the liver to clear normal amounts of bilirubin from the blood or to increased destruction of red blood cells with the degradation of hemoglobin and release of bile pigments.

The patient who is jaundiced has a yellowish cast to his skin and the whites of his eyes. He may experience severe itching over his entire body as a result of deposits of crystals on his skin. He may suffer from mental confusion and extreme irritability. Because the liver is concerned with the production of vitamin K, many patients with jaundice have a pronounced tendency to bleed readily because of impaired ability to form blood clots. In obstructive types of jaundice, the urine will be dark from bile pigments excreted by the kidney, and the stools light or clay-colored because of decreased amounts or absence of bile pigments normally in feces.

Nursing care includes skin care to relieve itching. This means frequent sponge baths with a starch or vinegar solution, followed by application of calamine lotion. The patient is watched closely for signs of bleeding internally or externally and any changes in his condition should be reported immediately so that hemorrhage can be averted. The patient's environment should be nonstimulating with avoidance of bright lights, noises or other stimuli which can aggravate his irritability.

PAIN

Pain is such a universal symptom, common to so many diseases, that it is difficult to be specific in regard to the physical illnesses it accompanies. Individuals vary in their response to pain and what might be simply annoying to one person will be unbearable to another. Emotions also affect the degree of tolerance to pain. The patient who is mentally at ease will suffer less from discomfort than one who is emotionally disturbed and fearful. The practical nurse must guard against an air of indifference to pain in others, and she should make no judgment as to its severity. Pain is a warning signal of distress within the body; the decision of whether it is real or not real rests with the physician.

In a sense, pain can be advantageous; in fact, we would have fewer people remaining ignorant of the early stages of disease if pain were always present at the beginning of an illness. Cancer rarely causes pain in its first stages of development. This is, of course, unfortunate, because by the time pain has entered into the clinical picture, there is usually very little that can be done to cure the patient of cancer.

It is extremely difficult for one person to evaluate and make a valid judgment about the extent and type of pain another person is experiencing. For this reason it is important that the nurse be as objective and specific as possible when assessing and reporting a patient's complaint of pain. Storlie suggests four indices for the assessment of pain: (1) severity, (2) duration, (3) possible precipitating event and (4) location.[14]

The nurse reports in the patient's own words his description of the pain he is feeling. He may use the words "cramping," "stabbing," "burning" or "crushing" to describe the pain. If he cannot be specific, but simply says that "it hurts," then this is how the nurse records his complaint. She also notes and records the patient's actions, his facial expression, posture in bed, whether he is thrashing about or lying rigidly in one position and any other visible signs of distress and discomfort.

Duration of pain is recorded according to the length of time given by the patient. He should be asked when the pain started and whether it has been constant or intermittent. If there is some particular action or event that brings on the episode of pain or increases its severity, this too should be noted. For example, lying in a certain position may increase abdominal pain, moving about may produce a headache or flexing the knee may cause discomfort in the hip.

The exact location of the pain should also be noted. Again the nurse asks the patient and helps him identify the source of his discomfort and whether it radiates to other parts of his body. An example of this radiating type of pain occurs in renal colic that accompanies the passage of kidney stones. The pain often originates in the flank and radiates down the inner side of the thigh.

In all the preceding statements about assessment of pain, we have looked to the patient as our source of information. This is an essential part of caring for a patient who is having pain. Studies have shown that it is helpful to the patient to talk about his pain and to know that others are aware of his suffering. A patient's ability to cope with pain depends to a large degree on what nurses do when he is uncomfortable.[9] His anxiety is frequently relieved when the nurse simply stands quietly at his bedside or is willing to spend some time discussing his pain with him. Some patients respond favorably to a soothing touch or a well-timed back rub. Showing concern without overdoing expressions of sympathy, and winning the patient's confidence can be more valuable than a hastily prepared and administered analgesic drug.

The problems of drug abuse and addiction make all of us wary of administering narcotics and other analgesics too freely. Although there is some justification for such fears, it is not true that every patient who requires pain-relieving drugs is a potential addict. Many factors other than repeated use enter into drug addiction. The nurse is aware of the hazards of extensive use of narcotics but she must avoid the two extremes of giving a drug of this kind immediately upon request or withholding it "for the good of the patient." Many times a little extra time and effort spent in using simple comfort measures to help the patient relax can be more effective than administering analgesic medications according to a rigid schedule.

CLINICAL CASE PROBLEMS

1. A young adult male is brought to the Emergency Room by the local police. He was found lying on the street in a comatose condition. Nothing is known about his illness, and there is no available information about his past history or how he became unconscious.

What are some observations the nurse might make regarding this patient?

If the patient is found to have a subnormal temperature, what are some possible causes? What nursing measures can be used to restore normal body temperature?

What events should be reported immediately if they should occur during the rewarming procedure?

2. Mrs. Clarke is a 42-year-old patient with an elevated temperature and dehydration. She has had a fever for three days prior to admission.

What are the nursing implications for Mrs. Clarke's care?

3. Mr. Alonzo is a 57-year-old patient with severe dyspnea. His physician has ordered oxygen by nasal prongs.

How can the nurse help relieve Mr. Alonzo's respiratory difficulty?

What observations would be of value to the physician in his diagnosis of the cause of Mr. Alonzo's dyspnea?

If Mr. Alonzo is troubled by large amounts of mucus in his air passages, what can be done to assist him in the removal of these secretions?

REFERENCES

1. Beland, I. L.: *Clinical Nursing: Pathophysiological and Psychosocial Approaches,* 2nd edition. New York, The Macmillan Co., 1970.
2. Burgess, A. M.: "A Comparison of Common Methods of Oxygen Therapy for Bed Patients." Am. Journ. Nurs., Dec., 1965, p. 96.
3. Cashatt, B.: "Pain: A Patient's Point of View." Am. Journ. Nurs., Feb., 1972, p. 281.
4. Du Gas, B. W.: *Kozier-Du Gas' Introduction to Patient Care,* 2nd edition. Philadelphia, W. B. Saunders Co., 1972.
5. Flatter, P. A.: "Hazards of Oxygen Therapy." Am. Journ. Nurs., Jan., 1968, p. 80.
6. Guyton, A. C.: *Textbook of Medical Physiology,* 4th edition. Philadelphia, W. B. Saunders Co., 1966.
7. Hadley, F., and Bordicks, K. J.: "Respiratory Difficulty." Am. Journ. Nurs., Oct., 1962, p. 64.
8. Healy, E. A., and McGurk, W.: "Effectiveness and Acceptance of Nurses' Notes." Nurs. Outlook, March, 1966, p. 32.
9. McAfferty, M., and Moss, F.: "Nursing Intervention for Bodily Pain." Am. Journ. Nurs., June, 1967, p. 1224.
10. Nett, L. M., and Petty, T. L.: "Acute Respiratory Failure." Am. Journ. Nurs., Sept., 1967, p. 1847.
11. "Pain: Programmed Instruction." Am. Journ. Nurs., May and June, 1966, p. 1085, and p. 1345.
12. Shafer, K. N., et al.: *Medical-Surgical Nursing,* 5th edition. St. Louis, The C. V. Mosby Co., 1971.
13. Smith, D. W., and Gips, C. D.: *Care of the Adult Patient,* 2nd edition. Philadelphia, J. B. Lippincott Co., 1966.
14. Storlie, F.: "Pain—Describing It More Accurately." Nursing '72, June, p. 15.
15. Watson, J. E.: *Medical-Surgical Nursing and Related Physiology.* Philadelphia, W. B. Saunders Co., 1972.
16. "What's the Meaning of That Patient's Odor?" Nursing Update, April, 1971, p. 12.

SUGGESTED STUDENT READING

1. Cashatt, B.: "Pain: A Patient's Point of View." Am. Journ. Nurs., Feb., 1972, p. 281.
2. Cunningham, L. S.: "What Are You Noting?" Journ. Pract. Nurs., Oct., 1964, p. 28.
3. "Pain: Programmed Instruction." Am. Journ. Nurs., May and June, 1966.

OUTLINE FOR CHAPTER 3

I. Introduction

A. Ready and correct observation probably most vital of all nursing processes.

B. Nurse uses all her senses to detect signs and symptoms of illness.

II. Vital Signs

A. Signs of life most frequently used "yardsticks."

B. Extremes of body temperature—fever and hypothermia. Nursing measures aimed at restoring normal body temperature and preventing complications.

C. Pulse—disorders include arrhythmias and pulse deficit.

D. Blood pressure—disorders include hypertension and hypotension. Pulse pressure is difference between systolic and diastolic pressure. Nurse should be aware of postural hypotension.

E. Respiration—normal breathing dependent on many factors. Nurse most concerned with adequate oxygen supply and open airway.

    1. Patient with respiratory difficulty suffers from mental as well as physical distress.

    2. Nursing implications—proper positioning, intelligent observation, oral and nasal suctioning.

III. Convulsions

A. Are seizures of uncontrollable muscular contractions. Types include tonic, clonic and jacksonian.

B. Nursing care includes intelligent observation and protection of the patient from injury.

C. Frequently associated with epilepsy and with high fevers in children.

IV. Delirium (Mental Confusion and Disorientation)

A. Protection of patient and providing a non-stimulating environment are important factors in nursing care.

B. Often accompanies high fevers, alcoholism and drug addiction.

V. Incontinence (Inability to Control Functions of Elimination)

A. Nurse must approach problem with a positive attitude.

B. Keep patient clean, odorless and dry.

VI. *Jaundice*

A. It is a symptom rather than a disease; the result of increased bile pigments in the blood.

B. May be due to:
1. Obstruction of the flow of bile from liver to intestines.
2. Inability of liver cells to clear bilirubin from blood.
3. Increased destruction of red blood cells with degradation of hemoglobin.

C. Symptoms include yellowing of the skin and white of the eyes. In obstructive type the stools are clay-colored and the urine is dark.

D. Nursing care includes skin care to relieve itching (use starch baths or calamine lotion), observation for bleeding and provision of a quiet environment.

VII. *Pain (Extreme Discomfort)*

A. Nurse evaluates patient's pain on the basis of what he tells her.

B. Those in pain need sympathetic understanding.

4

The Patient
With Fluid and
Electrolyte
Imbalance

VOCABULARY

Buffer
Capillary
Halitosis
Impaction
Mastectomy
Peristalsis

INTRODUCTION

More than half (approximately 65 to 70 per cent) of the total body weight is composed of water which contains dissolved organic and mineral nutrients and waste products (see Fig. 4–1). Water is essential for transporting various substances to and from the cells, is necessary as a solvent for the electrolytes, and works to maintain the chemical balance needed for normal functioning of the cells. The taking in of nutrients and the excretion of waste products is a continuous, lifelong process internally, within the cells and tissues, just as it is externally with the total individual man. When something happens to disturb this internal process of intake and output, the chemical balance of the cell is upset, and if the situation is not relieved, death of the cells and tissues and eventual death of the body as a whole will result.

Even though the body fluids are continuously in motion, passing through cell membranes and the walls of the

blood and lymph vessels, physiologists consider these fluids to be compartmentalized. The fluid outside the cell walls is called *extracellular fluid,* and the fluid inside the cells is called *intracellular fluid.* The extracellular fluid may be in the tissue spaces between the cells, in which case it is called *tissue fluid* or interstitial fluid, or it may be within the blood and lymph vessels, in which case it is called *intravascular fluid,* or plasma (see Fig. 4–2). If one understands the meaning of the prefixes *intra-* (within) and *extra-* (outside of), it is easier to remember these terms.

Dissolved in the body fluids are substances which play an essential role in maintaining normal fluid balance and in promoting normal function of the cells. Among these substances are proteins and chemical compounds called *electrolytes.* As the name implies, once the electrolytes are dissolved in water, they are capable of conducting an electric current. When electrolytes are in solution, they break up into separate particles called *ions.* The positively

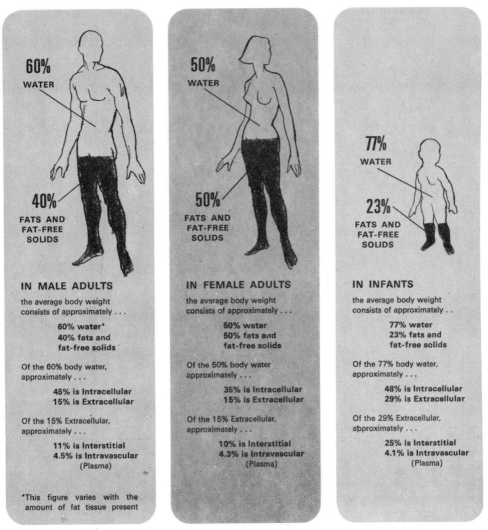

Figure 4–1. Relationship of body water and body solids to the body weights of the adult male and female and the child. (From *The Fundamentals of Body Water and Electrolytes—A Visual Review*. Travenol Labs, Inc., Deerfield, Illinois, p. 260.)

charged particles are known as *cations*, and the negatively charged particles are *anions*. An electric charge is created by these differently charged ions, and this charge, which develops across the cell membrane, allows nerves to transmit impulses, muscles to contract and glandular cells to secrete.

The electrolytes of significance to the nurse and the care of her patients are potassium, calcium, magnesium, sodium and chloride. Potassium, which is largely concentrated within the cells (in intracellular fluid), is important in the growth of cells, repair of tissue, transmission of impulses in nerves and muscles and many different aspects of metabolism. Calcium plays a vital part in the formation of blood clots and is essential to normal functioning of muscle tissue. Sodium, magnesium and chloride are essential to chemical changes necessary for normal body function. Sodium is especially im-

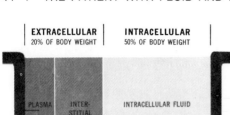

EXTRACELLULAR 20% OF BODY WEIGHT	INTRACELLULAR 50% OF BODY WEIGHT

Extracellular is subdivided into

PLASMA 5% of body weight	INTERSTITIAL 15% of body weight

Figure 4–2. "Compartments" or fluid spaces in the body. Based on estimate that 70 per cent of body weight is water. (From *The Fundamentals of Body Water and Electrolytes—A Visual Review.* Travenol Labs, Inc., Deerfield, Illinois, p. 27.)

portant in the maintenance of a normal fluid balance in the body.

The fluids within the various compartments contain differing concentrations of electrolytes. This difference in concentration accounts for the movement of water and electrolytes from one compartment to another. Through the principle of osmosis, water will move from the space with the less concentrated solution to that with the more concentrated solution. This principle is significant to the nurse caring for a patient receiving intravenous fluids. Pure water is not used as an intravenous fluid because it would rapidly move from the extracellular compartment into the cells and cause them to swell. A highly concentrated intravenous fluid solution (hypertonic solution) can cause the cell to lose its fluid and shrink as the fluid moves into the plasma fluid of the blood. Dextrose and sodium chloride are used as additives to water for intravenous administration so that the solution will be as near isotonic (equal to the concentration of body fluids) as possible and thus will not interfere with the normal movement of fluids among the compartments.

In a healthy person, the hormonal mechanisms which regulate the functions of the kidneys and lungs provide for a normal balance of fluids. Water is added to the body through oral intake and is eliminated through the skin, in the urine and stools and in expired air (see Fig. 4–3). When there is too much water in the body, the patient is said to have overhydration or edema. A deficiency of water produces dehydration.

THE PATIENT WITH EDEMA

An excessive amount of fluid within the interstitial spaces (tissue fluid), accompanied by swelling of the affected part, is referred to as edema. The tissue in which the swelling is apparent is called edematous tissue. The edema may be localized or generalized. An example of localized edema is swelling of a leg due to a clot obstructing a leg vein. Other causes of localized edema include obstruction of the flow of lymph through the lymphatic vessels, injuries due to extreme heat or cold and allergic reactions. Edema of the lungs (pulmonary edema) can also be localized without any outward sign of edema elsewhere in the body.

Generalized edema, involving all the body's tissue fluids, always results from failure of the kidneys to eliminate sodium from the body. This failure may be due to impairment of the function of large numbers of nephrons (as in kidney failure), or it may be caused by a decrease in the volume of intravascular fluid circulating through the body (as in congestive heart failure). In either case, the sodium is retained in the body, which in turn causes retention of fluid in the tissues.

Pitting edema is a condition in which a small depression or pit occurs when one presses his finger against an edematous area. This condition is caused by a shifting of the tissue fluid from the area beneath the pressure point to another nearby tissue area.

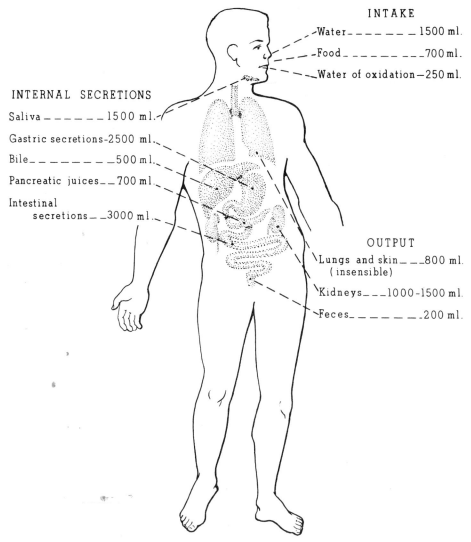

INTAKE

Water ------ 1500 ml.

Food -------- 700 ml.

Water of oxidation — 250 ml.

INTERNAL SECRETIONS

Saliva ------ 1500 ml.

Gastric secretions-2500 ml.

Bile -------- 500 ml.

Pancreatic juices -- 700 ml.

Intestinal secretions -- 3000 ml.

OUTPUT

Lungs and skin --- 800 ml. (insensible)

Kidneys --- 1000-1500 ml.

Feces ------- 200 ml.

Figure 4–3. Balance between intake and output. (From Jacob and Francone: *Structure and Function in Man,* 2nd edition, W. B. Saunders Co., Philadelphia.)

Pitting edema usually accompanies a disease of the kidney, liver or heart.

In *brawny edema,* the patient's skin is hard to the touch, and the fluid cannot be shifted from one area to another. An example of this type of edema affects the arm of a patient who has had axillary lymph nodes removed in a radical mastectomy.

Early signs of generalized edema can often be detected in the patient on bed rest by frequent checking of the sacral region and buttocks. The ambulatory patient or one who sits for long periods of time shows early edema in the feet, ankles and legs. This type of edema is called *dependent edema.*

Another early sign of generalized edema, other than obvious swelling, is weight gain. The accumulated water in the tissues causes a gain in body weight. The physician often requests that the patient be weighed daily when edema is present, so that he can determine the amount of body fluid being gained or lost.

When daily weight is ordered, the nurse must be careful to obtain as accurate a reading on the scales as possible. Ideally, the patient is weighed before breakfast and at exactly the same time every day. The same scales are used at each weighing, and the patient should be wearing the same type of clothing. The loss or gain of one or two pounds of body weight can be quite significant in the course of the patient's illness.

Another symptom of fluid retention is decreased urinary output. An accurate record should be kept of the fluid intake and output of the edematous patient. The intake record reflects all fluids taken into the body, whether orally, intravenously or any other way. Output includes all urine, vomitus, watery stools and unusual sweating. Recording these measurements is a nursing responsibility and should not be delayed until a physician's order is written for an intake and output record.

If the physician restricts the patient's fluid intake to a certain amount in a 24-hour period, the nurse plans the patient's schedule and arranges it so that the liquids are evenly spaced and he does not receive all the liquids in an 8- to 12-hour period.

When nursing a patient with edema, we must remember that the tissues and capillaries are not functioning normally, and the skin is stretched beyond its normal limits. Care must be taken to preserve the skin surface as much as possible. Bed linens are kept dry and smooth, and the patient is turned frequently to relieve pressure of the body weight on susceptible areas. In turning and moving the patient, it is necessary to be as gentle as possible and to avoid unnecessary friction against the skin. A break or abrasion of edematous skin can very rapidly develop into a large decubitus ulcer.

We know that sodium plays an important role in water retention and the development of edema. Because of this, the patient with generalized edema is nearly always placed on a sodium-free or low-sodium diet. This means that table salt is not allowed and that special attention must be paid to all foods and liquids consumed by the patient. There are many hidden sources of sodium in foods in their natural state as well as in those commercially prepared (see Table 4–1).

Diuretic drugs are often prescribed for the patient with edema. These drugs greatly increase the volume of urine and the frequency with which the patient must void. Such a situation can be tiresome and embarrassing for the patient. He should be assisted to the bathroom or with the urinal or bedpan as often as necessary, and he must be reassured that his frequent requests for assistance are not an inconvenience, but are expected. Diuretic drugs are discussed more fully in Chapter 15.

Excessive amounts of fluid in the body can affect the brain tissues and produce mental confusion or irritability. The nurse should be alert for possible hazards to the patient's safety, and she should provide a quiet, non-stimulating environment so that he can get adequate rest.

THE DEHYDRATED PATIENT

The term *dehydration* refers to the removal or loss of water. The patient who is dehydrated has a deficiency, or negative balance, of body fluids. Since these fluids are necessary for dissolving and transporting electrolytes, a depletion of fluids also means a disturbance in normal electrolyte concentrations in the body fluids.

The dehydrated patient will have skin that is very dry and wrinkled and that has lost its elasticity. The eyes appear sunken, and the mucous membranes lose their moisture. The patient appears weak and lethargic and may have increased pulse and respiratory rates. Other signs include decreased urinary output, highly concentrated urine, fever and mental irritability.

Dehydration often results from an

TABLE 4–1. WATER AND ELECTROLYTE IMBALANCES*

Substance	Major Functions	Effects of Too Little (Observable Symptoms)	Effects of Too Much	Primary Food Sources
Water	Dissolves electrolytes, other substances. Aids chemical changes. Affects body temperature. Acts as lubricant.	Highly concentrated urine, scant urine, thirst, fever, circulatory failure.	Dilute urine, polyuria, headache, confusion, nausea, vomiting, muscle twitching and cramps, coma.	All liquids, meat, vegetables, eggs.
Sodium	Maintains osmotic pressure. Affects muscle and nerve irritability.	Hypotension, nausea, vomiting, diarrhea, muscle weakness, abdominal cramps.	Manic excitement, tachycardia, edema.	Salt, meat, fish, cheese, most canned and preserved foods.
Potassium	Maintains intracellular fluid balance, heart rhythm, muscle and nerve irritability.	Apathy or anxiety, muscle weakness, nausea, tachycardia.	Muscle weakness, colic, diarrhea, changes in ECG.	Meat, fish, fruit juices (grape, apple, cranberry, orange, pear, apricot), bananas, tea, cola beverages.
Calcium	Maintains muscle contraction, normal heart rhythm, nerve irritability, blood clotting.	Numbness; tingling of nose, ears, finger tips or toes; tetany.	Few clinical problems.	Milk, cheese, broccoli, shrimp.
Magnesium	Maintains muscle and nerve irritability.	Hypotonic tetany, muscle twitching.	Few clinical problems.	Milk, cereals.
Chloride	Maintains osmotic pressure.	Symptoms occur only after prolonged vomiting. Few clinical problems.	Few clinical problems.	Salt, milk.
Phosphate	Aids in building bones and teeth, buffering system, transporting fatty acids, metabolizing fats and carbohydrates.	Poor mineralization of bones, rickets.	Tetany.	Milk, egg yolk, whole-grain cereals.
Bicarbonate	Maintains acid-base balance.	Ketosis, tendency to greater water and electrolyte losses.	Hyperglycemia, glycosuria, hepatic failure.	Eggs, meat, fish, beef and chicken broth.

*Copyright 1970 by Medical Economics Company. Adapted with permission, from RN Magazine, Vol. 33, No. 9, September, 1970.

excessive fluid loss from the gastrointestinal tract, as in prolonged vomiting or severe diarrhea. Overenthusiastic use of gastric suction can also rapidly deplete the electrolyte and fluid supply of the body. Unusual amounts of drainage from a surgical wound, as in ileostomy and colostomy, or from a traumatic wound, as in a severe burn, can also cause dehydration. Dehydration can result from any large blood loss, as well as from excessive perspiration and high fever.

The nurse's observations of the patient can be valuable in the detection of early dehydration and as a guide to the physician in prescribing treatment when dehydration is severe enough to require attention. An accurate record of fluid intake and output is essential. The character of the urine, whether dilute or concentrated, is noted and recorded because this is an indication of the state of the body fluids and the kidney's ability to function properly.

The patient's vital signs are checked frequently, and any rise in temperature or change in the rate and character of the pulse is reported. Special mouth care is especially important to avoid halitosis and painful cracking of the lips.

The body fluids and electrolytes may be replaced orally if the dehydration is not severe and the patient is able to cooperate. It is not unusual, however, for the physician to choose rapid replacement of the fluids and electrolytes by the intravenous route.

DISORDERS OF ELIMINATION

All the body's metabolic processes eventually produce waste products that must be eliminated from the body. If these substances are not eliminated properly, they can become toxic, causing serious illness. It is also possible for loss of fluids and electrolytes to occur when there is excessive vomiting or diarrhea or both.

Nausea. Nausea is a feeling of discomfort in the stomach region, with an urge to vomit. Extreme nausea is usually accompanied by vomiting, which is defined as expulsion of the contents of the stomach. The causes of nausea and vomiting are many and varied, including gastrointestinal disorders, radiation sickness, reaction to various drugs and chemicals swallowed or absorbed through the skin, anesthetics and pregnancy.

Relief of nausea and vomiting is usually best achieved by the administration of one or more of the antiemetic drugs. These drugs depress the vomiting reflex and also have a tranquilizing effect. They must be used with caution, since they can cause oversedation and lower the blood pressure.

Antihistamines such as dimenhydrinate (Dramamine), meclizine hydrochloride (Bonine), and trimethobenzamide hydrochloride (Tigan) are effectively used in the treatment of nausea. In postoperative patients and those with prolonged episodes of vomiting, other antiemetic drugs may be used. These include prochlorperazine (Compazine), promethazine hydrochloride (Phenergan), and perphenazine (Trilafon). These are the antiemetic drugs which are most likely to have the side effects of oversedation and hypotension mentioned earlier.

Nursing measures during a vomiting episode include having the patient lie down and holding his head so that it is turned to one side to prevent aspiration of the vomitus into the respiratory tract. An emesis basin should be held close to the side of the face. A cool, damp washcloth is used to wipe the patient's face, and a glass of ice water or mouthwash may be offered to the patient after vomiting, so that the mouth can be rinsed. The vomitus is observed for odor, color, contents and approximate amount. It is best for the patient to remain quiet and avoid oral intake during severe nausea. Physical activity or an intake of liquids or food can trigger further attacks of vomiting. When oral nourishment is allowed, it should initially consist of small amounts of liquids and gradually progress to solid foods. If the nausea and vomiting persist over a period of time, and dehydration is evident, intravenous therapy will be needed to replace the lost fluids and nutrients.

Diarrhea. Diarrhea refers to the passing of frequent, watery stools. The number of stools can range from 3 or 4 to as many as 15 to 20 per day. The consistency of the stools, rather than the number per day, is the factor that determines whether diarrhea is present. It is usually accompanied by cramplike pains in the abdomen, a result of hyperactive peristalsis and increased flatus.

Diarrhea may be a symptom of gastrointestinal diseases, such as infectious inflammatory processes or obstruction of the intestinal tract due to fecal impaction or neoplasms.

The strength of the patient with diarrhea is rapidly spent. Nursing measures should be aimed at rest and eventual replacement of fluids. In acute diarrhea, the stomach is kept empty for at least 24 hours to rest the intestinal tract. A soda water enema is sometimes given to remove irritating substances from the lower bowel. Oral feedings, when allowed, consist of liquids at first and gradually include more solid foods.

Medications prescribed for diarrhea depend on the cause of the disorder and the length of time the condition has been present. Mild cases usually respond well to kaolin and bismuth preparations (for example, Kaopectate) which coat the intestinal tract and make the stools more firm. Antispasmodic drugs such as belladonna or paregoric reduce the number of stools by decreasing the peristaltic rate and relaxing the intestinal musculature. If the patient with diarrhea shows signs of nervous tension and anxiety, sedatives or tranquilizers may be prescribed. Diarrhea that is caused by infections may be treated with drugs that are specific for the causative organism.

The nurse is responsible for noting and recording on the patient's chart the number of stools per day and the characteristics of the feces—the color, consistency and odor each time the patient has a bowel movement. If the stools are extremely watery, the patient can become dehydrated very rapidly. If the symptoms of dehydration appear, they should be reported immediately.

Chronic diarrhea is usually accompanied by anemia because there is often loss of blood with the frequent stools. Food passing through the intestinal tract too rapidly cannot be properly digested and absorbed, so malnutrition may also be present. The treatment in these cases consists of bland diet and vitamin and mineral supplements to help maintain adequate nutrition.

Diarrhetic patients are frequently nervous and embarrassed about their condition. These patients can be helped by a nurse who maintains a calm, dignified manner and provides a restful environment with privacy.

ACID-BASE BALANCE

Normally the body maintains a very delicate balance between acids and bases (alkalis) in the body fluids (see Fig. 4–4). This balance is maintained through complex chemical reactions that involve three major buffer systems. The buffers help regulate hydrogen ion concentrations and, in so doing, control the acid-base balance. Even slight changes in the chemical reactions in the cells can cause some reactions to speed up and others to slow down. These chemical reactions are vital to the life of the cell and occur in all organs of the body. When the chemical processes of the cells of an organ are accelerated or depressed, the functions of the organs are similarly affected.

A shift in acid-base balance can present a variety of symptoms, ranging from mild to severe or even fatal reactions. In general, it is found that the patient with uncontrolled acidosis will die in coma, and the patient with uncontrolled alkalosis will die in tetany or convulsions.

Acidosis. A shift of the body fluids toward acidity produces the condition known as acidosis. Such a condition can occur in uncontrolled diabetes mellitus and starvation (metabolic acidosis), or in respiratory disorders which interfere with adequate release of carbon dioxide from the lungs and thereby cause an accumulation of carbonic acid in the blood (respiratory acidosis). Symptoms of acidosis include dyspnea with deep, periodic breathing, a sweet-smelling odor of fruit on the breath, disorientation, coma and eventually death if the condition is not treated. Symptoms are relieved by the administration of sodium bicarbonate or sodium lactate orally or intravenously.

fruity breath

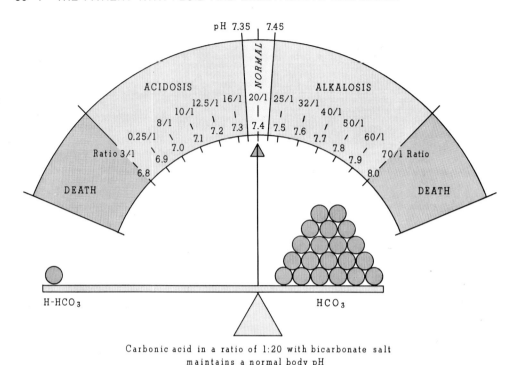

Figure 4–4. Acidosis and alkalosis showing ratio between carbonic acid and bicarbonate ion. (From Jacob and Francone: *Structure and Function in Man,* 2nd edition, W. B. Saunders Co., Philadelphia.)

Treatment is aimed at controlling the condition causing the acidosis.

Alkalosis. The opposite of acidosis is alkalosis, in which there are excess alkaline substances in the body fluids. Alkalosis can be caused by excessive vomiting or improper use of a gastric suction apparatus and by hyperventilation, when an individual breathes too rapidly. Symptoms include shallow respiration, a tingling sensation in the fingers, toes and lips, muscular cramps, tetany and convulsion. Respiratory alkalosis is relieved by administering carbon dioxide by mask or having the patient breathe into a paper bag or hold his breath. Severe alkalosis requires removal of its underlying cause.

INTRAVENOUS THERAPY

Whether or not the nurse is responsible for starting an intravenous infusion under the direction of a physician depends on the policy of the institution or agency for which she works. One must bear in mind, however, that all nurses have the responsibility of monitoring the intravenous fluids and observing the patient when they are caring for someone receiving intravenous therapy.

Intravenous therapy demands frequent checking of the apparatus to see that the rate of flow ordered by the physician is maintained and that no complication is developing in the patient. If the needle becomes dislodged, the solution will infiltrate into surrounding tissues, causing pain and damage to the tissues. A rate of flow that is too rapid can lead to an overloading of the circulatory system with excessive fluid in the intravascular compartment and eventually congestive heart failure or pulmonary edema. These complications and others are listed in Table 4–2. The primary

TABLE 4-2. POSSIBLE COMPLICATIONS OF IV THERAPY*

Complication	Cause	Symptoms
Air embolism	Air in IV setup	Cyanosis, hypotension, weak and rapid pulse
Circulatory overload	Too-rapid flow $\quad$ c HF	Headache, dyspnea, flushed skin, rapid pulse; congestive heart failure, pulmonary edema
Infiltration	Needle dislodged from vein	Edema at site of needle, discomfort, IV flow slows or stops
Nerve damage	Tightly bound arm board, compressed nerve	Numbness in little and middle fingers and in hand
Phlebitis	Irritating IV fluid or overuse of vein	Pain, redness, warmth and hardness along vein site
Pyrogenic reaction	Bacterial contamination in IV fluid or tubing	Rapid rise in temperature; severe chill 30 minutes after start of infusion

*Copyright 1970 by Medical Economics Company. Adapted with permission, from RN Magazine, Vol. 33, No. 9, September, 1970.

responsibility of the nurse in regard to these complications includes observing the patient and reporting immediately any evidence that a complication is developing.

All equipment from an infusion must be handled very carefully once it has been removed from the patient's vein. There is always the possibility that infectious hepatitis may be spread by way of contaminated intravenous equipment.

If the patient has had a "cut down" into the vein, the area must be treated with care and kept free from contamination during the treatment and after it is discontinued. A "cut down" is an incision into a vein for the purpose of inserting a needle or plastic tubing for administration of fluids. This procedure is necessary when intravenous therapy is continued for an extended period of time or when peripheral circulation is poor and the blood vessels have collapsed. Unless the incision is properly cared for, it may become contaminated, and thrombophlebitis can develop in the immediate area. Adequate cleansing around the area must be performed and proper dressings applied during fluid

therapy and should be continued until the area has healed completely.

Patients who are receiving continuous infusions require special mouth care, since they usually take no food or drink by mouth to stimulate the flow of saliva and keep the lips moist. If a patient is semiconscious or totally unconscious, he will breathe through his mouth most of the time, thus causing the mucous membranes to become dry.

TRANSFUSION OF WHOLE BLOOD

The word "transfusion" refers to the transfer of whole blood from one person to another. In earlier times, the only method used was by direct transfer. Today, blood is usually taken from the donor and stored in a blood bank until needed. With this modern method of transfusion and the use of blood banks for proper storage and typing of blood, there is less danger of reaction to blood transfusion than formerly. It is still a potentially dangerous procedure, and the patient must be observed carefully for signs of a reaction during and after the transfusion.

Before any unit of blood is administered, it must be properly identified and checked. The nurse who administers the blood inspects it for signs of clotting, hemolysis and contamination. If there is any discoloration or if gas bubbles are present, the blood should not be given. Two nurses work together to check the information on the unit of blood. They compare the blood type, Rh factor, serial number, patient's name and hospital number and any other information that is on the container with the written order for the blood transfusion.

Nurses must never become complacent about transfusions, no matter how many times they may see them safely administered without incident. Any symptoms observed or any complaint from the patient should be reported without delay. If any symptoms of a reaction become apparent, the nurse should stop the flow of blood, check the patient's blood pressure and notify the physician.

The word "reaction," when used in reference to the transfusion of blood or infusion of fluids, means a sensitivity to the blood itself or to preservatives or other substances added to the blood or fluids. The symptoms of a reaction may be so mild as to be unnoticed, or so severe that death is the eventual outcome. In milder cases, the patient develops a rash and complains of itching, or he may have chills and fever. In more severe cases, the patient may experience dyspnea, coughing, flushed face and restlessness. Eventually, collapse, coma and death will occur. Treatment of a reaction depends on its nature. If it is a simple allergic reaction, the physician may order antihistamines to relieve the symptoms. In severe reactions, epinephrine may be needed to prevent death from anaphylaxis.

CLINICAL CASE PROBLEMS

1. Mrs. Carlos, age 61, is admitted to the hospital with congestive heart failure. She is extremely edematous and obese. Mrs. Carlos is slightly confused upon admission, and though she is not on absolute bed rest, she tells you that she cannot get out of bed. She continues to refuse to get up or move about in bed the next morning, when you are assigned to care for her.

What type of diet do you expect would be prescribed for Mrs. Carlos? How would you explain to her the restrictions of her diet and the need for her to follow it?

How might you encourage Mrs. Carlos to get out of bed for her daily weighing?

If Mrs. Carlos's fluid intake is restricted, how would you schedule her fluid intake?

What problems might be presented by Mrs. Carlos's obesity and her inactivity?

2. Mr. Wong is a 35-year-old patient who has suffered a severe gastrointestinal upset producing nausea, vomiting and diarrhea. His physician has prescribed intravenous fluids.

List the observations you should make while caring for Mr. Wong.

What nursing measures might be taken to relieve his symptoms? What medications might you expect him to receive?

What are your responsibilities regarding Mr. Wong's intravenous therapy? Would you measure his intake and output? What electrolytes might he be deficient in?

REFERENCES

1. Berry, M. A., and Kerlin, C. B.: "The Drops of Life: Fluids and Electrolytes." RN, Sept., 1970, p. 35.
2. Burgess, R. E.: "Fluids and Electrolytes." Am. Journ. Nurs., Oct., 1965, p. 96.

3. Campbell, A. G. M.: "Electrolyte Imbalance in Infants: Implications for Nursing Care." Journ. Pract. Nurs., Dec., 1971, p. 20.
4. Child, J., et al.: "Blood Transfusions." Am. Journ. Nurs., Sept., 1972, p. 1602.
5. Downs, H. T.: "The Control of Vomiting." Am. Journ. Nurs., Jan., 1966, p. 76.
6. Durr, E. E., and Fierro, L. E.: "IV Therapy as a Nursing Responsibility." RN, Sept., 1970, p. 40.
7. Fenton, M.: "What to Do About Thirst." Am. Journ. Nurs., May, 1969, p. 1014.
8. Heath, J. K.: "A Conceptual Basis for Assessing Body Water Status." Nurs. Clin. N. Amer., Vol. 6, No. 1, 1971, p. 189.
9. "The Patient With Edema." Nursing Update, Jan., 1971, p. 1.

SUGGESTED STUDENT READING

1. Berry, M. A., and Kerlin, C. B.: "The Drops of Life: Fluids and Electrolytes." RN, Sept., 1970, p. 35.
2. Campbell, A. G. M.: "Electrolyte Imbalance in Infants: Implications for Nursing Care." Journ. Pract. Nurs., Dec., 1971, p. 20.
3. Durr, E. E., and Fierro, L. E.: "IV Therapy as a Nursing Responsibility." RN, Sept., 1970, p. 40.
4. Keusck, G.: "Bacterial Diarrheas." Am. Journ. Nurs., June, 1973, p. 1028.
5. Ledney, D.: "IV Therapy." Bedside Nurse, Aug., 1971, p. 17.

OUTLINE FOR CHAPTER 4

I. Introduction—65 to 70 Per Cent of Total Body Weight is Water

A. Body fluids present within the cells (intracellular fluid) and outside the cells (extracellular).
B. Interstitial fluid—that in the spaces between the cells.
C. Intravascular fluid—within the blood and lymph vessels.
D. Electrolytes—chemical compounds that conduct electric current when in solution.
E. Significant electrolytes are potassium, calcium, magnesium, sodium and chloride.
F. Body water volume and distribution are controlled by water-sodium gains and losses.
G. A balance between intake and loss of fluids and electrolytes is essential to good health.

II. The Patient With Edema

A. Definition—an excessive amount of tissue fluid with swelling of the affected area.
1. Localized—restricted to one area.
2. Generalized—involves all body tissues; results from failure of kidneys to eliminate sodium.
3. Pitting edema—depression occurs under area of pressure.
B. Signs of edema and their implications for nursing.
1. Dependent edema—early sign of generalized edema.
2. Weight gain—patient may be weighed daily.
3. Decreased urinary output—record kept of patient's intake and output.
4. Tissues and skin stretched—require special care to avoid decubiti.
5. Low-sodium diet—nurse explains diet to patient and reason for diet.
6. Mental confusion and irritability—safe, quiet atmosphere should be provided.

III. The Dehydrated Patient

A. Definition—removal or loss of water.
B. Causes include prolonged nausea, vomiting, diarrhea; unusual amounts of drainage from wounds; fever and excessive perspiration.
C. Nurse observes patient for early signs of dehydration, measures intake and output and observes character of urine. Special mouth care required.

IV. Disorders of Elimination

A. Nausea and vomiting—can lead to dehydration and electrolyte imbalance.
1. Antiemetic drugs relieve nausea.
2. Nursing measures—prevent aspiration of vomitus, apply cool cloth to face and supply liquid for rinsing mouth, keep patient quiet and restrict oral intake.
B. Diarrhea—determined by consistency of stools rather than number per day.
1. Medications protect intestinal lining and reduce peristalsis.
2. Nurse observes patient and records character of each stool;

reports signs of dehydration immediately.
3. Patient helped by calm, dignified manner and a restful environment with privacy.

V. Acid-Base Balance

A. A shift in acid-base balance can present mild or severe symptoms.
B. Acidosis—shift of body fluids toward acidity.
    1. Metabolic acidosis—starvation, uncontrolled diabetes mellitus.
    2. Respiratory acidosis—accumulation of carbon dioxide.
C. Alkalosis—opposite of acidosis.
    1. Causes include excessive vomiting, hyperventilation.
    2. Relieved by rebreathing or by administration of carbon dioxide by mask.

VI. Intravenous Therapy

A. Nurse must monitor flow of fluids and observe patient closely.
B. Possible complications include infiltration, too-rapid flow, pyrogenic reaction, air embolism and nerve damage.

VII. Transfusion of Whole Blood

A. Blood should be inspected and identification of unit and donor checked.
B. Patient is observed closely for signs of reaction during and after transfusion.
C. Symptoms of reaction should be reported immediately and transfusion stopped.

5

Diagnosis
of Illness

VOCABULARY

Antibiotic
Atom
Cauterize
Element
Fulguration
Oxidation
Radiopaque
Virulent

INTRODUCTION

The diagnosing of illness has always presented a challenge to the physician. It is the very cornerstone of medical practice, for once the diagnosis has been made, the course of treatment will be comparatively clear. The word "diagnosis" is derived from two Greek words: *dia*—through, and *gnosis*—knowing or recognition. Thus the word implies an ability to see through and detect facts not easily determined. In primitive times man resorted to witchcraft and superstitious practices in an effort to explain the symptoms of illness. When the modern physician diagnoses an illness, he is still seeking the "demons of illness," but he has the advantages of many instruments and laboratory tests to aid him in his search. In the past few decades, the use of laboratory tests as aids to diagnosis has become increasingly important, and it is expected that in future years the medical team will become more dependent on the chemist, physicist and radiologist in the battle against disease and illness.

PURPOSES OF SPECIAL DIAGNOSTIC TESTS

The physician uses information from laboratory tests in several ways: (1) As a method of determining the patient's general physical condition. Most patients will receive a complete blood count and urinalysis as a part of the initial examination in the physician's office or hospital, because abnormal findings in the blood and urine are common to many diseases. (2) As a means of determining the cause of disease, e.g., cultures grown in the laboratory to isolate the causative organism. (3) As a verification of the diagnosis the physician may have already suspected from other findings. An example would be the glucose tolerance test, which, if positive, would indicate the presence of diabetes. (4) As a guide to the physician in his method of treating a certain disease. Anticoagulant drugs such as Dicumarol, for example, are given only after the prothrombin time of the patient has been determined. This is done daily before each dose is ordered, so that the physician can adjust his treatment according to the progress of the patient.

It is sometimes confusing to the practical nurse when she finds an order for collection of a specimen from one system of the body as a diagnostic test for quite a different organ or system. A tubeless gastric analysis, for instance, requires that specimens of urine be gathered at intervals, even though this test measures the presence of free hydrochloric acid in the stomach. Urine samples may also be taken for tests done to obtain information about liver function. This is not too surprising, however, when we remember that all organs of the body are interdependent and interrelated and that the physician interprets the various findings in relation to the *total* physical condition of his patient.

NURSING IMPLICATIONS

The nurse plays an important role in carrying out diagnostic tests, even though the physician has the ultimate responsibility of establishing a diagnosis of the patient's illness. It is the nurse who gives support to the patient, preparing him for diagnostic procedures, explaining his responsibilities before, during and after the procedure or test and offering encouragement during tedious and sometimes painful examinations and procedures.

The general physical examination is a routine preliminary to diagnosis and treatment. The practical nurse learns to assist the physician with the physical examination early in her training because it is a basic procedure in nursing. She learns the proper draping, positioning and reassurance of the patient during the physical examination and the instruments the physician generally uses. Her efficiency in having the necessary equipment readily at hand is, of course, appreciated by the physician, but perhaps more important, she is not distracted from the care of the patient during the examination. She has more time to console him when necessary, to reassure him that the procedure is progressing and will soon be over and to let him know that he has not been forgotten.

Special laboratory tests involving the collection and examination of specimens are an equally important part of diagnosis, and the nurse has special responsibilities in this area. She is often the "connecting link" between the patient and the many aspects of the diagnostic tests he will require.[6]

In general the nurse is expected to (1) prepare the patient and bring the necessary equipment to the bedside; (2) label the specimens accurately and be sure they are sent to the proper laboratory promptly, with accompanying information sheet as required by the laboratory; and (3) collect specimens as required by the test.

Of all the nursing duties and responsibilities, none can be more exacting or more demanding than the proper preparation of a patient for diagnostic tests and the conscientious follow-through of the procedure to its completion. A spinal tap for diagnostic laboratory work cannot be considered finished until the specimen of spinal fluid has been placed safely in the laboratory technician's hands; a glucose tolerance test is not completed until the last specimen of urine has been collected, labeled and taken to the laboratory. When there are several departments of the hospital involved in a procedure, there is sometimes a tendency to let someone else worry about the details. This is inexcusable, however, and the nurse assisting with any diagnostic procedures must understand her responsibilities and accept them as she should.

URINALYSIS

The term "routine urinalysis" usually means the examination of a single specimen of urine collected after one voiding and under conditions of cleanliness. The amount of urine needed is usually 60 to 100 ml. (cc.), and the specimen should be fresh when examined. The doctor usually prefers that urine specimens be collected in the morning after a night's sleep. This is particularly true if the patient is an outpatient. In this case, the nurse should inform the patient of the doctor's wishes in regard to the time the specimen is to be collected and the time it should be brought to the office or clinic.

The composition of normal urine may vary from time to time; this is an indication of good kidney function and is no cause for alarm. However, abnormal substances in the urine are an indication of disease. These abnormal constituents include (1) numerous red cells, (2) pus cells, (3) bacteria, (4) albumin, (5) sugar, (6) acetone and (7) bile (see Table 5-1).

There are times when the nurse may need to collect a 12-or 24-hour specimen for Addis count. This laboratory procedure is a measurement of each of the cellular elements in the urine sample and involves a count of the number of casts, red cells and white cells present. The Addis count is high in active chronic nephritis and in acute and terminal nephritis.

The specific gravity of urine is helpful in determining the ability of the kidneys to dilute and concentrate urine. Specific gravity is measured in grams per milliliter. Since water weighs 1.000 gram per ml., it is used as a basis of comparison for other liquids. The normal specific gravity of urine ranges from 1.010 to 1.025 grams per ml. It is more concentrated than water and therefore "weighs" more and has a higher specific gravity. A highly concentrated urine (one with an increased specific gravity) occurs in acute nephritis, dehydration, and uncontrolled diabetes mellitus in which the urine contains large amounts of sugar. In chronic nephritis and diabetes insipidus, the urine is very dilute, and the specific gravity is lower than normal.

The acidity or alkalinity of urine is expressed by the symbol pH. The complete range of pH values is from 1 (extremely acid) to 14 (extremely alkaline). The normal pH of urine ranges from 4.5 to 7.5. The pH of urine is high in certain bacterial infections of the

TABLE 5–1. ABNORMAL CONSTITUENTS OF URINE

Substance Present	Conditions Indicated
1. Blood	Damage to tissues somewhere along the urinary tract.
2. Pus cells	Infection in the urinary system.
3. Bacteria or other infectious organisms	Local infection of bladder or urinary tract.
4. Proteins, mainly albumin	Kidney disease involving the glomeruli, hypertension, severe heart failure, toxic conditions or abnormal proteins in the blood.
5. Acetone	Diabetes mellitus, ketosis accompanying starvation.
6. Sugar	Diabetes mellitus or some other metabolic disorder.
7. Bile	Obstruction of bile ducts from liver or gallbladder, or liver disease which interferes with normal bile removal.

TABLE 5–2. COLOR OF URINE IN VARIOUS CONDITIONS*

Color	Source of Color	Pathologic Condition
Dark yellow to amber	Increase of normal pigments; concentrated urine	Acute febrile diseases
Milky	Fat globules; pus cells	Chyluria; purulent diseases of the urinary tract
Orange	Excreted drugs, such as santonin, chrysophanic acid, pyridine	
Red or reddish	Hemoglobin, red blood cells	Hemorrhage; hemoglobinuria; trauma
Brown to brown-black	Hematin, melanin, blood pigments	Hemorrhage; melanotic sarcoma
Greenish-yellow or brown, approaching black	Bile pigments	Phenol poisoning; jaundice
Dirty green or blue (dark-blue surface scum, blue deposit)	Excess of indigo-forming substances; methylene blue medication	Cholera; typhus (seen especially when urine is putrefying)

*Adapted from French: The Nurse's Guide to Diagnostic Procedures. 3rd edition. Copyright McGraw-Hill, Inc., 1971. Used by permission of McGraw-Hill Book Company.

urinary tract, in alkalosis and in potassium depletion. It is low in metabolic and respiratory acidosis, fever and certain disorders of metabolism. Sometimes the physician will deliberately alter the pH of the urine as a form of treatment for certain disorders. For example, some types of kidney stones can form in very acid urine, while other types form in alkaline urine. Controlling the pH of the patient's urine decreases the formation of the stones. There also are certain types of infections that respond more readily to treatment when the pH of the urine is controlled.

HEMATOLOGIC STUDIES

Recent advances in medical technology have greatly expanded the number and kinds of studies that can be made of blood samples. These advances bring us closer to realizing the dream that soon we will be able to diagnose disease in its earliest stages, perhaps before it even appears. Such screening techniques as the SMA-12 and electrophoresis provide the health team with a large volume of information about a patient in a relatively short period of time. They also can serve as a basis for comparison in ongoing studies of the patient and his status in the health-illness continuum.

The study of the elements and chemical components of blood is extremely complex, requiring much more information than can be included in a text of this kind. It is hoped, however, that the reader will gain some basic information about the ways in which hematologic studies aid the diagnostician and that such an understanding will serve as an incentive to seek and find more extensive sources when more detailed information is needed.

NURSING IMPLICATIONS. Hematologic studies involve detailed analyses of a specimen of the patient's blood. This means that in some way the patient must be subjected to an unpleasant procedure for withdrawal of the specimen. Those studies done on capillary blood require small amounts, such as, for example, blood from a finger prick. Many times, however, several studies are ordered at the same time, and 10 ml. or more of blood must be obtained from the patient.

Whether or not the nurse performs the venipuncture, she should be aware of the apprehension with which many persons view the withdrawal of blood from their veins. Such fears should not be taken lightly, and certainly the patient deserves an explanation of the reason for withdrawal of what appears to him to be a large and perhaps dangerous amount of blood. A few words of explanation and reassurance can do much to relieve the patient's anxiety and promote cooperation.

The responsibility for proper performance of the laboratory tests lies with the personnel in the laboratory, but the nursing staff must usually prepare the patient correctly to ensure valid testing. This preparation often involves restriction or limiting of food and fluid intake until after the blood is drawn and may also require administration of a drug or other pretest medication. The nurse is not expected to be able to recite from memory the preparation of each patient for each laboratory test. She must, however, utilize the resources at hand, such as a procedure manual or laboratory manual, to determine exactly what preparation is necessary. It is rather exasperating to the patient and the laboratory personnel to find that a test must be repeated because the patient was not prepared properly. Nevertheless, the patient who is able to understand directions and cooperate must accept some responsibility for following the directions given to him. If he has been told not to eat or drink after the evening meal and is given an explanation of why these restrictions are necessary, it is not unreasonable to expect him to comply with the directions.

Cell Count. A laboratory procedure that is frequently performed at the time of a patient's admission to the hospital is the RBC, or red blood cell count. Another frequently ordered test is the WBC, or white blood cell count. In each of these tests, the blood sample is diluted in the laboratory and the cells are counted and recorded in numbers per cubic millimeter (1/1000 of a cubic centimeter). The normal RBC range is 4.8 to 5.5 million per cu. mm. for men and 4.4 to 5.0 million per cu. mm. for women. The normal WBC is a total of 6000 to 9000 per cu. mm.

A differential white cell count determines the numbers of various kinds of leukocytes present in the specimen of blood (see Fig. 5–1). There is a distinction made between absolute and relative white blood cell counts, and the nurse should keep this in mind when reading reports on differential WBC's. An *absolute* count is the exact number of the specific type of leukocytes present in the blood sample. A *relative* count indicates the percentage of the specific type of leukocyte as compared to all other types present in the specimen being examined. For example, the absolute count of lymphocytes may be 2100 per cu. mm., while the relative count is 25 per cent.

The physician uses information about the absolute and relative counts of the different kinds of leukocytes in diagnosing specific diseases. In agranulocytosis, for example, there is a decrease in the number of granulocytes in the blood stream. In certain types of leukemia, there may be an increase in eosinophils or basophils, depending on the type of leukemia involved.

Platelets, also called thrombocytes, are minute particles suspended in the blood. As the name implies (*thrombo*—clot, *cyte*—cell), they are essential to the clotting of blood. Information about the number and different types of platelets is valuable in diagnosing a variety of diseases affecting or affected by the clotting of blood. The normal

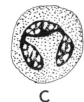

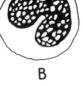
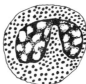

A

B

C

D

E

Figure 5–1. Various types of leukocytes that are counted and recorded in a *differential white cell count. A,* Lymphocyte. *B,* Monocyte. *C, D* and *E,* Granulocytes. *C,* Neutrophil. *D,* Eosinophil. *E,* Basophil. (From Manner: *Elements of Anatomy and Physiology,* W. B. Saunders Co., Philadelphia.)

range for a thrombocyte count is 200,000 to 350,000 per cu. mm.

Other Blood Elements and Values

Hemoglobin. Hemoglobin is a chemical compound of protein and iron. It is responsible for carrying oxygen in the blood and is the substance that gives red blood cells their color. A determination of the amount of hemoglobin in the red blood cells is important in the diagnosis of certain types of anemia. There are a number of different types of hemoglobin. The types are designated by letters, such as, for example, hemoglobin A, which is normal adult hemoglobin, and hemoglobin S, which is found in sickle cell diseases. The normal range for hemoglobin is 14.5 to 16.0 grams per 100 ml. of blood in men and 13.0 to 15.5 grams per 100 ml. of blood in women.

Hematocrit. A hematocrit is a test to measure the volume of blood cells in relation to the volume of plasma. When there has been a loss of body fluids but no cell loss, as in dehydration, the cell volume is high in proportion to the amount of liquid (plasma) in the blood stream. On the other hand, when either hemorrhage or anemia has depleted the supply of cells, the blood is "thinned," and the hematocrit, or cell volume, is low. The normal range for the hematocrit is 45 to 50 ml. per 100 ml. for men and 40 to 45 ml. per 100 ml. for women.

Erythrocyte Sedimentation Rate (ESR or Sed Rate). This test measures the length of time it takes the red cells in a sample of whole blood to separate from the plasma and settle to the bottom of a glass test tube. The blood cells of a person suffering from an infectious disease or some other disease such as rheumatic fever or arthritis will settle more rapidly than those of a healthy person. The test is used less frequently than formerly because it is not always reliable, does not specify the particular kind of infection or inflammation present and is now being replaced by more accurate and specific tests. It does have some value in determining the progress or regression of a disease and is more often used as an index to the success of treatment than as a diagnostic aid. Normal range for the ESR varies with the type of test done. It is recorded in millimeters per hour; for example, in the Cutler method, the normal range for men is 0 to 8 mm. per hour and for women it is 0 to 10 mm. per hour.

STUDIES IN HEMOSTASIS

In its broadest sense, the term hemostasis refers to the processes of blood coagulation and all factors affecting the formation of a clot. The advent of anticoagulant drugs has increased the frequency with which studies in hemostasis are now done.

Prothrombin Time. In the formation of a clot, prothrombin is converted to thrombin. If the prothrombin level is very low, the clot forms much more slowly than normal. The diseases most commonly associated with slow prothrombin time are liver diseases and vitamin K deficiency. There are times, however, when the physician wishes to slow down the clotting process of the blood, as in the treatment of diseases in which there is a pathologic formation of clots. Patients who have had coronary occlusions, for example, are often placed on anticoagulant therapy to decrease the probability of another occlusion due to a blood clot lodging in a coronary artery. For these patients, the physician usually orders a daily test of prothrombin time during hospitalization. The test is performed in the morning before the anticoagulant drug is given. The prothrombin level is kept within a safe range that avoids the danger of hemorrhage and at the same time decreases the probability of clot formation within a blood vessel. The normal range for prothrombin time is 12 to 15 seconds. If a control is used, the therapeutic range is approximately twice that of the control. Thus, if the control is 15 seconds, the reading should be 30 seconds for anticoagulant therapy.

Coagulation Time. This test measures the ability of the blood to clot (coagulate) in a given period of time. It incorporates all the factors involved in the clotting mechanism. A prolonged clotting time indicates a danger of hemorrhage or excessive blood loss. Some diseases involve a deficiency of one or more of the essential clotting factors. In the management of these diseases, a knowledge of the patient's clotting time can be of great importance. The normal range for clotting time depends on the method used in the laboratory. The safe range for coagulation time using the Lee-White method is 9 to 12 minutes.

BIOCHEMICAL EXAMINATIONS

In this day of computerized medicine, it is not surprising that there are sophisticated laboratory instruments capable of performing simultaneously a variety of blood chemistry tests on blood specimens from as many as 60 patients. Using 2.5 ml. of blood in each sample, the instrument called the SMA* (sequential multiple analysis) evaluates and records on a print-out sheet as many as 12 different readings on the chemicals in a sample of blood. The record is in the form of a graph. Shaded areas indicate normal ranges and a dark line shows the individual patient's reading (see Fig. 5–2).

The chemicals tested in an SMA-12 can vary, but they usually include the electrolytes, albumin, blood urea nitrogen, bilirubin, glucose and certain enzymes. The information obtained in this battery of tests is extremely valuable in detecting specific disorders and eliminating other suspected illnesses.

Another relatively new laboratory technique is concerned with an analytic study of the proteins in the blood. These proteins are essential to normal functioning of the body, particularly in maintaining normal osmotic pressure between the intravascular and extravascular fluid compartments. The analytic study of these proteins through a procedure called electrophoresis is of value in diagnosing many diseases affecting the protein levels in blood. The procedure derives its name from the use of an electric field

---

*SMA is the trademark of the Technicon Corp., Tarrytown, N.Y.

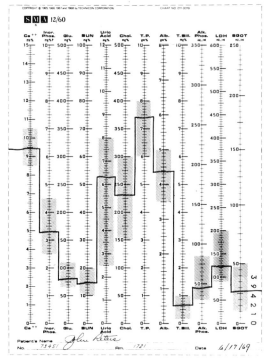

Figure 5–2. SMA™ 12/60 serum chemistry graph. Shaded areas on each column indicate normal ranges. Line indicates results obtained on patient's specimen. (Trademark. Technicon Corp., Tarrytown, New York.)

across which each blood protein moves in a characteristic manner. In this way the volume and activity of each protein can be distinguished from other proteins. This technique is also used to separate and identify various types of hemoglobin, such as the abnormal hemoglobin in sickle cell disease.

The normal range for total proteins in the blood is 6.5 to 8.0 grams per 100 ml. Of these proteins, the individual normal ranges are as follows:

Albumins—4.0 to 5.5 grams per 100 ml.
Globulins—2.0 to 3.0 grams per 100 ml.
Fibrinogen—0.2 to 0.4 grams per 100 ml.

ENZYMES

You will recall from your nutrition classes that enzymes are chemical agents that act as catalysts in the breakdown of complex substances into simpler substances. These enzymes are particularly important in the digestion and metabolism of food. Recent research has shown that when cells of the body are damaged by physical or chemical trauma, the injured cell membranes permit leakage of enzymes from the cell body into the blood stream. Because many enzymes are specific for the cells of the organs from which they escape, a determination of the level of specific enzymes in the blood can indicate which organ has been damaged and to what extent.

The names of enzymes are distressingly long and difficult to pronounce. For the sake of expediency, abbreviations are used. For example, damaged heart muscle cells release CPK, SGOT, LDH and GPT. The names for each of these enzymes are, respectively, creatine phosphokinase, serum glutamic oxaloacetic transaminase, lactic dehydrogenase and glutamic pyruvic transaminase. It is easy to understand why abbreviations are used.

The patterns displayed by the various enzymes can be of help in the diagnosis of disease of the liver, pancreas and heart; in detecting certain anemias and leukemias; in tracing the metastasis of malignant cells; and in monitoring and evaluating tissue rejection in organ transplants. Normal ranges vary with the testing method used.

X-RAY STUDIES

Normal sight depends on the response of the eye to light rays. In order for us to see an object, it is necessary for rays of light to be present. We know that ordinary light cannot penetrate some objects of certain density, and for this reason we are not able to see beyond or into these objects. When there is a complete absence of light rays, we are in total darkness and cannot see "our hands before our faces."

In the year 1895, a German physicist by the name of Roentgen discovered some unusually penetrating rays, which he produced by directing a stream of electrically charged particles onto a metal surface. He did not know or fully understand how these radiations or rays worked, so he called them x-rays ("x" being the symbol for the unknown quantity). As Dr. Roentgen experimented with these rays, he found that he could direct them through certain materials and their outline would be left on films placed behind them.

X-ray films are *negatives*. They are not pictures in the true sense of the word. When the x-rays pass through structures such as skin and fat, they do so readily and leave a dark area on the film. If, however, the rays strike a denser structure such as bone, they are slowed down in their progress and will make a much lighter mark on the film. Thus, objects of greater density appear lighter on the x-ray film, and objects of lesser density appear darker on the film. It is important that this be understood before one can fully realize the importance of removing flatus, etc.,

from the intestinal tract during x-rays of the abdominal area. If flatus or fecal material is present, it will cast dark and confusing shadows on the film, making the interpretation of the film difficult for the radiologist.

Hollow tubes and organs such as those in the intestinal tract and urinary system can be filled with barium or very dense radiopaque dyes containing iodine. Following the instillation of the opaque substance, x-ray films are taken. Obstruction from tumors, twisting or kinking and other abnormalities of the organ can then be readily diagnosed. The normal hollow organ will fill readily and can be outlined on the film, whereas obstruction of a tube or organ will prevent filling beyond that point and the exact location of the difficulty can be pinpointed. This is generally what occurs when a GI series, barium enema, gallbladder series, or pyelogram is done. These specific diagnostic tests are discussed more fully under diseases of their respective systems later in this text.

Fluoroscopy is a method of x-ray in which there are no "still pictures" taken. Fluoroscopy might be compared to a motion picture, whereas x-ray is comparable to a photograph, although neither is a picture in a true sense of the word. During fluoroscopy the physician can watch a particular organ at work—for example, the action of the heart or the flow of barium through the stomach and small intestine.

Preparation of the Patient for Diagnostic X-ray Films

The nursing procedures necessary for preparing the patient for x-ray will depend on the area being filmed and the purpose of the x-ray examination. In some instances, such as in x-ray studies of the lungs or bones, no special preparation may be necessary. In others, especially those employing a radiopaque substance to fill the hollow organs of the abdominal cavity, preparation of the patient is of primary importance. It can readily be understood that if even air has some density and will not permit the full penetration of x-rays, the patient's intestinal tract must be completely empty before successful diagnostic films of the abdomen can be taken. From our knowledge of gross anatomy, we are aware that the ureters are posterior to the intestines; thus, any fecal material or flatus left in the intestinal tract will prevent clear "pictures" of the ureters or kidneys. The same is true of x-rays of the intestinal tract because the presence of the flatus and feces can prevent complete filling with barium or can cause confusing shadows on the x-ray film.

The exact method of cleansing the intestines will vary according to the wishes of the radiologist in charge. Generally, however, the practical nurse can expect that examination of the upper intestinal tract by x-ray will be done on a fasting patient; the lower intestinal tract or other abdominal examinations will require catharsis and cleansing enemas. *Success or failure of the examination will depend greatly on how conscientiously the nurse carries out her responsibilities prior to the examination.*

ENDOSCOPIC EXAMINATIONS

An endoscope is a special instrument designed for inspection of the interior of hollow organs such as the stomach, bladder, esophagus and bronchi. The names of the various types of endoscopes tell us of their specific purpose. The bronchoscope is used in examination of the bronchi, the gastroscope is used for visualization of the stomach and the cystoscope for the urinary bladder. Each type of endoscope utilizes light and reflection via mirrors to inspect body cavities that would otherwise be inaccessible. The more recently designed endoscopes are made up of glass fibers. Each fiber acts as a mirror, thus allowing light to "go around corners" and permitting viewing in a variety of directions.

Although the endoscope is primarily used for diagnosis, it can be employed in various types of treatment, as in removing a foreign body from the trachea or bronchus, cauterizing polyps and fulgurating bladder tumors or ulcerations.

RADIONUCLIDE STUDIES

The term radionuclide is a combination of two words: "radioactive" and "nuclei." An element that is radioactive is one which gives off radiations, or streams of particles, that can be detected by special equipment. The suffix "nuclide" is derived from "nucleus" (plural, "nuclei"). The nuclei of the atoms of radioactive elements emit the particles of which alpha and beta "rays" or radiations are composed.

Another term that is often used in diagnostic studies using radioactive substances is radioisotope. Isotopes are different forms of the same element. For example, an isotope of iodine has the same chemical and physical properties as an atom of iodine, but it differs in the number of neutrons in its nucleus (mass number); it is, therefore, not exactly the same as an atom of iodine.

Most chemical elements are not radioactive. They possess a balanced ratio of protons to neutrons in their nuclei and do not give off any form of radiation. Those elements (such as radium) which do not have this balanced ratio are said to be unstable. All unstable elements try to achieve stability by altering the ratio of protons to neutrons. They do this by releasing with great energy particles from the nucleus. These particles form the rays which constitute radiation. Elements which are naturally stable and therefore not radioactive can be made unstable by bombarding them with large numbers of free neutrons in a nuclear reactor. Cobalt-59 is a stable, nonradioactive element. When atoms of cobalt-59 are

TABLE 5–3. RADIOISOTOPES IN CURRENT CLINICAL USE*

Isotope	Symbol	Principal Uses in Diagnostics
Iodine	^{125}I ^{131}I	As iodine for thyroid studies; with phenolphthalein for liver studies; with Hippuran for renal studies; with albumin for pulmonary studies.
Technetium	^{99m}Tc	In brain scanning; for study of hemodynamics; with sulfur to study reticuloendothelial system. Has replaced ^{203}Hg and ^{198}Au to a large extent.
Strontium	^{85}Sr	In bone scanning.
Selenium	^{75}Se	In pancreatic scans; may also be used in bone scanning and lymphoma.
Xenon	^{133}Xe	In studying either circulation or gaseous exchange in the lung and in studying circulation in the brain.
Chromium	^{51}Cr	To tag red cells to study hematologic disease and the spleen.
Cobalt	^{60}Co ^{57}Co	To study absorption and excretion of vitamin B_{12}; to study megaloblastic anemias.
Iron	^{59}Fe	To study ferrokinetics.

*Adapted from Nursing Update, Oct., 1971, p. 14

placed in a nuclear reactor, some of the atoms will absorb an extra neutron in their nuclei. This upsets the atom's balanced ratio of protons to neutrons, and each atom so altered becomes cobalt-60, a radioactive isotope of cobalt-59.

A radioisotope behaves in the body in the same way as its nonradioactive counterpart. This means it follows the same metabolic pathways and is concentrated in the same organs and tissues. Because the radioisotope gives off some form of radiation, it can be followed and located by an externally placed detector. This process then gives the diagnostician information about the function of an organ or tissue, or it can locate and give the type and degree of abnormality that may be present in the organ or tissue.

Radioactive iodine, for example, can be used in the diagnosis of thyroid disorders because the thyroid gland takes up and utilizes iodine in the synthesis of its hormone thyroxin. (See Table 5–3 for other radioisotopes used for diagnosis.) Some diagnostic procedures use radioisotopes for the sampling and radioactive counting of blood, urine and other body fluids and tissues. Counting gives an indication of the concentration or density of such substances.

The term *scanning* is used to describe a procedure whereby a detector moves slowly over a body area and produces a "picture" composed of a series or grouping of dots. The dots are produced by the rays or emanations from the radioisotope concentrated in the area (see Fig. 5–3).

Most diagnostic tests utilizing radioisotopes are done in an outpatient clinic. Some explanation should be given the patient as to what specific test is to be done and its purpose. Scanning requires that the patient remain almost motionless during the procedure so that a clear, well-defined picture can be

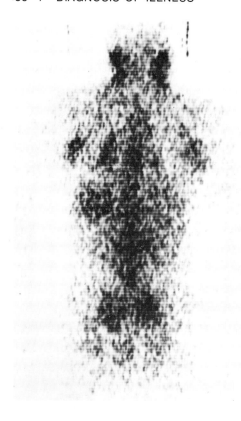

Figure 5–3. Whole body scan, using indium-111. (Courtesy of Dr. L. R. Bennett in James and Squire: *Exercises in Diagnostic Radiology—6. Nuclear Radiology.* Philadelphia, W. B. Saunders Company, 1973.)

obtained. This may be difficult for the patient unless he is positioned comfortably before the scanning is begun. In some cases sedation may be necessary. Although all radioactive materials require special handling and precautions, radioisotopes in the dosage used for most diagnostic tests do not require any special precautions once the test is completed. This also should be explained to the patient before he is dismissed from the clinic.

CLINICAL CASE PROBLEMS

1. Mr. Gordon, age 42, is admitted to the hospital for diagnostic tests. He is very apprehensive about his hospitalization, which is a new experience for him, and he is obviously upset about providing specimens of urine and blood.

What can you do or say to relieve some of Mr. Gordon's anxiety?

What observations might you make in regard to Mr. Gordon's urine specimen?

How would you describe an SMA-12 test to one of your classmates?

How would you describe electrophoresis?

2. Mrs. Lucas is scheduled for a diagnostic test involving the use of radioactive iodine.

What type of disorder is associated with this type of test?

How is the radioactive iodine used in the diagnostic study?

REFERENCES

1. Barnett, M. "The Nature of Radiation and Its Effect on Man." Nurs. Clin. N. Am. Vol. 2, No. 1, p. 11. Philadelphia, W. B. Saunders Co., 1967.
2. Deal, J.: "'Just Another Lab Spec'?" Bedside Nurse, April, 1972, p. 12.
3. French, R. M.: *The Nurse's Guide to Diagnos-*

tic Procedures, 3rd edition. New York, Mc-Graw-Hill Book Co., 1971.

4. Rodriguez-Antunez, A. et al.: "How They're Using Radioisotopes Today." Nursing Update, Oct., 1971, p. 11.

5. Sister Marie Louise: *The Operating Room Technician*. St. Louis, The C. V. Mosby Co., 1965.

SUGGESTED STUDENT READING

1. Deal, J.: "'Just Another Lab Spec'?" Bedside Nurse, April, 1972, p. 12.

2. Miller, R. E., and Gerard, S.: "The Nurse on the Radiological Team." Am. Journ. Nurs., July, 1964, p. 128.

OUTLINE FOR CHAPTER 5

I. Introduction

A. The chemist, radiologist and pathologist aid the physician in diagnosis of an illness.

II. Purposes of Special Diagnostic Tests

A. To determine the patient's general physical condition.
B. To find the cause of illness.
C. As a verification of diagnosis.
D. As a guide for treatment.

III. Nursing Implications

A. Nurse has supporting role and responsibilities to the patient.
B. Also responsible for collecting and proper labeling of specimens.
C. Proper physical preparation of the patient essential to diagnostic studies.

IV. Urinalysis

A. Abnormal constituents include red cells, pus cells, bacteria, albumin, sugar, acetone and bile.
B. Addis count—done on 12- to 24-hour specimen. Involves counting of cellular elements in urine.
C. Specific gravity—relative dilution and concentration of urine.
D. pH—expression of acidity or alkalinity.

V. Hematologic Studies

A. Recent advances in technology have increased number of tests.
B. Blood studies very complex.
C. Nurse responsible for preparation of patient, explanation of tests and reassurance.

D. Cell count—one of most common blood tests.
  1. Cells counted and recorded in numbers per cu. mm. of blood.
  2. Differential count determines numbers of various kinds of cells.
E. Hemoglobin—tested for amount and types.
F. Hematocrit—measures volume of cells in relation to plasma volume.
G. ESR—measures length of time it takes erythrocytes to separate from plasma.

VI. Studies in Hemostasis

A. Concerned with clotting of blood.
B. Prothrombin time—useful in diseases of liver and vitamin K deficiency. Also used in anticoagulant therapy.
C. Coagulation time—measures clotting ability of blood.

VII. Biochemical Examinations

A. Sequential multiple analysis (SMA) measures a variety of chemicals.
B. Electrophoresis—analytic study of blood proteins.

VIII. Enzymes

A. Damaged body cells leak enzymes into the blood.
B. Determination of specific enzymes in the blood can indicate which organ has been damaged and to what extent.

IX. X-ray Studies—Use of Roentgen Rays Which are Capable of Penetrating Soft Tissues

A. Proper preparation of patient essential to adequate studies.
B. Fluoroscopy—x-ray studies of organs in motion.

X. Endoscopic Examinations

A. Utilization of a special instrument that is inserted into hollow organs.
B. Bronchoscope, cystoscope and gastroscope are examples of instruments used.

XI. Radionuclide Studies

A. Useful in diagnosis because radioactive isotopes give off radiations that can be detected by special equipment.
B. Used in diagnosis of thyroid disorders to "count" blood, urine and body fluid concentrations and to help locate abnormal structure and function of certain organs.

6

The Surgical Patient

VOCABULARY

Apprehension
Diaphragm
Distention
Incoherent
Trauma

INTRODUCTION

The nursing care of the surgical patient is generally divided into three phases: (1) the preoperative period, (2) the operative and immediate postoperative period and (3) the period of convalescence and rehabilitation. The length of time each of these periods involves varies according to the type of surgery and the general physical condition of the patient.

The preoperative period includes physical, mental and emotional preparation for the surgical procedure. The operative period includes the time the patient is under anesthesia and recovering from the anesthesia. In most hospitals the patient is kept in a special area usually called the recovery room until this phase of surgery and anesthesia is completed. The postoperative period of convalescence and rehabilitation demands the attention of many members of the medical team and may include the occupational therapist, physical therapist and social worker.

PREOPERATIVE PERIOD

Emotional and Psychological Preparation

Preparation of the patient for surgery actually begins when the surgeon first decides that an operation is necessary and explains to his patient the need for surgery and the kind of operation which will be done. It is usually something of a shock to the patient and his family to learn that surgical treatment is necessary, and this change in the routine of their everyday lives will place some personal and financial burdens on them. For some patients, the surgery will alter their lives permanently, leaving them handicapped in some way and requiring an adjustment in their lives and the lives of their families. Others may expect to be greatly helped by the surgical procedure, but even they will have some fears and misgivings about the prospect of having anesthesia and surgery.

All of us fear the unknown. The surgical patient who has never had surgery before or is not familiar with hospital routine will have many questions about what is in store for him now that he realizes surgery is necessary. It is to the advantage of all concerned that these questions be satisfactorily answered and that the patient have a general idea of what he might expect before and after surgery.

We know that there should always be an effective means of communication between hospital personnel and the patient. What do we mean by good communication? Our first thought is usually communication by the spoken word. But the patient may not feel free to ask questions or to voice his apprehension about surgery and anesthesia. The first step, therefore, is to instill a feeling of confidence and trust in our ability, and to demonstrate by our attitudes and actions that we are sincerely interested in the patient as a person. When questions are asked of us, we must exercise extreme care in the answers we give. We are often as much misunderstood by what we *don't* say as by what we *do* say. It is far better, then, if the patient asks a nurse a question she is not qualified to answer, for her to say simply that she doesn't know but that the nurse in charge or the physician can tell him what he wishes to know. An example of this is a question such as, "Will the doctor remove my whole stomach or just the part where the ulcer is?" Obviously she is not qualified to explain the intentions of the surgeon. A general question, however, such as, "Will I wake up in my own room after surgery?" can be answered quite easily.

The patient should be encouraged to ask questions about certain aspects of his care that he does not understand, and he should be given answers promptly and accurately. It is extremely frustrating and a bit frightening for him when his questions are evaded or answered in a vague manner at a time when everything happening to him seems so important. And indeed it is

important to him and to his recovery. The relaxed and confident patient is under less strain physically as well as mentally and will recover more rapidly than one who is confused, angry or fearful.

We must not forget the patient's family in the emotional preparation for surgery. They should be informed of the usual routines, including the premedication the evening and morning of surgery, which will make the patient somewhat groggy and incoherent just before he goes to the operating room. It is also helpful if the family realizes that the length of time the patient is away from his room does not necessarily represent the length of the operation. There are sometimes slight delays in getting the procedure started in the operating room. And then, after surgery, most hospitals have a recovery unit where the patient is kept under close observation until he is considered out of immediate danger and awake from anesthesia. This simple explanation of what they can expect and how long they may have to wait to see the patient after the operation helps to prevent much unnecessary worry and anguish about their loved one.

It is also reassuring to the patient and his family if they have some idea of the treatments which may be necessary postoperatively. So many people associate the administration of oxygen, blood transfusions or IV fluids, and the presence of a Levin tube or other drainage apparatus, with a critical situation. If they understand that many of these treatments are commonplace in surgical procedures, they will realize these do not indicate the patient has "taken a turn for the worse."

The goals of the nursing staff in preparing a patient for surgery can be summarized as follows: (1) lessening of the fears and anxieties of the patient and his family, (2) assurance that the patient and his family accept necessary procedures and understand the purpose of equipment that will be used in his care and (3) optimum cooperation between the patient and the nurses who will care for him.[8]

Spiritual Preparation *important*

Since most of us have a justifiable fear of anesthesia and surgery, it is comforting to have some moral and spiritual support before surgery. The patient or his family may ask that a spiritual advisor be called in. This is a very important aspect of preoperative care and must not be overlooked in the many activities of physical preparation. The nurse who displays a sincere interest in every aspect of her patient's care will do all that she can to help him gain peace of mind.

Physical Preparation of the Patient for Surgery

Preoperative Examination. Before he undertakes surgery, the physician will try to have his patient in the best possible condition. In emergencies, of course, he cannot always manage this, but in planned surgery he may postpone the operation for days or weeks until the patient is physically able to withstand the rigors of anesthesia and major surgery.

On admission to the hospital, the surgical patient will have a hemoglobin test and a blood count ordered. If the laboratory reports indicate any abnormalities, measures will be taken to improve the general health of the patient before surgery is scheduled.

A urinalysis is also done to eliminate the possibility of an infection or other disease of the urinary system. Surgery puts an additional strain on the circulatory, urinary and respiratory systems. Thus the heart and lungs will be carefully examined for pathologic conditions. These are all the responsibilities of the physician, but the nurse may need to explain to the patient the need for these tests before surgery. Once the patient is confident that everything is being done to assure him of a safe and successful operation, he will become more relaxed and cooperative.

Preoperative Instruction. There are distinct advantages to teaching the patient certain procedures and practices that will benefit him postoperatively. Such instruction gives the patient an opportunity to participate in his care, obtains his cooperation in prevention of postoperative complications and works to reduce anxiety in the patient and his family. These preoperative instructions may vary from one institution to another, but they usually include deep breathing and coughing techniques, leg exercises and practice in moving about in bed and getting in and out of bed (see Fig. 6-1). *unless cor*

If it is expected that members of the patient's family will assist him during the postoperative period, they are included in the teaching sessions. In this way, the patient as well as his family gain confidence that they are all able to cooperate in helping the patient achieve a smooth and rapid recovery from the surgical procedure (see Figs. 6-2 and 6-3).

Preparation of the Skin. The skin and hair are both harborers of many microorganisms. It is not possible to make the skin completely sterile, but most of the organisms may be removed by shaving and scrubbing the area with green soap or hexachlorophene. The exact procedure for cleansing the operative area varies according to the wishes of the surgeon and the accepted procedure of the hospital. In some types of bone surgery, sterile towels or dressings are applied after the area is cleansed. However, some surgeons believe that dressings tend to increase perspiration, bringing deep-seated bacteria to the surface of the skin. When the nurse has no definite orders as to how the surgeon wishes the area to be prepared, she should ask for specific instructions from the nurse in charge. These instructions should designate the total area to be shaved and scrubbed as well as the method to be used.

to heal, don't say to prevent

PATIENT INSTRUCTION SHEET
FOR A BETTER RECOVERY AFTER YOUR SURGERY

Repeat the following exercise every 1-2 hours until you are up and around. Nurses will assist you if you have any difficulty or any questions.

DEEP
BREATHE

AND

COUGH! ! !

KEEP LUNGS FUNCTIONING PROPERLY! ! !   *prevent hypostatic pneumonia*
1. Inhale as deeply as you can.
2. Hold for a second or two.
3. Exhale completely.
4. Repeat several times. Then:
5. Inhale deeply.
6. Produce a deep abdominal cough (not shallow throat cough) by short, sharp expiration. (Incision may be splinted with hands or bedclothes. Flexing knees relieves strain on abdominal muscles.)

CHANGE

POSITION! ! !

MAINTAIN GOOD CIRCULATION! ! !
Lie on each side as well as on your back.

To turn easily:

1. Bend one knee, planting foot firmly on bed.
2. Lift opposite arm overhead (in direction of turn).
3. Roll onto side, pushing with bent leg (bedrails can be used to aid in turning).
4. If you need assistance, call one of the nurses.

To turn back again:

1. Bend knee of upper leg.
2. Place palm of top arm solidly on the side of the bed.
3. Push yourself over onto your back.

EXERCISE

FEET

AND

LEGS! ! !

PROMOTE GOOD CIRCULATION IN YOUR LEGS! ! !
Perform the following exercises *fairly slowly*, but with strong muscle contraction.   *prevent thrombophlebitis*

1. Push the toes of both feet toward the foot of the bed. Relax both feet. Pull toes toward the chin. Relax both feet.
2. Circle both ankles, first to the right; then to the left. Repeat three times. Relax.
3. Bend each knee alternately, sliding foot up along the bed. Relax.

prevent pulmonary embolism   OOB SOON AS DR ORDERS

Figure 6–1. Sample instruction sheet for surgical patients. (From Mezzanotte: American Journal of Nursing, January, 1970.)

if pt will have line

Restriction of Oral Intake. The surgeon will leave written orders regarding restriction of food and drink before surgery. It may be necessary for the nurse to explain to the patient that he is not allowed anything by mouth because of the danger of vomiting with subsequent aspiration of the vomitus into the air passages during or immediately after surgery. In some cases a gastric tube may be inserted into the stomach by way of a nostril and gastric suction started the evening or morning before surgery. This tube is to be clamped off and left in place just before the patient is taken to the operating room. It may reassure the patient if he understands that gastric suction eliminates much unnecessary distention, nausea and vomiting postoperatively, all of which place strain on the sutures and are exhausting and unpleasant for him.

Elimination. Surgery involving the abdominal cavity, rectum or perineum usually requires a cleansing of the lower intestinal tract by catharsis and/or enemas. This preparation will reduce the possibility of contamination of the operative area during anesthesia

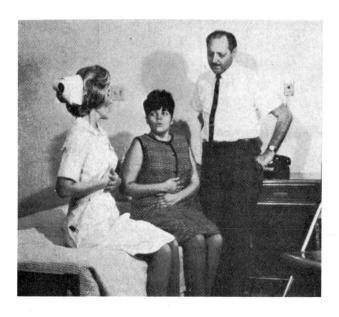

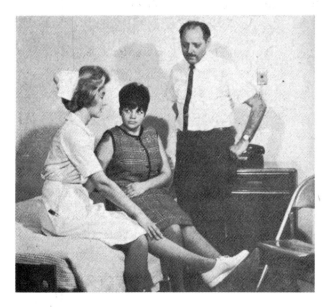

Figure 6–2. Deep breathing and leg exercises are demonstrated by nurse and practiced by patient. Family will help in postoperative care. (From Healy: American Journal of Nursing, January, 1968.)

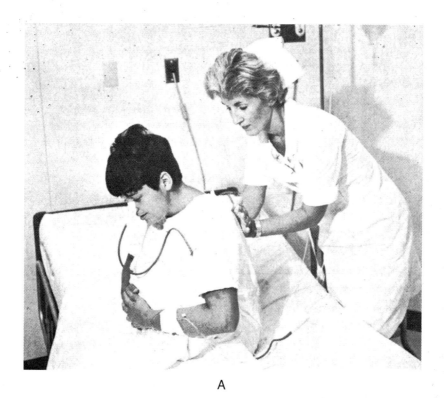

A

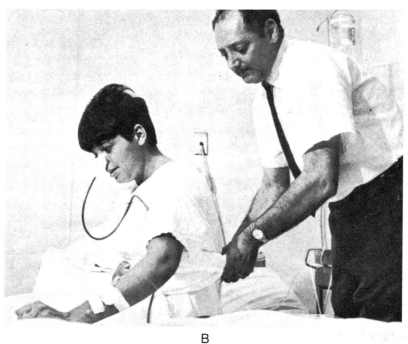

B

Figure 6–3. *A,* Coughing becomes more effective and less painful when the patient splints her operative site with a pillow and the nurse gives firm support to the patient's back. *B,* Bracing with a towel pulled snug on side opposite operative site during cough, then releasing its pressure for deep breathing, is another way to give support during coughing. (From Healy: American Journal of Nursing, January, 1968.)

when the sphincter muscles are relaxed and will also help to eliminate distention following surgery. Patients having rectal surgery or other operative procedures in which the surgeon does not wish the patient to have a bowel movement for several days after surgery often have "enemas until clear" ordered preoperatively. These are very exhausting and should be given slowly and with care, allowing the patient to rest between enemas.

Rest and Sedation. The body needs all of its strength and physical resources when coping with surgical procedures. Thus the patient should have a restful night with adequate sleep the night before surgery. A barbiturate is usually ordered, but this does not always guarantee that the patient will sleep well. The nurse should check frequently during the night to make sure the patient is sleeping. If he is awake and seems restless and fearful, she should stay with him for a while, answer his questions and try to allay his fears. It may be necessary to secure an order to repeat the sedation given at bedtime. If the patient is sleeping well, he should not be disturbed for routine procedures during the night and morning of surgery.

The Operative Permit. Before the surgeon can perform an operation, he must have written permission, signed by the patient or his guardian. This written permit protects the surgeon against "claims of unauthorized operations and protects the patient against unsanctioned surgery."[4] In most hospitals this permit is a printed form which the hospital will have the patient sign before surgery. This permit is then attached to the patient's chart and sent to the operating room with the chart (see Fig. 6–4).

Immediate Preoperative Care. The patient must wear a hospital gown to the operating room. The hair should be covered with a towel or cap, and in some hospitals surgical boots are put on the patient. Women with very long hair should have it combed and plaited into braids, and all hairpins must be removed from the hair. If the patient wishes to wear a wedding ring, it should be secured in place with a loop of gauze or tape slipped through the ring and tied to the wrist. Watches and other valuables must be removed from the bedside table and placed under lock and key according to the hospital policy. Dentures are usually removed, placed in a denture cup and kept in a designated place according to hospital policy. Sometimes the anesthesiologist will request that the dentures be left in place because they help maintain the contour of the face and facilitate the administration of inhalation anesthesia.

An identification bracelet or tag is attached to the patient's wrist to avoid any error or mix-up of patients in the operating room.

Unless there is a urinary catheter in place, preoperative patients are offered the bedpan or urinal just before going to surgery. As stated before, the sphincter muscles may become completely relaxed during anesthesia, and the patient might be incontinent and contaminate the operative field.

In the evaluation of the vital signs postoperatively, it is helpful to know the patient's blood pressure, pulse and respiration rate before he is sent to the operating room.

The preoperative medication must be administered at exactly the time ordered by the surgeon or anesthesiologist. This is essential because the amount of anesthesia and time of induction have been calculated according to the hour the premedication was expected to be given. A delay in the preoperative medication may cause difficulties for the patient and a great inconvenience to the person administering the anesthesia. All preliminary preparations should be done before the medication is given so that it will have maximum effect.

Preoperative medications are given to (1) promote rest and relaxation, (2)

AUTHORITY TO OPERATE

a.m.
Date............................ 19...... Time................p.m.

I hereby authorize the physician or physicians in charge of the care of

_____

(Name of Patient)

to administer any treatment; or to administer such anesthetics; and perform such operations as may be deemed necessary or advisable in the diagnosis and treatment of this patient.

Witness _____   Signed _____
(Patient or Nearest Relative)

Witness _____   _____
(Relationship)

Authorization must be signed by the patient, or by the nearest relative in the case of a minor, or when patient is physically or mentally incompetent.

Figure 6–4. Sample operative permit. These are used when surgical procedures are performed and must be completely filled out and properly signed before the operation is begun.

atropine

decrease secretion of mucus and other body fluids and (3) enhance the effects of the anesthetic. The sedatives that are usually used are barbiturates such as phenobarbital or Seconal. The drying agents may include atropine or scopolamine. Narcotics such as morphine or Demerol are given to supplement the anesthetic.

Many hospitals have a check list to be filled out by the nurse in charge before the patient is taken to the operating room. This eliminates the danger of omitting any part of the preoperative preparation (see Fig. 6–5).

ANESTHESIA

Anesthesia (the loss of sensory perception) came into use as an accepted part of surgical procedure in the 1840's. With the advent of drugs which safely produced anesthesia, the performance of surgical operations became a more widely accepted and successful means of treating disease and injury. Few of us would accept surgery without the advantage of being insensible to pain during the operation, and the modern surgical procedures requiring several hours would be impossible without adequate anesthesia.

The first anesthetics used were ether and nitrous oxide. It is interesting to note that these drugs were used as a source of entertainment and amusement before anyone considered using them in medical practice. Nitrous oxide, commonly called "laughing gas," was sometimes administered to a volunteer from the audience of a side

CLEARANCE RECORD FOR SURGICAL OPERATIONS

NAME   HOSP. NO.   DATE

	YES	NO	REMARKS
1. Written permission for surgery	✓		
2. Blood count and hemoglobin	✓		
3. Urinalysis	✓		
4. History and physical	✓		
5. Valuables			
a. Removed and placed in cabinet	✓		
b. Tied to patient's wrist			
6. Dentures removed		*none*	
7. Identification bracelet on patient	✓		
8. Vital signs 30 min. preoperatively			
a. BP *132/84*			
b. Pulse *90*			
c. Resp *18*			
9. Preoperative medication given			*at 7:45 a.m.*
10. Bleeding and clotting time (for T & As)			
11. Consultation sheet for sterilization for first Cesarean section			

Figure 6–5. Clearance record for surgical operations.

show for the purpose of watching the antics of the victim as he was transported into a state of euphoria and became hysterical with laughter. During the 1800's, ether "frolics" were also a source of entertainment (crude and dangerous as it may seem to us), in which medical students and other persons with access to the drug inhaled a small amount of ether and subsequently enjoyed a feeling of lighthearted gaiety. Today, both of these drugs are in common use in surgery and are considered to be among the safest and most effective anesthetics for major surgery.

There are three main objectives in the administration of an anesthetic: (1) to prevent pain, (2) to achieve adequate muscle relaxation and (3) to calm fear, allay anxiety and give forgetfulness.[2]

Types of Anesthesia

In order to achieve the objectives mentioned above, there are a variety of anesthetics available. The choice of anesthesia rests with the anesthesiologist and depends on the type of surgery to be performed, the age and physical condition of the patient and his ability to tolerate the anesthetic. The types of anesthesia may be classified according to the method of administration. They include inhalants, intravenous anesthetics, local anesthetics, spinal anesthetics and refrigeration anesthesia.

Inhalants. These include ether, nitrous oxide, trilene, cyclopropane, and methoxyflurane (Penthrane). Most of these gases and liquids are highly inflammable and demand extreme caution to guard against electric sparks in their presence. Ether causes an irritation of the mucous membranes, resulting in large amounts of mucus in the respiratory tract. Patients receiving ether will, therefore, need frequent suctioning while unconscious, and must be encouraged to take deep breaths and cough up the bronchial secretions once they have awakened. They will frequently have nausea and vomiting of the mucus which has collected in the stomach and esophagus.

Intravenous Anesthetics. The drug most commonly used for this type of anesthesia is Pentothal, a fast-acting barbiturate, which produces immediate unconsciousness when it is administered. A patient who has received this anesthetic must be watched closely during the immediate postoperative period for cyanosis, restlessness and dyspnea, which are signs of laryngeal spasm, a condition sometimes associated with the administration of Pentothal.

Local or Regional Anesthesia. In this type of anesthesia, only the area of the surgical incision and adjacent tissues are deadened to the pain involved, and the patient remains awake. This method is used most frequently for minor surgery, diagnostic tests and examinations. Drugs most commonly used are procaine, tetracaine and dibucaine. Newer drugs include mepivacaine (Carbocaine) and prilocaine (Citanest). Some hypersensitive individuals may suffer a severe reaction to the drugs used in local anesthesia, and circulatory failure and death may occur. The nurse assisting with procedures in which a local anesthetic is used should be alert for signs of hypersensitivity in the patient and be prepared for the administration of oxygen and an emergency drug such as Adrenalin in the event that a reaction

develops. Usually, if there is any possibility of an idiosyncrasy to the anesthetizing drug, the physician will do a skin test before injecting a local anesthetic.

TOPICAL ANESTHESIA. This is a form of local anesthesia in which the drug is applied directly on the surface of the area to be treated. It is used frequently in examinations or treatments of the eye, nose and throat.

Spinal Anesthesia. The spinal cord serves as a pathway for nerve impulses passing to and from the brain. By injecting a drug into the spinal cavity around the spinal cord, these impulses are blocked, and there is complete loss of feeling in all areas of the body below the site of injection. This is what is done when a spinal anesthesia is given. Obviously this type of anesthesia can only be used for surgery below the diaphragm, but it is very effective and produces complete muscular relaxation even though the patient remains awake during the operation.

The postoperative care of the patient receiving spinal anesthesia is basically the same as for a general anesthesia, although there are usually fewer gastrointestinal and respiratory complications to be guarded against following spinal anesthesia. On the other hand, the nurse must realize that respiratory difficulties and cardiovascular complications can develop when spinal anesthesia is given. If the anesthesia ascends beyond the point of injection, innervation of the respiratory muscles and blood vessels is effected. This produces depression of respiration and a lowering of the blood pressure. In case respiratory embarrassment occurs, artificial respiration by machine or the mouth-to-mouth method must be employed. Hypotension is treated by the administration of drugs such as ephedrine or methoxyl unless the lowered blood pressure is caused by blood loss. The patient may not be placed in shock position with the head lowered until at least 20 minutes after injection of the anesthetic.

As the anesthesia wears off, the patient may complain that he cannot move his legs and that they feel numb and heavy. This is to be expected at first and will gradually subside. The patient is kept flat in bed for a minimum of 8 hours, and longer if he experiences headache or dizziness. Some confusion and dizziness may be due to the preoperative drugs given; in this event, side rails are applied and the patient is watched carefully until he is no longer dizzy and confused. He may be turned from side to side unless there are specific orders to the contrary. The first few times the patient is allowed out of bed, there must be someone in attendance to protect him from falls and injury because he may experience some difficulty in maintaining his balance.

Refrigeration Anesthesia. This type of anesthesia is produced by lowering the temperature of a part (usually a lower limb) until the extreme cold retards the conduction of nerve impulses. It is sometimes supplemented by the administration of another anesthetic. Advantages of refrigeration anesthesia include minimal bleeding during and after surgery, less possibility of physical shock and elimination of the hazards of inhalation anesthesia for patients who are weak and debilitated.

This type of anesthesia is especially useful for amputations in the treatment of arteriosclerotic gangrene. The area to be anesthetized is packed in ice or wrapped in a special electric refrigeration unit. Tourniquets are applied to prevent chilling of the rest of the body. The length of time necessary for anesthetizing the area ranges from 1 to 3 hours, depending on the size of the area to be anesthetized and the type of equipment used. Duration of the anesthesia is about one hour.

HYPOTHERMIA

The term hypothermia refers to a reduction of body temperature. Its pur-pose in surgery is to lower metabolism and thereby decrease the need for oxygen. In many types of surgery involving the heart, blood vessels or brain, it is necessary to interrupt the flow of blood through the body. By lowering the body temperature to between 32°C. (89.6°F.) and 26°C. (78.8°F.), the metabolic needs of the vital organs are reduced, and they are less likely to be damaged by a decreased supply of blood and oxygen. Hypothermia may also be used in the treatment of diseases accompanied by a high fever.

There are several ways in which hypothermia can be achieved. In external hypothermia, the patient's body is wrapped in a cooling blanket, packed in ice or submerged in a tub of ice water. This is done after the patient has been anesthetized and immediately before the surgical procedure is performed.

In extracorporeal cooling, the patient's blood is cooled outside the body. It is removed from a major vessel, circulated through a refrigerant unit for cooling, and then returned to the body by way of another large blood vessel. This is the quickest way to achieve hypothermia and is usually the method used for patients undergoing surgery.

The reduction of body temperature by drugs which affect the heat regulating center in the brain is called internal hypothermia. The drug most often used is chlorpromazine hydrochloride (Thorazine) and it is given in combination with sedatives such as Demerol and Phenergan. Internal hypothermia usually reduces the body temperature by no more than three or four degrees.

During the rewarming process the patient's temperature is raised gradually. Care must be taken to avoid burns if warm baths or diathermy are used. The rewarming procedure is discontinued when the body temperature is within one or two degrees of normal. Observations during the rewarming include checking the pulse, blood pressure and respiration as well as the temperature.

Any sudden change must be reported immediately.

POSTOPERATIVE PERIOD

Immediate Postoperative Care

This is a critical period for the patient, one which demands close and constant observation by persons well trained and equipped to handle any emergency which may arise. The ideal situation is, as mentioned before, placing the patient in a special section of the hospital such as a recovery unit, where trained personnel may give him individual and constant attention until he is considered safely past immediate danger.

Every recovery room should have a clearly defined and well organized plan of care that is followed routinely by each member of the recovery room staff. The routine care plan is usually designed so that all aspects of patient care receive attention. An example of this kind of care plan is presented below. It is one that has been used at Norfolk General Hospital and is described by Burgess. The plan is as follows:

1. *Vital Signs.* These are checked every 15 minutes until they are stable and within the range noted on admission and also that recorded on the anesthetist's record.
    a. The *color* of the skin, lips, nail bed, and extremities is noted.
    b. The *body temperature* is checked. Does his body feel warm, cool, damp? Is he in shock?
2. *Respiration.*
    a. Is respiratory exchange adequate? Is oxygen needed?
    b. Is the airway patent?
    c. If an airway is not in place and if the exchange is inadequate, turn the patient on his side or insert an airway.
    d. Suction the trachea as necessary.

e. As soon as the patient begins to respond, encourage deep breathing every 15 minutes.
3. *Fluids.* If IV fluids are running, check the following:
    a. Is the needle or cannula still in the vein?
    b. Are the fluids running at the proper rate?
    c. If blood is being given, watch for a reaction. Don't overlook another chance to recheck the type and crossmatch level.
    d. Are more fluids to follow?
    e. Make sure the arm is positioned comfortably and secured.
4. *Site of Operation.* Check the following:
    a. Is the dressing dry? Is a drain in place? Should some drainage be expected?
    b. Carefully check all drainage tubing such as Levin, urinary, gallbladder, and chest tubes. Note the color and amount of drainage. Is the tubing properly positioned and secure, with no kinks? Connect the tube or leave it clamped, depending on the order given.
5. *Charting* (an art in itself). Clearly, briefly, and quickly record all observations pertinent to the particular operation and patient.
6. *The Patient's Needs.* As the patient begins to regain consciousness, orient him as to time, place and events. Give him reassurance as needed.
7. *Transfer from the Recovery Room.* This can take place when the patient is stable as to vital signs and bleeding points and responds to simple commands. All orders should have been read and understood.[3]

During the time that the patient is beginning to recover from the effects of anesthesia, the nurse must also give some attention to simple nursing measures which can relieve some of his discomfort. Because the patient has had nothing by mouth for 8 hours or more, he may experience severe thirst. If there are no contraindications, the nurse may offer him small sips of water; otherwise his lips can be moistened with a gauze square dipped in ice water. If he is receiving intravenous fluids, it is wise to restrain the arm loosely so that in his state of semiconsciousness he will not fling his arm about and dislodge the needle. Plastic armboards shaped to fit the arm are more comfortable than the straight armboards made of wood, but in either case, the bony prominences of the arm should be well padded and the hand supported so that it is not hanging off the edge of the board.

Many surgical procedures extend over a period of hours, which means that the patient has been lying motionless, in a fixed position, on a hard table for that length of time. No wonder, therefore, that the patient often complains of backache when he first wakes up. Turning the patient on his side and administering a gentle back rub will help. If he cannot be turned, the lumbar region may be supported with a small pillow or folded bath towel.

Nausea and vomiting following anesthesia are not uncommon. Supportive measures such as holding the patient's head or turning it to the side to prevent aspiration of the vomitus if he is not fully awake are most helpful and reassuring to the patient. He will also appreciate a few sips of water to rinse his mouth after the siege of vomiting is over.

While the patient is apparently still under anesthesia, the nursing staff and other persons within his hearing should be careful in their conversations. Many times the patient misinterprets the bits of conversation he hears and becomes unduly alarmed and disturbed. It is best to avoid talking except when absolutely necessary, and then the voice should be kept low unless the patient is being addressed. Whispering is inexcusable.

Other measures must include turning the patient every hour and encouraging deep breathing and coughing. This is necessary to improve circulation of the blood and expansion and aeration of the lungs. If the blood flow is allowed to become sluggish, there is danger that clots may form and give rise to a thrombus. The lungs must be expanded and secretions coughed up so that hypostatic pneumonia will not occur. In turning the patient, the nurse must guard against handling the patient too roughly or turning him too quickly. A sudden overstimulation might result in a drop in blood pressure.

Complications During the Postoperative Period

The two most common and serious complications of surgery are shock and hemorrhage. These two terms represent

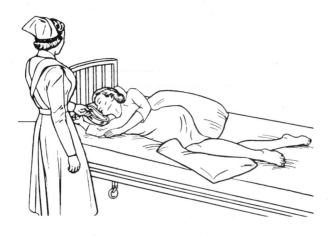

Figure 6–6. Position for immediate postoperative patient which permits drainage of mucus from the mouth and general relaxation. (From Winters: *Protective Body Mechanics in Daily Life and in Nursing*, W. B. Saunders Co., Philadelphia.)

separate and distinct complications, although hemorrhage, if unchecked, will rapidly lead to a state of shock.

Shock. The word "shock" actually represents a group of symptoms resulting from a failure of the blood vessels near the surface of the body to function properly. This collapse of the peripheral vessels leads to a serious decrease in the supply of circulating fluids to the vital organs. The pathological changes which occur internally lead to the following signs and symptoms: the skin is pale and clammy and cold, the temperature is subnormal, the pulse rapid and weak and the respiration rapid and shallow. The blood pressure during shock may drop to 90 mm. systolic pressure. If the pressure continues to drop and remains below 50 mm. for very long, there is permanent damage to the vital centers of the body.

TREATMENT AND NURSING CARE. The simplest form of shock is fainting. The more serious types of shock (for example, after severe trauma) may become extreme and result in death if the process is not quickly reversed by treatment. Because a surgical incision and major surgical procedure are unavoidably traumatic to the body, the postoperative patient must be watched very closely for symptoms of shock. The blood pressure, pulse and respiration must be taken at frequent intervals. Observation of the color and general condition of the skin are equally important, as is the patient's state of consciousness, because the patient may lose consciousness if shock is severe or prolonged.

Elevation of the foot of the bed by adjustment of the Gatch bed to Trendelenburg position or placing "shock blocks" under the foot of the bed will help increase the flow of blood to vital organs. Application of heat in the form of blankets or hot water bottles is no longer advocated because it is believed to bring the flow of blood to the peripheral vessels and thus further deprive the vital organs of their blood supply. It is sufficient merely to keep the body warm enough to protect the patient from excessive heat loss through the skin. Intravenous fluids, plasma or whole blood may be ordered by the physician to increase the blood volume. Other medications and treatments ordered for the patient in shock must be carried out with dispatch, as the loss of time due to inefficiency or apathy may lead to the loss of a life.

Hemorrhage. Hemorrhage (*hemo*—blood, *rrhage*—excessive flow) is the flow of blood from the body in amounts sufficient to endanger health and life. Postoperatively, hemorrhage might occur when a ligature slips off a vessel tied during surgery, or when a drainage tube causes erosion in the wall of a blood vessel. The patient suffering from hemorrhage, whatever the cause, must receive immediate treatment or death will eventually be the outcome.

Hemorrhage may occur internally or externally. External hemorrhage is, of course, much more obvious and easily determined, but in both types the patient's vital signs are of extreme importance in evaluating his condition. Generally hemorrhage is accompanied by a drop in blood pressure and an increase in pulse and respiration. The patient may become restless and complain of thirst and feeling cold. The skin will be pale and moist and the extremities mottled and cold to the touch. If the hemorrhage continues unchecked, the lips and conjunctiva will become extremely pale and the patient will complain of weakness, fatigue and spots before his eyes.

The treatment of hemorrhage is to stop the flow of blood and to replace by transfusion that which has been lost. In emergencies, the blood loss may be diminished by pressure dressings over the area, manual restriction of the blood flow to the area with tourniquets, or pressure on the so-called "pressure points" of the body. If the hemorrhage is postoperative, the patient may be taken back to the operating room and the bleeding vessel retied.

During the postoperative period, therefore, we can see the importance of checking the blood pressure, pulse and respiration at frequent and regular intervals to determine whether the patient is bleeding internally or going into shock. During this time and for several days or more postoperatively, the dressing must be carefully observed for signs of fresh bleeding. It is also important that all body excretions be closely observed for evidence of internal bleeding. This is also true for drainage from tubes or surgical drains.

If a patient does show signs of hemorrhage, the nursing staff must move quickly but with a minimum of excitement. The patient is usually frightened and partially aware of what is going on, and any unnecessary anxiety on his part will only aggravate the bleeding. Conversations among the nursing personnel must be kept at a minimum in his presence, and evidence of the hemorrhage, such as blood-soaked dressings or soiled linen and gown, should be quickly removed from sight. It will be necessary to reassure the patient frequently and demonstrate by a calm, efficient bearing that everything is under control and will turn out well.

Wound Infection. With the advent of antibiotics (the so-called "miracle drugs"), the word *infection* has become less frightening, and we have become more complacent about the need for precautions against wound infection following surgery. We must not use antibiotics as an excuse for careless nursing. In the first place, there are many microorganisms that have developed a resistance to the antibiotic drugs. This is particularly true of many strains of staphylococci which are capable of causing painful and stubborn infections. Secondly, even though the infection eventually may be overcome, the patient has been unnecessarily subjected to discomfort, inconvenience and added expense.

Prevention of wound infection begins before surgery and continues until the surgical wound is healed. It includes careful attention to rules of surgical asepsis and also entails the less glamorous cleaning chores that must continue from day to day. It is expected that table tops and other visible surfaces in the patient's room will be kept free of dust, but what about the lower rungs and wheels of beds, stretchers, chairs, etc.? Are we constantly aware of the fantastic rate of reproduction that is characteristic of pathogenic microorganisms, and do we realize that many are resistant to all but the strongest disinfectants? And what about handwashing? Each time the nurse begins any procedure involving direct contact with a postoperative patient, she should wash her hands for at least one full minute under running water.

One must never let familiarity with "routine" nursing procedures give her a feeling of complacency or security. Wound infection is a very real hazard which has become increasingly more prevalent in recent years, and it is all the more tragic because it can be prevented. That fact should make us more aware than ever of the need for applying the basic principles of cleanliness and sanitation.

CONVALESCENCE AND REHABILITATION

The period of convalescence from surgery has been greatly shortened by modern surgical techniques. Surgical procedures are less traumatic than formerly because of the development of improved surgical instruments and equipment. The practice of encouraging early ambulation and rapid return to physical activities has given the patients (and the nurses) a more optimistic view of surgical procedures and has helped the patient in his recovery and return to his former life.

TABLE 6-1. POSTOPERATIVE CARE

I. Control of pain	Nursing measures to provide maximum comfort and reassurance of the patient
	Analgesic drugs
II. Maintenance of drainage	Urinary catheters
	Gastric suction
	Thoracic drainage
	Bile drainage
	Drainage from surgical wounds
III. Maintenance of fluid and electrolyte balance	Intravenous fluids and minerals
	Oral intake
	Observation and recording of output
IV. Relief of abdominal distention, nausea and vomiting	Rectal tube
	Gastric suction
	Ice collar
	Antiemetic drugs
V. Prevention of complications:	
A. Shock	Close observation for signs of shock and hemorrhage
B. Hemorrhage	
C. Blood clots in vascular system	Frequent turning
	Early ambulation
D. Hypostatic pneumonia	Encourage coughing and deep breathing, and turn frequently
E. Decubiti	Frequent turning
	Skin care
F. Contractures	Proper positioning
	Exercise
G. Wound infection	Adherence to the basic principles of cleanliness and asepsis

Rehabilitation is the restoring of the patient to as near his former state of health and activity as possible. For the surgical patient, rehabilitation may include readjustment to a completely new and better way of life, as is necessary when the surgery is restorative and the patient is able to be more active physically than he formerly might have been. Other types of surgery will render the patient more handicapped and helpless to some degree. Surgical procedures which require the use of a prosthesis or special appliances (such as a permanent colostomy) demand much time and specially trained personnel to help the patient learn to live with his handicap. In rehabilitation, probably more than any other phase of nursing, we can see the advantages of a well-coordinated medical team. It is in this phase of care that the physiotherapist, occupational therapist, social worker and public health nurse can make their greatest contribution toward the care of the patient and his restoration to a life more productive and thus more bearable.

For further information on rehabilitation, the reader is referred to Chapter 8 of this text.

CLINICAL CASE PROBLEMS

1. Mrs. Smith, age 43, is admitted to the surgical unit of the hospital with a diagnosis of acute cholecystitis and obesity. She is the mother of five children and her husband has been dead for four years. Mrs. Smith works in a sewing plant to support her family. Her oldest son, age 19, also works to provide an income for the family.

This patient has never been hospitalized before, except for the birth of her last three children. She is extremely apprehensive about her illness and is worried about her children and the financial status of the family now that she cannot work.

Several days after her admission to

the hospital, the acute inflammation responds to treatment sufficiently to permit surgical removal of the gallbladder. The patient gives her consent to the surgery, but she is very frightened and seems to feel that she will never be well again.

What problems can you see in this situation?

How can you help reassure Mrs. Smith before surgery?

What preoperative instructions might you give?

In what ways might you help Mrs. Smith with her problem of obesity?

2. You are assigned to the care of a 20-year-old woman who has just returned from surgery for removal of a small tumor of the breast. You overheard the head nurse tell another staff nurse that the tumor was benign. In spite of the minor nature of the surgery, the patient has shown signs of shock in the recovery room and requires careful attention when she is returned to her room. When she recovers from the anesthesia the patient is very nauseated and uncomfortable.

What special observations should you make while caring for this patient?

How can you help relieve the nausea and vomiting?

If the patient asks you whether the tumor was benign or malignant, and you are not really sure because nothing has yet been recorded on her chart, what would your answer be?

3. This is your first day on duty on a surgical ward.

What specific policies and procedures are required by your hospital when a patient undergoes surgery?

Is there a clearance record or check list to be completed?

REFERENCES

1. Beland, I. L.: *Clinical Nursing,* 2nd edition. New York, The Macmillan Co., 1970.
2. Breckinridge, F. J., and Bruno, P.: "Nursing Care of the Anesthetized Patient." Am. Journ. Nurs., July, 1962, p. 74.
3. Burgess, M. G.: "A Nursing Care Plan for the Postoperative Patient in the Recovery Room and the Intensive Care Unit." Nurs. Clin. N. Amer., Vol. 3, No. 3, 1968, p. 499.
4. Harmer, B., and Henderson, V.: *Textbook of the Principles and Practice of Nursing,* 5th edition. New York, The Macmillan Co., 1960.
5. Healy, K. M.: "Does Preoperative Instruction Make a Difference?" Am. Journ. Nurs., Jan., 1968, p. 62.
6. Mezzanotte, E. J.: "Group Instructions in Preparation for Surgery." Am. Journ. Nurs., Jan., 1970, p. 89.
7. Minckley, B. B.: "Physiologic Hazards of Position Changes in the Anesthetized Patient." Am. Journ. Nurs., Dec., 1969, p. 2606.
8. Smith, D. C., and Fiedler, J. P.: "Fears, Facts and Fantasies about Pre- and Postoperative Care." Nurs. Outlook, Feb., 1970, p. 26.
9. Smith, D. W., et al.: *Care of the Adult Patient,* 3rd edition. Philadelphia, J. B. Lippincott, 1971.
10. Smith, R. B., et al.: "In a Recovery Room." Am. Journ. Nurs., Jan., 1973, p. 70.
11. Tantum, K. R., and Dripps, R. D.: "The Scope and Challenge of Modern Anesthesia." Nurs. Clin. N. Amer., Vol. 3, No. 4, 1968, p. 591.

SUGGESTED STUDENT READING

1. Breckinridge, F. J., and Bruno, P.: "Nursing Care of the Anesthetized Patient." Am. Journ. Nurs., July, 1962, p. 74.
2. Carneval, D.: "Preop Anxiety." Am. Journ. Nurs., July, 1966, p. 1536.
3. Clark, R. B.: "The Case for Spinal Anesthesia." Am. Journ. Nurs., Feb., 1967, p. 294.
4. Elder, F.: "Effective Support for the Preoperative Patient." RN, May, 1962, p. 47.
5. Healy, K. M.: "Does Preoperative Instruction Make a Difference?" Am. Journ. Nurs., Jan., 1968, p. 63.
6. Hickey, M. C.: "Hypothermia." Am. Journ. Nurs., Jan., 1965, p. 116.
7. Landis, E. M.: "Some Pointers on Postoperative Care." RN, July, 1962, p. 54.

OUTLINE FOR CHAPTER 6

I. Introduction

A. Nursing care divided into three phases: preoperative, operative and immediate postoperative, and convalescence and rehabilitation.

B. Length of each period varies with individual patient.

II. Preoperative Period

A. Emotional and psychological preparation:
1. Listen to patient and answer his questions to the best of your ability.
2. Prepare patient and family so that they will know what to expect during postoperative period.
B. Spiritual preparation for peace of mind.
C. Physical preparation:
1. Preoperative examination to determine patient's physical status.
2. Preparation of skin to reduce chance of postoperative infection.
3. Restriction of oral intake to avoid complications of nausea, vomiting and distention after surgery.
4. Cleansing of intestinal tract if ordered, to avoid contamination of operative site.
5. Rest and sedation to conserve strength and energy of patient.
6. Operative permit must be signed to avoid legal difficulties.
7. Immediate preoperative care is done according to hospital's policies and procedures and directions of the patient's physician. Medications must be given on time.

III. Anesthesia—Loss of Sensory Perception

A. Given to prevent pain, achieve muscular relaxation and allay anxiety.
B. Types include:
1. Inhalants.
2. Intravenous anesthetics.
3. Local or regional anesthetics.
4. Spinal anesthesia (drug is injected into spinal cavity, anesthesia achieved below point of injection).

5. Refrigeration anesthesia (temperature of a part is lowered so that conduction of nerve impulses is retarded).

IV. Hypothermia—Reduction of Body Temperature

A. Used in some types of surgery to lower metabolism and decrease the need for oxygen.
B. Methods:
1. External hypothermia: using ice packs or other forms of external cold.
2. Extracorporeal hypothermia: rerouting the blood outside the body, through a cooling unit and back into the body.
3. Administration of drugs.
C. During rewarming period, patient's vital signs are noted at frequent intervals.

V. Postoperative Period

A. Recovery room care—be sure to check:
1. Vital signs.
2. Open airway and adequate respiratory exchange.
3. IV fluids.
4. Operative site.
5. Charting.
6. Patient needs.
7. Transfer from recovery room.
B. Nursing measures:
1. Prevent aspiration during vomiting.
2. Avoid noise and conversation within patient's hearing.
3. Turn patient frequently to avoid circulatory stasis and respiratory failure.
4. Handle gently.
5. Complications to be watched for include shock, hemorrhage and wound infection.

VI. Convalescence and Rehabilitation

A. Length of time will vary depending on type of surgery and patient's reaction.
B. Ultimate goal is return of the patient to as near his former state of health and activity as possible.

7

Nursing Care of the Aged

VOCABULARY

Alveolar
Disorientation
Emollient
Fetid
Geriatric
Gerontology
Interdependent
Peripheral
Psychosocial
Stasis

INTRODUCTION

In 1900 one American in every 25 was 65 years old or older; by 1969 every tenth person was in that age bracket, and by 1985 the older population is expected to reach 25 million persons. This rapid increase in numbers within a segment of our population has stimulated interest in the aging process, extensive study of the special needs of the aged and a search for solutions to the problems associated with growing old.

The process of aging actually begins at the moment of conception. Barring fatal illness or accident, each of us will, as the days of our lives rush by, get nearer that stage in life referred to as old age. Yet we should know that the number of years one lives is not the only factor involved in deciding whether he is aged. A person's attitude toward life, his acceptance of new ideas, his variety of interests and zest for living, his opinion of himself and tolerance for the shortcomings of others all affect the way in which he bears the burden of increasing years. Plato said, "If man is moderate and contented, then age is no burden; if he is not, then even youth is full of cares."

To speak of the special needs of the aged is not to imply that all elderly persons are in need of continuous medical and nursing care. The goal of gerontology is not only to determine ways of prolonging life but also to improve the quality of life for older persons and to assure that their added years will be active and productive ones.[17] The specialty of geriatric nursing is relatively new and is based on a rapidly growing body of knowledge about the aged and the physiologic and psychosocial needs brought on by advancing age. Fortunately, the major focus on care for the aged is shifting from merely custodial care, with its emphasis on the infirmities of the aged, to preservation of aged patients' personal assets and maintenance of the highest level of function possible for each person. There are rich and rewarding experiences in store for those who dedicate themselves to this type of care. All the human qualities of warmth, love and understanding are required of the geriatric nurse, plus an extra measure of each for those individuals who have lived much but still have much to give.

ATTITUDES TOWARD THE AGED

It is difficult for many persons in the health professions to believe that at least 85 per cent of the population aged 65 years or older are essentially healthy and capable of leading vigorous and useful lives.[15] Because most of us engaged in providing health services become involved almost exclusively with elderly persons who are not well and exhibit some degree of dependence on us, we tend to think that all of the elderly are incapacitated in some way. Our opinions are, quite naturally, influenced by our personal experiences, so we erroneously think that the few active and vigorous old people whom we know about are exceptions rather than the rule. Such negative attitudes and the practice of prejudging individuals on the basis of age, sex or any other external characteristic can have the same detrimental effect on the elderly as it has on other groups in our society.

A nurse's feelings, prejudices or biases toward a group of persons have a direct bearing on the caliber of care she will give the individuals of that group. For this reason the practical nurse

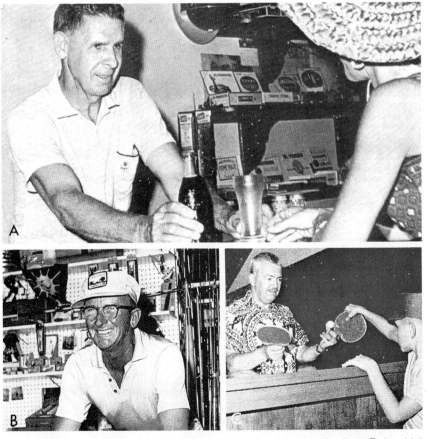

Figure 7–1. Most persons over the age of 65 lead vigorous and productive lives. To be old does not mean to be sick.

should evaluate her feelings toward old age. She should think of growing old in relation to herself and her future years when she too will be over 65. Does she dread this time of her life and put off thinking about it? Has she neglected to prepare for it by failing to develop hobbies and a variety of interests outside nursing? Sean O'Casey, the Irish author, wrote the following when he was 79 years old:

We must begin at school and college to learn to absorb life so that when we grow old we may be filled with its colors, thoughts, and sounds . . . If we don't, then the old seek relaxation in being a misery to themselves and a damned nuisance to others.

Many people have mixed feelings about elderly persons. They may be amused at first by the little idiosyncrasies and strange quirks that they attribute to the aged, but with constant and close association, the amusement is short-lived and the "cute" mannerism becomes a "disgusting habit." Actually old people are neither amusing nor disgusting—at least not any more or less than people of any other age. They are individual human beings and they long to be treated as such.

Perhaps the practical nurse has not been around the elderly long enough to have formed any definite preconceived ideas and opinions about them. Our culture and the society in which we live have not prepared many Americans for proper relations with the elderly. We have in America a clearly defined social pattern of idolizing youth, while in oriental cultures it is a compliment to a person if he is mistakenly judged to be older than his years. In these societies, old age signifies wisdom and is treated with reverence. There are reasons for the differences between the two attitudes: Ours is a comparatively young country, and our population has been predominantly young since the days of colonization. Another influence has been the movement of people from rural living

in family homes sheltering several generations, to city life in rented apartments or small houses. More than one fifth of our population changes its address at least once a year, and this increase in mobility has had its effect on the family unit, which no longer seems to include grandparents and elderly unmarried aunts and uncles. Many older persons feel that there is no place for them. They withdraw from society, losing their individuality and incentive for living.

In the preparation of their standards for practice in geriatric nursing, the American Nurses Association's Committee on Standards for Geriatric Nursing Practice recognized the need for a change in attitudes toward the elderly of our country. The tentative standard published in the *American Journal of Nursing* is quoted here in its entirety because it is of such importance in every aspect of geriatric nursing:

STANDARD #3: The nurse demonstrates an appreciation of the heritage, values, and wisdom of older persons.
Rationale: The nurse has some understanding and appreciation of the social and historic settings in which older people have developed, and how these factors may affect their behavior and values. This enables her to respect the older person as an individual and provides for enrichment of the nurse's life. Such an appreciation also provides ways in which the nurse can point out how the present generation has built on their foundation, thus helping to keep older persons in the present.
Examples: The nurse helps older persons share their experiences and talents with the present generation.
The nurse respects the older person's right to practice religion as he desires.
The nurse accepts the older person's desire to cling to a particular item, such as a piece of jewelry or a photograph. .
The nurse accepts the older person's right to wear the clothes he is accustomed to wearing, such as a night cap or long underwear.

A major challenge in geriatric nursing is to overcome the all too prevalent inclination for many people to confuse pediatric nursing with geriatric nursing. Perhaps it is because they lend credence to the expression "second childhood" that younger persons tend to treat the elderly as children. Nothing can be more destructive to human dignity and self-esteem than being treated as an infant or spoken to as if one were either deaf or stupid. Dr. Verwoerdt has written: "It is not uncommon practice to call aged patients by their first name, to speak loudly to them as if to shake them up, to talk about them in their presence, to smile or laugh at their oddities, and even to scold them for undesirable acts. On the other hand, it is not so difficult to combine *sincere respect* for the patient (in spite of his oddities) with considerate helpfulness (without infantilizing him)."[24]

Negative attitudes toward the elderly cannot be reconciled with our concept of ourselves as a humane and civilized society; nurses in particular should assume some responsibility for setting an example for others to follow. A recent headline in an Associated Press newspaper article read: "Indigent, Sick Elderly Dumped at Hospital Door." The text of the article explained that almost daily an elderly person in a wheelchair or on a stretcher is left at the doorstep of a large city hospital located in a southeastern state. Many of these helpless individuals have "Do Not Return" tags pinned to their clothing and are left by relatives or nursing home officials who feel that they are not receiving adequate funds from state and federal agencies to care for them. While we cannot make a judgment about a family's or agency's ability to cope with the financial burden of caring for the sick and elderly, we can wonder about our values and how we as a society can justify allowing the aged to become the victims of our indifference.

In contrast to the story cited previously, Dupuis's article, "Old is Beautiful," emphasizes the need for positive attitudes toward the care of long-term elderly patients, particularly in general hospitals. She concludes that unless newer ways are found to bridge the generation gap and make it possible and probable for youthful nurses to relate to elderly patients, we must face the fact that the majority of elderly patients will be admitted to hospitals in which most of the nursing personnel simply do not care. This problem is particularly disturbing when we realize that there are increasing numbers of elderly patients admitted to general hospitals (see Fig. 7-2).

MEDICARE

Medicare is a governmental health insurance program under Social Security which is designed to help pay the cost of health care for American citizens 65 years and older and many severely disabled persons under the age of 65. There are two types of insurance under Medicare: (1) a hospital insurance program which helps pay for the care received as a patient in a hospital and for certain followup care after hospitalization, and (2) a medical insurance program which helps defray the cost of physicians' services, outpatient hospital services, and many other medical expenses not covered under hospital insurance.

At the present time (1974) the services covered in a hospital or skilled nursing care facility include the cost of semi-private rooms and meals, including special diets. These services include those provided in regular nursing units as well as in intensive care units. The hospital insurance coverage also includes the cost of drugs, supplies, appliances, and equipment.

Services *not* covered by the hospital insurance program include doctor bills; private duty nurses; cost of the first three pints of blood needed during a period of hospitalization; convenience items, such as telephone and television; and care that is simply custodial.

All persons who are eligible for a social security or railroad retirement check either as a worker, dependent, or survivor automatically have hospital insurance protection when they reach the age of 65 years. Those who are not automatically eligible for hospital insurance can be covered by enrolling and paying a monthly premium as

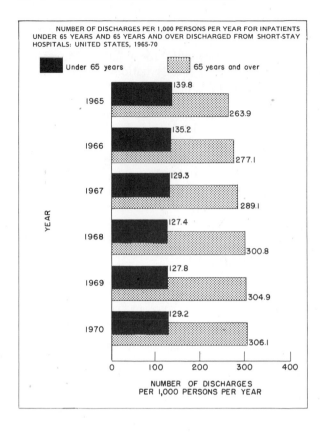

NUMBER OF DISCHARGES PER 1,000 PERSONS PER YEAR FOR INPATIENTS UNDER 65 YEARS AND 65 YEARS AND OVER DISCHARGED FROM SHORT-STAY HOSPITALS: UNITED STATES, 1965-70

■ Under 65 years   ▨ 65 years and over

Figure 7–2. Statistics comparing hospital discharges for younger and for older patients. (From National Center for Health Statistics, U.S. Department of Health, Education and Welfare.)

they would for any other health insurance. Those who buy Medicare hospital insurance also must enroll in the medical insurance program.

The medical insurance program under Medicare is available on a voluntary basis to all persons 65 years and over and to others who are disabled and qualify for the hospital insurance program. Effective July 1, 1973, aged persons who choose to enroll in the medical insurance program pay a monthly premium and the federal government provides matching funds from general revenues. The medical insurance program is a $60 annual deductible policy, which means that after the participant has paid the first $60 of his medical bills in a calendar year the insurance program covers 80 percent of the reasonable charges for physician fees, certain outpatient services, and medical equipment.

Nurses are involved in implementation of the Medicare program in many ways. Patients who could not afford even the most basic health needs now have an opportunity to share in the many advantages offered by modern medical science. By stimulating the expansion of such facilities as outpatient services, extended care in nursing and convalescent homes and home health programs, Medicare has provided a wider variety of job situations and greater challenges to practical nurses in all parts of the country. It has also increased the need for all types of personnel in the health field and granted recognition to the licensed practical nurse as an important member of the health team. By their education and experience, licensed practical nurses are highly qualified to meet the nursing needs of older persons effectively.[18]

The far-reaching effects of Medicare can be appreciated by the following facts compiled after 18 months of operation of the plan:

tion and physicians' care are estimated by the Department of Health, Education and Welfare to account for more than two-thirds of all expenditures for such services provided to the aged. During the fiscal year 1972, benefit payments amounted to more than $8.4 billion: $6.1 billion under the hospital insurance program and $2.3 billion under the supplemental medical insurance program.*

We can measure the number of persons helped and the amount of money spent in carrying out such a program, but it is difficult indeed to estimate its true value to the lonely and the desperate who have learned that there is a way in which they can be cared for and their health needs can be met. The nurse's task is to show that she not only cares *for* these persons, but that she truly cares *about* them.

*U.S. Department of Health, Education and Welfare, Social Security Administration. "Social Security Programs in the United States." U.S. Government Printing Office, Washington, D.C. 1973.

HEALTH NEEDS OF THE AGED

In the Code of Ethics for the Licensed Practical Vocational Nurse adopted by the National Association for Practical Nurse Education and Service (NAPNES) in 1971, the first two statements are concerned with conservation of life, prevention of disease and the promotion and protection of the physical, mental, emotional and spiritual health of the patient and his family. These statements reflect the newer and broader concept of total health care and are particularly relevant to the elderly, who are most often in need of services that provide assistance in preventing illness and treating chronic diseases in their early stages. For too long we have associated old age with institutional and custodial care, ignoring the fact that "only about 4 per cent of the elderly are in long-term care institutions and only about 16 per cent are so incapacitated as to be unable to carry out the major activities of daily living."[18] This does not mean that those

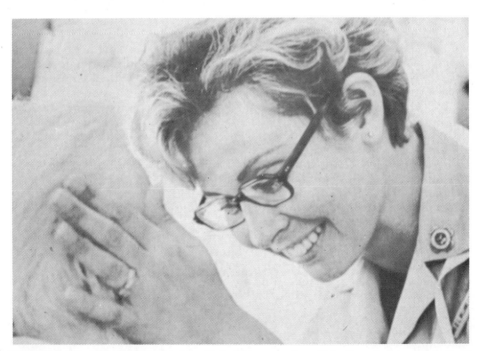

Figure 7–3. An LPN and her elderly patient. Old can be beautiful with mutual love and attention. (From: Bedside Nurse, April, 1972.)

who need skilled nursing should have less than their share of attention, but rather that the concept of health care must be expanded to include all of the factors that influence the quality of one's life and the status of his health.

Although the population within the age group designated as elderly has been rapidly increasing during the last 50 years, the health needs of this group have only recently begun to receive attention and services from health and welfare agencies in this country. A report published in 1961 by the White House Conference on Aging shows the far-reaching effect the health needs of the elderly have on the entire nation. The report points out that "prolongation of life and increasing numbers of people in the later stages of life aggravate problems of health and disease for both the members of the older population and the community." Chronic disease and the dependence and inactivity it produces are extremely expensive in time and money required for treatment and care, to say nothing of the cost to the patient in terms of personal loss of self-esteem. Through good health care and education, it is possible to avoid the more serious effects of the chronic disease and health problems of the elderly. It is also possible to improve the quality of their lives and to prolong them, as well.

There are some factors involved in the planning of health care which directly affect the success and effectiveness of any program designed to meet the health needs of the elderly. They are included here because they are basic to all aspects of geriatric nursing and fundamental to an understanding of the needs, fears and desires of the elderly. As Archer points out, they will "influence the types of laws, programs, and services provided for the aging person and the manner and extent to which they are used."

1. The most important point is that old age and illness are not synonymous. To be old does not mean to be ill.
2. It is common for older people to have more than one disease at the same time.

3. Symptoms of disease in elderly people are not as noticeable or may take different forms than in younger people.
4. Many older people tend not to seek help for poor physical condition or illness until it becomes an emergency for the following reasons:
   a. Belief that unpleasant symptoms are a normal part of growing old.
   b. Ignorance as to the correct place to seek help.
   c. Lack of finances and fear of accepting "charity."
   d. Lack of energy plus difficulty of transportation.[3]

There still remains a gap between what we know about the health needs of the elderly and what is being done to meet those needs. As the gap narrows and services become more readily available, nurses will be expected to accept (and should accept) the challenge to become increasingly involved in putting the principles of gerontology into practice.

PHYSIOLOGIC CHANGES AND PHYSICAL NEEDS

Standards. Although it is difficult to make a clear distinction between normal aging and pathologic aging and disease, it is nevertheless important to understand that the standards for measuring health needs in an elderly person cannot be identical with those used for young adults. The goal of the geriatric nurse should be to help her patient maintain a condition normal for his age. While he can never again have the health and strength of a 20-year-old, he can possibly become a healthy 70-year-old. Biologic deterioration and a gradual "wearing out" of tissues are inevitable consequences of aging. The rate at which these changes take place varies in each individual, and though we must be aware of the ways in which such changes affect each person's state of health, we must also not have a defeatist attitude toward the aging process and its physical consequences. It is best to think of the physiologic changes as leading to reduced friction of the organs and not necessarily as total loss of functional capacity.

Rest and Exercise. Among the more common physiologic changes occurring with age are those involving the musculoskeletal system. The joints become stiffer, the muscles become weaker, and motion becomes more of an effort when one is no longer young and agile. A regular program of exercises designed to meet the needs of the individual can do much to help him keep active and avoid the complications associated with limited physical activity. (Effects of immobility are discussed later in Chapter 8.) A large percentage of the elderly suffer from some degree of *osteoporosis,* a condition in which the bone cells are decalcified and the bones become porous. Osteoporosis is thought to be the result of insufficient weight supported by the bones. That is, the person confined to a bed or chair for long periods of time no longer uses his bones for support and motion and does not subject them to the normal stresses of weight bearing and exercises.

In his booklet, "Exercises for the Elderly," Dr. Kamenetz points out that exercise and overexertion are two different things. He advises the elderly to begin an exercise program slowly, gradually working up to a comfortable pace that will build up capabilities. The exercises recommended include those for the person in bed, sitting in a chair or standing.[14] The booklet is distributed as a service by Armour Pharmaceutical Co., P.O. Box 1022, Chicago, Illinois, 60690.

Whatever exercising routine is established for an elderly person, the best time for the exercises is in the morning when the joints should be loosened and the muscles stimulated, and in the evening to produce moderate fatigue so that the muscles are relaxed and sleep is more restful and effective. We must also consider the many other advantages to exercise, such as improved circulatory and respiratory function.

The sleep and rest patterns of the elderly are often erratic and sometimes quite disturbing to those who care for the elderly, if not to the elderly person himself, who may fail to understand why everyone gets excited about his frequent daytime naps and periods of wakefulness in the middle of the night. Unless his individual schedule of sleep and rest presents a very real danger to him or an intolerable inconvenience to others, it would be better to plan his care according to his needs rather than try to force him to conform to the rules of the institution. If the nurse realizes that the sleep pattern of the elderly is quite often very different from that of other age groups and that her older patient has little control over his periods of restlessness, perhaps she will be less likely to criticize him for getting out of bed at all hours of the night. She may also be more aware of the need for frequent checking at night to see if he wants to sit up in a chair for a while or would like to have someone keep him company for a short time.

Special Skin Care. Most nurses have been so thoroughly indoctrinated with the creed of the daily bath that they are shocked at the thought of not performing this essential part of morning care. So when 80-year-old Mrs. Thomas, hospitalized with a fractured femur, refuses her bath on the grounds that "I had a bath yesterday, I haven't stirred from this bed since then, I am not dirty and I do not need a bath," the nurse shakes her head at the strange ways of old ladies and then busily prepares the bath water.

But Mrs. Thomas is right! Her sweat and oil glands are no longer as active, she perspires little and the daily bath can actually do her thin and dry skin more harm than good. A condition, well named "bath itch," occurs frequently in the elderly. It invariably begins as small raw areas on the shins and spreads over the body. It is best prevented by limiting the complete bath to one or two weekly, using mild soaps or natural detergent solutions. Bathing between times should be arranged to insure personal cleanliness, especially in the incontinent patient. After the bath, and perhaps as a substitute on the days when a bath is not given, the skin may be gently massaged with lanolin or some oil-base lotion. If any kind of bath oil is added to the tub bath, one must be aware of the need to protect the patient from slipping and falling in the tub.

Prevention of decubiti in the elderly begins with good nutrition and careful handling of the skin, as though it might break down at any minute. In turning a patient, the nurse must be sure to avoid pulling the undersheet roughly against the skin. This error can best be avoided by turning the patient far enough to be able to pull the undersheet and tuck it securely without rubbing it across the patient's side or back. Because the skin is so sensitive to trauma from burns and friction, great care should be used in the application of heat and in the method of massage.

The term "pressure sores" is frequently used to designate decubiti. It is a good name, for pressure on any one area of the skin, with resulting accumulation of heat and moisture and accompanying deprivation of an adequate blood supply, will eventually lead to an ulcer (see Fig. 7-4). For relief of this pressure, frequent turning and proper positioning of the patient are necessary. This practice applies to all patients who are inactive but is particularly important in the aged.

Care of the Nails and Hair. The nails, especially the toenails, undergo changes which make them so brittle and thick that they should not be cut without first softening them by applying some type of emollient preparation such as liquid lanolin, mineral oil, castor oil, petroleum jelly or even vegetable oil if no other preparation is available. The practical nurse may feel confident about clipping the toenails of a patient who has no special problems with his feet and nails, but she should seek help from a physician or podiatrist when the patient has a thick, discolored, fungus-infested ram's horn nail or one that is inverted or ingrown. Many elderly persons attempt to diag-

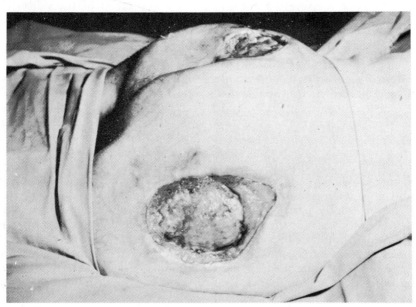

Figure 7-4. Decubitus ulcers of sacrum and right trochanter one week after admission. (From Line, R. E.: Nursing Clinics of North America, September, 1966.)

nose their own foot problems and may need instruction in proper care of the feet and nails, particularly in regard to nail trimming and the application of harsh medications such as iodine, salicylic acid or zinc preparations. If the patient has a problem with profuse or fetid perspiration of the feet, he should have his feet washed and dried thoroughly several times a day and massaged with an emollient. Clean socks should then be put on. Under no circumstances should the nurse allow the patient to trim corns or calluses or apply corn preparations or medicated plasters.[20]

It has been proved in mental institutions that even the most seriously deranged person will respond to an improvement in his physical appearance. Cosmetics and attractive clothing help the patient return more quickly to reality. An elderly person will have a similar reaction, his physical appearance greatly affecting his attitude toward himself and others. Male patients who are shaved and neatly manicured, with well-groomed hair, are more likely to welcome visitors and show some interest in getting up and out into a more active environment.

Dermatologists agree that most bases for powder and lipstick are not harmful to the skin of an elderly person, and the nurse may safely encourage her elderly female patients to "primp" a little, offering the assistance they need to make themselves more attractive. In cleansing the hair and scalp, scrubbing should be avoided. A shampoo for dry hair is the best and safest to use on an elderly person.

Nutritional Needs. The food likes and dislikes of the elderly often become a point of irritation to those who are striving so diligently to provide an adequate diet. It is futile, however, to try to change lifelong habits abruptly. One's only choice is to exercise patience and imagination in getting the patient to eat what he must have to maintain his health and to provide a

relaxed and sociable atmosphere at mealtime, remembering that food is a treat, not a treatment. Recent studies have shown that a glass of wine or beer benefits many elderly patients at mealtime, giving the meal a festive air and producing a feeling of relaxation and sociability.

In spite of claims to the contrary, there is no special diet that will guarantee long life or continued health in old age. The needs of the aged are basically the same as those for any other age group, except that the aged may need fewer calories as they become less active, and some modification of the food may be necessary because of chewing and digestive difficulties. Such factors as habit, ignorance of what constitutes a well-balanced diet, economic and emotional insecurity, cultural differences, and poorly fitting dentures or absence of teeth all contribute to the malnutrition that occurs in most persons over the age of 60.

The greatest difficulty with wearing dentures has been identified as "poor fit." Symptoms of this condition include sore and inflamed mucosa along the alveolar ridge, burning of the tongue or palate, dryness of the mouth, soreness at the corners of the mouth and painful chewing. When these symptoms are observed in a patient who also has a nutrition problem, one must recognize the possibility that a combination of poorly fitting dentures and vitamin deficiencies may be the cause.[5]

In addition to vitamin deficiencies in the elderly, there is usually poor absorption of calcium into the tissues, so ways of increasing the calcium intake must be devised. Unfortunately, most old people do not like milk. Substitutes such as cheese, ice cream or custards and foods cooked with milk will help make up for the lack of calcium in the diet of those who refuse to drink milk. Sometimes it is necessary to increase food intake, but older persons may resist attempts to increase the amount of solid foods they eat. If so, nutritious liquid feedings may be planned for them. It is usually better to give frequent small feedings than to adhere to the routine of three large meals a day.

Older persons may also suffer from *achlorhydria,* a condition in which free hydrochloric acid is no longer present in the stomach. This absence of hydrochloric acid hinders digestion and interferes with the absorption of iron. For this reason, anemia is often present in the elderly. In addition, muscular actions of the digestive tract slow down with age, and the intestinal mucosa is easily irritated by excessive bulk and rough residue.

An understanding of these changes which directly affect the appetite and digestion should make the nurse more aware of the special nutritional needs of the elderly and assist her in solving the feeding problems of the elderly.

Whenever possible, the patient should be allowed to feed himself. If he has great difficulty with liquids and hard-to-manage foods, the nurse can thoughtfully offer assistance without taking away the patient's sense of dignity and self-esteem. No mention should be made of the mess he might make in attempting to feed himself. The important point is to make sure he has an adequate intake of food and that utensils are designed and arranged on his plate so that they can be handled without difficulty. Some patients will not be able to feed themselves. When feeding an elderly person, it is best to elevate his head and shoulders slightly, with his spine straight and his shoulders back. This position will aid digestion and prevent difficulties in swallowing. The gag reflex may not function very well in an elderly person, creating dangers of aspiration during eating and drinking. The elderly must be allowed ample time to chew their food thoroughly and swallow it completely, and each meal should be a pleasurable and leisurely experience. Above all else, the nurse must show that she cares. Offering food and shar-

ing our daily bread are expressions of love and outward signs of our belief in the brotherhood of man. Frequently, therefore, one of the first signs of withdrawal from society is a refusal to eat. The basic principles of serving food attractively and lovingly, providing appetizers and an atmosphere conducive to eating and selecting foods with as much consideration for preference and taste as is practical are no less important for the aged.

Elimination. Constipation in the elderly is generally a result of a slowing down of intestinal tract movement compounded by decreased physical activity and poor eating habits. Because it is irritating to the intestinal mucosa, extremely rough bulk cannot be used as a means of correcting constipation. The diet should include such vegetables as carrots and potatoes, which do not require much chewing when adequately cooked, and some whole grain cereals. Both of these food groups contain "soft" bulk that is not unduly irritating.

Laxatives and frequent enemas should be avoided, even though it is typical of elderly persons to be overly concerned about their bowels. Such practices can quickly lead to excessive potassium loss, which in turn produces mental confusion and a potentially dangerous electrolyte imbalance. It is for this reason that stool softeners that make defecation less difficult are preferred to laxatives and enemas. Diarrhea is frequently a symptom of fecal impaction, and its occurrence should be reported to the physician or nurse in charge so that the impacted feces can be broken up manually and an oil retention enema given.

Benign prostatic hypertrophy, so common in elderly men, is discussed elsewhere in this text. However, this is by no means the only genitourinary problem to be considered in the elderly. Urinary incontinence, for one reason or another, frequently occurs, particularly after an injury or acute illness. Following either of these events, the aged person becomes temporarily confused and fearful. He doesn't feel comfortable using a bedpan or urinal and isn't quite sure they won't leak or run over. A simple, tactful explanation with assurance of privacy may be all that is necessary to gain his cooperation and save him needless embarrassment. Sometimes the "incontinent" patient isn't incontinent at all. He may just not get the impulse to void in time to call for a bedpan or urinal. All muscles of the aged lose some of their tone: this includes the sphincter muscles of the urinary and rectal outlets. For this reason, the nurse may find she can prevent accidental and embarrassing bedwetting and unnecessary work for herself by offering the elderly patient a bedpan or urinal at frequent and regular intervals. The practice of getting a patient out of bed regularly often has surprising results in the control of incontinence.

In spite of these techniques, urinary and fecal incontinence will persist in some patients. There are several appliances available for the collection or control of the flow of urine in the incontinent male patient. Although the problem is less easily solved in the female, there are measures that can be taken to keep the patient dry and socially acceptable. The kind of nursing care he receives will have a direct bearing on his ability to maintain dignity and avoid anxiety about the body functions over which he no longer has control.

Vision and Hearing. The U.S. National Health Survey revealed that in the 65 years and over age group, 40 per cent of the men and 60 per cent of the women must wear glasses to correct vision. One type of visual disturbance common to elderly persons is the gradual loss of peripheral vision, which results in "tunnel vision." In tunnel vision, the affected person is able to see only what is directly in front of him. The nurse who is aware of the problem will remember to stand in front of the patient when she is talking to him and to avoid handing objects to him from the side. She will also bear this special problem in mind when arranging articles in his immediate vicinity, so that he will not stumble over them or topple them over as he moves about.

A good many elderly persons wear the same glasses for years without having their eyes reexamined and their glasses updated. Perhaps because of economic reasons, inability to get to an optometrist or ophthalmologist, or an unawareness of the need to do so, they will often not obtain good eye care for preservation of their vision. They also tend to wear a relative's glasses, to buy glasses at a variety store or to use a magnifying glass for reading, all of which delay proper attention to their visual difficulties and in many cases prevent early treatment of conditions that can lead to blindness.

Hearing usually becomes less acute as one grows older. Studies have shown that elderly persons have most difficulty hearing high frequencies. This evidence suggests that the nurse wishing to make herself heard by her elderly patients should pitch her voice lower and, as stated previously, stand directly in front of them when speaking. It is only good manners to enunciate words clearly and to speak slowly to those who have difficulty understanding our speech, but our speech should not be exaggerated, and the problem is certainly not a license to shout. Not all elderly persons have a hearing loss. Because of nervous system changes, some may have a delayed reaction time and are unable to respond quickly to the spoken word. The best approach, therefore, is to slow our speech and pace our conversations so that the elderly have time to respond.

Hearing aids can present some very real difficulties for the elderly patient who needs this type of device. The parts of a hearing aid are small and difficult for some patients to handle, and batteries are not always readily available should one need to be replaced. The nurse is not expected to know all the intricacies and inner workings of a hearing aid, but she should certainly be aware of the problems her patient may be having with one. When such a problem develops, she should enlist the aid of a qualified expert. Most states have a hearing aid society whose members are more than willing to assist a person in need of professional advice and assistance.

Environmental and Safety Needs. The physical environment of the aged, particularly the home and community environment, has only recently received the long overdue attention required to help elderly persons live their last years in comfort and safety. There has been particular concern for the aged poor, those referred to by Frances Storlie as a powerless, voiceless group in our society.[22] Although it is not within the scope of this text to explore all the environmental needs of the aged, it is apparent that no one can give "total nursing care" to an aged patient without knowing something about how this person has lived, what stresses he has adjusted to through the years and what realities of life he will be asked to face in his final days. In the future, there will be more of a shift toward home care, with nursing care delivered in the patient's home or neighborhood senior centers. The principles of environmental safety for the aged will be important in any nursing care setting, and the practical nurse must develop an awareness of her role to protect and support the aged wherever they may be.

Geriatric Nursing Standard #5, as proposed by the ANA Committee for Geriatric Nursing Practice, reads as follows: "The nurse protects aged persons from injury, infection and excessive stress and supports them through the multiplicity of stressful experiences to which they are subjected." Every year 25,000 elderly persons die as a result of accidents and another 3 million are injured. Falls are the largest

single cause of accidental deaths among the elderly. Such statistics clearly show that there is a crying need for measures to protect the elderly from safety hazards.

We are all products of our environment to some degree, from the moment of conception to our last day on earth. No one denies that during the early years of life, the infant and child have the right to a safe and healthy environment. Can we be any less concerned about the elderly? If an elderly patient falls, do we say the accident happened because he is just clumsy and shouldn't have been up and about, or do we recognize our shortcomings in leaving something in his path? If he is burned by a hot water bottle, do we excuse ourselves by saying that he insisted it was not warm enough the first time it was filled, or do we acknowledge that we should have known that elderly persons have decreased sensitivity to heat and cold and therefore must be protected from extremes of temperature? And when we find him wandering through the halls of the hospital, do we make belittling remarks about his mental status? Perhaps we would be more honest if we agreed with Ujhely when she says that within the institution, "the elderly person frequently finds himself to be an isolated dot in a sea of vast corridors and identical rooms, all painted uniform white, so that it takes more skill than he could possibly have at his disposal to orient himself."[23]

Consideration of the special environmental needs of the elderly cannot be limited to buildings and furnishings. We must also take into account the many other aspects of their lives. For example, elderly persons take more medications than persons of other ages. These medications include prescription drugs and those bought over the counter by elderly persons who attempt to medicate themselves with patent medicines. When the elderly patient is receiving medications in the hospital, he must be observed more closely than other adults because the aged do not excrete drugs as rapidly and cannot detoxify them as well as younger adults. All physiologic processes slow down with age and can lead to an accumulation of a drug which exceeds the limits of the maximum dose. It is also possible that elderly persons will not react to a drug as expected and may, in fact, have results exactly opposite to those expected. This type of reaction frequently occurs with barbiturates and opiates, so that the nurse who has given an elderly patient a sedative to quiet him may find that the drug has made him restless, disoriented and uncooperative. Or she may, after having given the drug for several evenings, find that the patient is showing signs of oversedation as the drug accumulates in his body.

If an elderly person is expected to administer his own medications after leaving the hospital, the nursing staff should make every effort to help him understand the schedule for his various medications. He may, for example, need a clearly marked calendar telling him at what hour and on what days he should take each of the drugs. He should know why each drug has been prescribed, how it is supposed to affect him and what may happen if he fails to take his medications as prescribed. It is also important for him to have a simple method for identifying each drug and distinguishing one from the other. Studies have shown that without such assistance there will be a dangerously high incidence of drug errors when elderly persons must administer their own medications.[25]

Generally speaking, the special environmental and safety needs of the elderly are concerned with pace and atmosphere. We must slow down our actions, give elderly persons time to respond physically and mentally to the many demands made of them, protect them from needless worry and harm and provide an atmosphere of trust, confidence and security. Whenever the nurse uses her knowledge of gerontology to protect and care for her elderly patient, she has the satisfaction of knowing that her actions and concern have enhanced his physical condition, bolstered his self-esteem and increased his ability to cope with the realities of life.

PSYCHOSOCIAL CHANGES AND EMOTIONAL NEEDS

Introduction. Man, being a social animal, cannot escape the effects of society or deny the influence of social pressures on his behavior. Many of the behavioral changes that are attributed to mental deterioration in the elderly are the result of the negative attitudes of society mentioned earlier in this chapter. This statement is not meant to deny that there are organic changes in the brain that are associated with old age. To deny such changes would be less than honest and would pose a serious obstacle to understanding and working with the elderly. There is a slowing of the mental processes, some loss of memory for recent events and a tendency toward confusion and disorientation when an elderly individual is exposed to sudden change or unusually stressful situations. Important points to remember are that such changes in mental capacity vary greatly from one person to another, and that an elderly person may not always react as usual when placed in a situation different from the one to which he has become accustomed. It would be a rash person indeed who would state that the mental faculties decline at a steady rate after a given age and thus conclude that all old people are stupid and forgetful.

We do not have adequate tools yet for diagnosing senility. We do not know why some elderly persons regress more rapidly than others. It is agreed, however, that factors contributing toward staying young mentally include *a variety of interests in life, physical fitness, a feeling of being needed and the companionship of others.*

Working With the "Confused" Elderly Patient. There has been so much said and written about confusion in the elderly, that we must be wary of labeling all elderly people "confused," and we must know that when confusion does occur in the elderly patient, it is not the same as irreversible senility. We should also be honest enough to admit that there are times when it would be more accurate to say that it is ourselves who are confused and not the elderly patient. Weymouth points out that "what we actually need to distinguish is who is confused about which part of the communication or behavior."[27] Differences in cultural educational and social backgrounds can cause difficulties in communication, and the fact that such difficulties exist may be due to our failure to understand rather than to the patient's confusion.

Many elderly persons with a chronic illness or disability manage fairly well in their home environment, but when they must be hospitalized, they become confused and disoriented. In the new environment, away from familiar surroundings and persons whom he knows, the patient may be less able to think clearly and express himself properly. He may show signs of forgetfulness, wandering about his ward or room hopelessly lost, or resort to belligerence to express his frustration. He may also show signs of extreme tension, anxiety or anger that produce insomnia and further aggravate his confusion.

Mental health and emotional stability depend to a great degree on meaningful communication with others. The patient who is prematurely diagnosed as senile or confused often cannot have helpful conversations with others for the simple reason that they do not treat him as if he were rational. It has been proved that so-called confused elderly patients can become reoriented rather quickly if they are given appropriate clues and handled as if everyone expects them to be clear-headed and alert. Davis points out that elderly persons tend to adopt very quickly whatever role is expected of them, and that the expectations of those around them can undoubtedly account for the childish, dependent or erratic behavior of elderly persons.[10] If we expect them to behave as eccentric and childish nuisances, they are quite capable of living up to those expectations.

What do these statements mean to the nurse? How can she contribute to the mental well-being of her elderly patients? Burnside suggests that we provide clocks and calendars that can be used by the elderly for orientation to time.[6] Other time-orienting aids could include radio and television, visitors from the outside and hospital personnel who are willing to work at keeping the elderly patient in tune with the world around him. It is not a kindness to "go along with" the elderly patient who has you confused with his grandchild. You should tactfully remind him of your name and why you are there to help him. Nicknames such as "Granny" and "Pop" do not help him remember who he is, nor do they help him maintain his dignity and individual personality. Ignoring his obviously confused request to go to bed in his room at home when he is in an institution does not help him keep in mind where he is and why he is there. Many of our patronizing acts performed in the name of kindness have served only to confuse our elderly patients further and have added to their anxieties.

Nurses may also be guilty of other acts that contribute to mental confusion. When the nurse assists an elderly patient from a lying or sitting position and forces him to stand up too quickly, there can be a sudden drop in his blood pressure with resultant mental confusion. If she prepares a tub bath that is too hot, this too can cause a drop in blood pressure and result in mental confusion. Many patients accused of being confused and consequently restrained "for their protection" become more cooperative and less disoriented when the restraints are removed.

These are only a few of the things we

have learned about the elderly and their special needs created by mental changes. As we learn more about the aging process, we can become more proficient in caring for the aged, but while we are learning, let us not be too quick to judge or too anxious to act in haste.

Emotional Changes and Social Needs. Our emotions and our ability to handle them are closely linked with how we see ourselves and the ways in which others show that they see us. Isolation and alienation can be extremely damaging to one's self-image and can directly affect one's physical and emotional well-being. Elderly persons often have difficulty expressing their emotions appropriately. They are also frequently placed in a position of helplessness with little or no control over what happens to them or how they are treated by others.

Old people need friends and contact with persons of all ages to keep themselves alert and mentally and emotionally happy. They respond to youth and are very much interested in what young people are doing today. Conti recalls that a group of senior citizens with whom she was working complained that everyone in the group was old and had the same complaints. They asked that special parties and gatherings be arranged with groups of young people so that they could enjoy their companionship.[9]

This account should tell us something about the social needs of the elderly and that we must do more than give them "something to do." The younger nurse should not be shy about talking with elderly persons, and if she is at a loss for a topic of conversation, she would do well to remember that all people enjoy talking about themselves and that elderly persons particularly enjoy talking about their youth, which they usually remember with amazing clarity. No one likes to look back over his life and remember it as dull. We can sometimes get an elderly person away from an often-told tale by asking him

about some detail in the story. If, for instance, Mr. Thompson, for the tenth time, launches into his favorite account of the day half his home town burned down, one might ask him how fire alarms were spread in his day or what methods were used to extinguish the blaze. This type of question will show genuine interest and give Mr. Thompson something more to talk about. The important point is to let the older person set the pace in the conversation or activity in which *he* is interested.

Sometimes, when we try so hard to meet the social needs of the elderly patient by engaging him in lengthy conversations, we forget his need for rest and periodic naps. The author remembers a young student nurse who was determined to socialize with an elderly patient. They talked for quite a long time, and finally the patient asked her why she was spending so much time with him. She responded by saying that she was there to "meet his needs." His reply was, "Well, young lady, what I need most now is a little rest." Again we are reminded of the need to know each patient as an individual and to develop a sensitivity to him and his needs.

The kind of hospital care that is bound to a routine that meets the needs of the institution rather than the needs of the patients can do much to harm and little to help the geriatric patient. Physical illness can be exaggerated by isolation and loneliness. Anderson cites a study that was done with geriatric patients in a public mental institution. The patients on the unit were "encouraged to participate in a wide range of social, recreational and educational activities." When data from the study were evaluated, it was found that "the discharge rate on this unit was three times higher, and the mortality rate one third lower, than rates in a control group receiving traditional care."[2]

Perhaps it would be well to point out that not all old people need constant activity. Some prefer and enjoy periods of solitude. Again it is a matter of adjusting our nursing care to meet the individual needs of the patient. A story is told of an elderly woman who wrote daily in her diary for a full year the following entry: "No one came." A group of people concerned about the welfare of the elderly in their community were saddened when they heard of the woman's loneliness. They set out to contact other isolated persons and to one elderly woman they told the story of the diary. The second elderly woman responded with her own point of view, which was, "From another old lady who writes in her diary: No one came—thank goodness."[9]

We can conclude, therefore, that elderly persons, like all others of varying ages, are persons. We cannot know their needs, their likes and their dislikes until we know them as persons, and we cannot know them as persons until we treat them as such.

CLINICAL CASE PROBLEMS

1. Mrs. Dalton, age 78, is admitted to the hospital for treatment of a fractured femur. After surgical fixation of the fracture, she becomes very confused and is incontinent of feces and urine. She also refuses to eat or to try to help herself in any way. Her husband is still living, and they had managed to care for one another in their farm home before Mrs. Dalton's accident. They have only one child, a son who is married and lives in another city about 80 miles away. He is a successful lawyer and the father of four children. He comes to see his mother occasionally while she is in the hospital and would like to have his parents come to live with him, but his wife does not feel there is room in their home for the elderly couple.

What nursing problems can you see for Mrs. Dalton while she is in the hospital?

What factors will influence Mrs. Dalton's reaction to her accident?

What other problems aside from nursing have been created by her accident? How can they be solved? What resources might be available for help for the elderly couple?

2. Mrs. Petrone, age 74, is admitted to the hospital for diagnostic studies. She is very weak and apathetic and seldom speaks to the hospital staff. You are assigned to care for Mrs. Petrone, but when you enter her room, she tells you in very broken English that she does not want to eat or bathe and that you should go to other patients who are young and able to be well again. When you finally coax Mrs. Petrone into allowing you to give her morning care, she begs you not to remove the religious medal that she wears on a heavy chain around her neck.

What relationship do you see between Mrs. Petrone's situation and the ANA's proposed Geriatric Standard #3?

What are some possible causes of Mrs. Petrone's attitude toward the hospital food? Toward her future and her ability to recover from her illness?

Mrs. Petrone's daughter, with whom she has been living, tells you that she does not know how she can ever pay the medical bills and that since her mother was born in a foreign country she is sure that government aid would not be available to her. How would you explain Medicare to her?

What might be some possible reasons for Mrs. Petrone's failing to seek help for her physical condition until it became an emergency?

3. Mr. Fogarty, age 84, fell in the hall at 1:00 A.M. and sustained a laceration on his forehead. The following evening at 10:45, he was brought to the nursing station by a male attendant who found him wandering through the

halls on the floor below his room. The attendant commented that Mr. Fogarty should be called "Mr. Foggy," because he does not know who he is or where he is. Mr. Fogarty's chart is full of recorded incidents indicating his confusion and disorientation.

What might be some attitudes of the hospital staff that contribute to Mr. Fogarty's confusion?

What are some positive steps that might be taken to help this patient and to protect him from further injury, both physical and psychological?

REFERENCES

1. Amburger, P. I.: "Environmental Aids for the Aged Patient." Am. Journ. Nurs., Sept., 1966, p. 2017.
2. Anderson, C. J.: "Alienation in the Aged: Implications for Psychiatric Geriatric Nursing." Am. Journ. Nurs., Dec., 1967, p. 2581.
3. Archer, S. K.: "Health Maintenance Programs for Older Adults." Nurs. Clin. N. Amer., Vol. 3, No. 4, 1968, p. 729.
4. Burchette, D. E.: "Factors Affecting Nurse-Patient Interaction in a Geriatric Setting." Am. Journ. Nurs., Dec., 1967, p. 2581.
5. Burnside, I. M.: "Accoutrements of Aging." Nurs. Clin. N. Amer., Vol. 7, No. 2, 1972, p. 291.
6. Burnside, I. M.: "Clocks and Calendars." Am. Journ. Nurs., Jan., 1970, p. 117.
7. Butler, R. N.: "The Crises of Old Age." RN, Oct., 1969, p. 47.
8. Carlson, S.: "Communication and Social Interaction in the Aged." Nurs. Clin. N. Amer., Vol. 7, No. 2, 1972, p. 269.
9. Conti, M. L.: "The Loneliness of Old Age." Nursing Outlook, Aug., 1970, p. 28.
10. Davis, R. W.: "Psychological Aspects of Geriatric Nursing." Am. Journ. Nurs., April, 1968, p. 802.
11. Dupuis, P.: "Old is Beautiful." Nursing Outlook, Aug., 1970, p. 25.
12. Hodkinson, M. A.: "Some Clinical Problems of Geriatric Nursing." Nurs. Clin. N. Amer., Vol. 3, No. 4, 1968, p. 675.
13. Jennings, M., et al.: "Physiologic Functioning in the Elderly." Nurs. Clin. N. Amer., Vol. 7, No. 2, 1972, p. 237.
14. Kamenetz, H. L.: "Exercises for the Elderly." Am. Journ. Nurs., Aug., 1972, p. 1401.
15. Lane, H. C.: "Foreword—Symposium on Care of the Elderly." Nurs. Clin. N. Amer., Vol. 3, No. 4, 1968, p. 649.
16. Lawton, A.: "Accidental Injuries to the Aged." Gerontologist, Vol. 5, 1965, p. 96.
17. Moses, D. V.: "Assessing Behavior in the Elderly." Nurs. Clin. N. Amer., Vol. 7, No. 2, 1972, p. 225.
18. Robins, E. G.: "Understanding the Health Needs of the Elderly." Journ. Pract. Nurs., June, 1972, p. 16.
19. Schwarz, D.: "Problems of Self-care and Travel Among Elderly Ambulatory Patients." Am. Journ. Nurs., Dec., 1966, p. 2678.
20. Simko, M.: "Foot Welfare." Am. Journ. Nurs., Sept., 1967, p. 1895.
21. Stone, V.: "Keeping Up with Geriatric Nursing." Nursing '72, April, p. 32.
22. Storlie, F.: "The Aged Poor." Nursing '72, May, p. 29.
23. Ujhely, G. B.: "The Environment of the Elderly." Nurs. Clin. N. Amer., Vol. 7, No. 2, 1972, p. 281.
24. Verwoerdt, A.: "Psychological Factors in Geriatric Nursing Care." Journ. Pract. Nurs., Feb., 1967, p. 24.
25. Watson, J. E.: Medical-Surgical Nursing and Related Physiology. Philadelphia, W. B. Saunders Co., 1972.
26. Weg, R. B.: "Physiologic Changes with Age that Affect Patient Care." Journ. Pract. Nurs., Oct., 1971, p. 34.
27. Weymouth, L. T.: "The Nursing Care of the So-called Confused Patient." Nurs. Clin. N. Amer., Vol. 3, No. 4, 1968, p. 709.

SUGGESTED STUDENT READING

1. Burnside, I. M.: "Clocks and Calendars." Am. Journ. Nurs., Jan., 1970, p. 117.
2. Calloway, A. B.: "Social Needs of the Geriatric Patient." Journ. Pract. Nurs., March, 1968, p. 34.
3. Carlson, S.: "Communication and Social Interaction in the Aged." Nurs. Clin. N. Amer., Vol. 7, No. 2, 1972, p. 269.
4. Conti, M. L.: "The Loneliness of Old Age." Nursing Outlook, Aug., 1970, p. 28.
5. Dupuis, P.: "Old is Beautiful." Nursing Outlook, Aug., 1970, p. 25.
6. Gerbaukas, D.: "A Nurse's Guide to Medications for the Geriatric Patient." Journ. Pract. Nurs., Aug., 1971, p. 22.
7. Hardy, F.: "Care of the Geriatric Patient." Journ. Pract. Nurs., Sept., 1970, p. 33.
8. Hutchins, M. H.: "The Geriatric Patient: 'Help Me.'" Nurs. Clin. N. Amer., Vol. 6, No. 4, 1971, p. 795.
9. McCarthy, M.: "Old Men in a Hospital," from "The Old Men" in Cast a Cold Eye. New York, Harcourt, Brace & World, Inc., 1950. Reprinted in Nurs. Clin. N. Amer., Vol. 1, No. 3, 1966, p. 523.
10. Rasmussen, S.: "Medicare and the Practical

Nurse." Nursing Outlook, June, 1966, p. 62.

11. Stone, V.: "Keeping Up with Geriatric Nursing." Nursing '72, April, p. 32.

12. Storlie, F.: "The Aged Poor." Nursing '72, May, p. 29.

13. Thompson, P. W.: "Physiological and Psychological Aspects of Aging." Bedside Nurse, June, 1970, p. 13.

14. Verwoerdt, A.: "Psychological Factors in Geriatric Nursing Care." Journ. Pract. Nurs., Feb., 1967, p. 24.

15. Volpe, A., and Kastenbaum, R.: "Beer and TLC." Am. Journ. Nurs., Jan., 1967, p. 100.

16. Warner, B. A.: "The Processes of Aging." Nurs. Clin. N. Amer., Vol. 1, No. 3, 1966, p. 407.

17. Weg, R. B.: "Physiologic Changes with Age that Affect Patient Care." Journ. Pract. Nurs., Oct., 1971, p. 34.

OUTLINE FOR CHAPTER 7

I. Introduction

A. The rapid increase in numbers of older people in our population has stimulated interest in the aging process, special needs of the aged and solutions to the problems caused by aging.

B. Aging process varies with individuals.

C. Goal of gerontology is to prolong life and improve the quality of life for the elderly.

D. Goal of geriatric nursing is preservation of each individual patient's personal assets and maintenance of highest possible level of function for him.

II. Attitudes Toward Aging

A. Negative attitudes are detrimental to welfare of the aged. At least 85 per cent of all elderly persons are, in fact, essentially healthy and leading active and useful lives.

B. Nurses need to evaluate their feelings and attitudes and understand how attitudes toward the elderly are developed. They should "demonstrate an appreciation of the heritage, values and wisdom of older persons."

III. Medicare—A Governmental Health Insurance Program Designed to Meet the Health Needs of the Elderly

IV. Health Needs of the Aged

A. Concept of health care for elderly expanding beyond institutional care.

B. Health needs of the elderly have far-reaching effect on the entire nation.

C. Factors involved in health care planning:

    1. To be old does not mean to be ill.

    2. Older persons often have several diseases at one time.

    3. Symptoms may not be as noticeable in the elderly.

    4. Many older people do not seek medical help until an emergency arises.

V. Physiologic Changes and Physical Needs

A. Standards for measuring health needs in an elderly person cannot be the same as for younger adults.

B. Rest and exercise—joints become stiffer, muscles weaker

    1. Exercises should be modified for elderly.

    2. Complications that can be avoided by exercise include osteoporosis, joint stiffening, circulatory and respiratory stasis.

    3. Sleep and rest pattern for elderly person often erratic and unsimilar to patterns considered normal for younger adults.

C. Special Skin Care—oil and sweat glands less active.

    1. Skin becomes dry and easily damaged.

    2. Daily bath may be harmful; emollient massage recommended.

    3. Prevention of decubitus ulcers especially important.

D. Care of Nails and Hair.

    1. Nails become brittle and thick. Emollients used to soften.

    2. Many elderly persons tend to diagnose their own foot problems. Harsh medications, corn plasters, self-trimming of nails, corns and calluses can be very dangerous.

    3. Elderly respond favorably to their personal cleanliness and good grooming.

E. Nutritional Needs—No special diet to prolong life. Needs are the same except for possible reduction in calories.

    1. Malnutrition common in the elderly. Possible causes include

chewing and digestive problems, ignorance of what constitutes a well-balanced diet, economic and emotional insecurity, life-long habits of nutritionally inadequate diet.

2. Greatest difficulty with dentures is "poor fit," which makes chewing difficult.

3. Vitamin deficiencies and poor absorption of calcium frequently present.

4. Achlorhydria may lead to anemia.

5. Feeding an elderly patient requires patience and tact.

6. Food should be a treat, not a treatment.

F. Elimination—Constipation not uncommon because of slowing down of intestinal activity, decreased physical activity and poor eating habits.

1. Elderly typically overconcerned with their bowels.

2. Laxatives and frequent enemas can lead to serious potassium loss.

3. Urinary problems in males frequently caused by benign prostatic hypertrophy.

4. Incontinence may be controlled by regular schedule for offering bedpan and allowing patient out of bed when possible.

G. Vision and Hearing—Some degree of visual and hearing loss present in many elderly persons.

1. Glasses may be out-of-date or nonprescription glasses.

2. Tunnel vision a common disorder—can be a safety hazard.

3. Hearing aids may cause problems that require expert advice.

4. Communication with elderly improved by speaking slowly, in low-pitched voice, and standing directly in front of them when talking.

H. Environmental and Safety Needs— "The nurse protects aged persons from injury, infection and excessive stress. . . ."

1. Accidents account for death of 25,000 elderly persons every year and injury to another 3 million.

2. Medications can be hazardous to the elderly.

3. Special needs—slower pace and atmosphere of trust.

VI. Psychosocial Changes and Emotional Needs

A. Introduction—Many behavioral changes in the elderly caused by negative attitudes of society.

1. There is a slowing of the mental processes, some loss of memory for recent events and a tendency toward confusion when subjected to sudden change.

2. Mental changes vary widely among individuals.

3. Factors contributing toward staying young mentally include variety of interests, physical fitness, feeling needed and companionship of others.

B. The So-called Confused Elderly Patient.

1. We need to determine who is confused—it may not be the patient.

2. Not a kindness to "go along" with confused patient. He needs help to orient himself.

3. Time-orienting devices such as clocks and radios helpful.

4. Elderly patients very good at adopting whatever role is expected of them.

5. Nurses may be guilty of acts that cause drop in blood pressure and mental confusion.

C. Emotional Changes and Social Needs.

1. Elderly may have difficulty expressing emotions appropriately.

2. Old people need friends and contact with persons of all ages.

3. Isolation can aggravate physical ills.

4. Some may prefer periods of solitude.

8

The Chronically Ill

"If I am ugly, I am not ugly only in my own eyes, I see myself in the looking-glass of your eyes as ugly too. You are the witness of my ugliness. In fact, insofar as ugliness is relative, if you and everyone else saw me as beautiful I might be ugly no more."

R. D. Laing, *Interpersonal Perception*

Part One. Care of the Patient With a Chronic Illness or Disability

INTRODUCTION

In the early 1900's, the main causes of death and disability in this country were the infectious diseases such as pneumonia, septicemia and influenza. With the perfection of immunization techniques, the discovery of newer drugs for combating infections and the improvement of sanitation practices, the health-illness pattern of the nation changed. Today the major health problems in the United States are chronic disease and disability. In the 1970's, the National Center for Health Statistics estimates that 27.6 million persons have definite or suspected heart disease, 13 million have arthritis, 6 mil-

lion are mentally retarded, 1 million have severe visual impairment and 0.25 million are deaf. These are only a few of the statistics for chronic illness and disability; they do not begin to give the whole picture of the human misery and financial burden imposed by disorders of this kind.

The Bureau of Census predicts that by 1980 there will be 39.5 million *more* people with chronic disease than there are at present. The increase does not mean that our population is any less healthy than it was formerly. The statistics reflect an expected increase in population as a whole and improvement in our methods of detecting chronic illness in its early stages. They indicate advances in medical technology which have allowed more efficient treatment and control of diseases that formerly were fatal. The figures also show the results of increased life span, because those persons who live to reach their 70's and 80's almost invariably have some type of chronic disorder, even though it may not prevent them from leading active lives.

The U.S. Public Health Service lists more than 40 diseases as chronic or long-term illnesses. As the preceding figures show, heart disease is the most common affliction, with the arthritides (plural for arthritis) ranking second. Other chronic diseases include metabolic disorders, malignant growths, paraplegia and quadriplegia, various neuromuscular diseases and visual and hearing difficulties, as well as chronic mental disorders.

Definition

The reader may well wonder about the difference between an acute illness and a chronic illness and how this difference might affect the type of care a patient will need. An *acute* illness is one that has a rapid onset, lasts only a relatively brief period of time and ends with complete recovery or death. A *chronic* illness has a more gradual beginning, with vague symptoms that become progressively more severe if treatment is not initiated. A chronic illness does not go away. The chronically ill person must learn to live with his illness, and he will need continued support throughout his lifetime. His care will involve a variety of individuals on the health care team. A chronic illness is rarely restricted to one system of the body, because of the interdependence of all systems for the maintenance of body function.

Although there is an inevitable degeneration of tissues and organs in a chronic illness and only partial recovery can ever be expected, these patients do not necessarily follow a steadily downward course. There may be times when the disease will lie dormant and present few symptoms. These times are called periods of *remission.* When the symptoms become more severe because of a flare-up of the disease process, the term *exacerbation,* or *acute phase,* is used. The acute phase may last a relatively short time, followed by another remission, or it may become progressively more critical and lead to the death of the patient.

It is important not to confuse an acute illness with the acute phase of a chronic illness. The patient with an acute illness will have needs that are quite different from those of the patient who is suffering an acute exacerbation of his chronic illness. Acute illness is an event that will temporarily interrupt an individual's pattern of living and cause his family some inconveniences that are not usually permanently disruptive. Chronic illness will create a need for long-term planning and coordination of individuals and agencies that are available to provide continuity of care throughout the chronically ill person's life. Such an illness will almost invariably have some lasting effect on the patient's family.

When we think of chronic illness, many of us have a mental picture of an elderly person who is totally dependent on others and unable to carry out the most basic activities of daily living. This is a common misconception, and a very damaging one to the many people who have a chronic illness or disability. Of the estimated 17 million persons in this country who have a chronic illness that imposes some limitation on their physical activity, about 5 million are under 45 years of age and another 6 million are in the 45 to 65 year age group.[22] It is obvious, therefore, that just as being old is not the same as being sick, being chronically ill is not always the same as being old.

We must also be careful about equating chronic illness with serious disability. More than half the chronically ill persons in this country have no limitation of their activity. They require periodic medical examinations and often need continuing treatment with drugs, dietary regimen or some other method of controlling their illness, but they do not think of themselves as disabled or handicapped, as indeed they are not. These facts are important to keep in mind because they have a direct bearing on one's attitudes toward chronic illness and the persons who suffer from disorders of this type.

Attitudes Toward the Chronically Ill

The patient who is disabled with a chronic illness or permanent handicap faces somewhat the same problems as the elderly person. Both must contend with society's negative feelings toward the aged and infirm. It is tragic to note that the National Commission on Chronic Illness found that the attitudes of the general public are shared by many in the health professions. The commission reported a study which showed rejection of the aged, chronically ill and disabled by the general public and professional persons as well, accompanied by a widespread feeling among health care personnel that long-term care is dull, depressing and almost nonproductive.

Admittedly, it is more dramatic and exciting to experience with a patient his quick and complete recovery from an acute and critical illness. Those who are privileged to share in such a recovery cannot help feeling truly heroic, knowing that their efforts have been productive and worthwhile. Does this attitude mean that there are no rewards for those who care for the chronically ill? Is it not possible that in nursing a patient with a chronic illness, one has more time for learning to care *about* the patient as she cares *for* him? The long periods of personal contact between nurse and patient can give very real meaning to the words *involvement* and *commitment.* Typically, the patient who is disabled with a chronic illness or permanent injury is faced with the

possibilities of loss of function, poor prognosis for cure and some adjustment to his manner of living and life expectancy. He needs supportive nursing care that is diligent, consistent and directed toward small gains that may be achieved only after long and tedious effort. If he cannot find such support from those who are supposedly dedicated to the care of the sick, he may well ask, "To whom can I turn? Where do I go to find someone willing to share her strength, knowledge and courage with me so I can have a better life? Who will accept me as I am and work with me to accomplish something better?"

It is imperative that a chronically disabled person find acceptance from the nurses who are in daily contact with him. Acceptance of the patient means accepting him *as he is,* taking the bad with the good, but with a vision of hope about his potential to become something more. He must know that he is perceived as a whole person and not as a paraplegic, an interesting case of diabetes or a rare neuromuscular disorder. Wolf reminds us that when we think of a person only in terms of his disability, we "strip him of his individuality and reduce him to the factor of his particular handicap . . . as if that were all there is to him."[23]

It is true that health professionals often have a tendency to focus on the disease or disability and ignore the "personhood" of the patient. Perhaps we do this as a protective measure against the hurt and heartache that can come from personal involvement with a patient. But if this detachment is what we seek, it is important to be honest and admit that we do not want to take the risk of becoming involved. We must not fool ourselves by making excuses that are not valid. Unless a patient is accepted as a whole person, he cannot be himself on his own terms; the reality of his existence is diminished when those around him do not take note of the fact that he does indeed exist as a whole person.

Those of us who are involved in the care of the sick and disabled must be careful that we do not make premature judgments about chronically ill or disabled patients. Many authorities in the field of physical rehabilitation share the notion that the physically disabled person is a member of an underprivileged minority as are Jews, Negroes, the poor and other members of groups that are "different" from the majority. They see him as a victim of prejudice and as restricted in his relationship with others because they have prejudged him before they have sufficient knowledge to make such a judgment. It is important that nurses realize the danger of prejudging their patients and that they avoid placing each patient in a neat and tidy category, satisfied that they know all there is to know about him.

In his autobiography, *To Race the Wind,* Harold Krents, who has been blind since birth, tells about his struggle to overcome the prejudice of others who were quick to assume that he was incapable of living a normal and active life. He refused to accept the role that society had cast for him and set out to prove that his capabilities far outweighed his disability. The story of his victories over the negative attitudes of society is recommended reading for anyone interested in dealing with the problems of chronic illness and disability in a positive and helpful way.

SPECIAL NEEDS AND THEIR NURSING IMPLICATIONS

Assessment of Needs

It is difficult if not impossible to make a complete and accurate assessment of a patient's needs without having extensive knowledge about him and his family and the community in which he lives. This assessment is particularly necessary for the chronically ill patient, who will have health and welfare needs that go beyond hospital

care and that will continue throughout his lifetime. We can make some general statements about types of problems that he may encounter and some ways of coping with and solving the problems, but we must emphasize that patient assessment is never static. It is an ongoing and continuous process, and as the patient's total situation is evaluated from time to time, some needs will take precedence over others.

The general areas in which an individual patient's needs will be assessed include (1) physical needs as dictated by the degree of impairment present, (2) general state of physical and mental health, (3) his home and community environment, (4) his financial situation, (5) his talents, aptitudes and interests in recreational and occupational activities, (6) his ability to relate to and socialize with others and (7) his motivation for self-care and adjustment to his illness.

Physical Needs

The chronically ill patient often requires a high level of physical care in the hospital as well as in the home after discharge. Of particular concern are the many hazards of immobility, which are an ever-present danger to these patients. The prevention of deformity and maintenance of the highest possible level of function in each of the major systems of the body require diligent care and determination. The human body is designed for motion. Studies have shown that even normal and healthy persons will suffer loss of function and damage to the body systems when they are forced to remain immobile over a period of time.

Cardiovascular System. It is now believed that the heart works harder when the body is in a resting, supine position. We can understand this idea when we realize that blood normally distributed in the legs when the body is in an upright position is released from gravity pressure when one lies down.

This means that the blood leaves the legs and enters the total blood volume to be redistributed in other parts of the body by the pumping action of the heart. In addition, a state of immobility leads to development of blood clots within the blood vessels. This situation is aggravated by allowing the patient to lie in one position too long so that the weight of the body causes continued pressure against the blood vessels and inhibits the flow of blood. When a patient is lying on his side with the weight of one leg resting on the other, he is quite likely to develop blood clots in the leg bearing the weight.

Nursing measures that can reduce the workload of the heart and increase circulation include turning the patient frequently, suggesting and helping with passive and active exercises of the muscles and, whenever possible, elevating the head of the bed or sitting the patient in a chair.

Respiratory System. Immobility can have three physiologic effects on the respiratory system. These are decreased movement of the respiratory muscles and diaphragm, decreased movement of secretions within the respiratory tree and a disturbance in the balance between carbon dioxide and oxygen.

The nursing measures to avoid these developments are not complicated; in fact, they are so simple that they are often overlooked. Obviously, some steps must be taken to exercise the muscles of respiration (the intercostals and the diaphragm) and to increase the flow of secretions. These measures include helping the patient with routine deep-breathing exercises and coughing. He must also be turned frequently and, if he is able, he must sit up and stretch or change position often so that there can be adequate expansion of the chest. If removal of secretions in the lower respiratory tract is extremely difficult, postural drainage and chest tapping may be necessary or treatment with a respirator may be indicated.

Gastrointestinal Tract. The inactive patient is subject to indigestion, loss of appetite, distention, diarrhea and constipation. The causes of these symptoms may be the stress and nervous tension produced by immobility, or they may result from poor muscle tone, absence of normal reflexes or failure of the patient to heed the defecation reflex. Constipation is a problem that may require considerable patience and individual planning to overcome. Strong laxatives and enemas are not recommended, since they are often abused and do not offer a permanent solution to the patient's problem. Stool softeners and exercises to strengthen the abdominal muscles are helpful. In addition, the patient should be instructed in the process of elimination and a routine should be worked out on the basis of each patient's individual need.

Musculoskeletal System. The muscles, bones and skin of an immobile patient are likely to deteriorate very rapidly. Even in normal, healthy individuals, a lack of activity will very soon lead to loss of muscle tone. Since about 40 per cent of the body is made up of muscle, it is imperative that some regimen of exercises be established. If the muscles are not exercised regularly, the muscle fibers lose their elasticity and their ability to contract and stretch. *Contractures* then develop, and the joints become fixed in one position, making motion impossible. Proper positioning of the patient and putting the joints through their full range of motion at least once daily will help prevent these complications (see Fig. 8–1). *Osteoporosis* (porous bone) is another hazard of immobility. It is the result of demineralization of the bone and occurs when the usual stress and strain of walking and moving about is no longer placed on the bones. This stress normally stimulates the process of building bone—that is, replacing old bone cells with newer, stronger ones. When activity ceases, the building process stops and the calcium, phosphorus and nitrogen that usually aid in the building process are removed from the bone. The bone then becomes soft and spongy and may easily be deformed or broken.

Decubitus ulcers (pressure sores) are a well-known problem to anyone who has cared for a bedridden patient. Cleanliness of the skin, frequent massage to stimulate circulation to pressure areas and a regular routine for turning to relieve pressure on bony prominences are necessary to prevent decreased blood supply to an area and the development of necrotic tissue.

Urinary Tract. The urinary system of man functions most efficiently when the body is in an erect position. The flow of urine out of the renal pelvis and through the urinary tract is greatly reduced when physical activity ceases and one remains in a supine position for a prolonged period of time. *Urinary stasis* (decreased flow of urine) leads to the formation of urinary calculi (stones) and the development of infection.

To avoid urinary stasis and its complications, one must realize the relationship between inactivity and decreased flow of urine. If at all possible, the nurse should establish some routine of physical activity for the patient, utilizing both active and passive exercises. In addition, she needs to keep an accurate record of intake and output, encouraging her patient to drink sufficient fluids to keep the urine dilute and checking the patient frequently for bladder distention. With continued pressure of urine against the bladder wall, the normal reflexes may become impaired. Nursing measures to induce voiding and moderate pressure of the hand against the lower pelvis to facilitate emptying of the bladder during urination often is sufficient to prevent bladder distention. Catheterization, unless carried out under ideal conditions, tends to introduce infection into the urinary tract and is not recommended for a chronically ill patient.

Emotional Needs

The emotional needs of the chronically ill or disabled patient are extremely complex, and it would be presumptuous to imply that a thorough discussion of the nurse's role in meeting these needs could be covered in a textbook such as this one. We can only hope to give some insight into the difficult psychologic and emotional adjustments demanded of the individual who strives to learn to live with his disability.

There is increasing evidence that the patient, and not his diagnosis, is most important in his reaction to his illness.[1] An individual's adjustment to chronic illness or disability will depend on such factors as age, cultural background, type of illness and the limitations it imposes, role in the family and emotional stability.

When the patient first learns that he has a chronic illness or permanent disability, he experiences an emotional upheaval and profound grief similar to that caused by death. This is because in some ways his old "self" is indeed dead, and he is faced with the task of building a new life around a new self. In order to do this, he must come to the realization that his illness does exist and that it is going to make a difference in many aspects of his daily life and in his relationships with his friends and relatives. Most patients find this realization extremely difficult, so the first step in the process of adaptation is one of denial. This denial that anything is wrong is simply a matter of self-protection. The patient is shocked by the fact that the illness is threatening his usual pattern of life. The nurse's reaction to such denials should be that of a quiet listener. She should not argue with him or insist that he is wrong in denying the illness; she can only allow him to express his feelings and show that she can be depended on to help him when he is able to admit that he needs her help.

Gradually the patient will begin to show that he has become aware of his

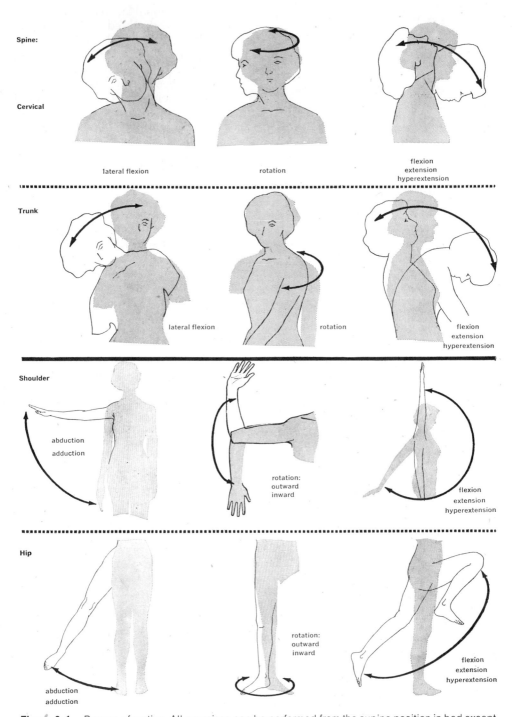

Figure 8–1. Ranges of motion. All exercises can be performed from the supine position in bed except hyperextension of the spine, hips, and shoulders and flexion of the knees, for which the person must lie prone or on his side. (From Kelly: American Journal of Nursing, October, 1966.)

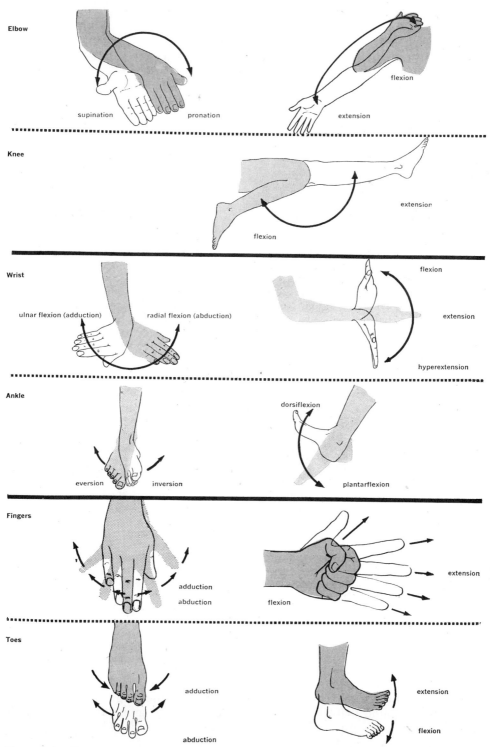

Figure 8-1. (Continued)

predicament. He may do this by trying to place the blame for his illness on someone who cares for him or is trying to help him. During this period of anger and resentment, the patient may make statements that indicate a lack of confidence in the physicians and nurses or anger toward his relatives and friends. Again the nurse must listen to the patient, but she should not argue with him. Her task is to follow the details of medical attention and nursing care scrupulously, showing by her attitude and actions that she considers every phase of his treatment important and that she is sincerely interested in doing everything possible to help the patient in his illness. During this stage, she may notice that the patient will become more and more dependent on her. If she can get across to him that she is available for help whenever it is needed, he will then progress to less dependence as he gains confidence in himself and the care he is receiving.

Finally, the patient must begin to reorganize his relationships with his friends and family. This process is necessary, because he is now a sick person with an illness that is not going to go away. Nothing can change that. Once he is able to admit that he is a different person because of his illness, he will be better able to live with it.

The role of the nurse is that of a guide. She must not force or push the patient into his new way of life or try to change him so that he "fits into" the world of the chronically ill. She must offer support and guidance to the patient as he moves toward a new and different kind of existence.

The family, friends and acquaintances of the patient may make a healthy contribution to his adjustment, or they may add to his emotional problems. A study by Jerome Siller identifies some common reactions of healthy persons to disfigurement or disability in others. He found that some persons feel guilt because they are able-bodied; others have a fear of developing a disability similar to that of the patient, or they see the patient as an unpleasant reminder of the precariousness of health. They may also be embarrassed or afraid of doing or saying the wrong thing in the patient's presence.

A certain type of disfigurement may be particularly repulsive to a person. The nurse who experiences some of these reactions in herself needs to understand that such feelings are not necessarily wrong and a reason for guilt. If she finds that she cannot overcome such reactions, she must recognize her inability to help the patient and avoid placing herself in a position to do him further emotional harm.

Social Needs

There is no one solution to the problem of providing healthy social relationships for a chronically ill or disabled patient. Some feel more secure and less threatened when they are among other persons with similar disabilities. They derive from the group a sense of identity and learn to overcome a negative self-concept. Others resent being isolated from the give and take of society and readily oppose any suggestion that they join a group composed of "fellow-sufferers." Such persons have a strong sense of personal worth and prefer to be seen as individuals who incidentally happen to have a disability.

Family and friends of the chronically ill or disabled person will require some support and encouragement prior to the patient's leaving the hospital and returning to his home and community. Almost invariably, they want to be helpful but do not know what to do for the patient and what to expect from him. Although the nurse cannot deal with these questions alone, she should be aware of the need for the family to express their concerns, and she must recognize their right to expect and receive advice and referral to qualified resource persons who are capable of helping them.

REHABILITATION

Definition

The term "rehabilitation" first became widely used after World War I, when wounded American soldiers returned home and ways were needed to help these veterans adjust to their physical disabilities. Today the concept of rehabilitation extends beyond physical care to include all aspects of the disabled person's life. The National Council on Rehabilitation defines it thus: "Rehabilitation means the restoration of the individual to the fullest physical, mental, social, vocational and economic capacity of which he is capable."

All the activities concerned with reaching the goals of rehabilitation are carried out by a variety of persons: physicians, nurses, physical therapists, public health workers, psychologists and vocational counselors.

Nurse's Role in Rehabilitation

The plan of nursing care for rehabilitation begins with admission of the patient to the hospital. This simply means that from the beginning the nurse must keep in sight the goal of returning the patient to his family and community in a condition that will allow him to realize his full potential within the limits of his capabilities.

There are four steps in the overall plan for nursing care and rehabilitation of the chronically ill and disabled: (1) preventive measures against complications and deformities, (2) early activities of self-care, (3) teaching the patient and his family how to manage his illness (4) referral to other professions and agencies for continuity of care.[19] These steps are not truly steps in the sense that one follows the other. They are all needed in almost all phases of patient care.

In the first step, the nurse brings to bear all the skills and ingenuity she can muster to prevent loss of function and further damage to the body systems. She also uses her "self"—her personality, love and attention, her hopes and dreams for the patient's future—to help meet his psychological and emotional needs as he adjusts to his new way of life. She emphasizes his abilities rather than his disabilities and directs his attention to the things he can do rather than the things he cannot do.

The simple tasks of eating, dressing, maintaining good personal hygiene and getting about from place to place are usually taken for granted by those of us who are well, but they can be extremely complex and frustrating activities for someone who has become limited in the kinds of movements he can make. Each patient will need specific instructions and continuous encouragement to help him regain some independence in self-care activities. The newly blind person, the patient who is paralyzed and the patient who has an amputated limb will all have special problems and individual needs.

The nurse in a general hospital can do much to help her patient achieve the goals of self-care within the limits of his disability. She should not give in to the tendency to do everything for her patient but allow him to care for himself as much as he is able. He must start as soon as he is physically able to begin relearning the tasks of self-care so that when he returns home or is transferred to another institution he will be prepared to accept some responsibility for his personal care.

There are numerous self-help devices and specially designed articles of clothing that are available to the disabled person (see Figs. 8–2 and 8–3). If the patient expects to use any of these articles, they should be brought to the hospital so that he can practice using them and become familiar with them before discharge. Each time he accomplishes another small task in feeding, dressing or bathing himself, he is one

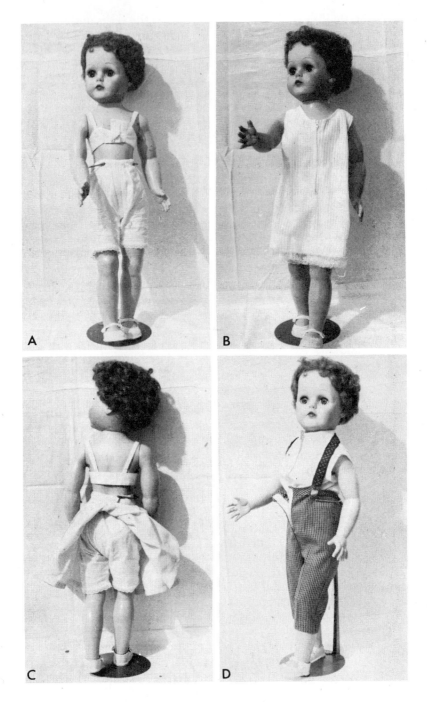

Figure 8–2. *A,* Patients with hemiparesis like front closing bras fastened with Velcro; all like elastic straps. Such bras are commercially available. Pettipants make slips unnecessary, are comfortable in wheelchairs and keep a urinal bag concealed even when a skirt hikes up during a transfer from car to wheelchair. *B,* Patients who have restricted shoulder movement find front-zippered slips convenient. *C,* Back-wrap skirts can be folded to the front when the patient sits in her wheelchair, avoiding pressure from folds of material. *D,* Halter made from half a pair of suspenders holds up the trousers adequately, lessens the danger of a patient's tripping when he raises his trousers after toilet. Velcro can replace the zipper as a fly fastening when necessary.

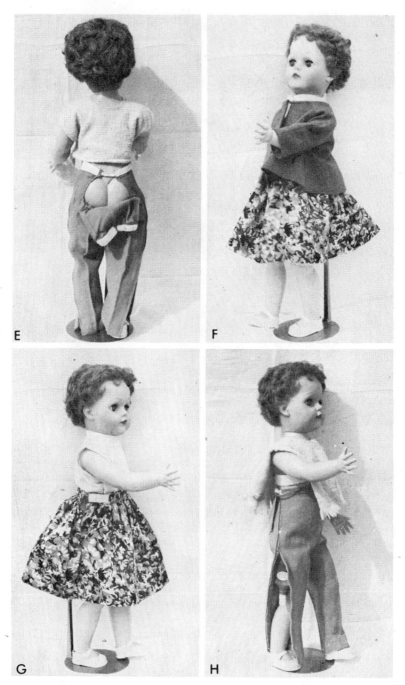

Figure 8–2. (Continued) *E,* Drop seat makes it possible to air skin over the sacral area without the patient's having to disrobe. *F,* A cape or coat with large armholes is just long enough to keep the patient's back warm, too short to create bulky folds under the buttocks. The front, like the waist band of the skirt above, is fastened with Velcro, manageable when buttons are a problem. *G,* Ambulant patients with limited hand dexterity like full skirts with a deeply overlapping placket that needs no zipper, just a small amount of Velcro fastening at the waistband. *H,* Side zipper from ankle to waist permits applying or removing leg brace or urinal bags without disrobing. Terry top, fastened with ties, Velcro, snap fasteners, grippers or whatever, is machine washable, needs no ironing. (From Smith: American Journal of Nursing, June, 1966.)

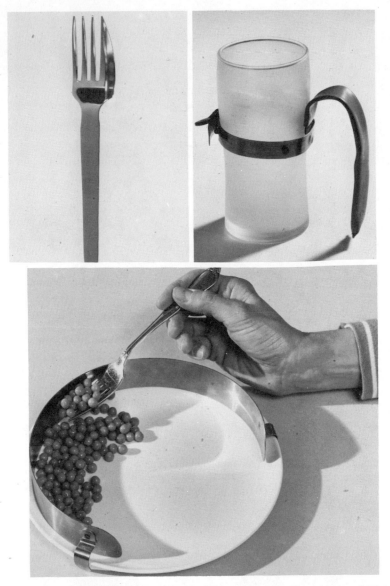

Figure 8–3A. Commonly used devices for eating: *A,* Knifork. *B,* Glass holder. *C,* Plate guard. (From Stryker: *Rehabilitative Aspects of Acute and Chronic Nursing Care.* W. B. Saunders Co., Philadelphia.)

step closer to restoring his feelings of dignity and personal worth.

The third step, teaching the patient and his family, is one that is too often neglected, especially in the hospital setting. For some reason, many nurses do not see themselves as teachers, and as a consequence, many patients and their families remain ignorant of good health habits and disease control. Numerous studies have shown that one of the greatest areas of need for the disabled or chronically ill patient and his family is that of instruction in managing the patient's illness after he has left the hospital or other type of health facility. If the practical nurse does not feel competent to teach the patient and

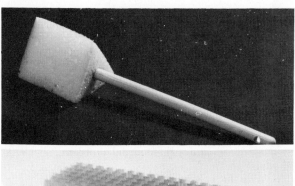

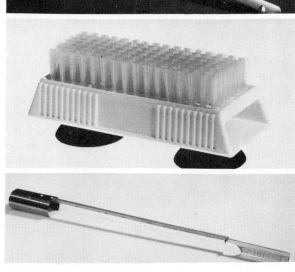

Figure 8–3B. (Continued) Commonly used devices for personal hygiene: *A,* Long-handled sponge for bathing. *B,* Hand brush on suction cups. *C,* Long-handled comb. (From Stryker: *Rehabilitative Aspects of Acute and Chronic Nursing Care.* W. B. Saunders Co., Philadelphia.)

his family (although she does this by example every time she gives nursing care), she should seek help from other sources. To be effective, good teaching, like good nursing, requires thoughtful planning. Almost every hospital has a department of staff development or in-service education whose staff is qualified to give assistance in patient teaching. There are also local and national governmental and voluntary agencies which can be excellent sources of help and information. Examples of resources of this type include the local public health department, Home Health Aides, homemaker services, the Council on Aging and societies and associations concerned with specific types of illness, such as the American Cancer Society and the American Heart Association.

Continuity of care refers to uninterrupted care of the patient throughout his illness and is directly related to referral of the patient and his family to professionals and agencies best prepared to meet his needs after discharge from the hospital.

Research has shown that there are serious difficulties imposed on the patient, and there is a tragic waste of effort by health workers when there are interruptions in the care of the patient with a long-term illness.[13] Losses such as these can be avoided by adequate coordination and a well-organized referral system. Although activities such as referral and coordination of all aspects of patient care may be beyond the scope of the practical nurse, as an important member of the health team she should be aware of her role in providing continuous and comprehensive care for chronically ill and disabled patients.

Stryker offers some pertinent and

useful questions that she refers to as the "key to continuity of care." The questions arc included here to give the practical nurse some insight into the kinds of problems that may be encountered by the patient and those concerned with his care:

1. Will the family and patient have an adequate opportunity to receive help while they are working out their initial problem of adjustment?

2. Will the family be able to adapt the physical environment to provide maximum independence for the patient?

3. What are the financial abilities of the family, and where can they obtain financial assistance? A social worker is essential in this area.

4. What equipment will be necessary for the patient?

5. What must he know in order to take care of himself?

6. What family teaching is essential to his care?

7. What additional resources must be sought—for example, an attendant? a housekeeper? a home health aide? school referrals? outpatient treatment? medical follow-up? vocational training? social organizations? recreational groups?

8. What members of the health team will be needed after discharge?

9. Where can the patient go to obtain further information?[22]

It is obvious that a chronic illness or permanent disability can create a multitude of needs for the patient and his family. We cannot ignore these needs and we must find ways to meet them; otherwise, we can expect to find that the patient will regress physically, emotionally and socially because of a lack of continuity in his care.

Part Two. Institutional Care of the Aged and Chronically Ill

INTRODUCTION

Nursing homes and convalescent care facilities in this country have changed in many ways in the past two decades. The dismal and dreary firetraps that once housed the aged and infirm are being replaced by modern buildings designed to meet the needs of the patients and staff. Perhaps more important than the change in outward appearance, however, is the gradual change in the philosophy of these institutions and in the goals of the persons who work in them. The modern nursing home is not a place to "put away," out of sight and out of mind, the hopelessly ill and aged but is an integral part of the entire health care system. Its chief purpose is the maintenance of or improvement toward the optimal level of function of each patient.

Nursing homes never should have been and certainly cannot now be a place of last resort where patients are more or less adequately fed, clothed and housed and then left to wait out their final days in an atmosphere of hopelessness. Such "custodial" and "terminal" care fosters dependence and subjects the patient to indignities that deprive him of his individuality and rob him of any hope for the future. It casts the patient in the role of a dependent child who is isolated from the mainstream of life and is, in effect, socially dead.

To change the whole concept of institutional care for the aged and chronically ill is a challenging task for the nurse. One goal should be a shift of emphasis from long-term care, which implies months, or even years of institutional living, to *transitional* care. The nursing home need not be a dead-end street but rather a detour by which the patient travels on his way from an acute care facility to his home. This may not be possible for every chronically ill patient, but it can become a reality for many as community resources become more readily available to families, assisting them in the home care of the aged and infirm.

We know that few people prefer living in nursing homes, and that the vast majority want to live in their own homes as long as possible. One has only to witness the response of a hospitalized patient when he is told that he is being transferred to a nursing home to realize the devastating effect of such a pronouncement. Many times he has no other choice, and he knows it. He must do what others have decided is "best" for him, and he often accepts the decision as one accepts a prison sentence. Such feelings toward nursing homes and the kinds of care they provide cannot be allowed to prevail. Society in general and nursing in particular have an obligation to offer something better to our sick and disabled. We have made a beginning. We look backward only to see the mistakes we have made and the harm we have done. Then we look forward to the future, to what can be done to assure the best possible care for those we wish to serve.

NURSING HOMES AND THE PATIENTS IN THEM

What are nursing homes really like today, and what kind of patient is being cared for in them? It is difficult to generalize about nursing homes because they vary so greatly in size, staffing, facilities provided and underlying philosophy of care. They may have fewer than 10 or more than 500 beds, and they may offer only the most essential medical and surgical services. Others have their own pharmacy, x-ray and laboratory facilities, and many have some type of equipment for physical therapy and recreational therapy.

The variety in nursing homes is not limited to bed capacity and the services and equipment available. Some facilities have an air of gloom and depression and invoke a pervasive and persistent feeling of despair that is evident as soon as one enters the building. Others may have a cheerful and hopeful appearance but do not have the adequately trained staff or sound nursing practices to fulfill the bright promise of comfort and happiness.

Laura H. Larson, an experienced nurse in the licensing and certification of nursing homes, devised a rating chart that includes all factors that she considers of importance in determining how good a nursing home really is (see Fig. 8–4). Ms. Larson attaches much importance to the philosophy of the institution and whether or not the practices of the personnel are consistent with the stated philosophy.[10] In judging a nursing home, one should also consider to what extent community resources are utilized by the institution and how much opportunity there is for the general public to observe and evaluate the kind of care being provided. Frances Storlie writes that the ideal nursing home is a fallacy and that care which we may label ideal may in reality seem unsatisfactory to those for whom it is intended. She suggests that we consult the patients themselves if we want to know how a nursing home measures up and how well it meets the needs of its patients.[21]

At the present time, the majority of patients in nursing homes are over 65 years of age. These patients suffer from a multiplicity of chronic physical ailments, and there are increasing numbers with mental problems. The latter have often been transferred from mental institutions that are shifting from long-term care of mental patients to acute care and community mental health centers for outpatient treatment. The disabilities of patients in nursing homes are not necessarily so severe that they prevent the patients from living at home, but because so few families are

RATE YOUR NURSING HOME

	AVERAGE MINIMAL	BELOW AVERAGE DEDUCTIONS	ABOVE AVERAGE CREDIT
1. Compliance With Standards			
Current *full* license	20		
Current provisional license		−10	
J.C.A.H. Accredited			+ 5
2. Location			
Easily accessible via public—private transportation. .	5		
3. Physical Environment			
Physical plant, equipment and maintenance meet minimum requirements	25		
If improper construction and maintenance standards, and objectionable and masking odors are noted. . .		−10	
If facilities are provided above requirements, i.e., beauty-barber shop; physical therapy room and equipment; occupations or arts and crafts room and equipment; innovative environmental assistive approaches as color coding doors, etc.			+10
4. Management Services			
Costs clearly identified in writing. Basic fee includes all costs for basic nursing, personal and dietary services. Meets minimum staffing requirements. (R.N. and L.P.N.)	50		
If additional charges are made for incontinent and/or bedfast patients or those requiring assistance with feeding.		−15	
If philosophy of administration is in writing and consistent with modern medical care and services to aged. Practices of personnel consistent with philosophy.			+10
Personnel employed beyond licensure requirement, Registered nurses			+10
Registered physical therapist (full or part time). . .			+ 5
Registered occupational or recreational therapist. .			+ 5
Dietitian			+ 5
Utilizes outside community resources (volunteers, service groups)			+ 5
Religious services—all faiths			+ 5
	100	−35	+60

*100 points —Average, meeting minimal requirements
Under 70 —Undesirable
Over 100 —Most desirable

Figure 8–4. A rating chart for nursing homes. Raters may adjust the numbers according to their own conceptions of a nursing home rating system. (From Larson: American Journal of Nursing, May, 1969.)

financially able or physically equipped to give adequate home care, the patients must be kept in nursing homes. Hopefully this situation will change as more health care services become available in the community. Families will then be able to utilize personnel and facilities in the community to help them care for their infirm and aged relatives at home.

The average length of stay in a nursing home is several months. Some of the patients will require long-term institutional care because of the severely disabling nature of their illness or simply because they have nowhere else to go. Others need only short-term convalescent care as an intermediate step before returning home. Many of the patients have visual problems or hearing loss or both, and almost all require some assistance with their personal care and other activities of daily living. Few are there because they have freely chosen to be admitted to the institution, but there are some patients who find security in this type of setting and do not wish to face the challenges and problems of daily living in the outside world. Usually the patients have been forced to enter the nursing home because of circumstances that make living alone at home or staying with relatives impossible. For example, they may have reduced income brought on by retirement, the death of a mate or loss of other close relatives and friends —events that change their former life style and leave them isolated and relatively helpless in today's society.

It is not fair to attempt to describe the "typical" nursing home patient. To do so would deny each patient's individuality and give the false impression that all patients are the same, having the same nursing needs and personal problems. It is safe to say, however, that all patients who are aged and infirm, or of any age and disabled with a chronic illness, have a basic need for love and human companionship and a right to live their lives with dignity.

NURSING CARE

Nurses who work in extended care facilities such as nursing homes and convalescent care centers must be constantly aware of the need to wage a continual battle against complications or further deterioration that might threaten the patient's chance for restoring or at least maintaining the status quo. There are three goals for care of patients in a nursing home or similar institution: (1) to help the patient maintain his present level of function and to contribute toward restoring his independence within the limits of his illness or disability, (2) to prevent further deformity or disability insofar as possible, and (3) to provide an atmosphere which is not too different from normal living conditions and that can serve as a substitute for the patient's own home.[15, 19]

In order to reach these goals, every member of the nursing staff and all other members of the health team involved with patient care in nursing homes should be thoroughly familiar with the basic principles of geriatric care and rehabilitative care. The needs of the aged as described in Chapter 7 of this text are pertinent to the care of the elderly wherever they may be found. They are no less important in the nursing home than in the hospital. Many of the points previously mentioned in Chapter 7 and in Part One of Chapter 8 in regard to physical, mental and social rehabilitation will become more meaningful and useful when applied to patients in nursing homes.

It is especially important to attend to the patient's environment and living conditions. If there is a good chance that a patient may eventually return to his home and community, we must be sure that we have provided him with a homelike environment that will make such a transition relatively easy. If there is little hope that he will ever leave the nursing home but must call the institution his home, arrangements should be made to assure him of some privacy and a homelike atmosphere. Since it is not always possible to have private rooms for every patient, some effort and imagination may be needed to provide a specific place he can call his own and into which others may not come unless invited to do so. A corner of a ward may be all the patient has, but everyone should respect his right to call it his own domain and allow him to keep there the few personal belongings that he treasures.

All of us have experienced some anxiety and apprehension when we have just moved from familiar surroundings and close friends to a strange city, neighborhood or perhaps dormitory, so we can understand the emotional shock and fear suffered by patients who are moved from their homes and away from their families into a long-term care facility. A survey was conducted to determine how newly admitted geriatric patients adjust to institutional living and what barriers to adjustment were significant to them. The top ranking indicator of good adjustment was the patient's enjoyment of mealtime, second was his interest in visits from family and friends and third was his interest in his own physical well-being. The barriers to adjustment included poor preadmission preparation of the patient, poor orientation to the institution when he was admitted, lack of family love and support, the staff's lack of interest in the new patient and difficulty in accepting the new routine.[4]

It is hoped that the results of this survey will have some meaning to the nurse working in a nursing home and will give her some guidance in finding out what she might do to make it easier for her newly admitted patients to adjust to and accept their new way of life. There are, of course, some factors such as family love and attention which she may not be able to control. Others, such as orientation to the institution, can be relatively simple to carry out, but they are extremely important to the patient and his feeling of being wanted.

There are many satisfactions and rewarding experiences in store for the nurse who chooses a nursing home in which to work. She must be a very special kind of person to give the emotional support and skilled nursing care her patients will need. Joan Hudson, a medical researcher who has a chronic disability that has required admission to a long-term care facility, believes it probable that "only the best of nurses are capable of standing up to the demands of a good nursing home today. Such a nurse must . . . be able to retain her own mental and emotional balance in prolonged relationships that few others are called upon to meet in hospitals, doctors' offices, or in private duty nursing."

It is true that many special and different kinds of demands are made of one who cares for the aged and chronically ill. It is also true that this type of nursing demands more than a warm and loving nature and calls for creative talents as well as nursing skills. It is for these reasons that many authorities feel that every nurse should have some experience in this type of nursing, either as a student or as a graduate, so that she can have an opportunity to use all of her knowledge and personal resources in the care of patients who need so much and ask so little of her.

CLINICAL CASE PROBLEMS

1. Mr. Rodriguez is a 59-year-old patient with diabetes. He had one leg amputated when he was 47 years old and is now admitted to the hospital with a large ulcer on the other leg. He has difficulty managing his diabetes and has recently lost his job because of his present acute episode. His wife appears anxious to help him, but she cannot read English and does not understand his diet and medication regimen. All of their nine children have moved away with the exception of one 19-year-old son who is a college student living at home.

How would you go about assessing the needs of this patient and his family?

What might be the social and psychological needs of this patient?

What are some steps involved in planning rehabilitation for this patient?

2. You and two members of your class are assigned to four weeks of experience in a skilled nursing home. You have never even visited in such a home and have had little personal experience with chronically ill persons.

What type of patient might you expect to find in the home?

How might you go about rating this institution?

Can you plan an imaginary day of caring for four patients in this home?

If there were few recreational and occupational therapy projects available at the home, can you think of some that might appeal to these patients?

One of these patients is 47 years of age and chronically disabled. She refuses to indulge in any physical activity, although she could develop some degree of independence if she had the will to do so. What kinds of complications might develop as a result of her immobility? How would you go about trying to motivate her and help her achieve more independence in the activities of daily living?

REFERENCES

1. Beland, I. L.: *Clinical Nursing: Pathophysiological and Psychosocial Approaches,* 2nd edition. New York, The Macmillan Co., 1970.
2. Commission on Chronic Illness: *Chronic Illness in the United States.* Cambridge, Mass., Harvard University Press, 1959.
3. Dahlin, B.: "Rehabilitation and the Assessment of Patient Need." Nurs. Clin. N. Amer., Vol. 1, No. 3, 1966, p. 375.
4. Fussell, M. A.: "Newly Admitted Geriatric Patient's Adjustment to Institutional Living." ANA clinical paper presented at regional conference, Atlanta, 1969.
5. Gaspard, N. J.: "The Family of the Patient with Long-Term Illness." Nurs. Clin. N. Amer., Vol. 5, No. 1, 1970, p. 77.
6. Harrison, C.: "The Institutionally-Deprived Elderly." Nurs. Clin. N. Amer., Vol. 3, No. 4, 1968, p. 697.
7. Hentgen, J. H.: "Dressing Activities for Disabled Persons." Nurs. Clin. N. Amer., Vol. 1, No. 3, 1966, p. 483.
8. Hudson, J. H.: "Decision." Am. Journ. Nurs., April, 1970, p. 768.
9. Johnson, J. B., Thompson. L. F., *et al.: "The Hazards of Immobility."* Am. Journ. Nurs., April, 1967, p. 781.
10. Larson. L. H.: *"How to Select a Nursing Home."* Am. Journ. Nurs., May, 1969, p. 1034.
11. Loxley, A. K.: "The Emotional Toll of Crippling Deformity." Am. Journ. Nurs., Oct., 1972, p. 1839.
12. Program Guide, Nursing Service: *Nursing Care of the Long-term Patient,* G-8, M-2, part v. Washington, D.C., Department of Medicine and Surgery, Veterans Administration, 1963.
13. Robischon, P.: "The Public Health Nurse and Chronic Illness." Nurs. Clin. N. Amer., Vol. 1, No. 3, 1966, p. 433.
14. Shafer, K., *et al.: Medical-Surgical Nursing,* 5th edition. St. Louis, The C. V. Mosby Co., 1971.
15. Shaughnessy, M. E.: "Nursing in Nursing Homes—Whose Responsibility?" Nurs. Clin. N. Amer., Vol. 1, No. 3., 1966, p. 399.
16. Siller, J.: *Structure of Attitudes Toward the Physically Disabled.* New York, New York University, School of Education, Nov., 1967.
17. Smith, E. G.: "Albianna Fashions—Wardrobe with a Purpose." Am. Journ. Nurs., June, 1966, p. 1320.
18. Sorenson, K. M., and Amis, D. B.: "Understanding the World of the Chronically Ill." Am. Journ. Nurs., April, 1967, p. 811.
19. Spain, R. W.: "Rehabilitative Nursing." Nurs. Clin. N. Amer., Vol. 1, No. 3, 1966, p. 355.
20. Stokes, A.: "Institutional Care of the Aged." Journ. Pract. Nurs., May, 1964, p. 24.
21. Storlie, F.: "The Aged Poor." Nursing '72, May, p. 29.
22. Stryker, R. P.: *Rehabilitative Aspects of Acute and Chronic Nursing Care.* Philadelphia, W. B. Saunders Co., 1972.
23. Wolfe, I.: "Acceptance." Am. Journ. Nurs., Aug., 1972, p. 1412.
24. Zeffaro, L.: "Nursing in a Long-term Care Facility." Journ. Pract. Nurs., Oct., 1970, p. 35.

SUGGESTED STUDENT READING

1. Calloway, A. B.: "Social Needs of Geriatric Patients." Am. Journ. Nurs., March, 1968, p. 34.
2. Hentgen, J. H.: "Dressing Activities for Disabled Persons." Nurs. Clin. N. Amer., Vol. 1, No. 3, 1966, p. 483.
3. Larson, L. H.: "How to Select a Nursing Home." Am. Journ. Nurs., May, 1969, p. 1034.
4. Rasmussen, S.: "Medicare and the Practical Nurse." Nurs. Outlook, June, 1966, p. 62.
5. Stokes, A.: "Institutional Care of the Aged." Journ. Pract. Nurs., Oct., 1967, p. 27.
6. Wolfe, I.: "Acceptance." Am. Journ. Nurs., Aug., 1972, p. 1412.
7. Zeffaro, L.: "Nursing in a Long-term Care Facility." Journ. Pract. Nurs., Oct., 1970, p. 35.

OUTLINE FOR CHAPTER 8

Part One   Patient Care

I.   Introduction—Chronic Illness and Disability: Major Health Problem in this Country

A.   Examples of chronic illness and disability include heart disease, arthritides, metabolic disorders, paralysis and mental disorders.

B. Definition—chronic illness is one that has gradual onset, progresses slowly, has acute episodes and remissions.
1. Rarely restricted to one system.
2. Creates a need for long-term planning, coordination of agencies for continuity of care and family involvement.
3. Not all of the chronically ill are aged.

C. Attitudes toward chronic illness—generally negative.
1. Health care personnel often view long-term care as dull, depressing and nonproductive.
2. Patient needs supportive care that is diligent, consistent and geared toward small gains.
3. Chronically ill patients must find acceptance: they are often victims of prejudice.

II. Special Needs and Nursing Implications

A. Assessment of needs based on knowledge of the individual patient.

B. Physical needs concerned with hazards of immobility and its effect on body systems.

C. Emotional needs extremely complex. Adjustment depends on patient's age, cultural background, type of illness, role in the family and emotional stability.
1. Acceptance of illness goes through stages.
2. Contribution of family and friends important to patient's adjustment.

D. Social needs depend on individual patient.

III. Rehabilitation

A. Definition—"restoration of the individual to the fullest physical, mental, social, vocational and economic capacity of which he is capable."

B. Nurse's role
1. Preventive measures against complications.

2. Early activities of self-care.
3. Teaching patient and family how to manage his illness.
4. Referral to other professions and agencies for continuity of care.

Part Two   Institutional Care

I. Introduction—Modern Nursing Home is an Integral Part of the Entire Health Care System

A. Custodial care fosters dependence.

B. Emphasis should be toward transitional care and eventual return of patient to his home.

II. Types of Nursing Homes and Patients in Them

A. Many different types of institutions.

B. "Ideal" nursing homes may not exist but there are factors to consider in rating an institution.

C. Majority of patients over 65 years of age.

D. Average length of stay is several months.

E. Few patients have freely chosen to be in the institution.

III. Nursing Care

A. Three goals:
1. To help patient maintain present level of function and contribute toward restoring his independence.
2. To prevent further disability.
3. To provide an atmosphere not too different from normal living conditions.

B. Barriers to patient adjustment to institutional living:
1. Poor preadmission preparation.
2. Poor orientation to the institution.
3. Lack of family love and support.
4. Staff's lack of interest.
5. Patient's difficulty in accepting new routine.

9

Care of the Patient With an Infectious Disease

VOCABULARY

Asepsis
Disinfectant
Immunity
Pathogenic
Susceptible

INTRODUCTION

In Chapter 2 we discussed infectious agents as possible causes of disease. These agents include bacteria, viruses, fungi, helminths (worms), protozoa and rickettsia. As one might suspect, the list of diseases that can be caused by these agents is quite lengthy and varied, but they can all be classified as *infectious diseases* (that is, those that are caused by specific pathogenic microorganisms). A *communicable disease* is one that can be transferred directly from one person to another or transmitted indirectly from an infected person or animal to a susceptible host. Some of the terms with which the nurse should be familiar are the following:

Contamination—the presence or possible presence of living pathogenic microorganisms in or on an article, a person or matter.

Carrier—an apparently healthy person who still harbors living pathogenic microorganisms and can spread them to others.

Disinfection—killing of infectious agents by chemical or physical means. *Concurrent* disinfection is the immediate destruction of microorganisms as they leave the body or immediately after they have contaminated objects in the infected person's environment. *Terminal* disinfection is the destruction of infectious agents that remain in the patient's environment after he is no longer considered a source of infection.

Epidemic—a temporary and significant increase in the occurrence of disease in a specific area at any given time.

Endemic—a disease of low incidence that is constantly present in a community.

Isolation—a technique used to separate or set apart the patient with an infectious disease for the purpose of preventing the spread of the disease.

Reverse Isolation—a technique which provides the patient with an environment that is as free from pathogenic organisms as possible. It is similar to surgical asepsis in many aspects, and its purpose is to avoid transmission

TABLE 9–1. INCUBATION PERIODS OF COMMUNICABLE DISEASES*

I. Incubation Period. Usually about 0 to 7 Days.

Disease	Incubation Period (Avg. and/or Range)		Isolation	Immunization
Anthrax	1-4	(1-7)	'Clean' technique	
Bacillary dysentery	2-4	(1-7)	Till stool neg.	
Chancroid	3-5	(1-12)	From sexual contact	
Cholera	3	(1-5)	Till stool neg. (quarantine)	
Dengue	5-6	(3-15)	Screen	
Diphtheria	2-5		Till nose & throat neg.	Toxoid/antitoxin
Epidemic diarrhea of newborn	6-7	(2-21)	Yes (quarantine)	
Erysipelas	0-2		'Clean' technique	
Food poisoning Staphylococcus Salmonella Botulinus	2-4 12 18-24	(1-6) hrs. (6-48) hrs. (2-48) hrs.	From food handling	Antitoxin
Gonorrhea	3-5	(1-14)	From sexual contact and children	
Impetigo contagiosa	< 5		From child contacts	
Infectious keratoconjunctivitis	5-7			
Influenza	1-3		Acute stage	Formalin virus
Meningitis, meningococcic	< 7	(2-10)	24 hrs., if treated	
Paratyphoid	1-10		Till stool & urine neg.	Vaccine
Plague	3-6		Till well	Formalin vaccine
Pneumonia, bacterial	1-3		Respiratory precautions	
Puerperal infection	1-3		Till well	
Relapsing fever tick	3-6	(2-12)		

*From Smith, Kline & French Laboratories: Pocket Book of Medical Tables. 17th revised edition. 1968.

Table 9–1 continued on opposite page.

TABLE 9–1. INCUBATION PERIODS OF COMMUNICABLE DISEASES* (CONTINUED)

I. Incubation Period. Usually about 0 to 7 Days. (continued)

Disease	Incubation Period (Avg. and/or Range)		Isolation	Immunization
Rocky Mountain spotted fever	3-10			Yolk-sac vaccine
Scabies	1-2		From school	
Scarlet fever	2-5		Respiratory pre- cautions	
Tularemia	3	(1-10)		
Yellow fever	3-6		Screen	Modified virus

II. Incubation Period. Usually about 7 to 14 Days.

Disease	Incubation Period (Avg. and/or Range)		Isolation	Immunization
Coccidioidomycosis	10-15	(7-21)	Till sputum neg.	
Equine encephalitis				
Infectious mononucleosis	11	(7-15)	Respiratory precautions	
Leptospirosis	9-10	(4-19)		
Lymphocytic chorio- meningitis	8-13			
Measles	9-14		Till 5 days after rash	Vaccine
Pertussis	5-9	(2-21)	From school & susceptibles	Vaccine
Poliomyelitis	7-14	(3-35)	First 2 weeks	Vaccine
Primary atypical pneumonia	11	(7-21)	Respiratory precautions	
Psittacosis	6-15		Till afebrile	
Relapsing fever louse	7	(5-12)	To delouse	
Scrub typhus	7-10	(7-14)		
Smallpox	12	(7-21)	Till scabs off (quarantine)	Vaccinia
Trichinosis	9	(2-28)		
Typhoid fever	7-14	(3-38)	Till stool & urine neg.	Vaccine
Typhus fever	12	(6-15)	To delouse (quarantine)	Vaccine

*From Smith, Kline & French Laboratories: Pocket Book of Medical Tables. 17th revised edition. 1968.

Table 9–1 continued on following page.

TABLE 9-1. INCUBATION PERIODS OF COMMUNICABLE DISEASES* (CONTINUED)

III. Incubation Period. Usually over 14 Days.

Disease	Incubation Period (Avg. and/or Range)		Isolation	Immunization
Amebic dysentery	21-28	(8-90)	From food handling	
Brucellosis	14	(6-30+)		
Chickenpox	14	(12-21)	Till skin clear	
German measles	16-18	(10-21)	First week	
Granuloma inguinale	10-90		From sexual contact	
Hepatitis, infectious	25	(15-35)	Stool disinfection for 3 weeks	Immune globulin
Hepatitis, serum	80-100	(60-180)		
Lymphogranuloma venereum	7-28		From sexual contact	
Malaria	10-17	(to 35+)	Screen	
Mumps	18	(12-26)	Till glands down	Vaccine
Q fever	14-21			Vaccine
Rabies	14-42	(10-180)	Aseptic technique	Attenuated vaccine
Rickettsialpox	10-24			
Syphilis	21	(10-90)	From sexual contact and children	
Tetanus	4-21			Toxoid
Tuberculosis	Variable		'Open' cases	BCG vaccine
Yaws	30-90		Desirable till treated	

*From Smith, Kline & French Laboratories: Pocket Book of Medical Tables. 17th revised edition. 1968.

of infectious agents to a patient who is unusually susceptible to and likely to suffer more than the usual consequences of an infection.

Nosocomial Infection—an infection which is acquired within the hospital or a similar institution.

THE NURSE'S ROLE AND RESPONSIBILITIES

In spite of the efforts of the medical sciences and the advances that have been made in the prevention and treatment of infectious diseases, these illnesses still take their toll in communities throughout the world. In industrialized countries, infectious diseases are no longer a major cause of illness and death, but they remain a threat to the health and welfare of all citizens. In the developing countries, infectious diseases account for most of the misery and death suffered by the population. Nurses must continue to work for eradication of infectious diseases and accept responsibility for the care of patients who are suffering from infectious disease.

In general, the nurse has as her goals (1) assisting in identification of the organism causing a particular type of infection, (2) controlling the spread of an infectious disease, (3) adequately protecting others against infectious diseases, (4) assisting the physician in controlling infection in specific patients and (5) providing physiologic support to the patient with an infectious disease as well as utilizing nursing measures to provide symptomatic relief.

Identification of the Causative Organism. Identifying the specific organism causing an infection and thereby establishing a definite diagnosis are essential to the patient's successful treatment and recovery. Laboratory procedures involving bacteriologic studies are of great value to the physician who seeks to determine the type of infection a patient has and the specific drugs which are best suited to destroy the causative organism. You may have noticed on a patient's chart the order for a specimen to be sent to the laboratory for "culture and sensitivity." The term "culturing" refers to encouraging the growth of an organism by placing it in an environment favorable to its growth. In a laboratory, the culture medium may be beef broth or some other substance which is nutritious to organisms and upon which they will grow rapidly. A sensitivity test determines the drug or drugs to which a

particular organism is most sensitive, i.e., the drug most likely to destroy it.

Specimens of urine, blood, spinal fluid or other body fluids which have been obtained for culture must be handled in a special way. Since the organisms must be alive and able to reproduce when they reach the laboratory for culturing, the specimen should be as fresh as possible. It should be sent to the laboratory promptly. Care must also be taken that organisms from sources other than the specimen do not get into the container used for collecting the specimen. The following rules must be adhered to in the collection of body excretions, exudates from lesions and other specimens intended for culture in the laboratory:

1. Use containers which are sterile and not cracked or broken.

2. Use standard tubes from the laboratory, and collect the specimen directly into the tube when possible.

3. Keep the inside of tube and the stopper of the tube free from contamination.

4. Do not use cotton plugs unless it is absolutely necessary. Cork stoppers are best. If cotton plugs are used, they must not be allowed to become wet, either from the contents of the tube or from outside liquids.

5. Place the plugs firmly in place, rotating them clockwise, after the specimen has been collected.

6. Be careful that the material is not spilled outside the container. If such material is spilled, report it immediately, and determine from the laboratory technician what antiseptic should be used to destroy the organisms. Warn others of the spilled material, and clean the area thoroughly as soon as possible.

7. Containers should not be filled more than halfway.

8. Containers must be kept in an upright position after the specimen is collected and should be taken to the laboratory at once. Avoid shaking the container.

There are other diagnostic tests that

TABLE 9–2. ACTIVITY OF SOME COMMON DISINFECTANTS*

Disinfectant	Vegetative Bacteria	Spores	Fungi	Viruses
Alcohol, ethyl, 70%–90%	Good	None	Fair	Fair
Alcohol, isopropyl, 70%–90%	Very good	None	Good	Fair
Alcohol, isopropyl, 70%–Iodine, 0.5%–2%	Very good	Fair	Good	Good
Benzalkonium chloride, 1:750–1:1000	Very good	None	Good	None
Chlorine (hypochlorites), 1%–5%	Very good	Fair	Fair	Good
Cresols, 1%–5%	Good	Poor	Good	Poor
Ethylene oxide gas mixture	Very good	Good	Good	Good
Formaldehyde solution, U.S.P., 37%	Good	Good	Good	Good
Formaldehyde, 20%–Alcohol, 50%	Very good	Very good	Good	Good
Glutaraldehyde, 2%	Very good	Very good	Good	Good
Hexachlorophene, 3%–4%	Fair	None	Good	Not known
Iodine (aqueous), 2%–5%	Very good	Poor	Good	Good
Iodophors, 1%	Good	Poor	Poor	Good
Phenols, 1%–3%	Good	Poor	Good	Fair

*From "Equipment Notes: Disinfection of Medical Equipment." Nurs. Clin. N. Amer., Vol. 2, No. 4, 1967, p. 799. Reprinted from The Medical Letter, Vol. 9, No. 7, 1967.

are useful in detecting certain infectious diseases. The *Schick* test detects susceptibility to diphtheria; the *Dick* test detects scarlet fever. A small amount of toxoid is administered intradermally on the inner aspect of the forearm. If a red, swollen area appears in 24 to 48 hours, the reaction is considered positive, indicating susceptibility or lack of immunity. Some patients do not exhibit a positive reaction until 3 to 5 days. For this reason, they should be instructed to return for a repeat reading if they notice the area becoming red or swollen.

A tuberculin test is done in a similar manner. A reaction indicates only that the individual has been exposed to the tubercle bacillus some time in the past, but it does *not* indicate that he has an active case of tuberculosis. An exception is a positive reaction in children under two years of age. In that case, a positive reaction can indicate active tuberculosis.

Control of the Spread of Infectious Disease. Although the environment of man is well populated with disease-producing microorganisms, there are methods of control that can be used to prevent their multiplication and their spreading to susceptible persons. The process by which an infectious disease is transmitted has been described as a circular chain.[3] Each link must be present and in logical sequence in order for the disease to spread (see Fig. 9–1).

This figure may serve as a guide to controlling the spread of infectious diseases. We begin with link #1, the causative organism. In order to remove this link in the chain, it is obvious that the causative organisms must be destroyed or rendered relatively harmless whenever they are in the environment of a susceptible host. Disinfection and sterilization should be familiar to anyone working in the health field. Autoclaving is considered the most effective means of killing bacteria and other harmful organisms. All living organisms can be destroyed by exposure to moist heat of at least 250°F. (121°C.) for 15 minutes. If the nurse is responsible for soaking inanimate objects in a sterilizing solution, she must always be sure that the articles are completely submerged in the solution. She must also know how strong the solution should be and the period of time recommended by its manufacturer for

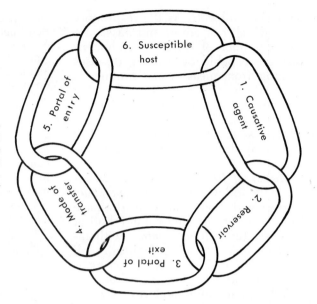

Figure 9–1. Each link of the infectious process must be present and in proper sequence in order to produce disease. (Adapted from Brunner, et al.: *Textbook of Medical-Surgical Nursing,* 2nd Ed., J. B. Lippincott Co., Philadelphia.)

adequate sterilization. One should bear in mind that not every kind of disinfectant destroys all types of microorganisms. The effectiveness of disinfection will depend on a number of factors, including (1) the type and number of organisms, (2) whether or not there is organic material such as mucus present on the object to be disinfected, (3) the type and strength of disinfectant and (4) the length of time the microorganisms are exposed to the disinfectant. Most importantly, the nurse should never rely on guesswork to determine whether or not an object has been sterilized. She must also remember that no disinfectant is a substitute for scrubbing with soap and water.

Reservoirs (link #2) of causative organisms are places in which the organisms thrive and reproduce. These may include the body tissues and wastes of humans, animals and insects. Reservoirs may also be food and water contaminated by the microorganisms. In the hospital, the patient with an infectious disease is isolated in order to remove from the chain this vital link. Also, the nurse must consider all patients in the hospital as possible sources of infection. That is why the nurse is admonished over and over again to wash her hands after contact with each patient, regardless of his diagnosis. All newly admitted patients should be observed for signs of infection such as boils, infected wounds or fever. If there is a sign of infection, it should be reported immediately so that proper precautions can be taken. Visitors and hospital personnel can also serve as sources of infection. Every student nurse usually knows that hospital dust, insects and vermin are all extremely likely to serve as reservoirs of infectious microorganisms. She must not, however, let familiarity breed complacency so that she becomes careless in maintaining an environment of cleanliness and order for her patients and herself.

The route by which a pathogen leaves the body of its host is called its *portal of exit;* the route by which it enters the body to establish infection is called the *portal of entry.* An example of a portal of exit is the intestinal tract through which the typhoid bacillus leaves in the patient's feces. The digestive tract serves also as a portal of entry when one eats food or drinks water that contains pathogens. Another portal of both exit and entry is the respiratory tract, which can admit and pass on a large number of different pathogens that are capable of causing diseases ranging from measles and mumps to tuberculosis and hepatitis. The skin and mucous membranes also can serve as portals of entry and exit, as in the transmission of syphilis, gonorrhea and many different kinds of skin disorders.

Modes of transfer of pathogens include the following: (1) *direct personal contact* with body excreta or drainage from an ulcer, infected wound, boil or chancre; (2) *indirect contact* with inanimate objects (called *fomites*) such as contaminated needles and syringes, drinking and eating utensils, dressings and hospital equipment; (3) *vectors,* such as fleas, flies, mosquitoes and other insects that harbor infectious agents and transmit infection to man through bites and stings; (4) *droplet infection,* or contamination by the aerial route through sneezing and coughing; and (5) *endogenous* spread of infection from one part of a person's body to another.

A group of student nurses investigated cross-infection hazards in the medical unit of a typical modern hospital. Their study was published in the October, 1967, issue of the *American Journal of Nursing.* Excerpts from their findings are quoted below.

Inadequate handwashing was the most serious error discovered. In the room of a patient on reverse isolation,* students counted eight people who entered in a one-and-one-half-hour period. Although all persons wore masks, dust was seen on the television set, newspapers, and boxes. Soot entered through an open window, and a vacuum cleaner stirred floor dust. The laboratory technician did not wash her hands before working with the patient, and a nurse handled the medicine tray and cards which were used for all patients on the floor and then gave medicines to the iso-

lated patient without washing her hands. Bed linen touched the floor.

Among the housekeeping personnel, a maid pushed down garbage with her bare hands in the utility room and then traveled down the hall touching various items without washing her hands. The vacuum cleaner, whose gusty exhaust blew floor dust about, was dragged from room to room including that of the patient on reverse isolation. The porter did not wash his hands throughout the morning as he performed his various tasks, and handled many items including the doctor's bag.

Utility room surveillance disclosed that when a bedpan was put into the flusher, it was considered contaminated and was replaced with a sterilized pan. However, rectal tubes did not appear to be cared for properly: an aide emptied a bedpan, helped make a bed, and then washed her hands; and trash cans were overflowing.[6]

Nurses making a similar survey in their own hospital units might find that they can do more than they thought possible to protect their patients and themselves from needless contamination.

The final link in the chain, the susceptible host, is sometimes the most difficult to eliminate. Many persons are susceptible by virtue of their age, poor state of health and poor living conditions. The nurse strives to protect these persons from exposure to infectious agents and also endeavors to improve their state of health and living standards by encouraging good health habits. She also works to see that all persons needing immunization will be properly immunized.

Immunization against specific diseases has greatly reduced the number of cases of a variety of communicable diseases in this country. The diseases most affected by such vaccines are smallpox, diphtheria, tetanus, whooping cough, typhoid fever, poliomyelitis, measles, mumps and influenza. This is quite an impressive list but we still, after more than one hundred years of immunization procedures, cannot consider any of these diseases completely eradicated.

---

*Reverse isolation refers to isolation of the patient to protect him from infectious agents.

Nurses must always encourage immunization whenever the opportunity presents itself. Unfortunately, the availability of a specific vaccine is not immediately followed by prompt removal of the disease. There remains a considerable gap between *application* of effective immunization and the rapid advances made in disease prevention. The nurse is in an excellent position to encourage immunization so that no person will needlessly suffer from an illness because of ignorance, poverty or lack of concern.

Although some infectious diseases are virtually disappearing, others are emerging as major health problems. For example, hepatitis is one of the more serious communicable diseases at the present time in the United States. In fact, viral infections of all types seem to be destined to play a major role in morbidity and mortality statistics in the future.[9]

Because of the nature of viruses, particularly their ability to change characteristics so readily, immunization against viral diseases is not so easily accomplished. It is hoped that with continued research we will eventually be able to provide immunity against a greater number of viral infections.

Another type of infection that became notorious during the 1950's was that due to staphylococci—the dread "staph infection" that received so much publicity at the time. During the mid-1960's, staphylococcal infections became less troublesome, and we are now faced with a variety of gram-negative bacteria which, according to the National Communicable Disease Center, account for over 60 per cent of all hospital-acquired infections. Since infections acquired within a hospital are due in some degree to the carelessness of the hospital staff, the nurse should be particularly aware of her responsibility to avoid the spread of such infections. Studies have shown that, in some hospitals, up to 20 per cent of the patients who die there have an infection acquired in the hospital.

Although these infections were not necessarily the direct cause of death, they have materially contributed to the death of the patient.[9] It has been conservatively estimated that 5 per cent of *all* patients admitted to hospitals in the United States develop nosocomial infections.

SPECIFIC NURSING MEASURES TO CONTROL THE SPREAD OF AN INFECTIOUS DISEASE

Isolation. The term *isolation* probably is not the best to use in reference to the practice of separating the patient from others so that he will not continue to spread his infection. The word isolation has several psychological disadvantages for the patient and his family. A newer term, *barrier technique,* has been suggested because it does not imply that the patient is dirty or unacceptable to others.[10] Whichever term is used by the hospital staff, one must be very careful not to give the patient the impression that he is being isolated because he is a nuisance or a social or moral threat to others. His physical separation is quite a burden to him, too, and he will need more than the usual amount of explanation about the nature of his disease and a good bit of emotional support and psychological bolstering while he is isolated from others.

If the nursing staff has advance warning that a patient with an infectious disease is to be admitted, all unnecessary equipment and upholstered furniture should be removed from his unit before he enters the room. Once he has entered the room, everything in his immediate environment must be considered contaminated and will require either concurrent or terminal disinfection. He should have his own thermometer, tray for food, eating utensils, water pitcher and drinking glass.

Visitors are restricted to members of the family and designated friends approved by the physician, and all persons entering or leaving the patient's unit must follow the procedure outlined by the hospital to prevent the spread of disease.

While giving nursing care to the patient in isolation, the nurse must remember that whenever possible she should touch only "clean to clean" and "contaminated to contaminated." This means, for example, that she uses clean paper towels as "technic papers" to handle objects when her hands are contaminated. Once a clean object has come in contact with a contaminated article, both must be considered contaminated. A student nurse once remarked that she felt less likely to contaminate her hands if she imagined herself wearing spotless white gloves while in the isolation unit. The nurse must be careful not to spread infectious agents through careless use of her hands.

Handwashing. The term *medical asepsis* refers to the destruction of microorganisms *after they leave* the body of the patient. This is in contrast to *surgical asepsis,* which refers to destruction of microorganisms *before they enter* the body of the patient. This distinction is important to handwashing technique when one is caring for a patient with an infectious disease, because in this situation the nurse must consider part of herself contaminated and part of herself clean. Her hands contain microorganisms that must be destroyed after they have left the patient's body. She must therefore be very careful to wash her hands thoroughly after each contact with the patient and even during the immediate care of the patient when she realizes that her hands are grossly contaminated. It also means that during the handwashing procedure she must keep her hands *below the level* of her elbows (see Fig. 9–2). The hands should be washed under running water for at least one full minute. Friction between the hands is necessary to remove microorganisms from the lines and crev-

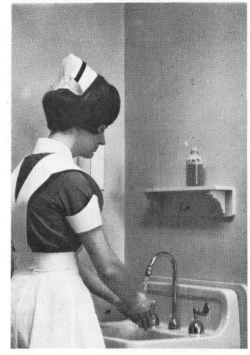

Figure 9–2. During a handwash for medical asepsis, the hands are kept lower than the elbows to keep microorganisms away from the elbows. (From Du Gas: *Kozier-Du Gas' Introduction to Patient Care,* 2nd Ed., W. B. Saunders Co., Philadelphia.)

ices of the skin. The fingernails should be given careful attention and be well lathered and rinsed. If bar soap is used, it is kept in the hands throughout the entire handwashing until the final rinsing of the hands. It is best to use foot pedals to control the flow of water, but if these are not available, a paper towel is used to turn off the water because the faucet handles are considered contaminated.

Using a Gown. When there is a possibility that the nurse's uniform may become contaminated while she is attending the patient with an infectious disease, she must wear an isolation gown for protection. The gown should have long sleeves and a high neck and should tie at the back of the neck and waist. It should be long enough to cover the nurse's uniform completely.

The gown is kept in the patient's room and should not be worn outside the room. If it is worn only once and discarded, there is no special procedure for donning and removing the gown. If it is to be worn again, it must be put on and taken off in a certain way because the outside is considered to be contaminated and the inside clean. Figure 9–3 shows how this is to be done.

Using a Face Mask. The face mask is of most benefit when the infectious disease can be transmitted via the respiratory tract. There is a distinction between a surgical mask and a mask used for medical asepsis. During surgical procedures the nurse wears a mask primarily for the patient's protection. In medical asepsis she wears it for her own protection.

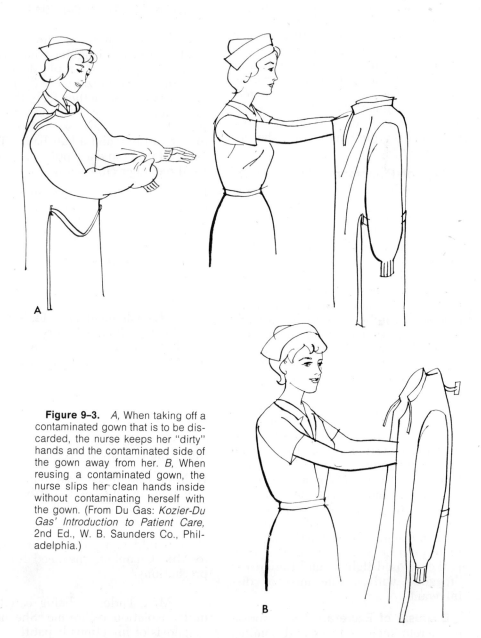

Figure 9–3. *A,* When taking off a contaminated gown that is to be discarded, the nurse keeps her "dirty" hands and the contaminated side of the gown away from her. *B,* When reusing a contaminated gown, the nurse slips her clean hands inside without contaminating herself with the gown. (From Du Gas: *Kozier-Du Gas' Introduction to Patient Care,* 2nd Ed., W. B. Saunders Co., Philadelphia.)

There are a variety of masks available for use, and each has its advantages and disadvantages. The disposable masks are probably the most widely used in medical asepsis because they are relatively inexpensive and require no handling by persons other than the ones wearing them. The mask should fit snugly and cover both the nose and the mouth. It should be worn for no longer than one hour because it becomes contaminated in that period of time and it is not effective once it becomes wet. When the mask is removed, only the ties are handled, as they are the least contaminated part of the mask. The hands are washed *before* the mask is removed, so that the wearer's hair and neck will not be contaminated by the hands when the ties are untied.

Care of Equipment. Dishes, trays and eating utensils are kept in the patient's room for reuse unless they are disposable. The patient's food and liquids are transferred from the "clean" tray held at the door by a "clean" nurse to the patient's tray that is kept in his room. Solid left-over food may be wrapped in newspaper and discarded in the incinerator. Liquids may be flushed down the toilet in the patient's room. Disposable equipment and soiled dressings are also wrapped in paper and placed in a specially marked bag that is taken to the hospital incinerator and burned.

Medicine glasses, syringes and other nondisposable equipment should be soaked in a disinfectant solution and then autoclaved after use. Linen from the patient's unit is placed in a special laundry bag marked "contaminated" or "isolation," and it is autoclaved before it is sent to the laundry. Other equipment such as furniture, bedding and suction machines is left in the patient's room until he is discharged. His room is then closed tightly, and the area is "fogged" with a fine mist of disinfectant.

Disposal of Excreta. The disposal of excreta such as feces and vomitus usually can be accomplished by flushing them down the hopper. In some communities where sewage treatment is not considered adequate for destruction of certain infectious agents, the excreta must be disinfected with chlorinated lime before it is discarded in the hopper.

CLINICAL CASE PROBLEMS

1. A friend of yours who lives in a rural area has a daughter who has infectious hepatitis. Her physician has said that hospitalization will not be necessary if the mother feels that she can safely care for the child at home. They live in a house with three bedrooms and one and a half baths. They use well water and a septic tank. There are three other children in the family.

How could you help this mother plan for the care of her daughter so that the other members of the family would not become infected with the virus?

What special precautions would be necessary in regard to dishes, linen and disposal of excreta?

2. Mrs. Chambers, age 44, is admitted to the hospital for a hemorrhoidectomy. During the admission procedure, you notice a large, draining boil in the patient's axilla. She also has a temperature of 100° F. and tells you that she has not felt well for the past few days.

What would be your course of action following this discovery?

If Mrs. Chambers was found to be infectious because of a possible staphylococcal infection, what precautions would be necessary?

How would you go about explaining to Mrs. Chambers the need for such precautions?

3. Mrs. Tudor is being cared for under isolation technique. She has a diagnosis of infectious hepatitis.

Identify each of the links in the chain of processes that take place in the spread of infectious hepatitis.

REFERENCES

1. Ager, E. A.: "Current Concepts in Immunization." Am. Journ. Nurs., Sept., 1966, p. 2004.
2. Beland, I. L.: *Clinical Nursing: Pathophysiological and Psychosocial Approaches,* 2nd edition. New York, The Macmillan Co., 1970.
3. Brunner, L. S., et al.: *Textbook of Medical-Surgical Nursing,* 2nd edition. Philadelphia, J. B. Lippincott Co., 1970.
4. Du Gas, B. W.: *Kozier-Du Gas' Introduction to Patient Care,* 2nd edition. Philadelphia, W. B. Saunders Co., 1972.
5. Evans, M. J.: "Some Contributions to Prevention of Infections." Nurs. Clin. N. Amer., Vol. 3, No. 4, 1968, p. 641.
6. French, J. G.: "Students Study Cross-contamination." Am. Journ. Nurs., Oct., 1967, p. 2104.
7. Gallivan, G. J., and Torey, J. D.: "Isolation for Possible and Proved Staph." Am. Journ. Nurs., July, 1967, p. 1048.
8. Garner, J. S., and Kaiser, A. B.: "How Often Is Isolation Needed?" Am. Journ. Nurs., April, 1972, p. 733.
9. Gregg, M. B.: "Communicable Disease Trends in the United States." Am. Journ. Nurs., Jan., 1968, p. 88.
10. Kozier, B. B., and DuGas, B. W.: *Fundamentals of Patient Care.* Philadelphia, W. B. Saunders Company, 1967.
11. Lentz, J.: "The Nurse's Role in Extending Infection Control to the Community." Nurs. Clin. N. Amer., Vol. 5, No. 1, 1970, p. 165.
12. Morrison, S. T., and Arnold, C. R.: "Patients With Common Communicable Diseases." Nurs. Clin. N. Amer., Vol. 5, No. 1, 1970, p. 143.

SUGGESTED STUDENT READING

1. Ager, E. A.: "Current Concepts in Immunization." Am. Journ. Nurs., Sept., 1966, p. 2004.
2. Baker, B. H.: "Infection Control. Parts I and II." Bedside Nurse, Oct. and Nov., 1972.
3. Barham, V. Z.: "How I Wanted to Be Treated." Nursing Outlook, Jan., 1971, p. 48.
4. Brachman, P. S.: "The New NCDC Isolation Manual." Nurs. Clin. N. Amer., Vol. 5, No. 1, 1970, p. 175.
5. French, J. G.: "Students Study Cross-contamination." Am. Journ. Nurs., Oct., 1967, p. 2104.
6. Gregg, M. B.: "Communicable Disease Trends in the United States." Am. Journ. Nurs., Jan., 1968, p. 88.
7. Rigor, L.: "Isolation." Journ. Pract. Nurs., June, 1970, p. 46.

OUTLINE FOR CHAPTER 9

I. Introduction

A. Nurse should know commonly used terms in communicable disease nursing; e.g., infections, communicable, contamination, carrier, disinfection, isolation.

II. Nurse's Role and Responsibilities

A. Goals are:
1. Identifying causative organism.
2. Controlling the spread of infectious disease and protecting others from them.
3. Caring for specific patients with infectious diseases.

B. Aids in obtaining specimens for culture.

C. Assists with diagnostic tests.

D. Conscientiously follows rules of cleanliness, sanitation and disinfection for destruction of infectious microorganisms.

E. Recognizes importance of mode of transfer and portals of entry and exit in spread of infectious diseases.

F. Encourages good health habits and immunizations to decrease susceptibility to infectious disease.

III. Specific Nursing Measures

A. Isolation—separation of the patient from others until he is no longer considered a source of infection.
1. Has psychological disadvantages of which the nurse should be aware so that she can reassure the patient and family.
2. Once patient has entered the unit, all equipment in the unit must be considered contaminated and will require concurrent or terminal disinfection.
3. Visitors are restricted. All persons entering and leaving the room must follow hospital procedures.
4. Once a contaminated object has come in contact with a clean object, both are considered contaminated, so one should touch only "clean to clean" and "contaminated to contaminated" objects.

B. Handwashing.
1. Hands are held under running water and washed for one full

minute, keeping them below elbow level.

2. Bar of soap is held in the hands throughout procedure until final rinsing.

3. If foot pedals are not available use paper towel to turn off water faucet.

C. Gown—used to protect nurse's uniform from contamination.

1. Kept in patient's room and should not be worn outside the room.

2. If to be worn again, it must be hung so that outside is exposed. Inside is considered clean and should be handled so that it does not become contaminated.

D. Face mask—worn for the nurse's protection against pathogens.

1. Should fit face snugly and cover both nose and mouth.

2. Should not be worn for more than an hour, at which time it is discarded and a new one put on.

A wet mask is considered contaminated.

3. Wash hands before removing mask.

E. Care of equipment.

1. Disposable objects are wrapped and burned.

2. Some objects can be soaked in a disinfectant; others are autoclaved.

3. Liquid waste may be flushed down hopper.

4. Laundry is placed in specially marked bag and autoclaved before laundering.

5. During terminal disinfection equipment that cannot be disinfected in any other way is left in patient's room and "fogged."

F. Disposal of excreta.

1. May be flushed down hopper if local sewage treatment is adequate; if not, excreta must be treated with chlorinated lime before disposal.

10

The Cancer Patient

VOCABULARY

Diffusion
Excision
Lymphatic
Penetration
Synthesis
Therapeutic

INTRODUCTION

Cancer is not new; it has been with us since the beginning of time. We hear about so many cases of cancer today because diagnostic tests are more accurate now than formerly, and as a result more correct diagnoses are being made. We must also remember that cancer is primarily a disease of the older age group and is more likely to develop in persons over 50 years of age. Since more persons now reach this age group, we can expect the incidence of cancer to increase (see Fig. 10–1).

In spite of the wealth of information

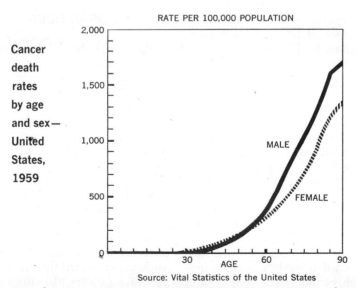

Cancer death rates by age and sex— United States, 1959

RATE PER 100,000 POPULATION

Source: Vital Statistics of the United States

Figure 10–1. Cancer death rate increases with age. Ninety per cent of cases of cancer occurs in persons over 40 and 50 per cent in persons over 60. (From American Cancer Society: *A Cancer Source Book for Nurses.*)

distributed to the public on the subject of cancer, there are still many persons who associate malignant growths with severe pain and inevitable death. The practical nurse and all the other members of the health team have an obligation to assist in public health education about cancer. It is important that lay people understand that cancer is not hopeless, that malignancies are curable in the early stages and that prolonged suffering and death are not inevitable companions of cancer.

According to the American Cancer Society, persons cured of cancer are those who "are without evidence of the disease at least five years after diagnosis and completion of treatment." In "The Hopeful Side of Cancer," a booklet published by the American Cancer Society, it is stated that over 1,300,000 Americans have been cured of cancer, and 183,000 patients are saved each year. Today, one out of every three persons with cancer is cured. Progress is being made in the fight against this disease.

Cancer is a neoplastic disease, which means that it is characterized by the reproduction and growth of new cells. We know that the human body is continuously manufacturing new cells for the maintenance of life and the repair of damage done by illness and injury. Most of the time this process of reproduction goes on in a normal fashion, and healing takes place without incident. Sometimes, however, the new cells become abnormal in their structure, and they cannot function properly. They grow too rapidly so that there is not sufficient nutrition for them, they cannot perform the work expected of them, and eventually they become extremely wild and disorganized. These pathologic changes in the cells occur in the beginning stages of cancer.

Later, if the new growths are not destroyed completely, they become necrotic in the center because they are starved for nutrition, and the cells in the outer edge of the mass break off and begin to spread through the body.

This spreading of the malignant cells is called metastasis.

There are five routes by which malignant cells may be transferred from the original site of the tumor to other parts of the body: (1) by direct extension, (2) by growing along the lymphatic vessel, (3) by embolism through the lymphatic stream to the lymph nodes, (4) by embolism in the blood vessels and (5) by invasion of the fluid within a body cavity, especially the abdomen and chest. Figure 10–2 illustrates these five routes of metastasis.

At the present time, intensive research is being conducted to learn more about cancer. The American Cancer Society lists the following as the principal goals of cancer research: "(1) the discovery of cellular trigger mechanisms that start malignant cell growth; (2) a means of checking metastasis; (3) chemicals effective in selectively killing or halting division in cancer cells; (4) understanding of possible immune defense mechanisms that may work against cancer; and (5) learning if viruses are a cause of some forms of cancer in human beings."[1]

CAUSES OF CANCER

It is now believed that there is no one specific cause of cancer, but rather that malignancy is the outcome of a number of conditions. These conditions merge to produce many different diseases that come under the heading of "cancer" or malignancy. The discovery of the exact molecular structure of the nucleic acids, deoxyribonucleic acid (DNA) and ribonucleic acid (RNA), has begun a whole new field of study of cells— abnormal and normal. This interest in the structure of cells and the ways in which they reproduce will, it is hoped, increase our knowledge of factors that increase or retard the reproductive and invasive powers of malignant cells.

Chemical Carcinogens. The word "carcinogen" means cancer-producing.

Cancer spreads by several routes:

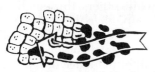

1. By direct extension into neighboring tissue

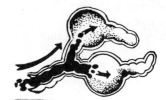

2. By permeation along lymphatic vessels

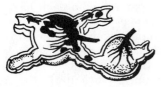

3. By embolism via lymphatic vessels to the lymph nodes

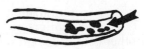

4. By embolism via blood vessels

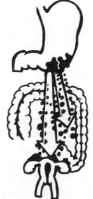

5. By invasion of a body cavity by diffusion

Figure 10–2. Routes by which cancer is spread to other parts of the body. (Modified from American Cancer Society: *A Cancer Source Book for Nurses.*)

Carcinogenic agents are substances which can cause the development of cancer cells. Almost 200 years ago, Sir Percival Potts linked the occurrence of cancer with a substance in man's environment when he observed that cancer of the scrotum was common among the chimney sweeps of London. He attributed this high incidence of cancer to repeated accumulations of soot on the skin of these young men whose occupation required continuous contact with the coal soot in the chimneys they cleaned. Since that time, over 400 different carcinogens have been identified.

Many of the cancer-producing substances in man's environment are related to occupations which involve repeated exposure to certain substances which the workers in these occupations handle or inhale. For example, cancer of the skin is often related to the handling of pitch, asphalt, crude paraffins and petroleum products. Lung cancer may be linked to irritating substances in the air, such as tobacco smoke from cigarette smoking and pollution of the air by chemical wastes from industry and automobiles. Cancer of the bladder is associated with certain substances in aniline dyes which are in the environment of workers in that industry. These are but a few of the many agents that can contribute to the development of cancer in man.

Chronic Irritation. In one of the earliest theories, cancer was attributed to long-term irritation of the skin and mucous membranes. Although this factor may be a contributing cause of cancer, chronic irritation alone usually does not lead to malignancy. There must be other conditions present, such as a mole or exposure to a chemical carcinogen.

Radiation. The high incidence of cancer, particularly leukemia, among the early experimenters with x-ray, radium and other radioactive substances led to the theory that exposure to large amounts of radiation produces cancer. With an increased awareness of the dangers of radiation and improved methods of protection against its harmful effects, the occurrence of cancer that is produced by radiation has decreased.

Viruses. Experiments in laboratory animals have demonstrated a clear-cut relationship between viruses and the development of cancer in these animals. Such experiments have sparked an increased interest in the linking of viruses and cancer in humans. There is, however, no positive proof that any one of the many types of malignant disease in man is definitely caused by a specific identifiable virus.

Internal Factors. Race, sex, age, hormonal balance and familial tendency are some of the forces at work in affecting a person's ability to resist the development and spread of cancer cells in the body. No definite pattern of hereditary relationship in the development of cancer has been established, but genetic factors cannot be com-

pletely eliminated. It is believed that some persons are lacking adequate defense mechanisms to prevent the growth and development of malignant cells, while others, through their genetic make-up, have the ability to destroy or at least localize cancer cells. The basis for this theory is the comparatively high incidence of malignancy in individuals whose parents develop cancer. It is estimated that the person born of parents who each have or develop cancer is approximately four times more likely to develop cancer himself than the person whose parents remain free of cancer.[9]

Hormones, particularly the sex hormones, are related to the development of cancer in the breasts, cervix and prostate. Recent studies have shown a definite link between estrogen and the development of breast tumors and cervical cancer.

It is hoped that with continued study of cancer cells, their reproductive activity and man's natural defense mechanisms, a means of preventing cancer through artificial immunity will eventually be discovered. In the meantime, the discovery of new diagnostic techniques and the development of more effective methods of treatment offer encouragement in man's struggle against the second leading cause of death in this country.

SYMPTOMS OF CANCER

Cancer begins very quietly and is capable of stealthily creeping up on an unsuspecting individual. It can cause considerable damage in the body before its victim is aware he has been attacked. Because the disease is so insidious, no one can afford to ignore the early symptoms of cancer, nor is it sensible to put off seeking expert advice from the physician when there is the slightest suspicion that cancer is present.

Cancer is sometimes called the "great masquerader" because it is capable of imitating the symptoms of a great variety of diseases. Since it may strike any part of the body and spread to any other organ (sometimes far removed from the original site), cancer is capable of producing an untold number and variety of symptoms in its later stages. Our main interest in the symptoms of cancer lies in the very early signs. They are included here for the purpose of reminding the practical nurse that they are extremely important and that she should be able to recite them from memory.

THE DANGER SIGNALS OF CANCER

1. Any sore that does not heal.
2. A lump or thickening in the breast or elsewhere.
3. Unusual bleeding or discharge.
4. Any change in a wart or mole.
5. Persistent indigestion or difficulty in swallowing.
6. Any change in normal bowel habits.
7. Persistent hoarseness or cough.

DIAGNOSIS OF CANCER

Physical Examination

Fortunately, the diagnosis of cancer is usually not difficult. The problem is getting the general public educated to the importance of regular physical examinations so that early cancer can be detected and treatment begun. New growths located near the surface of the body can very easily be felt by palpation. It is reported that whenever the movie, "Self-examination of the Breast' (distributed by the American Cancer Society), is shown to a group of women, several women in the audience visit their physicians within a few days because they have discovered nodules in their breast tissue. In many cases these nodules prove to be early malignancies, and the patient has an excellent chance of being cured of the cancer.

Skin cancer is easily seen by the naked eye, and with special instruments such as the vaginal speculum or proctoscope, cancer of the cervix or rectum can be seen by the examining physician. Other internal growths may be visualized with x-rays.

Biopsy

When the physician discovers a new growth, he immediately sets out to determine whether the growth is benign or malignant. This is done by biopsy, which is the removal of a sample of living cells from the growth. The cells may be removed by surgical excision of a small part of the tumor or by aspiration of the cells through a needle introduced into the growth (see Fig. 10–3). The specimen is sent to a specially trained pathologist who examines the cells and determines the type of growth they represent. Because of the danger of spreading the malignancy when a biopsy is taken, most surgeons prepare their patients for extensive surgery at the time the biopsy is done. Then, if the growth proves to be malignant, immediate steps may be taken to remove all traces of the growth.

Papanicolaou Smear

At the very beginning of the development of cancerous growths, it is possible to find cancer cells in the secretions from the body tissues adjacent to the site of the malignant growth. A physician, Dr. Papanicolaou, developed a technique for collecting samples of body secretions and examining them for malignant cells, thereby detecting the presence of cancer long before any other symptoms appear. This technique has saved the lives of countless people who have had Papanicolaou smears done as a routine diagnostic test at the time of regular physical examinations. Many cases of cancer of the cervix have been cured because of the ability to detect the disease in the early stages through the use of the "Pap" smear.

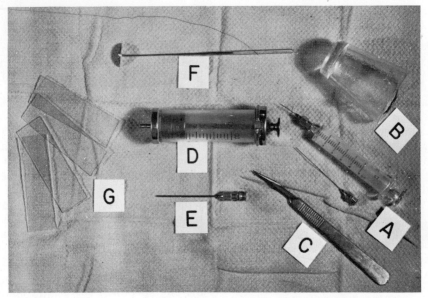

Figure 10–3. Aspiration biopsy set. *A*, 5 cc. hypodermic syringe with short and long needles for Novocain infiltration. *B*, Sterile medicine glass for Novocain solution. *C*, Scalpel with No. 11 Bard-Parker blade. *D*, 20 cc. Record syringe. *E*, 18 gauge needle with obturator. *F*, Instrument for raking out tissue from barrel of syringe. *G*, Glass slides for smears of aspirated material. (From Wolf: Nursing Clinics of North America, December, 1967.)

TREATMENT OF CANCER

At the present time there are several different forms of treatment for cancer. These include (1) surgery, (2) radiation therapy and (3) chemotherapy.

Because these methods may be used singly or together, there may sometimes be confusion in the minds of cancer patients as to which form of treatment will produce the best results. Actually, no one method is better or more effective than another except in relation to the location and type of malignancy present and the reaction of the particular type of growth to treatment. The physician chooses the method of treatment on the basis of many factors and in the best interest of the individual patient.

Surgery

Surgical removal of growths is the oldest method of treatment. It works very well for tumors which are readily accessible and located in areas where adjacent tissues, such as muscles, lymph nodes and lymph vessels, may also be excised. This radical cutting away of apparently normal tissue may seem unnecessarily drastic and mutilating to the lay person who does not fully understand the metastasis of cancer cells, but it has been proven that simple excision of the malignant tumor alone will not eliminate rapid spread and recurrence of the growth in adjacent tissues.

Radiation Therapy

This is a type of treatment that utilizes penetrating rays or emissions from an x-ray machine or radioactive substances. There are many types of radiations in our environment, for example, ultraviolet rays from the sun, light rays that we can see, radio waves that we can hear and infrared or heat rays that we can feel. The types of rays used for therapeutic purposes are alpha, beta and gamma rays and x-rays. These rays vary markedly in their composition and in their ability to penetrate matter. *Alpha rays* are composed of large particles which are highly charged and thus are not capable of traveling long distances or penetrating very deeply. *Beta rays* are smaller with less electric charge and have a longer range, making them capable of deeper penetration. *Gamma rays* have no mass and no charge. Like *x-rays*, they can travel long distances in the air and can completely penetrate the tissues of the body.

Radiation is harmful to living tissue and when delivered externally in comparatively large doses can cause disturbances in cell functions and interfere with growth and reproduction. When determining the "radiation dose" for each individual patient, the radiologist takes into account the age and general condition of the patient, his response to treatment, the size, location and depth of the tumor and the type of radiation that is available.[18]

The aim of radiotherapy is permanent destruction of the malignant cells in the growth. Unfortunately, there is nearly always some degree of damage to normal tissue in the process of reaching the underlying abnormal tissue. In addition, the patient may suffer from radiation sickness or a local reaction, either of which can interfere with the administration of an effective dose.

The damage to normal tissue can be kept at a minimum in x-ray therapy through accurate adjustment of dosage or degree of penetration and by aiming the rays from several different angles. The technique of using a variety of "ports" for entry of the rays into the body increases the concentration of the rays in the area of the tumor with a minimum of damage to overlying tissues. This is called the rotation method and can be applied with both x-ray therapy and teletherapy. In this technique the patient or the apparatus revolves slowly while the rays are aimed at the tumor (see Fig. 10–4).

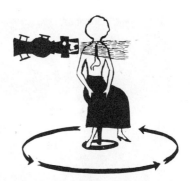

Figure 10–4. Rotation method of radiation therapy. (Modified from American Cancer Society: *A Cancer Source Book for Nurses.*)

Methods of Radiation Therapy.

The methods that may be used in therapeutic radiation include x-ray therapy, teletherapy, and interstitial therapy. *X-ray therapy* is administered by an x-ray machine that is of a higher voltage than the kind usually used for diagnostic procedures. The x-ray beam is aimed directly at the tumor and is delivered in a series of treatments planned for each individual patient.

Teletherapy is a procedure in which the source of radiation is a radioactive element that is housed in a shielded unit and located at a distance from the patient (see Fig. 10–5). The beam of radiation is controlled and directed by heavy shutters and special shielding that localizes the area of radiation. It should be remembered that gamma rays from a radioactive substance cannot be entirely absorbed by the shield, and there is no way to "turn off" a teletherapy unit; therefore one should spend as little time as possible in the teletherapy room with a patient.[18]

Interstitial therapy involves placement or implantation of a radioactive substance directly into the tissues of a malignant growth. The element used may be radium, cobalt-60, cesium-137, iridium-192, gold-198, or iodine-131. Radium is naturally radioactive; the other elements are isotopes of normally stable atoms that have been made unstable (radioactive) in a nuclear reactor. All of these radioactive elements emit gamma rays that are capable of pene-

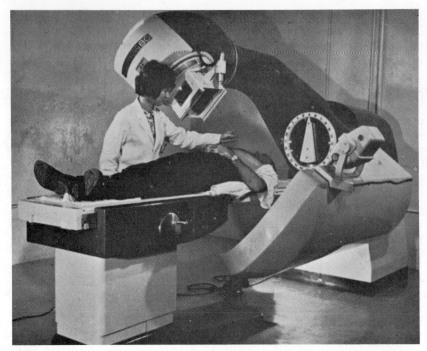

Figure 10–5. Patient treated with cobalt-60 teletherapy. (From Walker: Nursing Clinics of North America, March, 1967.)

trating tissue and destroying cells. There are a variety of forms of radioactive materials for implantation; they may be implanted as needles, tubes, seeds, wires or capsules.

Radiation Protection. Those who work with patients receiving radiation therapy must become familiar with the hazards of each type and source of radiation. Alpha and beta rays, being low in penetration, present primarily internal hazards when they are accidentally ingested, inhaled or otherwise taken into the body. Gamma rays and x-rays can readily penetrate the tissues of the body, so they present external hazards.

The effects of radiation may be divided into short-term and long-term effects. Short-term effects result from relatively large doses received for a short period of time and include localized skin burns, fever, hemorrhage due to destruction of bone marrow, diarrhea, fluid loss and central nervous system effects. The long-term effects may appear years after exposure and usually occur in individuals who have received small doses over a long period of time. These effects include shortening of the life span, predisposition toward leukemia and other malignancies and development of cataracts; when radiation is directed at the gonads, genetic mutations may arise.[2]

When considering the hazards and effects of radiation, one must avoid the extremes of complacency and total panic or paralyzing fright. After all, man has always been exposed to radiation in his environment. We are constantly being bombarded with cosmic rays from outer space, and there are naturally occurring radioactive materials in the earth and therefore in the foods we eat and water we drink. This does not mean we should be content with poor protection from radiation or complacent about the hazards when radiation is used therapeutically. Nurses simply must put these dangers in their proper perspective. We know that oxygen supports combustion and creates a fire hazard when it is administered to a patient, but we take the necessary precautions during oxygen therapy so that the patient may enjoy its benefits.

In general, the amount of radiation a nurse might receive while caring for a patient being treated with radioactive elements depends on three factors: (1) the distance between the nurse and the patient, (2) the amount of time spent in actual proximity to the patient and (3) the degree of shielding provided.[5]

Distance is an important factor in reducing exposure to radiation. By doubling one's distance from a radioactive element or x-ray beam, the exposure is reduced by one fourth, and tripling the distance reduces it by one ninth (see Fig. 10–6).[16]

Time spent near the source of radiation can be controlled by the nurse who plans her nursing care carefully so that she can spend less time with the patient without sacrificing the quality of care given. The occasions for application of this principle will most often be those in which the patient is hospitalized for implantation of a radioactive element.

Shielding from radiation exposure must take into account the type of rays being emitted. The more dense the shielding material, the less the possibility of penetration by the rays and the better the protection. A lead shield that is 1 cm. thick offers the same amount of protection as 5 cm. of concrete or 30 cm. of wood (see Fig. 10–7). Portable lead shields can be used to provide some protection for the nurse caring for a patient who is confined to bed for implantation therapy (see Fig. 10–8). Lead aprons give protection

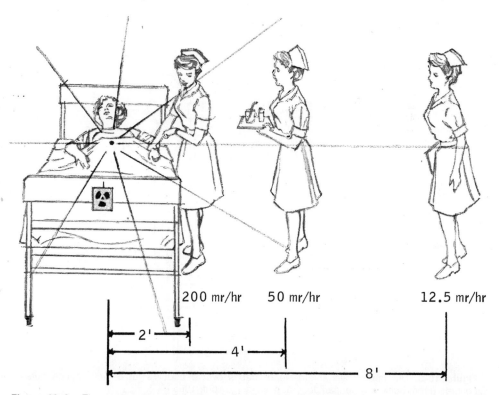

200 mr/hr   50 mr/hr   12.5 mr/hr

2'

4'

8'

Figure 10–6. The nurse nearest the source of radioactivity (the patient) is more exposed; at 2 feet, exposure is almost 15 times that at 8 feet. (From Boeker: American Journal of Nursing, April, 1965.)

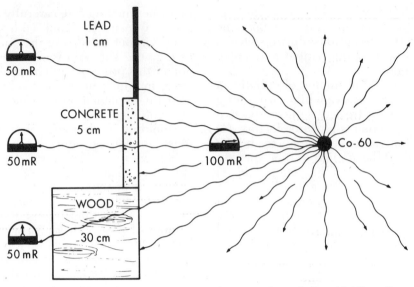

Figure 10–7. Comparison of efficacy of various materials for radiation shielding. (From Boeker: Nursing Clinics of North America, March, 1967.)

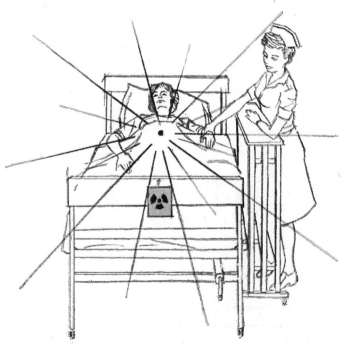

Figure 10–8. An improvised shield—lead drapes over a bedside table—will reduce personnel exposure . (From Boeker: American Journal of Nursing, April, 1965.)

from diagnostic x-rays but do not provide adequate protection from the gamma rays emitted by radium, cesium-137 or cobalt-60.

If the nurse understands good isolation technique in the care of a patient with an infectious disease, she will have no difficulty in avoiding contamination from radioactive isotopes used therapeutically. Dressings, bed linens and other articles that may be contaminated by solutions containing radioisotopes or excreta from the patient's body are treated as radioactive waste, and their disposal is carried out according to the policies of the institution in which the nurse is working. Since radioactive isotopes vary in their degree of penetration and the ways in which they can present internal and external hazards to nursing personnel, all persons concerned with the care of patients receiving radioisotopes as therapy should know exactly what precautions are necessary for each individual patient and how these precautions are to be carried out.

Radiation Sickness. Patients who have received large doses of therapeutic radiation sometimes suffer from a generalized systemic reaction known as radiation sickness. Symptoms of the reaction may vary from mild discomfort and malaise to severe nausea, vomiting and headache. Nursing measures that may help relieve these symptoms include providing adequate rest, encouraging the patient to eat small, nutritious and easily digested meals, and reassurance that such a reaction is temporary and will subside when the treatments have been completed. If the patient understands that such a reaction is a temporary discomfort similar in some ways to that experienced after surgery, he may accept the situation more readily and with less apprehension. Since most people associate radiation sickness or any other reaction to radiation with nuclear bombs and other destructive situations, the nurse must try to explain that radiation sickness is not unusual and will not permanently harm the patient.

Chemotherapy

The administration of specific drugs for destroying malignant cells or inhibiting their reproduction is particularly useful in the treatment of certain kinds of malignancies. Leukemias and lymphomas have been especially responsive to chemotherapy, and malignancies involving the reproductive system of the male or female are also amenable to treatment with specific hormones.

The drugs used in the treatment of cancer are, in general, and with the exception of hormones, toxic agents which destroy rapidly multiplying cells. While this destruction is beneficial in suppressing the growth and spread of malignant cells, it can affect certain types of normal cells which also multiply rapidly. The ultimate goal of this type of chemotherapy is maintenance of a delicate balance between malignant cell destruction and protection of normal cells. Because these drugs are so toxic to rapidly multiplying cells, their effect on bone marrow and the digestive tract have a direct bearing on the amount of drug that can be given to a particular patient.

The nurse caring for patients receiving these therapeutic agents should be aware of the need to watch for signs of extreme toxicity. Severe nausea and vomiting, diarrhea, loss of appetite and stomatitis (inflammation of the mucous membranes of the mouth) should be reported should they occur. Unusual bleeding and skin lesions should also be watched for and reported. If the drug is administered intravenously, it is especially important that the needle or catheter remain in the vein and that none of the drug be allowed to escape into adjacent tissues, since an accident of this kind will cause severe necrosis of the tissues.

Administration of the drugs used for cancer chemotherapy may be administered by any of a number of routes: (I) orally, (2) intravenously or intramuscularly or (3) intra-arterially, i.e., through an artery leading directly to the cancerous area. The last method is referred to as isolated perfusion or isolated infusion.

The drugs administered are usually classified according to their specific action. Some are cellular poisons which are known to be toxic to rapidly multiplying cells. These are called alkylating agents and include mechlorethamine (nitrogen mustard, Mustargen), chlorambucil (Leukeran) and cyclophosphamide (Cytoxan, Endoxan). Maximum toxicity to these drugs may occur as long as 2 to 3 weeks after the last dose has been administered.

The antimetabolites interfere with the synthesis of essential cell components and stop the process of cellular development by substituting false building blocks for the cells. Drugs of this type include Methotrexate, 5-Fluorouracil (5-FU) and 6-Mercaptopurine (6-MP and Purinethol). Toxic effects of these drugs include oral and digestive tract ulceration and bone marrow depression.

Antibiotics, such as actinomycin D, are sometimes given in conjunction with other drugs in cancer chemotherapy. The steroid compounds such as androgen, estrogen and ACTH are also included in the battery of anti-cancer drugs. In fact, the use of hormones in the treatment of prostatic cancer was one of the first significant developments in the field of chemotherapy.

NURSING CARE OF THE CANCER PATIENT

Physical Aspects of Cancer Nursing

Malignant growths reproduce cells so rapidly they soon use up all available nutrition. As they continue to multiply, many of the cells cannot be supported by the body and they die, bringing about ulceration and necrosis of the cells within the growth. The area is then susceptible to hemorrhage and secondary infections. These characteristics are common to all types of cancerous growths and require continued and conscientious nursing care in order to ensure as much comfort for the patient as is possible under the circumstances.

Many of the discomforts, obnoxious "sores," and "odors," commonly believed to be a necessary part of cancer, can be eliminated by dedicated application of the basic principles of cleanliness and medical asepsis. Any ulcer, regardless of its cause, will exude unpleasant odors and drain purulent material and make the patient very uncomfortable if he is not properly cared for. The basic treatment for elimination of these side effects of necrosis is regular and frequent irrigations. According to authorities, "The liberal use of wet dressings and irrigations is more important than what is put into the water." Thus we can see that continuous care and diligent cleansing of the area, with frequent changing of the dressings as needed, will greatly add to the comfort of the patient and make him feel more acceptable to others.

Hemorrhage does not occur very often, even in untreated cancer, unless the growth extends into the wall of a large blood vessel. Hemorrhage following surgery or radiotherapy is quite possible, however, and does occur occasionally. The symptoms and treatment for this type of hemorrhage are the same as for bleeding from other causes. The situation calls for close observation and prompt reporting of any signs that hemorrhage is occurring.

Emotional Aspects

Regardless of the type of cancer involved or its location in the body, the patient suffering from this disease has some emotional problems that other patients do not have. There is often fear of incapacitating surgery and prolonged treatments, expensive hospitalization and eventually a slow and painful death. The fact that none of these necessarily accompany cancer is not known to him, and he is frequently depressed and despondent to the point of total despair. The practical nurse must be aware of these problems and prepare herself for them so that she is able to offer comfort and moral support to the patient and the family without giving them false hopes. She must evaluate her own attitudes and feelings toward cancer, and continue to study and learn the new treatments which can offer cancer patients relief from symptoms and a longer life expectancy.

Any nurse who has close contact with a cancer patient must know whether or not the *patient knows* he has cancer. Some patients suspect that they have cancer, but they do not want to be told, and the doctor will, of course, respect their wishes. In this case, the nurse must also avoid a discussion of cancer in the presence of the patient, and under no circumstances is she to take it upon herself to "set him straight" about his diagnosis. Other patients know that they have cancer but refuse even to discuss the disease or any aspect of the treatments necessary. These too must be treated according to their wishes. The fact that the patient cannot discuss his illness frankly and face it squarely should indicate to the nurse how very frightened the patient is and how much he will need her sympathy and understanding.

There are some deeply religious and well-adjusted individuals who can accept their illness and will strive to learn to live with it. Just because these patients are less demanding of the doctors' and nurses' time does not mean that they are less in need of reassurance and support than those who cannot, or will not, adjust to the emotional shock suffered when they learn they have cancer. *All* patients with such a serious illness need and deserve continued encouragement and help in solving their many problems.

The Surgical Patient

The patient having surgery for the treatment of cancer is in many ways no different from a patient having surgery for any other reason. The preoperative and postoperative care of the patient having a gastrectomy requires certain procedures and nursing measures regardless of whether the operation is done to relieve the symptoms of a gastric ulcer or to remove a malignant growth. In addition to these basic principles of surgical nursing, there are certain special aspects of nursing care which must be considered in the care of the cancer patient who has surgery.

Usually the preoperative preparation of the patient with cancer includes detailed instruction of the patient and planning for his rehabilitation after surgery. The type of extensive surgery demanded by cancerous growths frequently involves permanent alteration of some of the usual functions of the various organs of the body and requires full explanation of the type of prosthesis or appliance the patient must adjust to after surgery.

The patient who has his larynx removed must be prepared for the use of the laryngectomy tube. During the postoperative period, he will receive special instructions in learning to talk without his larynx. This may be accomplished through "esophageal speech" or the patient may be fitted with an artificial larynx.

The patient who has a permanent colostomy, or the patient having a mastectomy, will also need preparation for his postoperative period, and plans must be made for rehabilitation and his return to society.

In general, the postoperative period for a cancer patient is longer than is expected for other conditions of illness because of his need for adjustment to his physical limitations. The nurse is not expected to accept the responsibility of teaching the patient everything he will need to know in order to return to his former life. She will, however, need an understanding of the problems he is facing in his struggle for a normal life, and she must assist him in any way she can through sympathetic understanding and encouragement.

Nursing Care of Patients Having X-ray Therapy

We know that use of x-rays for the destruction of malignant cells must necessarily be accompanied by some degree of damage to normal overlying tissues. It is, therefore, extremely unwise for the nurse to use the terms "x-ray burn" or "radiation burn" when speaking of reactions to radiation of the area involved. These terms imply a careless overdose or an amateurish handling of the case. In addition to the local reaction from radiotherapy, there is also usually a general feeling of malaise, nausea and loss of appetite (see the previous discussion of radiation sickness). These side effects from the use of x-ray are only temporary, and much of the patient's discomfort can be relieved by good basic nursing care.

The following outline is included in order to help the practical nurse understand the need for special care of patients receiving x-ray therapy. Most hospitals have their own procedures written specifically for the care of such patients, and these must be followed very carefully.

1. Preparation of the skin before the series of treatments is begun includes thorough washing of the area with soap and water to remove any ointments or dressings. This is followed by an alcohol rub.

2. The "ports," or areas of entry for the roentgen rays, are marked on the skin by the radiologist, and care must be taken that these marks are (not) washed off once the treatments are begun.

3. During the course of treatments, these "ports" are not washed nor rubbed with alcohol. Any pressure or friction of the skin will increase the irritation. Thus the patient is instructed not to lie on the area, and his clothing should be loose. The skin of these "ports" is very fragile and will break easily. Dusting with starch instead of powder will help relieve the itching.

4. If the skin becomes very irritated and dry before the treatments are completed, permission may be obtained from the physician to apply lanolin or petroleum jelly to the area. It is important that (no) other powders or ointments containing metals, such as zinc, be used because these absorb the rays and increase the damage to the skin.

5. Should blistering become severe during the treatments, the application of any dressing or medication must be done only on the order of the physician.

6. The internal mucosa reacts in much the same way as the skin when exposed to radiation. The treatments used consist of hourly irrigations of the mouth and gargles with a saline-bicarbonate solution when this is the area affected. It is helpful if the irrigations are followed with mineral oil as a mouth rinse to relieve drying and cracking of the mucosa.

7. The diet in such cases is usually a high-caloric liquid diet. If swallowing is impossible, the diet may be administered by gavage.

Nursing Care of Patients Receiving Interstitial Therapy

The nurse who is in any way concerned with the care of the patient who has had radium or radioactive cobalt substances injected into a malignant growth must first familiarize herself thoroughly with the special precautions and policies of the institution in

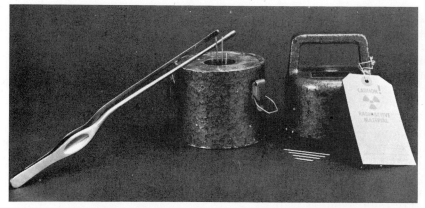

Figure 10–9. Lead container (pig), radium needles, forceps and caution sign, for use with radium therapy. (From Boeker: Nursing Clinics of North America, March, 1967.)

which she is working. Aside from the fact that radium is very expensive, it must be remembered that radioactive substances are also potentially dangerous to the patient and to those who come in direct contact with the patient. The radiologist usually assumes the responsibility for insertion, removal and storage of these substances. These materials must never be touched with the bare hands.

A few of the precautions used in the care of these patients are listed below. It cannot be emphasized too strongly that extreme care and strict observance of the rules of the hospital in regard to these patients must be scrupulously followed.

1. All linens, dressings, bedpans, or emesis basins are routinely checked before they are taken from the patient's room to see if the radium containers have been accidentally lost from the tissues.

2. Most of these patients are placed on bed rest and instructed to remain in certain positions so that emanations from radium will reach the desired area.

3. The patients are usually allowed no visitors. If visits are allowed, they should be limited to five minutes.

4. The nurses caring for the patient should not remain in the patient's room any longer than necessary at one time.

CARE OF THE PATIENT WITH TERMINAL CANCER

In the treatment of a patient in the last stages of cancer, good nursing is of primary importance. The doctor's orders are usually limited to medications for the control of pain, and the main burden of care rests on the shoulders of the nurse. It is difficult to state exactly what specific procedures are required for these patients because each patient will react in a different way to his illness. Generally it can be said that the primary concern of the nurse is the physical comfort and emotional support of the patient when the diagnosis is terminal cancer.

Rest and conservation of the strength of the patient must be regulated according to the wishes of the patient. He should be encouraged to be as active as his condition will allow and to participate in recreational activities as much as possible.

Adequate nutrition may be extremely difficult if the upper digestive tract is affected, and in some cases tube feedings may be necessary. Loss of appetite is aggravated by unpleasant odors or "bad taste" in the patient's mouth. Good oral hygiene and frequent mouthwashes with a mild, pleasant-tasting, antiseptic solution can eliminate this difficulty. Small feedings, properly spaced and attractively served, can provide adequate nutrition and are more likely to be accepted by the patient than large meals prepared without consideration of the patient's preference and tastes.

The *skin* must receive extra care because there is always danger of secondary infection and impaired healing in the cancer patient. Massage with lotions containing lanolin and frequent turning of the patient help to prevent pressure sores and add to the general comfort of the patient, as well.

The *control of pain* is one factor which concerns many lay people when they think of cancer. As stated before, uncontrollable pain does not necessarily accompany cancer and is, in fact, very unusual. It is best for the nurse to try simple comfort measures and mild sedatives rather than to administer large doses of drugs which can have undesirable side effects. The heavily sedated patient is likely to have little appetite and is inclined to develop incontinence and hypostatic pneumonia. If powerful drugs are administered early in the disease, they may lose their effectiveness by the time they are needed.

The nurse must bear in mind that the patient and his family will face many problems as they adjust to the fact that death is approaching. She must remain sympathetic and understanding even though their demands on her time and energy may sometimes seem unreasonable.

Because the patient with terminal cancer often presents such a hopeless picture, one who nurses these patients must find deep within herself a personal philosophy and attitude that can serve as a source of strength for herself and her patients. Dr. Cecily Saunders in an article printed in the *American Journal of Nursing* has written:

It seems to me that the way to find a philosophy that gives confidence and permits a positive approach to death and dying is to look continually at the patients, not at their need but at their courage, not at their

dependence but at their dignity. Doctors and nurses who have fought hard to save life or relieve dying rightly comfort themselves with the knowledge that they have done all they could. But those who realize how well the patient himself played his part can find consolation for loss and courage to face the future.[15]

Care of the terminally ill patient is discussed in more detail in Chapter 11.

CLINICAL CASE PROBLEMS

1. An acquaintance tells you that she has had a mole on her back for several years and it appears to be getting larger and darker. She admits that it could be malignant, but she argues that there is no point in going to a physician because there is nothing to be done for cancer, and she does not want to burden her family with doctor bills and hospital bills which will not accomplish anything.

What is your obligation as a nurse in regard to encouraging this person to see a physician at once?

What is your own attitude toward cancer and the treatment of the disease? *listen answer? refer to dr when necessary*

2. Mrs. Allgood went to her physician for a regular physical checkup and was found to have malignant cells in the cervical secretions obtained for a Papanicolaou smear. She was admitted to the hospital for a biopsy of the cervix, and this, too, proved to contain malignant cells. Radium was implanted in the cervix, and Mrs. Allgood was kept isolated during the treatment.

If you were assigned to give A.M. care to this patient, what special precautions should you take?

What special observations should you make?

3. You have been assigned to the care of Mr. Long, a 50-year-old man with terminal cancer of the throat. The

treatment is chiefly symptomatic because the disease was in the advanced stage before Mr. Long sought medical advice. The lesions of the throat and mouth are necrotic and draining. Mr. Long refuses foods by mouth and must be tube-fed.

What nursing measures can be used to eliminate some of Mr. Long's symptoms?

Why do you think Mr. Long waited so long to seek medical advice even though he suspected that he had cancer for some time?

REFERENCES

1. American Cancer Society: *A Cancer Source Book for Nurses.* New York, 1963.
2. American Cancer Society: *Essentials of Cancer Nursing.* New York, 1963.
3. Barnett, M.: "The Nature of Radiation and Its Effect on Man." Nurs. Clin. N. Amer., Vol. 2, No. 1, 1967, p. 11.
4. Beland, I. L.: *Clinical Nursing: Pathophysiological and Psychosocial Approaches.* 2nd edition. New York, The Macmillan Co., 1970.
5. Boeker, E. H.: "Radiation Safety." Am. Journ. Nurs., April, 1965, p. 111.
6. Fitzpatrick, G.: "Care of the Patient with Cancer of the Cervix." Bedside Nurse, Jan. and Feb., 1971, p. 11.
7. Fox, S. A., and Bernhardt, L.: "Target: Cancer. Chemotherapy Via Intra-arterial Infusion." Am. Journ. Nurs., Sept., 1966, p. 1966.
8. Hilkemeyer, R.: "Nursing Care in Radium Therapy." Nurs. Clin. N. Amer., Vol. 2, No. 1, 1967, p. 83.
9. Hopps, H. C.: *Principles of Pathology,* 2nd edition. New York, Appleton-Century-Crofts, 1964.
10. Kendall, E. B.: "Care of Patients Treated with Sealed Sources of Radioisotopes." Nurs. Clin. N. Amer., Vol. 2, No. 1, 1967, p. 97.
11. Livingston, B. M.: "Cancer Chemotherapy Research." Am. Journ. Nurs., Dec., 1967, p. 2547.
12. Lunceford, J. L.: "Leukemia." Nurs. Clin. N. Amer., Vol. 2, No. 4, 1967, p. 635.
13. Moore, G. C.: "Cancer—100 Different Diseases." Am. Journ. Nurs., April, 1966, p. 749.
14. Rummerfield, R. S., and Rummerfield, M. J.: "What You Should Know About Radiation Hazards." Am. Journ. Nurs., April, 1970, p. 780.
15. Saunders, C.: "The Last Stages of Life." Am. Journ. Nurs., March, 1965, p. 70.
16. Sellars, J. H.: "Special Nursing Care of Patients Receiving Liquid Radioisotopes." Nurs. Clin. N. Amer., Vol. 2, No. 1, 1967, p. 61.
17. Shafer, K. N., et al.: *Medical-Surgical Nursing,* 5th edition. St. Louis, The C. V. Mosby Co., 1971.
18. Walker, E.: "Responsibilities of the Hospital Nurse in the Clinical Use of Radiation." Nurs. Clin. N. Amer., Vol. 2, No. 1, 1967, p. 35.
19. Watson, J. E.: *Medical-Surgical Nursing and Related Physiology.* Philadelphia, W. B. Saunders Co., 1972.
20. Welsh, M. S.: "Comfort Measures During Radiation Therapy." Am. Journ. Nurs., Sept., 1967, p. 1880.

SUGGESTED STUDENT READING

1. Boeker, E. H.: "Radiation Safety." Am. Journ. Nurs., April, 1965, p. 111.
2. Fitzpatrick, G.: "Care of the Patient with Cancer of the Cervix." Bedside Nurse, Jan. and Feb., 1971, p. 11.
3. Fox, J. E.: "Reflections on Cancer Nursing." Am. Journ. Nurs., June, 1966, p. 1317.
4. Kautz, H. D., et al.: "Radioactive Drugs." Am. Journ. Nurs., Jan., 1964, p. 124.
5. Korsos, R. C.: "Nursing Care of the Patient with Radiation Sickness." Journ. Pract. Nurs., Oct., 1964, p. 24.
6. Saunders, C.: "The Last Stages of Life." Am. Journ. Nurs., March, 1965, p. 70.
7. Welsh, M. S.: "Comfort Measures During Radiation Therapy." Am. Journ. Nurs., Sept., 1967, p. 1880.

OUTLINE FOR CHAPTER 10

I. Introduction

A. Improved diagnostic techniques have found more cases of cancer; it is not a new disease.

B. A cancer patient is considered cured if there is no evidence of the disease at least five years after diagnosis and completion of treatment.

C. Metastasis (spreading of malignant cells to other parts of the body) occurs:
1. By direct extension.
2. By growing along lymphatic vessels.
3. By embolism through lymphatic system.
4. By embolism through blood vessels.
5. By invasion of the fluid within a body cavity.

II. Causes of Cancer

A. Malignancy is probably the result of more than one factor or condition.

B. External factors—those in man's environment.

    1. Chemical carcinogens, e.g., coal tars, polluted air, aniline dyes.

    2. Radiation—linked with leukemia.

    3. Viruses—specific identifiable virus or viruses not yet identified.

    4. Hormones—related to cancer of reproductive organs.

III. Symptoms

A. Capable of producing a great variety of symptoms.

B. Seven danger signals:

    1. Any sore that does not heal.

    2. A lump or thickening in the breast or elsewhere.

    3. Unusual bleeding or discharge.

    4. Any change in a wart or mole.

    5. Persistent indigestion or difficulty in swallowing.

    6. Any change in normal bowel habits.

    7. Persistent hoarseness or coughing.

IV. Diagnosis of Cancer

A. Physical examination.

B. Biopsy—removal of a sampling of cells for microscopic study.

C. Papanicolaou smear—a technique for collecting samples of body secretions or fluids and examining them for malignant cells.

V. Treatment of Cancer

A. Surgical excision of malignant growth and adjacent tissue.

B. Radiation therapy—use of radiation to penetrate and destroy malignant tissue.

    1. Methods of radiation therapy:

        a. X-ray therapy: the x-ray beam is aimed directly at the tumor in a series of treatments.

        b. Teletherapy: a radioactive element is housed in a shielded unit that is located at a distance from the patient.

        c. Interstitial therapy: placement of a radioactive substance directly into the tissues of a malignant growth.

    2. Radiation protection.

        a. Short-term effects of radiation exposure include localized skin burns, fever, hemorrhage due to destruction of bone marrow, diarrhea and central nervous system disorders.

        b. Long-term effects (appear years after exposure) include shortening of the life span, predisposition to leukemia and other malignancies and development of cataracts. When the radiation is directed at the gonads, genetic mutations may arise.

        c. Amount of radiation that a nurse might receive will depend on (1) distance between nurse and patient, (2) amount of time spent in actual proximity to the patient and (3) degree of shielding provided.

    3. Radiation sickness—a generalized systemic reaction to radiation.

        a. Symptoms are temporary and may vary from mild discomfort and malaise to severe nausea, vomiting and headache.

        b. Nursing measures include providing adequate rest, encouraging small, frequent feedings rather than large meals and reassurance that the condition is temporary.

C. Chemotherapy—use of drugs.

    1. Drugs may be administered orally, IV or IM, or intra-arterially by perfusion.

    2. Examples include alkylating agents, antimetabolites, antibiotics and hormones.

    3. When toxic agents are used, patient must be observed for damage to cells of bone marrow and digestive tract.

VI. Nursing Care

A. Frequent irrigations can relieve unpleasant odors from discharges that are present in some forms of cancer. Frequent changing of dressings may be necessary. Patient should be observed for signs of hemorrhage.

B. Emotional aspects of malignancy should be considered and the patient's wishes in regard to discussing his condition accepted.

C. Surgical patient will require general nursing care as for any surgical patient and often needs rehabilitation.

D. Patient having x-ray therapy will require special attention to skin and mucous membranes to avoid a breakdown and introduction of infection.

1. Do not wash off markings made for identifying "port of entry" for x-rays.
2. Never use powders or ointments containing zinc or other metals, and always have written orders for lotions, alcohol or other medications used on the patient's skin.
3. Instruct patient not to lie on inflamed area.
4. A high-caloric liquid diet may be necessary if patient has irritated lips and mouth.

E. Patients with implants of a radioactive element can serve as sources of radiation to those in close contact with them. Nurse must know and strictly adhere to rules and regulations of the hospital or clinic in regard to care of these patients.

VII. Terminal Cancer

A. Care of the patient involves attention to the emotional aspects of the disease and requires maturity and mental stability on the part of the nurse.

B. Physical aspects include adequate rest and conservation of the patient's strength, adequate nutrition, good skin care and control of pain.

11

Terminally Ill and Dying Patients

VOCABULARY

Euthanasia
Identification
Moral
Rationalization

INTRODUCTION

The topic of death and dying is one that most of us tend to avoid, preferring to dwell on life and the joys and happiness it can bring. We have been conditioned by our society to think of death as "the Grim Reaper," the intruder into life and the enemy of the living. Within the past decade, however, there has been a growing interest in the study of death and the dying process as a part of life rather than as an event that is in some way directly opposed to the concept of life. This does not mean that one should dwell upon the subject of death and become morbidly concerned with dying to the exclusion of understanding life, but rather that each of us should give some thought to the meaning of death and its relationship to health, illness and the many other factors that affect our lives.

It is especially important that nurses and other persons in the medical field be aware of the increasing interest in *thanatology*—the study of death and dying—and that they develop an understanding of the impact that these processes have on the terminally ill patient, his family and those caring for him in the last stages of his life.

In 1965 Dr. Elisabeth Kubler-Ross, a recognized authority on the subject of death and dying, was approached by four theology students of the Chicago Theological Seminary for assistance in a research project on death as a major crisis in human life. The subsequent interviews with patients and conclusions drawn from the data obtained during the study led to the book *On Death and Dying,* written by Dr. Kubler-Ross and published in 1969. Within a short time, a large number of articles and books have been written about death and dying. Seminars, conferences and college courses are now available in many communities to help interested persons explore the subject.

It is commendable that this previously neglected subject has been brought out of the shadows of fear and silence into the light of study and discussion, but the research and literature on the process of death and the lessons learned from the dying will be of little significance if they are ignored by nurses, physicians and other persons who care for and about the terminally ill.

When she first began her study of the phenomenon of death and its impact on the dying person and those in contact with him, Dr. Kubler-Ross and her coworkers were met with open hostility, denial and rationalization on the part of the staff in the hospital in which they conducted their study. In some mistaken idea of kindness to the dying patients, nurses and doctors refused to admit that there were patients who were approaching the ends of their lives. There seemed to be some thinly veiled conspiracy to ignore the dying and to protect them from anyone who wished to confront the issue of death.

Dr. Kubler-Ross writes that she was hopelessly naïve when she first entered the wards of the terminally ill seeking interviews with the patients. It was her purpose and that of the students under her direction to find persons who were terminally ill and to ask them how they felt, how they were being treated and how they would like to be treated so that their final days would be more meaningful and less frightening. The researchers were to find, however, that when they began their study in a 600-bed hospital, not one member of the hospital staff could or would direct them to a single dying patient.

Other studies similar to those conducted by Dr. Kubler-Ross have verified that, in general, nurses, physicians and other medical personnel tend to isolate the dying, withdrawing from them and gradually decreasing the amount of time spent with them. There are, of course, many reasons for this attitude on the part of the members of the medical-nursing team, but it is impossible to deny the fact that such isolation and abandonment of the patient deprives him of the personal attention and communication with others that he needs and wants when he realizes that death is approaching.

It is hoped that with increased understanding of the needs of the dying person and his family, and changing attitudes of our society toward discussion of death and dying, the health professions will recognize their responsibilities in granting each individual the right to die in peace and dignity. Although death is a very personal and emotional process, each person should have an opportunity whenever possible to share this final experience with persons of his own choosing and in surroundings that are familiar and comforting.

STAGES OF DEATH AND THEIR IMPLICATIONS FOR NURSING

When an individual realizes that he is approaching the final days of his life, he often uses certain coping mechanisms to adjust to this realization and to resolve the conflicts that arise. These series of stages through which the dying patient may progress are similar in some ways to the types of mechanisms that are used to resolve other personal conflicts. For example, in basic psychology one learns about identification, rationalization, projection and other defense mechanisms whereby an individual copes with the problems that arise when there is a conflict between what he wants to do and what others in his society expect or demand from him.

The stages of death are also similar to the process described in Chapter 8 of this text. That discussion deals with how a person copes with problems that arise when he realizes that he is permanently disabled with a chronic illness or injury. The ways in which he adjusts to the "death" of his former self and the emergence of a new person different from the former self are not unlike those experienced by the dying patient.

In general, the person who knows that death is near experiences five stages of adjustment. There are no time limitations on these periods, nor are they as clearly defined as the following discussion might indicate. It should be noted that every patient is unique, and not every one will go through an orderly progression of the stages as he faces death. The stages of adjustment are presented as guidelines for the nurse who wishes to understand what is happening to the dying patient and is anxious to provide comfort and consolation to him and his family.

Denial. The first stage in the coping mechanism is that of denying that death is imminent. Most patients initially refuse to face the issue, and the typical response to the news that they have a terminal illness is, "No, not me. It's not possible." This denial of one's death is usually only temporary, and the patient progresses on to the next stage. A small percentage, however, continue to the very end to deny that they are dying.

If the patient feels that family, friends and hospital staff expect or need him to continue his denial, that they are not willing to discuss death with him and that they prefer to ignore the issue, he will be much less likely to proceed to the next stage. The result is that the patient is denied the privilege of talking about his feelings and expressing his fears and anxieties about his death. He is also cheated of the opportunity to take care of unfinished business or financial matters and to "set his house in order." He is not given a chance to express to his loved ones certain feelings that he may want to express about them and his life with them and, finally, he loses some control over what happens to him in the final days of his life.

It is inevitable that nurses, who are devoted to the preservation and improvement of the quality of life, will often have difficulty finding the appropriate words and attitudes needed to help a patient through the first stage of the coping process. The nurse may have a strong desire to encourage the patient in his denial, telling him that he is going to be all right, and agreeing with him that he is not dying. She may consider such actions helpful in making it easier for the patient to pass through the final days of his life.

While it may seem a kindness to support the patient in his denial, such support is in reality a serious obstacle to his progress toward a dignified and peaceful resolution of his conflicts with the reality of death. This is not to suggest that the nurse or anyone else should force on the patient an acceptance of his state or indulge in arguments with him when he denies the fact that he is dying. In all instances, the patient is *assisted through* the stages of his coping process and helped to face the issue as honestly as he can.

Anger. A second common and important response to the knowledge that one's life is ending is that of frustration and anger. The patient no longer denies the fact that he is dying, but then asks, "Why me?" It all seems so unfair to him, and he retaliates by becoming belligerent, uncooperative and critical of those with whom he comes in contact. Visiting relatives and friends irritate him; they visit too often, not enough or at the wrong time. The physician is not prescribing the right medicines and treatments and may, in fact, be seen by the patient as the one who is responsible for his impending death.

Nurses, too, come in for their share of abuse and criticism from the patient. Efforts to employ such comfort measures as a back-rub or straightening the bed linen might be met with an angry outburst or a surly, "Get out of here and leave me alone." One is tempted, of course, to take the patient at his word and leave him alone, isolated in his room and left to his own devices. Or one may feel that the only sensible response is one of reciprocal anger toward the patient, giving him exactly what he asked for. Neither of these responses to his anger will be of much help to the patient. He does not intend his remarks to be taken personally. The anger he feels is not directed toward any one person but toward 'circumstances and events over which he has no control and against which he is helpless. When a dying patient wants to express his anger and rage, it is best to let him do just that—say what he feels, cry, curse, scream or do whatever he needs to do to release his pent-up feelings.

It is interesting to note that the very things nurses sometimes do or say in an effort to help their patients can be the most annoying to the patient who is terminally ill. For many of them the efficient, smiling, healthy nurse who bustles about the room serves only as a reminder that they are invalids unable to escape the confines of the hospital, perhaps physically unattractive to others and devoid of the energy to perform the simplest tasks. Again we must remember that the resentment toward the healthy and cheerful nurse should not be taken personally. Instead, the nurse should be aware that certain things may annoy the patient and that he deserves the opportunity to tell her what annoys him and contributes to his feeling of anger.

Bargaining. The third stage, that of bargaining, comes close on the heels of anger. The patient says, "Yes, me, but . . ." and then he sets out to work some kind of deal whereby he gives something to gain more days of life. Dr. Kubler-Ross observes that most bargaining is done with God, and that it often involves a promise, an exchange for prolongation of life. For example, the patient may promise to change his way of life, to become more generous or kinder, to give up something valuable to him as payment for a few more months or years.

The classic example of bargaining given by Dr. Kubler-Ross is that of a terminally ill patient who suffered severe pain requiring medication around the clock. One day she asked if it would be possible for her to leave the hospital to attend her son's wedding.

Permission for the day's leave of absence was granted, and the patient went to the wedding, remained free of pain during the entire day and returned that evening. As soon as the patient saw Dr. Kubler-Ross, she said, "Don't forget, Dr. Kubler-Ross, I have another son." Dr. Kubler-Ross cites this as the briefest, quickest example of the bargaining stage that she can give.

Depression. In the fourth stage, the patient drops the "but" and recognizes facts as they are. "Yes, me . . ." he says. He means that he knows he must prepare to take his leave of all that is near and dear to him on earth. He becomes depressed and, as expected, begins to grieve for all that he knows he will soon lose. When he has the courage to admit these feelings and to face the reality of his loss, he has earned the right to grieve and to mourn his loss.

Many patients become silent in this stage. They sit quietly, tears rolling down their faces, or sob uncontrollably when they are alone. And many do prefer to be alone in their grief, asking that visitors not come to call because they do not want to talk with anyone. The patient who is silently grieving may be more difficult to cope with than the one who is venting his anger. There seems to be so little one can say to comfort him and so little one can do to console him. The nurse can do no more than allow him to express his grief in his own way without fear of reprimand or ridicule. She strives to maintain communication with the patient, letting him know by her presence that she is aware of his suffering and that she is concerned for him. She gives him an opportunity to withdraw from others, accepting as a natural process his efforts to cope with the problem.

Acceptance. Finally, the patient accepts his imminent death and finds some degree of peace within himself. Dr. Kubler-Ross insists that we recognize acceptance as completely different from resignation or resentful giving in to the inevitable forces of "fate." In acceptance, the patient is not happy, but he at least appears to have won his struggle with fear and grief. He seems to be saying that he knows that death is near and that it is all right.

In the stage of acceptance, the patient may choose only one person with whom he wishes to spend his remaining time on earth. He wants only the comfort of being with a loved one or someone he trusts. He appreciates having a time of togetherness that does not necessarily involve extensive conversations or expression of his feelings. Although his depression may appear profound, it is a natural state and should not be cause for alarm or indication of a need for psychiatric help.

It might be well to repeat the admonition that the stages of the coping mechanism as just described are not clearly defined in every patient who is dying. The limits of time have little relevance to these stages; some patients may not have sufficient time to progress to full acceptance of the reality of their death. Others may rapidly progress through all of the stages within a very short period of time, sometimes within hours. Still others may skip over some of the steps and may or may not reach the final stage of acceptance. The stages have been presented here only as guidelines for the nurse who wishes to be helpful when dealing with a dying patient. With further study and contemplation of the process of death, she should become more capable and effective.

HOPE AND THE DYING PATIENT

It may seem contradictory to mention hope in regard to the dying person, but those who have studied the emotions and attitudes of the dying tell us that hope persists through all stages of the process. Even those patients who have accepted the reality of their death will seldom deny the possibility of a last-minute reprieve by a newly discovered drug or treatment.

The hope expressed by these patients serves to lift their spirits during difficult times and gives some meaning to the suffering they endure. This does not mean that these patients should be encouraged to seek false hopes about their condition, but rather that we understand their need for optimism and the relief that hope gives to them. In most instances, the patient interprets this allowing for hope as a sign that he is not being abandoned by those caring for him, that they have not "given up" on him, and that they will stick with him to the very end.

The hope that dying patients feel can change in nature, but it is almost invariably present. At first the patient may hope that his illness is not serious or that a wrong diagnosis has been made. Later he may hope that a treatment will be found that will cure his illness or at least prolong his life. Finally, he may hope that there is more to his existence than the life he has experienced in this world and that he will in some way continue to have life after death. Not every person can accept the concept of man having an immortal soul. For many the words "everlasting life" have little meaning until they are confronted with the reality of their own death, and even then they may question its relevance to their situation. Whatever the individual patient chooses to believe and rely on as his source of hope, he has the right to this belief and to the assistance of others in maintaining his hope. In this way, he can gain comfort and consolation as he approaches death.

COMMUNICATION WITH THE DYING PATIENT

We know that communication is a two-way process involving a sender and a receiver, and that there are times when one is in the mood for talking and times when he would rather remain silent. The patient who wants to talk about his feelings and frustrations one day may want to discuss more pleasant subjects at another time. He should be allowed the privilege of choosing the time, the topic and the person with whom he wishes to communicate. This implies that someone must "be there," available to him when the mood strikes him. It also means that the listener should be a person in whom the patient is willing to place his trust and confidence. The nurse who has avoided spending time with a terminally ill patient because he is a "hopeless" case that cannot benefit from her care cannot expect to be of much help to the patient when he needs to communicate his feelings. It is much more likely that he will choose the nurse who has had frequent personalized contact with him and has conveyed by her words and actions that she is interested in him.

Communication can be more than talking with the patient; just the presence of someone can be a comfort. Perhaps all the patient wants is a caring person sitting by his side, communicating with a touch of the hand the gentleness, kindness and strength that he needs to see him through his ordeal.

All members of the health team should share in the responsibility for discussing with the patient the seriousness of his condition. The hospital chaplain, social worker, psychologist or other team member might be the patient's choice for communication. It is, however, generally agreed that the responsibility for telling the patient that he is dying rests with the physician. In any event, the patient does have a right to know about the nature of his illness. It is also important that all persons in contact with the patient know what has been told to him. If he senses that some persons are not being entirely honest with him and are evading his questions, he will withdraw from them, thus breaking the thread of communication that could be a source of great comfort to him.

The controversy over whether or not the patient should be told that he is dying is still unsettled. There is a growing conviction that the patient who states a desire to know the truth, no matter how difficult it may be to accept, has the right to honest and straightforward answers to his questions about his condition. Those who defend the patient's right to know justify their position by saying that it is only fair to give him an opportunity to maintain some control over his life, to formulate plans for his survivors, make peace with his family and his God, and settle his business and financial affairs while he is still able to do so.[7]

Others feel that if the family and the patient prefer to avoid the issue and pretend that all is well, that should be their decision, and the hospital staff should abide by their wishes. In this case, there can be little or no meaningful communication with the patient about his condition and the nature of his illness. The essential point is the comfort and consolation of the patient and the needs that he feels as an individual. One must be careful not to close off all lines of communication with him, as he may change his mind about avoiding the subject of death. If and when he expresses a desire to talk with someone about his situation, the very least one can do is provide him with a good listener and an opportunity to communicate his feelings.

THE FAMILY OF THE TERMINALLY ILL PATIENT

It is not possible to exclude the effects of a terminal illness on the members of the patient's family. They, too, will experience some coping mechanisms as they react to the knowledge that their loved one is dying. Their words and actions also will have an impact on the patient's ability to handle his emotions and proceed through the stages to acceptance of his condition. Ideally, plans for helping the patient prepare for and cope with the crisis of death should include the physician, nursing staff, minister or rabbi and other available members of the health team. This type of consultation and planning is not always possible, however, and may be undesirable if too many persons become involved. It is essential, however, that we not ignore the family and that we recognize their need to express their feelings and find comfort and consolation during this trying time.

In her article, "Dealing with the Grieving Family," Kalish suggests some guidelines for the nurse who is dealing with the family once death has occurred. These are as follows:

1. Tensions and feelings that have been held in check before the patient's death may be suddenly released when the patient dies. The nurse can help by arranging for privacy so that pent-up emotions can be released more easily.

2. A family that is grief-stricken often needs to talk about its grief.

3. It is not uncommon for one or more members of the family to feel guilt and resentment when the patient dies.

4. It may be helpful to the family if the nurse shares with them her own feelings of loss and grief over the death of the patient.[12]

As all of the guidelines imply, the nurse who is most helpful to the family is one who demonstrates to them that she is a warm, concerned and feeling person who understands the family's grief, provides them with an opportunity to express that grief and shares with them their shock and. bewilderment at the loss of someone close to them all.

Most authorities on death and dying agree that the time for family members to talk about death and dying and their feelings about this event in their lives is long before the eventuality becomes a reality. Plans should be made and personal preferences should be expressed openly. Unnecessary heartbreak and guilt can be avoided if a parent, spouse, brother or sister has clearly stated how he wants to be treated should a fatal illness occur. Some insist that they want all possible help to live as many hours, days or months as medical science can sustain them. Others do not wish their lives prolonged by mechanical means and life-support measures when such efforts merely provide additional days of misery and suffering for all concerned.

The Euthanasia Council,* which is concerned with the right to die with dignity, has made available a document entitled "A Living Will." Since it is self-explanatory, it is presented here in its entirety:

To My Family, My Physician, My Clergyman, My Lawyer—If the time comes when I can no longer take part in decisions for my own future, let this statement stand as the testament of my wishes:

If there is no reasonable expectation of my recovery from physical or mental or spiritual disability, I (name) request that I be allowed to die and not be kept alive by artificial means or heroic measures. Death is as much a reality as birth, growing, maturity and old age—it is the one certainty. I do not fear death as much as the indignity of deterioration, dependence and hopeless pain. I ask that drugs be mercifully administered to me for terminal suffering even if they hasten the moment of death.

This request is made while I am in good health and spirits. Although this document is not legally binding, you who care for me will, I hope, feel morally bound to follow its mandates. I recognize that it places a heavy burden of responsibility upon you, and it is with the intention of sharing that responsibility and mitigating any feelings of guilt that this statement is made.

The preceding document gives evidence of the concern that many individuals feel about the right to live and the right to die. We are now confronted with the legal, moral and ethical implications of euthanasia and whether allowing someone to die is the same as "mercy killing." Just as we cannot ignore the many problems inherent in legalized abortion, we cannot avoid the issues of positive euthanasia in which a life is deliberately ended, and negative euthanasia, in which one is allowed to die when there is no hope for recovery. There are no simple, pat

*250 W. 57th St., New York, N.Y., 10019

answers to the questions arising from such issues. Every person involved in the care of the sick and injured has an obligation to study the subject, to discuss it with others and to develop within himself a philosophy and set of moral principles upon which to base his actions. The nurse who has not prepared herself to deal with the issues of life and death according to her own conscience and who has not resolved her own personal feelings about these matters cannot make a real and lasting contribution to the terminally ill patient and his family.

PHYSICAL COMFORT FOR THE DYING PATIENT

Nursing measures that can be used to lessen the physical discomfort of the terminally ill patient are no less important than the moral support and psychological understanding discussed on the preceding pages. From first-hand experience with terminally ill persons or friends and relatives, most of us know that a subtle change often occurs in the attitude of the hospital staff when a patient is diagnosed as terminally ill. Nurses tend to avoid contact with the patient and to regard his care as less rewarding than the care of patients who are recovering. These are not entirely unreasonable reactions to a very difficult situation.

For many nurses, death and dying are indications of failure on their part. Some experience feelings of guilt, and others are very personally and deeply affected by the knowledge that a patient is going to die in spite of anything they can do. Others are upset by the many decisions that must be made while caring for a patient who is in pain and dying. For example, should medication be withheld because it is "not time yet" for another dose? How much time should be spent with the "hopeless" cases when others who can recover are also demanding the nurse's time? How ethical or moral is it to continue doing anything for the patient that will prolong his life?

Quint tells us of one nurse who expressed her feelings about providing physical care for terminal cancer patients:

When the patient is completely mentally competent, you really want to get them in order. If the patient is comatose, you really let them go. Sometimes the crucial factor is the family's presence—you do it for the family.[21]

The nurse's feelings are understandable but no less regrettable from the patient's point of view. Whatever his state of consciousness, he has some degree of awareness, and it is not unlikely that he knows how repulsive he must seem to some persons and how they must dread giving him personal care.

The simplest of comfort measures that ensure cleanliness and good personal hygiene, provide adequate rest and allow for sufficient nutrition may be much more valuable to the dying patient than all the complicated life-sustaining machinery available. Sometimes, too, the nurse may be tempted to use these "things" to serve as a kind of barrier between herself and the patient. It may be easier for her to tinker with the oxygen mask and tubing and check the oxygen gauge than to lower the head of the bed, fluff the pillow and straighten the patient's pajama top so he can breathe more easily. The oxygen apparatus won't ask embarrassing questions about its condition, or make any requests for further attention or look pleadingly into the nurse's eyes and silently beg for just a few more minutes of her time.

It has been suggested, and rightly so, that nurses who are continuously exposed to terminally ill patients while on duty would benefit from a periodic transfer to another nursing unit, such as the obstetric unit, where death is a rare occurrence. The nurse also needs an opportunity to "blow off steam" once in a while, to talk about her feelings and to release emotions that she may have held in check for too long. In any event, she should try to understand her own attitudes and feelings about her role in caring for the dying. In so doing, she may be better prepared to use her imagination and skills to provide physical comfort and solace to the dying patient who depends on her for care.

CLINICAL CASE PROBLEMS

1. You are assigned to care for Mr. Roberts, age 38, who is terminally ill. His wife is a nurse who is unable to be with him more than a few hours a day because of her responsibilities at home and at work. Mr. Roberts is very difficult to care for because of his belligerent attitude. He refuses to eat and insists that he does not need A.M. care or any other kind of attention. The other nurses on duty do not go into Mr. Roberts' room except when absolutely necessary because "he has asked to be left alone, we are busy and, anyway, it is depressing to be around him. He is so young to die."

What stage of adjustment do you think Mr. Roberts is experiencing?

How can you help him?

Why do you think the nurses tend to ignore him?

2. The husband of a patient with terminal cancer refuses to accept her diagnosis and insists that she be kept alive at all costs. The patient has accepted her condition and wishes to talk about her feelings about her approaching death. She asks that you contact a minister but that you not tell her husband about the request. She also asks how you feel about using heroic measures to keep someone alive when they are hopelessly ill and willing to accept death.

What would you do about notifying the minister?

How would you answer her second question?

REFERENCES

1. Beland, I. L.: *Clinical Nursing: Pathophysiological and Psychosocial Approaches,* 2nd edition. New York, The Macmillan Co., 1970.
2. Bergeron, J. H.: "Tell Me, I Need to Know." Am. Journ. Nurs., Aug., 1971, p. 1572.
3. Blewlett, L. J.: "To Die at Home." Am. Journ. Nurs., Dec., 1970, p. 2602.
4. Brimigion, J.: "Living with Dying." Nursing '72, June, p. 23.
5. Burnside, I. M.: "You Will Cope, Of Course. . . ." Am. Journ. Nurs., Dec., 1971, p. 1354.
6. Davidson, R. P.: "To Give Care in Terminal Illness." Am. Journ. Nurs., Jan., 1966, p. 21.
7. Drummond, E. E.: "Communication and Comfort for the Dying Patient." Nurs. Clin. N. Amer., Vol. 5, No. 1, 1970, p. 155.
8. French, J., and Schwartz, D. R.: "Home Care of the Dying in Two Cultures." Am. Journ. Nurs., March, 1973, p. 502.
9. Gordon, D. C.: *Overcoming Fear of Death.* New York, The Macmillan Co., 1970.
10. Gullo, S. V.: "Thanatology." Bedside Nurse, May, 1972, p. 11.
11. Hamilton, S. M.: "The Dying Patient." Journ. Pract. Nurs., May, 1971, p. 25.
12. Kalish, R. A.: "Dealing with the Grieving Family." RN, May, 1963, p. 81.
13. Keisl, C. R.: "Thoughtful Care for the Dying." Am. Journ. Nurs., March, 1968, p. 550.
14. Kelly, H. S.: "The Sense of an Ending." Am. Journ. Nurs., Nov., 1969, p. 2378.
15. Kubler-Ross, E.: "Learning from Dying Patients." Am. Journ. Nurs., Jan., 1971, p. 54.
16. Kubler-Ross, E.: *On Death and Dying.* New York, The Macmillan Co., 1969.
17. Maxwell, Sister Marie: "A Terminally Ill Adolescent and Her Family." Am. Journ. Nurs., May, 1972, p. 925.
18. Mervyn, F.: "The Plight of Dying Patients in Hospitals." Am. Journ. Nurs., Oct., 1971, p. 1988.
19. Prattes, O. R.: "Helping the Family Face an Impending Death." Nurs: '73, Feb., p. 17.
20. Quint, J. C.: "Obstacles to Helping the Dying Patient." Am. Journ. Nurs., July, 1966, p. 1668.
21. Quint, J. C.: "The Dying Patient: A Difficult Nursing Problem." Nurs. Clin. N. Amer., Vol. 2, No. 4, 1967, p. 763.
22. Switzer, D. K.: *The Dynamics of Grief.* New York, Abingdon Press, 1970.
23. Tennyson, H., and Hautval, A.: "Who Shall Live? Who Shall Die?" Intellectual Digest, Vol. II, No. 7, p. 52.
24. VanderBergh, R., and Davidson, R.: "Let's Talk About Death." Am. Journ. Nurs., Jan., 1966, p. 71.

SUGGESTED STUDENT READING

* 1. American Friends Committee: "Who Shall Live? Man's Control Over Birth and Death." Am. Journ. Nurs., July, 1971, p. 1444.
2. Bergeron, J. H.: "Tell Me, I Need to Know." Am. Journ. Nurs., Aug., 1971, p. 1572.
3. Brimigion, J.: "Living with Dying." Nursing '72, June, p. 23.
* 4. Fletcher, J.: "Ethics and Euthanasia." Am. Journ. Nurs., April, 1973, p. 670.
5. Gullo, S. V.: "Thanatology." Bedside Nurse, May, 1972, p. 11.
6. Hamilton, S. M.: "The Dying Patient." Journ. Pract. Nurs., May, 1971, p. 25.
* 7. Hoffman, E.: "Don't Give Up on Me." Am. Journ. Nurs., Jan., 1971, p. 60.
8. Kalish, R. A.: "Dealing with the Grieving Family." RN, May, 1963, p. 81.
9. Mervyn, F.: "The Plight of Dying Patients in Hospitals." Am. Journ. Nurs., Oct., 1971, p. 1988.
*10. Prattes, O. R.: "Helping the Family Face an Impending Death." Nursing '73, Feb., p. 17.
*11. Weber, L. J.: "Ethics and Euthanasia— Another View." Am. Journ. Nurs., July, 1973, p. 1228.
*12. "When Death Strikes the Child." Nursing Update, Aug., 1971.

OUTLINE FOR CHAPTER 11

I. Introduction

A. There is growing interest in thanatology—the study of death and dying.

B. Dr. Elisabeth Kubler-Ross, one of the pioneers in researching the processes of dying and death.

C. Nurses, physicians and other medical personnel tend to isolate the dying and withdraw from them and their families.

II. Stages of Death and Their Implications For Nursing

A. These stages are fairly typical of the coping mechanisms used to resolve conflicts presented by dying and death.

B. There are five stages; however, not every patient will go through the process in an orderly manner.

   1. Denial—"No, not me. It's not possible."

   2. Anger—"Why me?"

   3. Bargaining (usually with God)— "Yes, me, but. . . ."

   4. Depression—"Yes, me. . . ."

   5. Acceptance—patient is not hap-

*Should be required reading for all students.

py, but he at least appears to have won his struggle with fear and grief.

III. Hope and the Dying Patient

A. The hope expressed by the dying patient may change, but it is almost always present.

B. Patient may hope that:

   1. His illness is not serious.

   2. A new cure will be discovered in time to save his life.

   3. There is more to his existence than the life he has experienced on earth.

IV. Communication With the Dying Patient

A. Patient should feel free to talk and should have someone to whom he can express his feelings.

B. Communication can be more than talking.

C. There is still some controversy over whether the patient should be told of his condition.

   1. Usually it is the physician's responsibility to tell the patient.

   2. Wishes of the patient should be respected in regard to discussion with him of his condition.

V. The Family of the Terminally Ill Patient

A. Family's attitudes and effects of patient's condition on them must be considered.

B. Family may feel guilt or resentment.

C. Family will need an opportunity to relieve tension, release pent-up emotions.

D. Family often appreciates nurse sharing her sense of loss and grief over the death of the patient.

E. Family may have strong feelings about the right to live and the right to die.

VI. Physical Comfort For the Dying Patient

A. Nurse may tend to neglect physical care of the dying.

B. Many different decisions may be necessary.

C. Comfort measures, adequate rest and good nutrition no less important for the dying patient.

12

The Patient Requiring Intensive Care

VOCABULARY

Cessation
Deprivation
Distortion
Electrode
Monitor

INTRODUCTION

The patient whose condition demands intensive nursing care is critically ill and in a crucial situation; he is often at the crossroads of life and death. He will usually require some assistance in maintaining one or more vital functions such as breathing, adequate circulation and fluid and electrolyte balance. And, finally, one or more of his vital functions may be monitored by relatively new and sophisticated equipment.

The duties of the nurse caring for the critically ill patient encompass many roles. She must be a skilled bedside nurse, intelligent observer, accurate reporter, friend and confidante and student. The practical nurse working in the intensive care unit or caring for an acutely ill patient in any other area of the hospital must give the best she has to offer in bedside nursing. She must follow all the principles of nursing care that she has been taught, she must discipline herself to watch her patient closely without being distracted, and she must perform each of her many tasks with complete accuracy. There is no room for compromise in nursing a

patient whose very life may depend on intelligent observation, good judgment and quick action.

Since critically ill patients do not always recover from their illness, death is a relatively frequent occurrence in the intensive care unit. The nurse must, therefore, be emotionally mature, with a firm philosophy of life that will sustain her in trying times.

There is often a profusion of complicated equipment surrounding the critically ill patient. This equipment can be frightening to the patient, and he may feel that he is losing his individuality and identity as a human being in such an environment. The nurse must guard against giving the impression that she is more concerned with care of the equipment than with care of the patient. Most intensive care units have a ratio of at least one nurse per patient; usually there are more nurses than patients on these units. This means that the practical nurse can and should get to know her patient intimately; she should use her time to establish a good relationship with him. By treating her patient as a person, she can gain his respect and cooperation.

Finally, and perhaps more im-

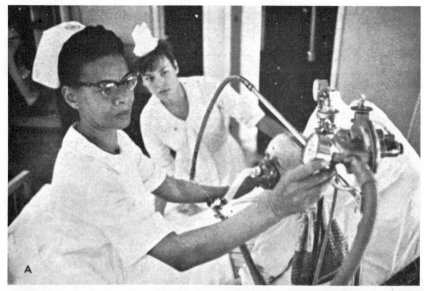

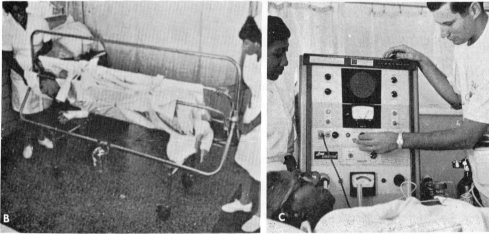

Figure 12–1. *A,* Under the watchful eye of the head nurse, LPN Edna Feamster operates oxygen equipment for ICU patient. *B,* Two LPN's in the Neurology ICU turn patient on Stryker frame. Patient is almost totally paralyzed following an automobile accident. *C,* LPN Rosa Blocker assists Dr. John Harris as he operates the cardiac monitor machine which notes any irregularities or changes in pattern of heart beats. The monitor is used on patients who have just had heart attacks. The LPN must let the doctor know of any changes in the patient's condition. (From Bradford: Journal of Practical Nursing, November, 1966.)

portant, the role of the nurse caring for the critically ill patient is that of a student. She must always be eager to learn and willing to study, and must actively participate in the in-service education programs provided by the hospital. The truly educated person knows how much he doesn't know. The rapid development of new techniques and new equipment used in pa-

tient care demands continuous study from those who wish to keep pace.

INTENSIVE CARE UNITS

Within the past few years, there have developed special care units within the hospital where patients can receive around-the-clock nursing care of the most detailed kind. These intensive care units (ICU's) are designed so that patients who require maximum nursing care and constant observation can be located in one specific area where special equipment, drugs and personnel will be readily available. They are usually planned so that all beds are visible from the nurses' station. The visitors' room is usually separate from the unit so that the family and friends may be near the patient but will not disturb him or interfere with his care.

Special equipment in the intensive care unit usually includes the following: (This may vary, however, according to the type of patient admitted to a specific unit.)

1. Cardiac monitor for the heart patient. The monitoring equipment is attached to the patient for the purpose of relaying continuous electrocardiographic information on an oscilloscope. In this way, the heart rhythm is continuously observed.

2. An artificial pacemaker that stimulates the heart by a series of electric shocks.

3. Respiratory resuscitative equipment that is used to reinstate breathing and maintain adequate exchange of gases in the lungs.

4. Reverse isolation set-up which protects the patient from contamination. It is used frequently for patients with extensive burns or for those who have lowered resistance to infection.

5. Oxygen apparatus, usually a wall unit.

6. Suction machine, also usually a wall unit.

7. Hypothermia blanket for control of body temperature.

8. Circolectric bed, Stryker frame or other equipment for patients who cannot be turned easily.

9. Special drugs that are used in acute illnesses, for example, heart stimulants, diuretics, vasodilators and vasodepressors.

The patient in the intensive care unit and his family, who are all concerned about the kind of care he is receiving,

rightfully expect a high caliber of nursing care the entire time the patient is in the unit. Many hospitals establish specific standards of care for the patient in the ICU. These standards are used by the staff as guidelines for their performance and as a means of determining what is expected of them by their employers and by the patient and his family.

One such list of standards is presented here to provide the reader with an overall understanding of the Intensive Care Unit and the quality of care that should be provided in a unit of this kind.

A Continuum of Standards for Care in an Intensive Care Area*

When the patient contracts for nursing care from the Special Care Unit, he can expect skilled and intensive efforts on his behalf to:

1. Restore and preserve cardiac function and corporeal circulation.
2. Restore and preserve respiratory function.
3. Restore and preserve chemical-fluid balance.
4. Maintain nutritional processes.
5. Prevent musculoskeletal deterioration.
6. Prevent sensory overstimulation or deprivation.
7. Prevent personal injury and maintain a safe environment.
8. Protect his privacy and provide for his comfort.
9. Recognize and support his dynamic dependent-independent state and relationships.
10. Provide for his knowledge and understanding about those forces affecting his situation.
11. Demonstrate concern and acceptance of the individual and his family.[10]

As one can see from the above statement of standards for one special care unit, it is not possible in this limited space or in a textbook of this kind to

---

*Standards of Care for the Special Care Unit, Good Samaritan Hospital, Phoenix, Arizona.

discuss in detail the many aspects of the care of a critically ill patient. The practical/vocational nurse working in such a unit cannot expect to know all of the nursing procedures and medical techniques for monitoring the patient's condition and delivering nursing care. She must, however, determine what is expected of her while working in the unit. She must also never underestimate the value of the basic nursing skills learned in the classroom and perfected at the bedside. Such skills are no less important to the well-being of a critically ill patient and may very well be the kind of care he will most appreciate.

MONITORING EQUIPMENT

In this age of automation, it is not surprising that a variety of equipment can continuously determine and record many vital activities in the human body. The monitoring equipment is not meant as a substitute for the observant nurse but simply as *an extension* of nursing observation. Machinery, as well as humans, is subject to error or breakdown, and no machine can replace the personal human warmth and concern that are so important to the emotional well-being of the patient.

Cardiac Monitoring. The cardiac monitor is becoming increasingly more familiar to all of those interested in health care. Even the average layman who watches television shows about hospital and emergency care can rather accurately describe the instrument that looks somewhat like a television screen across which wavering lines make peaks and valleys and from which comes a steady "beeping" sound. Perhaps they cannot explain the purpose of the monitor or exactly how it works, but most realize it has something to do with the heart. And they are right, of course, because the cardiac monitor does record the activity of the heart.

The monitor operates on the same principle as an electrocardiograph. Extremely weak electrical forces are generated in the heart with each contraction of the heart muscle. These impulses are transmitted outward through "leads," so called because they lead the impulses to the electrocardiograph. The impulses are amplified and their energy recorded on a graph as vertical lines. In an electrocardiogram, the electrical impulses are displayed on a paper strip; when a heart monitor is used, the impulses are displayed on a screen or *oscilloscope.* Other basic parts of a cardiac monitor are as follows:

A *sweep speed adjustment* which slows or speeds up the rate at which the electrocardiograph tracing moves across the oscilloscope.

A *pulse rate meter* which marks each heart beat with a sound (beep) and a flash of light. In this way, the pulse can be counted with accuracy.

An *alarm system* which alerts the observer that the heart rate has increased or decreased outside limits that have been pre-set on the pulse rate meter.

Electrodes which provide direct contact with the patient's skin so that electrical impulses from the heart can be transmitted to the oscilloscope.

There are several factors that can influence the efficiency and usefulness of the monitor. These are presented here so that the nurse giving bedside care to the patient may be aware of them and avoid doing anything that would interfere with successful monitoring. These factors are not by any means all that is involved in cardiac monitoring. The nurse wishing to learn more about the care of the patient on a monitor should seek additional training and on-the-job supervision.

First, the cooperation of the patient should be obtained whenever this is possible and an explanation given to him in words he can understand. He should be warned against sudden and vigorous movement. The cardiac monitor has no way of distinguishing between electrical impulses generated by skeletal muscle and those coming from the heart. For this reason, a sudden movement by the patient will activate the alarm system of the monitor, causing a false high rate alarm.

Another false alarm can be triggered by improperly placed or incorrectly attached electrodes. In either case, the monitor is not picking up the full force of the electrical impulses, so it interprets and records the situation as little or no heart activity, and the low rate alarm is sounded. To avoid this problem, it is necessary to: (1) be sure that there are adequate amounts of conductive medium (paste, jelly or cream containing salt) on the electrodes where they are in contact with the skin, (2) establish close contact between the skin and electrodes with straps or other types of fasteners and (3) be sure the electrodes are in correct position on the patient's body.

Electrical interference from the leakage of 60-cycle alternating current from wall sockets can produce a distortion of the tracing on the oscilloscope. Such leakage can be a nuisance and is also an electrical hazard to the patient and personnel. Improper grounding of the electrical equipment in the area is usually the cause of electrical interference, but whatever the cause, it should be located and corrected as soon as it occurs. The reader is referred to Suggested Student Reading #5 at the end of this chapter for further information on electrical hazards.

Cardiac monitoring equipment is extremely delicate and easily damaged. The careful handling of the equipment and a skilled, observant nurse who recognizes both the limitations and the potential of cardiac monitoring are perhaps the most important factors in successful use of the cardiac monitor for improvement of patient care.[6]

Arterial and Venous Monitoring.

Arterial monitoring is done for the purpose of providing a constant recording of the patient's blood pressure. A catheter is inserted approximately three inches into an artery and its distal end attached to a monitor which indicates the blood pressure on the monitor scope.

Venous monitoring measures the amount of pressure exerted by the blood in the vena cava or the right atrium of the heart. It is done for the purpose of determining whether a patient is in a hyper- or hypovolemic state; i.e., whether the fluid volume in the blood vessels is too high or too low. In central venous pressure (CVP) monitoring, the catheter is inserted into a vein and threaded through the superior vena cava into the right atrium of the heart (see Fig. 12–2).

CVP is used as a guide to administration of replacement fluids intravenously, particularly in patients with congestive heart failure and pulmonary edema. Normally, the right ventricle will accommodate an additional fluid load without an increase in central venous pressure. If, however, the right ventricle is failing to contract properly, it cannot handle additional fluids given rapidly into the circulatory system, and the CVP will rise. A high venous pressure may indicate heart failure, increased blood volume, cardiac tamponade (heart unable to fill), or vasoconstriction. A low venous pressure indicates low blood volume. In general, if administration of intravenous fluid does not increase the CVP, the patient will not develop pulmonary edema. Congestive failure and pulmonary edema are discussed in detail in Chapter 14.

In both arterial and venous pressure monitoring, the catheters are inserted under strict sterile conditions and, to prevent infection, the site is given careful attention until it is completely healed. After the catheter is inserted, there should be no tension to or on the tubing to which it is connected.

The patient with a venous pressure line and monitor may have infiltration of the fluid into adjacent tissue. A reddened, swollen or painful area at the

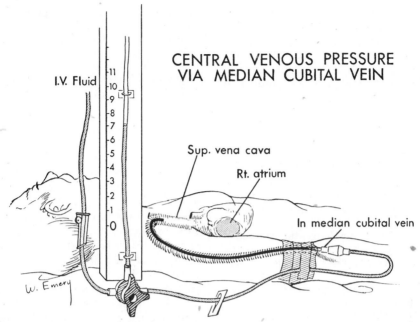

CENTRAL VENOUS PRESSURE
VIA MEDIAN CUBITAL VEIN

I.V. Fluid

Sup. vena cava

Rt. atrium

In median cubital vein

W. Emery

Figure 12–2. Note that the zero point on the manometer is at the level of the right atrium. A change in the patient's position requires resetting of the zero point. (From Gilb.: "Nursing Assessment of Circulatory Function." Nurs. Clin. N. Amer., Vol. 3, No. 1, 1968.)

site of insertion should be reported to the physician immediately. The apparatus should also be watched for obstruction to the flow of intravenous fluid. In general, the principles mentioned in Chapter 4 under intravenous fluid administration are applicable to the care of the patient and the apparatus used for central venous pressure monitoring.

NEUROLOGIC ASSESSMENT

Neurologic injury from trauma, infection, neoplasms or any one of a host of conditions affecting the central nervous system frequently demands specific nursing measures and observations on the part of the staff in a special care unit. One of the groups of signs and symptoms that is frequently used in assessing the condition of a patient with a neurologic condition is "neurologic vital signs." In most hospitals, a list of these signs will include (1) assessing the patient's level of conscious-

ness, (2) checking the pupils for reaction to light and equality of size, (3) checking the extremities for movement and strength and (4) determining the blood pressure, pulse, respiration and temperature.[7]

Of these neurologic signs and symptoms, the least familiar to the reader and the most difficult to measure is probably assessment of the patient's level of consciousness. The word "unconscious" is actually a relative term because there are varying levels of consciousness. To be fully conscious is to be aware of one's surroundings and to respond to various stimuli in a normal manner. If one is totally *unconscious* or *comatose*, there will be a total absence of any response to stimuli, and even the involuntary reflexes will not be present. The *semicomatose* or semiconscious patient will respond to painful stimuli, but he is usually unaware of his environment most of the time, and will only briefly show signs of wakefulness before sinking back into a deep sleep.

A suggested outline for the nurse who is assessing a patient's state of consciousness is presented below. The author does not present it as an exhaustive listing of the assessment process, but comments that it can be modified by individual patients. The items on it are not presented in order of priority.

Patient's Response to Auditory and Visual Stimuli*

1. Is the patient easily aroused when called by name? How easily?

2. How readily does he respond to the spoken word? In what manner?

3. Does he acknowledge the assessor's presence by verbal, nonverbal (moving eyes, head) response? Is he quiet or restless?

4. Is he unusually distracted by usual environment stimuli during the assessment? How shown?

5. Does he return to the pretesting state when stimulus is withdrawn?

6. What is the nature of his verbal response? (Groans, muttering, yes, no, etc.)

7. Does he respond to loud auditory stimuli? To bright lights? How? Is he withdrawn or combative?

8. Is he able to follow simple, first-level commands, such as "Raise your right hand"? Are his responses correct or distorted? Is he able to respond to second-level and third-level commands in proper sequence? (For example, "raise your right hand," "pick up the pencil on your bedside table," "put that pencil in your left hand.")

Patient's Response to Tactile Painful Stimuli

1. Does he react to gentle shaking? Does he move away from the source of movement? Are movements accompanied by a facial grimace or audible response?

2. Are his movements purposeful? For example, does he move voluntarily in bed to change position automatically? Does he respond when the blood pressure cuff is applied? Is it a helpful gesture or a with-

drawal? Does he attempt to protect himself from repeated stimuli?

3. Does he withdraw when painful stimuli are introduced—for example, pinching the biceps or Achilles tendons or stimulation of the sole of the foot? Is the withdrawal prompt and purposeful? Is the response selective to the area or is there general body withdrawal? Is the withdrawal accompanied or followed by abnormal movements or rigidity? Is there a pattern to his withdrawal? Is the response equal on both sides of his body?

Persons who are comatose, or are apparently unconscious and unable to respond, must have continued observation of their vital signs and accurate reporting of any change in these signs as long as they are unable to respond normally. There is one important point in the care of the unconscious patient which cannot be stressed too often, and which must be clearly understood by those who care for him. *His ability to hear and fully understand what is being said in his presence cannot be determined by outward appearance of his state of consciousness.* It is best to assume that the patient can always hear you, whether he gives any indication of hearing you or not. The nurse must explain all procedures and treatments to the patient at all times, just as though he were mentally and physically able to respond.

Whispering is always in bad taste and is especially annoying to the person who is the subject of the whispered conversation. If it is necessary to speak with the patient's family or other members of the nursing staff, it is best to talk with them in a low voice outside the patient's room. Caution must also be used in the conversations held within the patient's hearing. It is a fact that some patients who have been thought to be totally unconscious, and therefore unable to hear, have later repeated to the attendants or family the conversations they heard during their illness. This should be warning enough to use care in the things we say when caring for the supposedly unconscious patient.

---

*Reprinted from American Journal of Nursing: "Responsiveness as a Measure of Consciousness," M. A. Gardner, May, 1968, page 1034.

Perhaps it should be mentioned at this point that the eyes of the unconscious or comatose patient require special care to prevent damage. Often these patients do not close their eyes completely, even though they may not be able to respond to external stimuli. When this situation occurs, it is recommended that warm boric acid solution or normal saline be used to rinse the eyes several times a day. A drop of mineral oil in each eye after the rinsing will stimulate lacrimation and protect the eye from lint and dirt. Some physicians request that moist compresses be applied to the eyes several times a day. Without some type of special care for the eyes of the unconscious patient, it is possible for the cornea to become excessively dry, a condition which can eventually lead to blindness.

THE PATIENT IN AN ISOLATOR

The isolator is a specially designed unit that is used for the purpose of providing a physical barrier against microorganisms in the patient's environment. Fig. 12–3A and B shows the "Life Island" isolator, which was originally designed for the care of adult leukemia and tumor patients who were part of a research program.

In the case of these patients and others who have a greatly reduced resistance to infection, the isolator provides for "reverse" isolation and minimizes patient contact with harmful bacteria and other microorganisms. Isolators similar in principle to the Life Island isolator are sometimes used in the care of patients with severe burns or skin disorders which interfere with the normal function of the skin as a barrier to infectious agents.

As in any type of isolation, the patient may experience some emotional shock from his separation from others. Man, being a social animal, suffers from a lack of human contact and socialization. It is important, then, for the nurse to plan frequent "visits" to the patient and to recognize his need for personal attention. The exact procedure for serving meals and administering medications and treatments will depend on the type of isolator and the purpose for which it is being used. The reader is referred to a procedure manual in the hospital for details of care of a patient in an isolator and is encouraged to seek additional information and guidance before caring for such a patient.

CARDIOPULMONARY RESUSCITATION

The term "cardiopulmonary resuscitation" is a rather lengthy tongue twister that is usually abbreviated "CPR." The letter C stands for _cardio (heart)_, the P for _pulmonary_ (lung) and the R for _resuscitation_ (revival). Thus, CPR means reviving or re-establishing heart and lung action once it has suddenly stopped. Every person employed in a hospital, nursing home or similar agency should be able to perform this life saving technique. Through the efforts of the American Heart Association, programs are available in most communities for teaching CPR to firemen, policemen, Boy Scouts and Girl Scouts and any other group or person interested in learning this technique. There are many causes of sudden cessation of breathing and circulation, varying from electric shock to drowning to heart attack and cardiac arrest.

Prompt action is vitally important to the success of CPR. When a person stops breathing and his heart stops beating, "clinical death" has occurred. Within 4 to 6 minutes, the cells of the brain, which are most sensitive to lack of oxygen, begin to deteriorate. If the oxygen supply is not restored immediately, the patient suffers irreversible brain damage, and "biological death" occurs (see Fig. 12-4).

There are three signs that are used to indicate that clinical death has indeed occurred and that CPR is necessary.

A

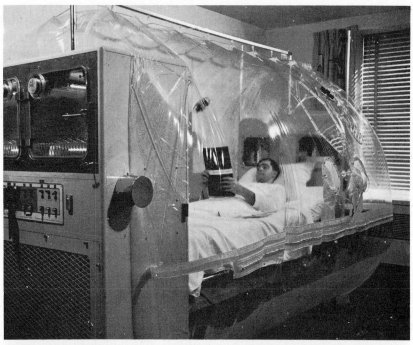

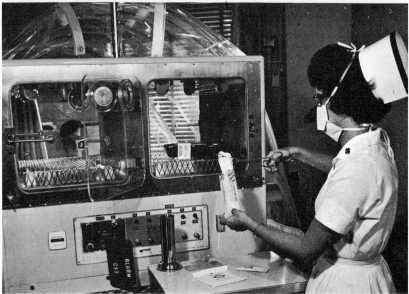

B

Figure 12–3. *A,* The Life Island isolator. The master console is at the foot of the bed with two ultraviolet lighted pass-through locks, a control panel, and air filtering system. All items enter and leave the isolator through the pass-through locks. *B,* All items (except oral medications) entering the isolator are sterile. Aseptic pass-through technique is used by the nurse. (From Seidler: Nursing Clinics of North America, December, 1966.)

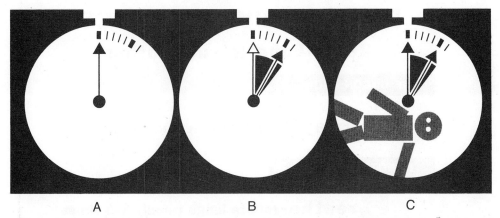

Figure 12–4. *A,* Clinical death: no breathing, no circulation. *B,* Biological death: irreversible cell damage. *C,* Signs of clinical death: no pulses, not breathing, not conscious, pupils dilating. (From Deal: Bedside Nurse, February, 1971.)

Since the technique of CPR is not without some danger to the patient, it is used only when necessary. The three signs that must be present before CPR is begun are: (1) absence of pulse, (2) absence of respiration and (3) dilated pupils that do not react to light. The pupils are used as an indication of the need for CPR because failure of the pupils to constrict in the presence of light indicates lack of oxygen supply to the brain cells.

The two major components of CPR are artificial respiration and external cardiac compression (heart massage). The mouth-to-mouth technique for artificial respiration is the type recom-

mended and should be used unless it is contraindicated by the patient's condition. In cardiac compression, the heart is squeezed against the spine, and in this way, blood is forced out of the heart and into the general circulation (see Fig. 12-5). Cardiac massage is contraindicated when the chest is surgically opened or when the patient has suffered severe injury to the chest wall.

As an aid to remembering the steps in CPR, the American Heart Association suggests using the ABC's. The letter A reminds one of "airway," B for "breathe" and C for "circulation" (see Fig. 12-6). The first step, therefore, is to be sure that the airway is open and can

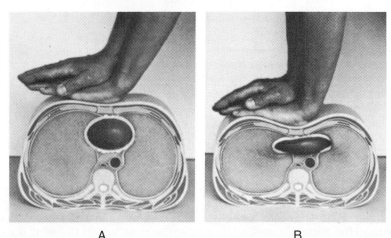

Figure 12–5. *A,* Thorax cutaway shows spine with ribs encircling chest, and sternum above the heart. *B,* With chest compression the heart empties. (From Deal, J.: Bedside Nurse, February, 1971.)

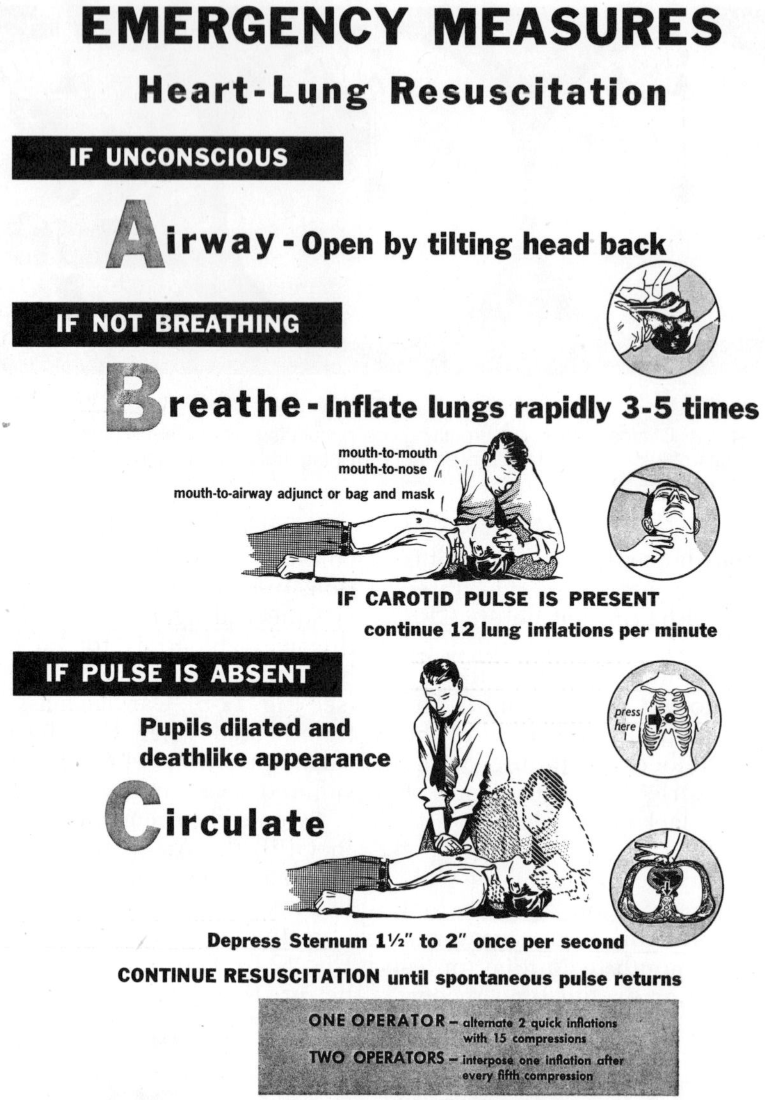

EMERGENCY MEASURES
Heart-Lung Resuscitation

IF UNCONSCIOUS

Airway - Open by tilting head back

IF NOT BREATHING

Breathe - Inflate lungs rapidly 3-5 times

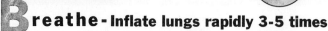

mouth-to-mouth
mouth-to-nose
mouth-to-airway adjunct or bag and mask

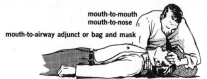

IF CAROTID PULSE IS PRESENT
continue 12 lung inflations per minute

IF PULSE IS ABSENT

Pupils dilated and
deathlike appearance

press here

Circulate

Depress Sternum 1½" to 2" once per second

CONTINUE RESUSCITATION until spontaneous pulse returns

ONE OPERATOR – alternate 2 quick inflations
with 15 compressions
TWO OPERATORS – interpose one inflation after
every fifth compression

Figure 12–6. Steps A, B and C of heart-lung resuscitation emergency treatment. (Prepared by the Committee on Cardiopulmonary Resuscitation, American Heart Association.)

allow for the passage of air into the bronchi. This step involves clearing the mouth of dentures, mucous or any other material that may interfere with the flow of air into the bronchi. After being sure that the mouth is clear, tilt the head back and pinch the nostrils with one hand. With the other hand lift up and extend the patient's neck so that the chin points upward (see Fig. 12-7).

After the airway is clear, make an airtight seal with your mouth over the patient's mouth and blow forcefully until the chest rises. If the patient is an infant or small child, less force is used, and small "puffs" of air are sufficient to inflate the lungs. After blowing into the patient's lungs, move your head away to take another deep breath and at the same time watch to see if the patient's chest is falling into a relaxed position and that air is being exhaled. The cycle

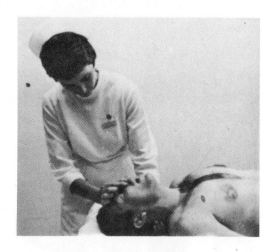

Figure 12–7. Pinch nostrils shut, lift up under the neck, push down and back on the head to hyperextend the head. (From Deal: Bedside Nurse, February, 1971.)

of blowing into the lungs and allowing air to be exhaled is repeated once every five seconds or about twelve times a minute.

It is obvious that oxygen in the lungs will be of little benefit if it cannot be transported from the lungs to the heart and from there to the tissues of the body. The transportation of oxygenated blood from the heart to the rest of the body is the purpose of cardiac compression. An effective squeezing of the heart is extremely difficult, if not impossible when the patient is lying on a soft surface that will move downward each time the chest is compressed. If the patient is lying on a soft mattress, place a board, food tray or any similar device under the patient's chest before cardiac compression is begun.

The first step in cardiac compression is location of the lower half of the sternum. This step is very important because improper positioning of the hands for pressure on the heart will not circulate the blood and may damage ribs and internal organs. If the hands are too far right or left, ribs may be fractured; if they are too high, a collarbone may be fractured; and if they are too low, the liver may be damaged. The lower end of the sternum can be found by pressing on the upper abdomen. The abdomen is soft and the sternum is hard. The point at which

they come together can be found rather easily. After locating the proper point at which pressure is to be applied place the heel of one hand on this point and the heel of the other is placed over the first. The fingers of both hands are held as high as possible, so that contact with the ribs is avoided (see Fig. 12-8).

The person giving external heart massage should position himself directly over the patient so that he can apply pressure downward vertically, thus using the weight of his upper body to compress the heart. Apply firm, heavy pressure, keeping the arms straight. The amount of pressure varies with the anatomy of the victim, but the goal is to push the sternum down 1½ to 2 inches in order to squeeze the heart against the spinal column. The sternum is pressed down and held about one-half a second and then rapidly released. The heel of the hand is not removed from the sternum, and *the rhythm is not interrupted.* Compression is applied once every second, or 60 to 80 times per minute, for adults. Children and infants require a faster rate of 100 to 120 times per minute.

The question of how one person can give CPR without assistance often arises. To perform CPR alone, he first blows into the victim's lungs three times. Then, quickly shifting position, he applies pressure to the sternum fif-

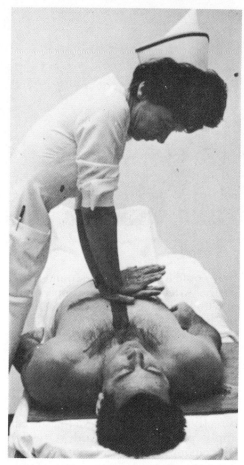

Figure 12–8. Get straight up above the patient and keep fingers up. (From Deal: Bedside Nurse, February, 1971.)

teen times. He then starts a cycle of two breaths to fifteen compressions. When there are two persons available to give CPR, the first rescuer immediately clears the airway and blows into the lungs three times. The second person immediately begins cardiac compression. When two persons are working together, the one giving artificial respiration blows into the lungs between every fifth and sixth compression. He also periodically feels for the carotid pulse to determine whether blood is being circulated by the compression. If resuscitation efforts must be prolonged, the two giving CPR can

switch positions so that neither one becomes unduly fatigued.

Many hospitals have some type of code name by which they alert personnel to the need for CPR. The reader is urged to become familiar with the procedure for a code of this type and with her responsibilities should the code be called in the hospital in which she is working. There is no excuse for ignorance in a matter that is so vital to the welfare of patients, whether they are in a special care unit or in any other department of the hospital.

EMOTIONAL ASPECTS OF NURSING THE CRITICALLY ILL

Nurses devote their lives to preserving life and restoring to health those who are sick and injured. It sometimes happens, therefore, that when a nurse is faced with the death of a patient she has tried so hard to save, she is overcome with a sense of failure. If she has performed her duties faithfully and well, there is actually no justification for such an attitude. Each of us must face grief and death; it is a part of every life, and our only recourse is to provide ourselves with a mature philosophy which will give some meaning to the unhappiness which life brings.

When a patient is critically ill, he is close to death. He may overcome his illness, or he may succumb and die, but in either case, he and his family need and deserve as much moral support as it is humanly possible to give them. The practical nurse, by the very nature of her role in nursing, is often very close to the patient and his family. She often spends more time at the bedside than other members of the nursing team, and the patient and his family may find it easier to confide in her than in others with more authority. When grief and fear overcome the patient or his family, it is often the nurse to whom they turn for moral support and spiritual strength. When this happens, the nurse has an obligation to provide whatever comfort she is able to give, even though it may be easier to leave them alone and become as little involved with their problems as possible.

There are no pat answers to these problems of grief and despair. The nurse's ability to conduct herself with composure and tact must come from deep within herself. She must be a mature person emotionally and spiritually, and she must be dedicated to the task of fulfilling her obligations to those she has pledged to serve in *all their needs.*

CLINICAL CASE PROBLEMS

1. Mr. Espana, age 52 years, was admitted to the coronary care unit one week ago with a diagnosis of myocardial infarction. It is now believed that he has some congestive heart disease. Since his heart attack, which occurred while he was working as a construction engineer, he has been very apprehensive and is especially concerned about the cardiac monitor and other equipment being used at his bedside. Mr. Espana does not understand English very well, but is very articulate in Spanish, which you understand and can speak with ease.

How could you relieve some of Mr. Espana's anxiety?

What would you tell him about the cardiac monitor? About the central venous pressure apparatus?

2. You are asked to observe Mandy, a 14-year-old accident victim who has suffered a severe head injury.

What are neurologic vital signs, and how would you observe Mandy?

3. As you enter Mrs. Galt's room to help her with her lunch, you see her clutch at her chest and then slump over in bed.

What is the *first* thing you would do?

If CPR is indicated, what would you do, and in what order would you carry out your actions?

REFERENCES

1. American Heart Association: *Cardiopulmonary Resuscitation.* 1967.
2. Brown, C., et al.: "Body Function Monitoring." Nurs. Clin. N. Amer., Vol. 1, No. 4, 1966, p. 569.
3. Deal, J.: "CPR and the ABC's." Bedside Nurse, Feb., 1971, p. 17.
4. Gilbo, D.: "Nursing Assessment of Circulatory Function." Nurs. Clin. N. Amer., Vol. 3, No. 1, 1968, p. 55.
5. Hammes, H. J.: "Reflections on Intensive Care." Am. Journ. Nurs., Feb., 1968, p. 339.
6. Jenkins, A. C.: "Successful Cardiac Monitoring." Nurs. Clin. N. Amer., Vol. 1, No. 4, 1966, p. 537.
7. Korte, M. L.: "Intensive Care of the Neurologic Patient." Nurs. Clin. N. Amer., Vol. 7, No. 2, 1972, p. 335.
8. Pinneo, R.: "Cardiac Monitoring." Nurs. Clin. N. Amer., Vol. 7, No. 3, 1972, p. 457.
9. Seidler, F. M.: "The Nurse and the Isolator." Nurs. Clin. N. Amer., Vol. 1, No. 4, 1966, p. 587.
10. Spicer, M. R.: "What About the Patient?" Nurs. Clin. N. Amer., Vol. 7, No. 2, 1972, p. 313.
11. Walker, P. H.: "Detecting Electrical Hazards in the Hospital." Bedside Nurse, March, 1973, p. 11.

SUGGESTED STUDENT READING

1. Bradford, C. M.: "The Intensive Care Unit and the LPH." Journ. Pract. Nurs., Nov., 1966, p. 35.
2. Brown, C., et al.: "Body Function Monitoring." Nurs. Clin. N. Amer., Vol. 1, No. 4, 1966, p. 569.
3. Hammes, H. J.: "Reflections on Intensive Care." Am. Journ. Nurs., Feb., 1968, p. 339.
4. Thomson, L. R.: "Sensory Deprivation: A Personal Experience." Am. Journ. Nurs., Feb., 1972, p. 266.
5. Walker, P. H.: "Detecting Electrical Hazards in the Hospital." Bedside Nurse, March, 1973, p. 11.

OUTLINE FOR CHAPTER 12

I. Introduction

A. Critically ill patient requires assistance with maintenance of one or more vital bodily functions.

B. Standards for care ensure high caliber of care for patient.

C. Basic nursing skills essential to good care of critically ill.

II. Monitoring Equipment—Serves as Extension of Nursing Observation, not as Substitute

A. Cardiac monitoring—continuous recording of electrical activity of the heart.
  1. Basic components are: sweep speed adjustment, pulse rate meter, alarm system, electrodes.
  2. Electrical interference can produce distortion.
B. Arterial and venous monitoring.
  1. Arterial monitoring provides continuous recording of patient's blood pressure.
  2. Venous monitoring records pressure exerted against wall of a vein.
  3. Central venous pressure used as a guide for intravenous administration of replacement fluids.
  4. Catheters inserted under strict sterile conditions.
  5. Patient observed for signs of infiltration and infection at site of insertion.

III. Neurologic Assessment

A. Neurologic vital signs.
B. State of consciousness.
  1. Unconscious or comatose patient gives no response to stimuli.
  2. Semiconscious patient responds to painful stimuli but shows only brief periods of wakefulness.
C. Eye care of unconscious patient necessary to prevent blindness.

IV. The Patient in an Isolator

A. Used to provide physical barrier against microorganisms. A type of "reverse isolation."
B. Patient will need frequent contact with others to avoid emotional problems of isolation.

V. Cardiopulmonary Resuscitation

A. Re-establishment of heart and lung action.
B. Prompt action essential to prevent biological death.
C. Three signs indicate need for CPR:
  1. Absence of pulse.
  2. Absence of respiration.
  3. Dilated pupils.
D. Artificial respiration given by mouth-to-mouth technique.
  1. Clear airway.
  2. Breathe into patient's mouth about 12 times per minute.
E. Cardiac compression—applied to lower half of sternum.
  1. Press downward to squeeze heart against spinal column.
  2. Press *without interruption* 60 to 80 times per minute.

VI. Emotional Aspects

A. Patient and family require support and understanding.
B. Nurse must be emotionally mature and base her actions on a well-thought-out philosophy of life and death.

13

Nursing Care of Patients With Disorders of the Skin

VOCABULARY

Debilitated
Exudate
Necrotic
Nodular
Occlusive
Transmitted

INTRODUCTION

The skin that covers our bodies is actually an organ, and like the liver or heart, it is one of the most essential for the maintenance of life and good health. The skin functions very much like a built-in suit of armor and is our first line of defense against invasion by the hordes of pathogenic bacteria living in our environment. The skin also protects us against loss of body heat by acting as a layer of insulation against changes in the temperature of our environment, and as a cooling system that reduces the body temperature through the process of evaporation of moisture from the skin's surface. In addition, the skin functions as a container for body fluids and helps in the disposal of some of the body's waste products.

When an area of the skin is destroyed by disease or trauma, its protective functions are immediately impaired, and the body is susceptible to infection. If very large areas of skin are destroyed, as in an extensive burn,

there is a disturbance in the water and electrolyte balance and loss of body heat.

DIAGNOSTIC TESTS AND EXAMINATIONS

Visual Examination

The physician must make his initial diagnosis of a skin disease by visual examination of the skin. This is not quite as easy as it would seem and requires much experience and training because there are such a wide variety of skin diseases and types of lesions. In addition to examining the lesions under a strong light, the physician also palpates the lesions to determine whether they are raised or nodular. He must also determine the subjective symptoms the patient has experienced, such as pain, itching (pruritus), burning or loss of sensitivity to heat and cold.

The diagnosis may be even more

185

difficult if the patient has tried to treat himself with patent medicines or homemade remedies before finally consulting a doctor. These treatments may completely change the appearance of the skin lesions. Many chronic diseases of the skin could have been prevented if only the individual had sought the aid of a physician when the skin lesions first appeared.

Nurses are often asked by friends, relatives and neighbors to diagnose a skin condition and are expected to suggest some simple remedy. This can put the nurse in an awkward position, but she should avoid the mistake of telling the questioner that the condition is probably "just the hives" and that it will go away when he calms down, or that it is "just a birthmark or mole" that is harmless. Very few skin disorders are caused by emotional upheaval, and the birthmark or mole may become malignant. No skin disorder should be treated lightly, particularly those which have not been disgnosed by a physician.

The hospitalized patient's skin is usually much more closely observed by members of the nursing staff than by the physician. One should always be alert for signs of skin disorders. They should be reported immediately and accurately (see Table 13-1 for name and description of common skin lesions).

It is especially important that the nurse watch for drug reactions, since almost all drugs can produce abrupt skin eruptions in some patients. Drug allergy or reaction can produce eruptions that imitate a long list of diseases, including measles, chickenpox, fungus infections, skin cancers and psoriasis. Loss of hair can also be the result of a drug reaction.[5] Intelligent observation of the patient and prompt reporting of a skin eruption can do much to avoid the more serious skin reactions to drugs.

CONTAGIOUS SKIN LESIONS. Since only 2 to 5 per cent of all skin lesions are not contagious, it is wise to use caution when caring for a patient with

TABLE 13–1. CLASSIFICATION OF SKIN LESIONS

Name of Lesion	Example	Description
Macule	Freckle, purpura	A discolored spot or patch on the skin. Usually is not elevated or depressed and cannot be felt.
Papule	Present in measles	A solid elevation of skin. May vary from size of a pinhead to that of a pea. Usually red, resembling small pimples without pus.
Pustule	Acne, smallpox	A small elevation of the skin or pimple filled with pus.
Vesicle	Blister	A small sac containing serous fluid.
Bleb	Common in pemphigus	A large elevation of the skin filled with fluid.
Excoriation	Friction burn, chemical burn	An injury caused by scraping or rubbing away a portion of the skin.
Wheal	Insect sting, hives, nettle rash	An area of local swelling usually accompanied by itching.

an undiagnosed skin lesion. Those which are contagious include all lesions containing pus and those of viral origin, such as fever blisters and warts. Herpes zoster (shingles) is also mildly contagious. Dressings, linens or other contaminated objects should be handled with care and properly disposed of. Handwashing is particularly important, especially immediately after patient contact.

History.   In the diagnosis of allergic skin diseases, contact dermatitis or infectious diseases of the skin, the history of the patient is of great importance to the physician making the diagnosis. He will need to know when the patient first noticed a change in the skin, where the lesions first appeared on the body and whether or not the patient has ever had these lesions before. If the lesions have occurred in the past, the doctor will want to know under what conditions the lesions appeared. An example is the development of a rash every time a certain soap is used, or perhaps there may be a relationship between certain foods eaten and the appearance of skin lesions. The cooperation of the patient and his family is very important in the type of detective work necessary for the correct diagnosis of many skin diseases.

Skin Tests.   There are two methods of testing for individual sensitivity to specific substances. The skin may be scratched slightly so that no blood appears, and a sampling of pollen, food or bacterial proteins is applied to the scratch. In the other method, the sampling is injected just below the first layer of skin. In a positive reaction, a small, dime-sized wheal appears at the site of contact with the sampling. This would indicate that the specific substance used in the test may be causing the disease. To prove the skin test further, the patient may be exposed to large amounts of the substance suspected and then watched carefully for the development of the skin disease.

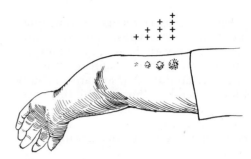

Figure 13–1.   Positive skin tests. Positive reactions are characterized by a wheal surrounded by erythema. The severity of the reaction frequently is described as ranging from 1+ to 4+.

Elimination Diets.   This type of test involves simply eliminating from the diet certain substances suspected of causing the skin disease. It is essential that the patient cooperate fully with the doctor in this test, making sure that he has completely removed the substance from his diet.

Cultures and Sensitivity Tests.   In the case of infectious diseases, especially boils and carbuncles, the physician may need to know the causative organism. A sampling of exudate is taken directly from the lesion and sent to the laboratory for culture. Once the organism has been isolated and identified, it may then be tested for sensitivity to certain antibiotic drugs. These tests take the guesswork out of treating the skin disease and very quickly establish the antibiotic which will most effectively destroy the organism causing the trouble.

PREVENTION OF SKIN DISEASE

Cleanliness.   The ritual of the daily bath is almost an obsession with the average American, and nurses are perhaps guiltier than most in their insistence on good, strong soap and plenty of hot water. No one will quarrel with the value of cleanliness, but it can be overdone, and the method of cleansing the skin deserves some thought and consideration.

First, we must recognize that there are various skin types. Some individuals have very delicate skin which requires special care to prevent drying and irritation. These are usually blondes and redheads. On the other hand, brunettes usually have skin that is considerably more oily and less susceptible to excessive drying and irritation.

If the skin appears dry and scaly, frequent bathing with strong soaps and water will only aggravate the condition. There are several oils and creams available which will cleanse the skin quite effectively and help replace the natural oils at the same time. The person with oily skin will need to clean the skin frequently, using a liberal amount of soap and water and avoiding the application of additional oils to the skin.

Diet. Adequate intake of vitamins and minerals is essential to the maintenance of healthy skin. Even borderline deficiencies in these nutritious elements will cause the skin to take on a sallow and dull appearance. Severe deficiencies lead to a breakdown of the skin and the development of sores and ulcers. Many teen-agers who are so concerned with their physical appearance that they refuse to eat properly for fear of gaining weight fail to realize that they are robbing themselves of one of the sources of real beauty; that is, a healthy and radiant complexion.

Age. Young people are not the only ones who should be concerned with the care of their skin, however. As we grow older, our skin undergoes certain changes which easily lead to irritation and breakdown of the skin if proper care is not given. The oil and sweat glands become less active as age advances, and the skin has a tendency to become dry and scaly. It also loses some of its tone, making it less elastic and more fragile. Frequent cleansing of the skin becomes unnecessary as the skin ages, and alcohol and other drying agents must be used sparingly if at all. As we grow older, we should establish a regular routine of massaging oils, creams or oily lotions into the skin, if not for the sake of vanity, at least for the sake of preserving a very important organ of our bodies.

Environment. There are several factors in the environment of an individual which may have a direct effect on the health of the skin. These include prolonged exposure to chemicals, excessive drying of the skin from repeated immersions in water or contact with soap and excessive burning of the skin by strong sunlight. Some of these factors are occupational hazards and may necessitate changing jobs to eliminate the causative factor (see Fig. 13-2).

The current fad of acquiring a "tan" by deliberately exposing the skin to strong sunlight for long periods of time is foolish when carried to extremes because it does lead to excessive drying of the skin if not actually burning it. The parts of the body exposed become wrinkled and age much more rapidly than those parts which are shielded from the sun. We must also remember that the incidence of skin cancer is highest among those who must work out in the sun (for example, farmers) and is usually located on the neck and face, where exposure is greatest.

GENERAL NURSING CARE

The word "dermatology" refers to the specialized study of diseases of the skin. A *dermatologist* is one who specializes in the treatment of disorders of the skin. Many dermatologists have some standing orders or written instructions they wish followed in the care of their patients who have been admitted to the hospital. If there are no specific instructions to follow, however, the nurse must use caution until she determines the wishes of the physician. Some general rules in the care of the patient with skin disease may be

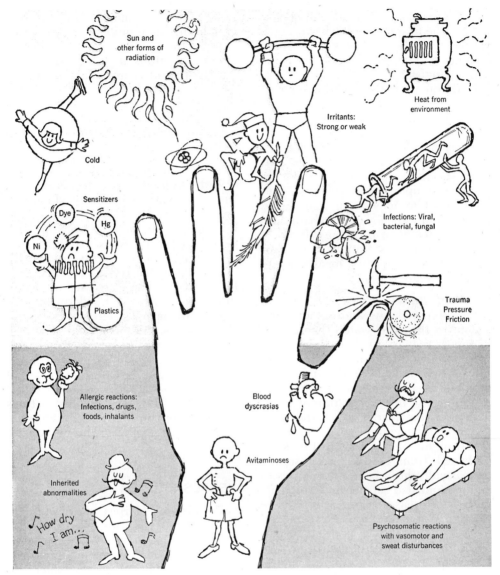

Figure 13–2. Factors that cause or complicate dermatitis. (From Goldman: American Journal of Nursing, March, 1964.)

helpful as a guide until specific orders are obtained. These are as follows:

1. Bathing with soap and water is usually contraindicated in all inflammatory conditions of the skin.

2. Dressing covering the lesions should not be removed when the patient is admitted unless there are specific orders to do so.

3. Do not attempt to remove scales, crusts or other exudates on the skin lesions until the physician has had an opportunity to examine the patient.

4. Observe the skin very carefully at the time of the patient's admission and record your observations on the chart or report them to the nurse in charge.

5. Avoid excessive handling or rubbing of the skin against the sheets and bedclothes when changing the bed.

6. Lotions and alcohol generally used in the hospital for back rubs, etc., are never applied to the skin of these patients without permission from the dermatologists.

7. If you are not sure about any part of the nursing care considered to be routine for all patients, ask before you act.

Once the physician has determined the type of lesions present, he will order specific treatments to relieve the patient's symptoms and promote healing. The two most commonly used treatments are special colloid baths and wet compresses or dressings. In addition, there may be lotions, salves or ointments to be applied locally at frequent intervals.

Colloid Baths. These are special baths prepared by adding soothing agents to the bath water. These may include starch, oatmeal or other cereals and sodium bicarbonate. The substances to be added will depend on the type of skin disease to be treated. For procedures in the preparation of a colloid bath, the reader is referred to a textbook in basic nursing.

During the bath, the patient must be protected from chilling because the bath usually lasts from 30 minutes to an hour and also because most patients with skin diseases have less resistance to cold. When the patient is removed from the tub, the skin is dried by patting rather than by rubbing. If medication is to be applied locally, it should be put on as soon as the bath is completed, so as to keep pruritus at a minimum.

The medicated bath has a very soothing and relaxing effect on the patient and also helps relieve the itching and burning so commonly associated with skin diseases. The nurse should encourage her patient to rest in bed and perhaps take a short nap after each bath.

Laundering. The bed linens and gowns used for patients with severe skin diseases may need special laundering to eliminate all traces of soap. In the hospital, this requires specific instructions to the personnel in the laundry and careful labeling of the linen to be used for the patient. If the patient is to be cared for in the home, vinegar may be added to the rinse water to neutralize the soap. The proportions used are one tablespoon of vinegar to each quart of water.

Wet Compresses or Dressings. There are various ways in which wet dressings may be applied to the skin, but the two general types are *open dressings* and *closed dressings.* In the open type, the compresses must be changed constantly and are never allowed to dry. These are used in certain diseases in which the dermatologist wishes to have air circulating to the skin lesions. In the closed type, the dressings are thoroughly soaked with the prescribed solution and wrapped in an airtight, waterproof material (see Fig. 13-3). It is recommended that the nurse obtain specific instructions from the dermatologist before applying wet dressings to any lesions of the skin.

HERPES SIMPLEX

Definition. Herpes simplex is the medical term used for fever blisters or cold sores. These lesions are caused by a virus and may occur alone or with other systemic diseases such as pneumonia, influenza and meningitis.

Symptoms. The vesicles of herpes simplex are found on the lips and inside the mouth. Sometimes the lesions may be found on the genitalia. Usually the lesions themselves are not considered to be serious, even though they may cause some discomfort and slight disfigurement.

Treatment. The symptoms of burning and itching which accompany herpes simplex may be relieved by the

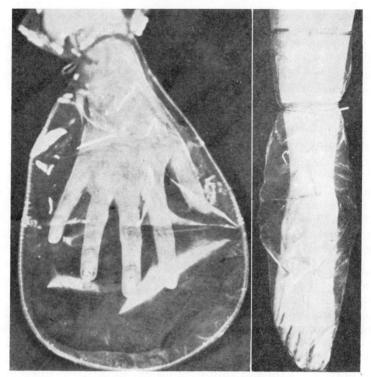

Figure 13–3. Plastic "mitt" and "sock," which may be used to hold "closed" wet dressings in place and maintain adequate degree of moisture to dressings. These may be improvised from plastic bags or the plastic wrapping available in most stores. (From Stryker and Grindon: Journal of the American Medical Association, July 13, 1940.)

application of warm compresses to the sores, followed by the local application of tincture of benzoin or spirits of camphor to aid in drying and healing the lesions. Antiseptic mouthwashes have been used with success in treating some mild cases.

For persistent cases in which there is frequent recurrence of the lesions, herpes simplex may be treated with smallpox vaccinations. This treatment is based on the fact that the virus that causes smallpox has some relationship to the one causing herpes simplex.

Some authorities feel that there may be some connection between certain foods eaten and the development of the lesions. Large amounts of orange juice or chocolate have been known to cause the development of these lesions on the lips and mouth.

HERPES ZOSTER

Definition. Another name for herpes zoster is shingles, probably because the scaly appearance of the skin does bear some resemblance to the material used to cover roofs. Herpes zoster is a viral disease of the skin and the peripheral sensory nerves that lie just below the surface of the skin.

Shingles is caused by a virus similar to the one that causes chickenpox and is usually found in older persons who had chickenpox in their childhood.

Symptoms. Herpes zoster begins with vague symptoms of chills and low-grade fever and possibly a gastrointestinal disturbance. About 3 to 5 days later, small groups of vesicles appear on the skin in the area of the spinal cord. The vesicles increase in number and spread around the trunk of the body, following the nerve pathways that lead from the spinal cord to the skin. The skin lesions change from small blisters to a scaly appearance, and there is pain and itching in the area. The skin lesions usually occur only on one side of the body; rarely is there involvement of both sides, and there is no foundation for the superstitious belief that the patient will die if the shingles "meet" as they progress around the body.

Pain is an outstanding symptom of shingles and may be quite severe, persisting for several days after the skin lesions are completely healed.

Treatment and Nursing Care. There is no specific treatment to cure herpes zoster, and the condition may continue for several months, especially in older and debilitated patients. One attack usually confers immunity.

The symptoms may be relieved by medication to reduce pain and antibiotic drugs to prevent bacterial infection of the skin lesions. If pain is severe and difficult to control with drugs, deep x-ray therapy may be of some benefit.

Fortunately, even though herpes zoster may seem to be very difficult to cope with while it is running its course, there are rarely any serious complications from the disease. In the rare cases that are very severe, the patient may suffer from extreme exhaustion, and death can occur as a result.

IMPETIGO CONTAGIOSA

Definition. Impetigo contagiosa is, as its name implies, a highly contagious disease of the skin. It is a very common skin disease occurring most often in infants and small children and may rapidly spread through an entire nursery or family. It is caused by a form of staphylococcus or streptococcus.

Symptoms. The disease begins with small vesicles which rupture and exude a pustular, honey-colored material that dries and forms a crust over the lesion. Impetigo is often mistaken for ringworm because of the round patches it forms (see Fig. 13-4).

The itching that accompanies impetigo brings about scratching and contamination of the hands with the

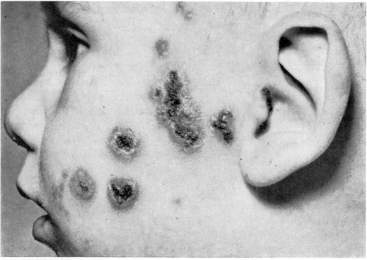

Figure 13–4. Impetigo contagiosa. Circular lesions are covered with dried crusts. Other lesions in early stages at hairline show blisters before they have ruptured. (From Top: *Communicable and Infectious Diseases,* 4th Ed., The C. V. Mosby Co., St. Louis.)

exudate from the lesions. The exudate is a source of infection, and thus the disease is spread to other parts of the body or to other persons.

Treatment and Nursing Care. Because the exudate is a source of infection, the crusts should be removed daily and the lesions thoroughly cleansed. An antibiotic ointment may be applied locally on the lesions several times a day; however, antibiotics by mouth are more effective. The patient or his family, in the case of small children, must be cautioned against spreading the disease by careless use of equipment used to cleanse the sores or failure to wash the hands thoroughly after each treatment.

PEDICULOSIS AND SCABIES

Definition. The parasites that cause pediculosis and scabies are found throughout the world in all types of climates, and they can infest anyone, no matter what his station in life. They are particularly troublesome, however, wherever people live under crowded conditions and are negligent in their personal hygiene. The occurrence of pediculosis and scabies in this country has recently increased significantly because of communal living and other "more natural" lifestyles chosen by some of the younger generation.

There are three basic types of lice which infest human beings: the head louse, *Pediculus capitus;* the body louse, *Pediculus corporis;* and the pubic or "crab" louse, *Phthirus pubis.* In addition, human beings may also be infested by the *Sarcoptes scabiei,* the mange mite that produces scabies. All types are acquired by contact with infested persons, their clothing, bed linen and bedding. Dogs have also been known to carry lice and the scabies mite.[16]

Symptoms. The most prevalent symptom of lice infestation is severe itching. The resultant scratching can lead to excoriation of the skin and secondary infection. If the lice infest the eyelids and eyelashes, the eyelids become red and swollen. Swelling may also occur in the lymph glands of the neck of a person heavily infested with head lice. The body louse can transmit typhus fever, trench fever and some other diseases. The other types of lice are not known to be transmitters of any other disease.

The scabies mites burrow under the top layers of the skin and live their entire life cycle there. They are more likely to be found in the skin between the fingers and toes, in the groin and other areas where there may be folds of skin. Excretions from the mites produce irritation with intense itching and blistering. Secondary infection is not uncommon with scabies.

Treatment and Nursing Care. The drug most commonly used and considered most effective against lice and scabies is 1 per cent gamma benzene hexachloride (Kwell).[16] It is available in a cream and a lotion which is applied to the infested area and surrounding tissues. It is left on the area for 12 to 24 hours and then removed completely with soap and water. If needed, the treatment may be repeated once more 24 hours later.

The medication is also available as a shampoo for head lice. The shampoo lather is rubbed on the hair and scalp for at least four minutes and then removed by thorough rinsing with water. A fine-toothed comb is then used to remove the nits (eggs) that may have remained on the hair.

Clothing, bedding and other contaminated articles should be cleaned thoroughly in order to decontaminate them. If decontamination is not possible, they should be burned. Isolation of the patient and protection from reinfestation of himself or contamination of others is similar to that for any patient with an infectious disease.

CONTACT DERMATITIS
(ALLERGIC ECZEMA)

Definition. Dermatitis is an inflammation of the skin. A contact dermatitis is an inflammation of the skin resulting from exposure to, or contact with, some substance in a person's environment. The substance may be animal, mineral or vegetable in origin and must be a substance to which the person has developed a sensitivity. In other words, contact dermatitis is an allergic reaction (see Fig. 13-5).

The word "eczema" is generally used to describe an external reaction to an allergen and is most often found in children who will eventually outgrow the eczema only to develop hay fever or asthma.

Symptoms. The inflammation of the skin usually begins with patches of redness on the skin followed by the formation of small vesicles which rupture and become scaly. Pruritus is very common in contact dermatitis.

Examples of contact dermatitis are reactions to poison ivy, poison oak or sumac, cosmetics, or drugs.

Treatment and Nursing Care. The basis of treatment is the determination of the specific allergens causing the dermatitis and removal of the offending substance from the patient's environment. In persistent cases, the doctor may "desensitize" the individual by exposing him to small amounts of the substance until he has built up an immunity.

The symptoms may be relieved by colloid baths to soothe the inflamed skin and lotions to reduce the occurrence of scaling and peeling. Antihistamines may be given to help control the itching.

Emotional factors play an important role in the development of skin disorders, especially those related to the allergies. The patient's anxiety and restlessness, aggravated by itching and the constant sight of his physical condition, make this type of illness a challenge to the nursing staff. There is a need for sustained reassurance of the patient and extreme patience and perseverance in carrying out the long list of treatments and nursing care necessary every hour or so.

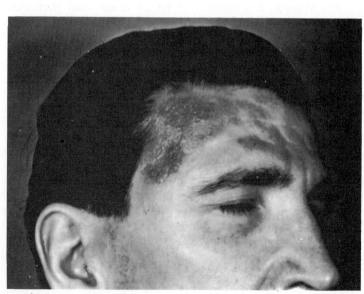

Figure 13–5. Dermatitis caused by allergy to the dye in a hat band. (Courtesy of Medichrome-Clay-Adams, Inc., New York.)

ACNE

Definition. Acne is a disorder of the skin characterized by eruption of papules and pustules over the face, back and shoulders at puberty (see Fig. 13-6). There are two kinds of acne: *acne vulgaris* and *acne rosacea.* Of the two, acne vulgaris is probably the most common, and it has been estimated that nine out of ten adolescents have this skin disease to some degree.

Acne rosacea usually affects persons over 25 years of age and may be more difficult to contend with because there is often some deep seated emotional problem associated with the disease and there is also little possibility of the patient's outgrowing the disease. The term "rosacea" is used to designate this type of acne because the skin around the pustules is very red.

Symptoms. The symptoms of acne vulgaris are familiar to most of us. We have observed the large blackheads *(comedones),* raised pustules, and

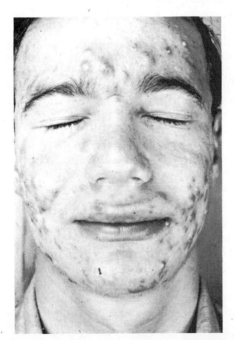

Figure 13–6. Typical appearance of acne. (Courtesy of Medichrome-Clay-Adams, Inc., New York.)

eventual pitted scarring that so frequently signals the onset of puberty and the beginning stages of adulthood. The relationship between the development of the disease and the adolescent phase is a result of the increase in hormonal activity which occurs at this time of life. The hormones apparently have some effect on the pores of the skin, blocking the flow of secretions through the pores and setting the stage for the formation of blackheads. The blackheads become infected with bacteria and thus lead to the development of pustules on the skin. It is believed that the hormonal activity varies among individuals, and this accounts for the fact that some persons are more likely to develop acne than others.

Treatment and Nursing Care. There is no specific treatment that will guarantee a cure for acne. Each patient must be treated on an individual basis because each case will react differently to certain medications or treatments. It is very important to instruct the patient about the nature of acne and the need for faithful adherence to the prescribed treatment. He should understand that treatment not only controls unsightly blemishes while the disease is active but also prevents permanent pitting and scarring of the skin.

An adequate diet with well-balanced meals has been shown to be very important in the management of acne, and while it does not guarantee absolute prevention of the development of the skin lesions, it does have some effect on the severity of the disease.

Cleanliness also plays an important role in controlling acne; however, there is no basis for the belief that acne is actually caused by improper cleansing of the skin. The purpose of frequent washing of the face and hands is to remove accumulated secretions and prevent secondary infection from bacteria that collect on the skin. The soap used should be a mild face soap and the method of cleansing restricted to gentle application. "Scrubbing" the skin must be avoided because it frequently damages the skin and causes greater irritation and inflammation. The hands are carriers of bacteria, and not only must they be kept scrupulously clean, but the patient must be instructed to keep his hands away from his face.

The pricking and squeezing of pustules seems to be a common temptation for the patient with acne, and he must be warned of the danger involved in such practices. There is serious danger of spreading the infection on the face and even getting the bacteria into the blood stream. It is also likely that squeezing and pressing the skin cause more scarring than necessary because the underlying tissues are damaged.

Blackheads that are not infected may be removed if they are soaked with hot compresses for 15 minutes and then removed with a specially designed instrument. The dermatologist usually wishes to instruct the patient thoroughly before allowing him to remove his own blackheads.

It is unfortunate that acne occurs during adolescence, because the patient is already undergoing some emotional strain during this period of adjustment without the added burden of a disfiguring skin disease. The nurse and the family of the patient must do all they can to offer moral support and understanding to the young person with acne.

PSORIASIS

Definition. Psoriasis is a chronic and recurring skin disorder that is characterized by papules covered with adherent silvery scales that produce pinpoint bleeding when they are removed. Its exact cause is unknown but it is a relatively common condition. For some unknown reason, it tends to subside and then flare up again. In some cases, the skin eruptions are accompanied by rheumatoid arthritis in the fingers and toes (see Fig. 13-7).

Treatment. Treatment may be both topical and systemic, depending on the severity of the symptoms. There is no known cure for psoriasis. However, by using the old reliable remedies such as mercury and coal tar ointments and the newer drugs such as the corticosteroids, the condition can be kept under control.

FUNGAL INFECTIONS

Introduction. Fungal infections of the skin are called *mycoses;* systemic fungal infections of the lungs and other internal organs are systemic mycoses. Relatively few fungi are pathogenic to man, and such infections are rarely fatal if they involve the superficial tissues; nevertheless, mycotic infections are exasperating because they progress slowly, are difficult to diagnose and are often resistant to treatment.

The most common types of fungal infections involving the skin are *epidermophytosis* (athlete's foot or dermatophytosis), *tinea of the scalp* (commonly known as ringworm) and *tinea barbae* (barber's itch). *Moniliasis* (thrush) is a fungal infection that can attack the mucous membranes of the mouth, rectum and vagina. All surface fungal infections produce itching, some swelling and a breakdown of tissue. Since fungi thrive in warm, moist places, a tropical climate or other environmental factors that produce prolonged heat and moisture can encourage the development of fungal infections.

Epidermophytosis. Epidermophytosis most often affects the feet, particularly in the areas between the toes. The infection may spread and cause blistering, peeling, cracking and itching of the entire foot. If it continues unchecked, it can spread to other parts of the body. The condition can be complicated by a severe bacterial infection.

Treatment of epidermophytosis consists of keeping the area dry, clean and

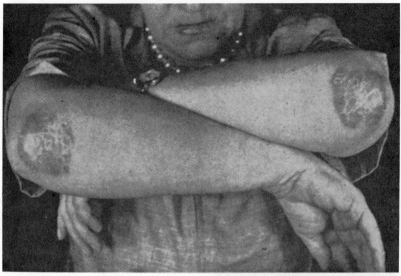

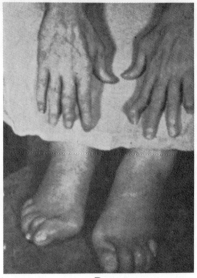

Figure 13–7. *A,* Classic lesion in psoriasis is the silvery scaling plaque found most frequently over the extensors of the extremities. The scalp is another commonly affected site. *B,* Rheumatoid changes in the distal interphalangeal joints may occur in association with psoriasis. Nails also show changes. (From Wechsler: American Journal of Nursing, April, 1965.)

A

B

exposed to the air and sunlight as much as possible. Clean cotton stockings should be worn every day and the affected areas between the toes should be separated by gauze or cotton. There are some medicated powders such as Desenex which work to keep the feet dry and also help control growth of the fungi. Other medications called *antifungals* or *fungicides* are effective in treating this condition.

Since most cases are contracted and spread in swimming pools, showers and other public facilities of this type, one should be careful to wash one's feet and dry them thoroughly after using such facilities. It is difficult to destroy the fungi causing athlete's foot by any method other than by boiling contaminated articles or by use of a strong disinfectant such as 0.1 bichloride of mercury or 0.2 creosol.

Ringworm. The term *ringworm* is often used to designate tinea of the scalp and beard. Actually, the term ringworm is incorrect and confusing.

The skin lesions do not necessarily appear in rings and they very definitely are not caused by a worm. If the infection is located on the scalp *(tinea capitis)* the hair falls out in patches and there are small, reddish lesions of the skin. Tinea capitis primarily affects children. Because it is highly infectious, any child with this condition should be kept from school until he is no longer a source of infection. His contaminated clothing should be boiled or destroyed to prevent the spread of the infection, and he should wear a stocking cap or surgical cap to protect his scalp during treatment.

Tinea barbae is called barber's itch because it affects the area of the face where the beard grows, and it is most often spread by carelessness in sanitary measures in a barber shop. The lesions produce a boggy swelling of the skin, soften the hairs of the beard and involve the lymph glands.

In both types of tinea, the infected hairs are removed by the tedious process of pulling them out one by one or by deep x-ray therapy performed by a skilled technician. *Griseofulvin* (Fulvicin or Grifulvin) is the fungistatic antibiotic that is most often used in the control of ringworm of the scalp and face.

CANCER OF THE SKIN

Introduction. Skin cancer is often neglected because there is no pain associated with it, and patients often fear that treatment will involve extensive or mutilating surgery. It has been estimated that each year 68,000 persons discover they have skin cancer and 4000 of these cases are fatal because of inadequate treatment. Almost all of these deaths could have been averted through early diagnosis and treatment.[4]

Causes and Susceptibility. There are several factors that predispose one to the development of skin cancer. Among these are internal changes within the cells themselves that may be due to hereditary factors, and external influences such as chronic exposure to chemicals or other irritants in the environment. Since children tend to inherit their skin characteristics from their parents, susceptibility to skin cancer tends to run in families. Blue-eyed blondes seem to be most susceptible, probably because they lack sufficient pigment to protect the skin cells from outside irritants. The incidence of skin cancer in Negroes is very low.

Irritants that can lead to the development of skin cancer include industrial dyes and chemicals, ultraviolet rays, as from the sun, and radiations from x-ray machines or radioactive elements. Repeated irritation of a mole, ulcer or other precancerous lesion also can lead to malignant changes within the lesion.

Treatment. Removal of cancerous skin tissue will depend on the type of malignancy present. In all but the most extensive growths, treatment is relatively simple and completely successful. Although benign precancerous lesions do not inevitably develop into malignancies, the most advisable course of action is to remove them when they are first diagnosed, before they become malignant. The nurse often is in a position to notice these lesions in their early stages and she should do her best to persuade the person with such a lesion to seek prompt medical attention.

The three main types of skin malignancy are basal cell epithelioma, squamous cell epithelioma, and melanocarcinoma.

Basal cell epithelioma usually appears first as a small, scaly area that tends to become larger as it progresses. It occurs most often on the faces and trunks of adults. As the scales shed, there will be a small amount of bleeding and the formation of a scab. As the scab is shed, the affected area becomes wider, and it is bordered by a waxy, translucent, raised area. This process of spreading may continue very gradually

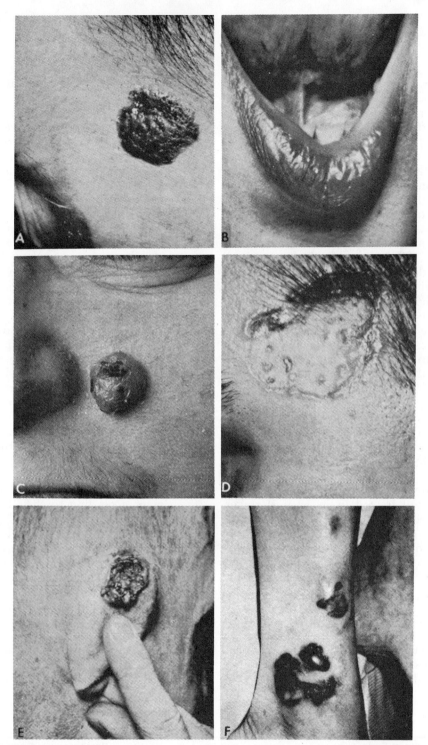

Figure 13–8. *A,* Precancerous keratoses such as this one on the temple are caused by chemical irritants and should be destroyed when they appear. *B,* Precancerous leukoplakia, white patch on the floor of this 26-year-old woman's mouth, developed after eight years of heavy smoking. *C* and *D,* Basal cell epitheliomas had been present on both these patients from 1½ to 2 years; were removed by local surgery; did not recur. *E,* Squamous cell epithelioma behind ear, a typical site. Local surgery destroyed it. *F,* Melanoma, here an ankle, metastasizes rapidly; starts as tiny dark papule or nodule. (From Cipallaro: American Journal of Nursing, October, 1966.)

over a period of several months or years. Even though these malignancies do not metastasize, they can invade underlying tissues, and death can result from complications such as infection, hemorrhage, or exhaustion. Smaller lesions can be removed under local anesthesia in a doctor's office. Larger lesions respond well to x-ray or radiation therapy.

Squamous cell epithelioma usually begins on the mucous membranes and can metastasize to other areas of the body. The tumor begins as a small nodule with rapid development of ulceration. Treatment must begin early if the condition is to be relieved before extensive damage is done. Surgical procedures must involve total removal or destruction of the lesions and surrounding tissues that have been invaded. Radiation therapy is advised for patients who are poor surgical risks or who are fearful of surgery.

Melanocarcinomas often originate in moles that have been subjected to repeated irritation or which have been incompletely removed. This type of skin cancer is highly malignant and requires radical treatment, especially if it is not treated in its earliest stages. The course of treatment depends on the stage of malignancy and the extent to which it involves other areas.

BURNS

Definition and Classification. Burns are injuries to the skin caused by exposure to extreme heat, electrical agents, strong chemicals or radiation. The classification of burns is based on the *depth* of the lesion and the *extent* of the body surface that has been burned.

Depth of burns is classified as first degree, second degree and third degree. A *first degree burn* involves only the outer layer of skin (epidermis); the underlying tissues are not injured. There is redness, tenderness, pain and some edema but no blistering with a first degree burn.

A *second degree burn* is deeper and involves both the upper and lower layers of the skin. In addition to the symptoms of redness and pain, there is blistering with a second degree burn. There is usually complete regeneration of the layers of the skin and little or no scarring.

A *third degree burn* is much deeper, with destruction of both the epidermis and dermis and some damage to the underlying tissues. There is no blistering, and after the initial severe pain, the patient usually does not complain of pain in the area of a third degree burn because the nerve endings have been destroyed. The surface of the skin may appear charred, or it may be white and lifeless in appearance.

The extent of a burn is calculated by the doctor according to the "Rule of Nines" (see Table 13-2). The depth of the burn is more difficult to determine because there are various gradations of injury in a major burn. The physician must make an estimate of some kind as to depth, however, because the patient's systemic illness and his prognosis are directly related to the amount of tissue destroyed. Since third degree burns destroy all layers of the skin, there can be no epithelialization. This means that eventual grafting will be

TABLE 13-2. RULE OF NINES

Area of Body	Percentage of Body Surface
Head and neck	9
Anterior trunk	18
Posterior trunk	18
Upper limbs	18
Lower limbs	36
Genitalia and perineum	1

necessary for adequate coverage of the area.

There are some terms that are relatively new in the field of burn therapy. These should be familiar to the nurse caring for a burned patient. *Partial-thickness wounds* are those in which the epidermal appendages (sweat and oil glands and hair follicles) are not destroyed, and the wound may heal without grafting. A *deep dermal* wound is a partial-thickness wound that is deeper, but resurfacing of the wound is possible if infection does not destroy the epidermal appendages. *Full-thickness wounds* involve all layers of skin, and the epidermal appendages are destroyed. Wounds of this type will require grafting if optimal function is to be restored.

The *crust* is the dry, scab-like covering that forms over a superficial burn. *Eschar* is a hard leathery layer of dead tissue that results when there has been a full-thickness injury. The eschar can act as a protective covering over the wound, serving as a barrier against infectious agents. *Slough* is the moist necrotic tissue of a burn.

Emergency Treatment. All burns should be considered potentially dangerous, and even the most minor ones should be cared for as aseptically as possible. Most authorities now recommend submerging the burned area in ice water or applying cold compresses as emergency first aid for less extensive burns. This helps to relieve pain and reduce edema. Under no circumstances should salves or ointments be applied to a burned area if there is any doubt as to the depth and extent of the burn. The removal of greasy substances is very painful, and the patient will suffer unnecessarily because of haste or poor judgment on the part of the person who gave improper emergency care. (First aid for major and minor burns is discussed in Chapter 23 of this text.)

As soon as the physician evaluates the depth and extent of the burn, he begins treatment aimed at combating shock and preventing infection.

The two most important measures used to combat profound shock in a burn patient are replacement of lost fluids and electrolytes and the relief of pain and mental anxiety. The loss of fluids and electrolytes is a result of the sudden shifting of the blood plasma and tissue fluids from their normal site to the area of the burn. The fluids are then lost by seepage through the open wounds where the skin has been destroyed by burns.

It is necessary to replace these fluids immediately; otherwise there will be collapse of the blood vessels and a resulting profound shock which may be fatal to the patient. Plasma, fluids and electrolytes are given intravenously, often through an incision into a vein, because there will be a need for

TABLE 13-3. GUIDES FOR ESTIMATING DEPTH OF INJURY*

Factor	Second Degree Burn (Partial Thickness)	Third Degree Burn (Full Thickness)
Cause	Hot liquids, flashes, flames	Flames, electricity, chemicals
Skin		
Color	Pink or mild red	Pearly white or charred
Surface	Vesicles are weeping	Dry
Palpation	Soft	Leathery
Response to pin prick	Painful	Anesthetic
Layers involved	Dermis	The fat or subcutaneous tissue

*From Larson and Gaston: American Journal of Nursing, February, 1967. Reprinted with permission.

continuous replacement of fluids until a normal fluid and electrolyte balance is established. In a severely burned patient, intravenous therapy may be necessary for several days or longer.

Measures to relieve pain include the administration of morphine or Demerol as soon as possible after the burn has occurred. Later the physician may choose to order other pain-relieving drugs which are less likely to lead to addiction, because of the long period of recovery which is usually associated with severe burns.

The nurse must use gentleness and care in handling the patient as she turns him or administers other treatments. Not only does this reduce the amount of pain the patient must suffer, but the less the patient is handled, the less danger there is of contaminating the wounds.

Even though there is not usually much pain involved with third degree burns, most patients who have such burns also have areas of second degree burns which are very painful long after the initial pain at the time of the accident. Added to this extreme discomfort is the patient's realization that he has been badly injured and is in serious condition. He no doubt thinks of all the horrifying sights and smells associated with burned flesh and suffers much emotional shock from such an experience.

The nurse assisting in the emergency care of the burn victim in the hospital should assemble the equipment that she can expect the physician to need. This equipment usually includes the following:

1. Intravenous fluids and apparatus for administering fluids and whole blood.

2. A catheterization tray and a No. 18 Foley catheter with tubing and drainage bottle. Specimen cup for urine specimen.

3. A tray containing equipment for withdrawing a blood sample and appropriate test tubes for blood typing, crossmatching, blood count and electrolyte analysis.

4. A tracheostomy tray.

5. A cutdown set with No. 16 tubing, suture material and skin antiseptic.

6. An instrument set and special dressings such as small gauze flats, gauze rolls, Ace bandages, adhesive tape, towels, gloves and sterile Vaseline gauze.

7. Surgical gowns and masks for those attending the patient during emergency care.

The nurse should also be prepared to administer tetanus antitoxin and one or more antibiotics as ordered by the physician. Since some preparation should be made on the unit to which the patient is to be admitted, the nurse should notify the unit of his impending admission and inform them of the need for a Stryker frame or Circolectric bed if the physician prefers one of these to a regular hospital bed for his patient.

General Treatment and Nursing Care

Treating the Wound. The past decade has seen a gradual revolution in the treatment of burns. In the early 1960's, most patients with third degree burns over 50 per cent of the body did not survive. Today, because of improved care to prevent infection and promote healing, many patients do survive such extensive burns.

Infection remains the major cause of death in burns. The necrotic tissue serves as an excellent breeding ground for microorganisms, and they multiply rapidly in the wound. Gram-positive microorganisms such as streptococci and staphylococci are usually well controlled by penicillin and methicillin. The gram-negative microorganisms also respond fairly well to antibiotics. The most recent hazard is *Pseudomonas aeruginosa.* It is a particularly virulent microorganism that has taken the place of the "staph" infections of the '50's. It is hoped that a vaccine against Pseudomonas will soon be available for patients who have developed this type of infection.[7, 10]

Topical applications to prevent infection have been used with some degree of success in recent years. In the mid-1950's, 0.5 per cent silver nitrate solution for soaks was introduced and gained widespread use in the 1960's. Although this method does control surface infection of the burn wound, it leads to a loss of chloride. The patient's electrolyte must, therefore, be carefully monitored.

One of the most widely used topical creams for burns is Sulfamylon acetate cream 10 per cent. It has a deeper penetrating effect than most other types but has the disadvantage of causing a severe stinging sensation when applied. It can also produce metabolic acidosis, and many patients develop an allergy to the drug. A combination of a sulfa drug and a silver salt, silver sulfadiazine, is also a relatively new topical agent that is used today.

In general there are two methods that may be used in the treatment of a burn wound: the *open method* and the *closed method.* In the open method, the burned area is left uncovered and exposed to the air. In the closed method, the area is covered with bulky dressings consisting of many layers and is then wrapped snugly with elastic bandages. There is no one "best" way to treat burns. Each patient must be evaluated according to his age, physical make-up and type of burn and then treated on an individual basis.

OPEN METHOD. When this method of treatment is used, the nurse must guard constantly against infection. Usually the serous fluid which exudes from the burns will harden and cover most of the burned area, but there are cracks in this exudate through which bacteria may enter. The bed linen is sterile, and a bed cradle or some other device is used to support the weight of the top covers and keep them off the burned areas. Those in attendance usually wear sterile caps and gowns and gloves while caring for the patient (see Fig. 13-10). In recent years, some hospitals have set aside special units in which burned patients are treated by the open method. These units are staffed with personnel specially trained in the care of the burned patient. For further details, the reader is referred to reference 4 under Suggested Student Reading at the end of this chapter.

Aside from preventing infection, the nurse must also provide additional warmth when the open method of treatment is used. Much body heat is lost through the parts of the body where the skin has been destroyed, and the patient is chilled easily. Heat lamps or small electric bulbs installed under the device used to hold up the top covers will usually provide the extra warmth needed.

Wet compresses or soaks to cleanse the area and remove excess exudate and drainage must be done with extreme care and under sterile conditions in order to minimize the danger of infecting the wound. An exception is the silver nitrate method, in which it is usually not considered necessary for the attendants to follow rigid isolation technique with masking and gowning.[17]

CLOSED METHOD. The closed method of treating burns presents fewer problems for the nursing staff because there is less danger of infection. There is also the added advantage of having the burned areas covered so that the patient does not have a constant visual reminder of his injuries. It is also true that patients who have pressure dressings are freer to move about and do things for themselves than those who do not have their wounds covered. The main disadvantage of the closed method is the need for frequent changing of the dressings, which may require administration of a general anesthetic and also involves some trauma to the regenerating tissue each time the dressings are removed. Other disadvantages of bulky dressings are that they provide a culture medium for the growth of bacteria,

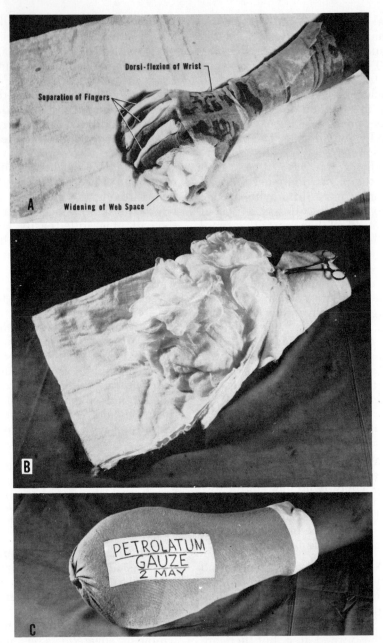

Figure 13–9. *A,* Initial step in applying an occlusive dressing to a burned hand. A layer of lightly impregnated gauze is placed over the burned area. The hand and forearm are put on two large abdominal pads. Fluffed gauze is placed on the palm of the hand in such a way that there is dorsiflexion of the wrist and acute flexion of metacarpophalangeal. joints. The fingers are separated with gauze and special attention is given to maintaining the width of the webbed space between the index finger and the thumb. *B,* Additional fluffed gauze is placed over the hand to make a large, absorptive dressing. It may or may not be necessary to put a plaster splint in the dressing to maintain dorsiflexion of the wrist. *C,* The entire dressing is wrapped with even compression by means of an elastic bandage. Stockinette is placed over the dressing. Then the type of treatment and date applied are noted on the dressing. (From Artz and Moncrief: *The Treatment of Burns,* 2nd Ed., W. B. Saunders Co., Philadelphia.)

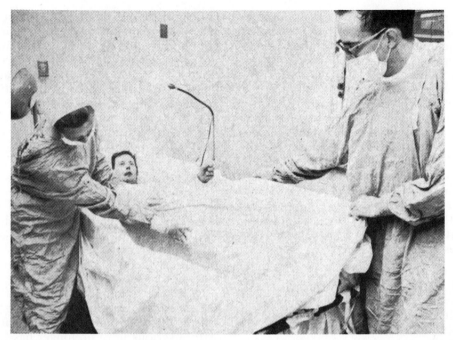

Figure 13–10. Two nurses wearing sterile gowns and gloves change the linen of a burned patient's bed. The patient is lying on a flotation mattress used to minimize pressure on burned areas. (From Noonan & Noonan: American Journal of Nursing, February, 1968.)

are difficult to apply properly to areas such as the face and perineum, may increase fluid loss and heat retention and can mask hidden bleeding.

Debridement and Grafting. Debridement involves removal of the eschar and necrotic material from underlying tissues. This must be done with great care so that bleeding is kept at a minimum and healthy tissues are disturbed as little as possible. Some physicians prefer the method of soaking off eschar by placing the patient in a tub containing a temperature-controlled, balanced salt solution. The bath water is gently agitated to facilitate the debridement process. Patients do not object to the bath as they do to other methods of debridement because the bath is soothing and relaxing, less painful for them and they can exercise more freely in the water.

Grafting of skin is done as early after the initial injury as possible. The physician usually waits until granulations

have begun to form and there is no gross necrotic tissue on the surface of the wound. The donor skin is best taken from the patient *(autogenous skin graft),* but when this is not possible, the skin of another person can be used *(homograft).* For further information on skin grafts, the reader is referred to Student Reading Reference No. 2.

Record of Intake and Output. This is one of the most important aspects of nursing a patient with burns. We know that many fluids and essential minerals are lost through the burned areas of skin, and these must be replaced so that a normal fluid and electrolyte balance is maintained. This loss of fluids results in a decrease in the amount of blood flowing through the kidneys, which may in turn lead to damage of the cells of the kidney.

The physician will depend on the nursing staff to keep an accurate record of the patient's intake and output of fluids and will use this information to determine the need for additional fluids or minerals. He may also order frequent laboratory tests of the blood to determine its electrolyte content.

In addition to keeping a careful record on the intake and output, the nurse must also observe the urine carefully for color and concentration. Blood in the urine may indicate damage to the kidneys; therefore, any unusually dark or abnormally colored urine should be reported. A large amount of very light colored urine frequently indicates overhydration and possible loss of essential minerals through the urine, while concentrated urine usually indicates dehydration.

Diet. During the period of healing and convalescence from the burn, the patient's diet is very important. The protein content is usually increased to several times that of a regular diet in order to assist the body as it rebuilds tissue. Dietary supplements for the severely burned patients usually include vitamins, especially vitamin C, minerals such as iron and electrolytes such as sodium, chloride and potassium.

The odor of the burn and the patient's despondency over his predicament may greatly contribute to a loss of appetite. Every device and trick known must be used to encourage the patient to eat all the meals and between-meal feedings prepared for him.

Emotional Aspects. We have mentioned the emotional shock of a severe burn and the understandable depression of the patient once he realizes what has happened to him. The nurse can surely understand that she must give the burn patient moral support and at the same time avoid having him become too dependent on the nursing staff. As is true in most long-term illnesses, there is a danger of complete boredom and apathy with a loss of the will to live unless diversional and occupational therapy are provided.

There is also a possibility of overdependence on drugs to relieve pain and anxiety if the nursing staff does not or will not attempt to make the patient comfortable through the use of simple nursing measures before administering drugs. The nurse must realize that a "p.r.n." order for a narcotic or sedative means the administration of the drug only as a last resort after all nursing measures have failed to make the patient comfortable.

Complications of Burns. Aside from the complications of pulmonary disease and circulatory stasis which are hazards for all patients confined to bed over a period of time, the burn patient must also be protected from the complications of infection of the wounds and contractures.

Of all the functions of the skin, that of protection from pathogenic organisms is the most important. The patient with a serious burn no longer has that protection, and so all exposure to possible sources of infection must be kept at a minimum. It is not possible to keep the environment completely free of bacteria, but ordinary precautions may greatly reduce the possibility of contaminating the wounds. These precautions include frequent and thorough washing of the hands, keeping all pressure dressings dry and clean and handling the dressings or open wounds as little as possible.

Another complication to be avoided in the severely burned patient is the development of *contractures.* These are a shortening of muscle tissue with loss of elasticity and resistance to stretching, leading to loss of motion in the affected part.

The development of contractures may be traced directly to improper positioning of the patient and lack of attention to exercises for the patient confined to bed. Burn patients are particularly susceptible to contractures because motion is often painful, and they tend to guard against this pain by staying in a fixed position unless encouraged to do otherwise.

If pressure dressings are used, the

nurse must see to it that parts which cannot be moved because of the dressings are at least kept in a position of optimum function so that foot drop and wrist drop are prevented. The parts of the body which can be moved must be exercised regularly. This is extremely difficult to accomplish if the nurse is overly sympathetic or the patient is insistent in his demands to be left alone. A common-sense approach must be used to solve the problem. Both the nursing staff and the patient must be fully aware of the crippling and permanent deformities which may result if the joints are not kept in motion and muscle tone is not maintained.

Rehabilitation should never be postponed until after the deformities occur. The long-range view must be taken so that the deformities are prevented rather than treated. Painful as the motion may be, the muscles must be gently stretched and used every day if they are to be kept in a good state of tone and functioning normally.

CLINICAL CASE PROBLEMS

1. As you are bathing a child in the pediatric ward one day, you observe some small blisters on her legs. Some of these blisters appear to have burst, and there is a honey-colored crust over them. These skin lesions were not reported to you when you assumed care of the child that morning, and there is no record of there having been any lesions present when she was admitted a week ago.

What are your responsibilities in regard to your observations?

If these lesions are diagnosed by the physician as impetigo contagiosa, what special nursing care will this child require while she is in the pediatric ward?

2. Mrs. Nation, age 32, is admitted to the ward with a diagnosis of severe contact dermatitis. Both her legs and arms are covered with a rash which causes much itching and burning.

What nursing measures can you use to help relieve her discomfort?

What effect will you expect the patient's mental attitude to have on her physical condition?

How can you help her to relax?

3. Martha M. is a 12-year-old child who was badly burned when her clothing caught fire while she was helping her mother cook hamburgers on an outdoor grill. She has second and third degree burns over her abdomen and chest and down the front of both of her legs. When you are assigned to care for Martha, she has been in the hospital for two weeks and has received much attention from her family and friends. She has become somewhat spoiled by all this attention and is very uncooperative when you attempt to do anything for her. In spite of the fact that she has no pressure dressings on her lower legs, she refuses to sit up and help herself in any way. She has refused most of her diet and prefers the soft drinks, candy bars and fruit that have been showered on her since her accident.

How can you help this child without arousing resentment and without offending her well-meaning family and friends?

REFERENCES

1. Beland, I. L.: *Clinical Nursing: Pathophysical and Psychosocial Approaches,* 2nd edition. New York, The Macmillan Co., 1970.
2. Ciporallo, A. J.: "Cancer of the Skin." Am. Journ. Nurs., Oct., 1966, p. 2231.
3. Conway, H., and Nayer, D.: "Skin Grafts: The Techniques, The Patient." Am. Journ. Nurs., Nov., 1964, p. 94.
4. Corliss, S.: "Improving Care of Severe Burn Wounds." Nursing '72, April, 1972, p. 6.
5. Derbes, V. J.: "Rashes: Recognition and Management." Nursing '73, March, 1973, p. 45.
6. Goldman, L.: "Prevention and Treatment of

Eczema." Am. Journ. Nurs., March, 1964, p. 114.
7. Jacoby, F.: "Current Nursing Care of the Burned Patient." Nurs. Clin. N. Amer., Vol. 5, No. 4, 1970, p. 563.
8. Judd, E.: "Herpes Zoster—A Nursing Challenge," Journ. Pract. Nurs., Nov., 1969, p. 27.
9. Larson, D., and Gaston, R.: "Current Trends in the Care of Burned Patients." Am. Journ. Nurs., Feb., 1967, p. 319.
10. Law, E. J.: "New Developments in Burn Care." Journ. Pract. Nurs., Oct., 1971, p. 24.
11. Minckley, B. B.: "Expert Nursing Care for Burned Patients." Am. Journ. Nurs., Sept. 1970, p. 1888.
12. Noonan, J., and Noonan, L.: "Two Burned Patients on Flotation Therapy." Am. Journ. Nurs., Feb., 1968, p. 317.
13. Samwitz, M. H.: "The Industrial Dermatoses." Am. Journ. Nurs., Jan., 1965, p. 79.
14. Shafer, K. et al.: Medical-Surgical Nursing, 5th edition, St. Louis, Mo., The C. V. Mosby Co., 1971.
15. Wechsler, H. L.: "Psoriasis." Am. Journ. Nurs., April, 1965, p. 85.
16. Wexler, L.: "Gamma Benzene Hexachloride in Treatment of Pediculosis and Scabies." Am. Journ. Nurs., March, 1969, p. 565.
17. Wood, M., et al.: "Silver Nitrate Treatment of Burns." Am. Journ. Nurs., March, 1966, p. 518.

SUGGESTED STUDENT READING

1. Argamaso, R. V., and Argamaso, C. A.: "Topical Sulfamylon—Current Adjunct in Burn Therapy." Bedside Nurse, Jan., 1971, p. 22.
2. Conway, H., and Nayer, D.: "Skin Grafts: The Techniques, The Patient." Am. Journ. Nurs., Nov., 1964, p. 94.
3. Henderson, J.: "An Odd Name for Odious Pain." Journ. Pract. Nurs., Dec., 1962, p. 30.
4. Horgan, P. D.: "How They Battle to Save the Badly Burned." RN, Feb., 1963, p. 46.
5. Judd, E.: "Herpes Zoster—A Nursing Challenge." Journ. Pract. Nurs., Nov., 1969, p. 27.
6. Law, E. J.: "New Developments in Burn Care." Journ. Pract. Nurs., Oct., 1971, p. 24.
7. "Case History of a Burned Seven Year Old." Journ. Pract. Nurs., Jan., 1968, p. 34.
8. "Taming the Sun." Journ. Pract. Nurs., April, 1963, p. 37.

OUTLINE FOR CHAPTER 13

I. Introduction

A. Skin protects against invasion of bacteria in the environment.
B. Helps regulate body temperature.
C. Holds in body fluids.

II. Diagnostic Tests and Examinations

A. Visual examination.
B. History—allergies, familial tendencies and environmental factors are important in determining cause of skin disorders.
C. Skin tests to determine an individual's sensitivity to specific substances.
D. Elimination diets—removal of foods that are suspected of causing the skin disease.
E. Cultures and sensitivity tests to determine pathogen causing a skin infection and to find an effective drug against it.

III. Factors in Prevention of Skin Disease

A. Cleanliness.
B. Good nutrition.
C. Age (older persons suffer from dryness of skin and loss of elasticity).
D. Environment—irritants such as chemicals and strong sunlight and other forms of radiation can lead to breakdown of skin.

IV. General Nursing Care

A. Rules for care include intelligent observation, careful handling of the skin and avoidance of alcohol, lotions or other skin applications not specifically ordered by the dermatologist.
B. Colloid baths—those in which soothing agents are added to the bath water. Avoid chilling the patient. Pat, do not rub, the skin dry after the bath.
C. Bed linens may require special laundering to remove all traces of soap.
D. Wet compresses or dressings are often used.

V. Herpes Simplex

A. Cold sores or fever blisters.
B. Caused by a virus similar to the one causing smallpox.

VI. Herpes Zoster ("Shingles")

A. A viral disease of the skin and peripheral sensory nerves.
B. Symptoms include blistering followed by scaling of the skin, skin lesions along nerve pathways, severe pain and itching in the affected area.

VII. Impetigo Contagiosa

A. A highly contagious bacterial infection of the skin.

B. Treatment consists of removal of crusts, thorough cleaning of the lesions and application of antibiotic ointments or administration of oral antibiotics.

VIII. Pediculosis and Scabies

A. Three general types of pediculi: head lice, body lice and pubic lice. Scabies is caused by the mange mite.

B. Most prevalent symptom is intense itching.

C. Treatment consists of application of 1 per cent gamma benzene hexachloride. The medication is left on the skin for 12 to 24 hours and then removed by thoroughly washing with soap and water. Also available as shampoo for head lice.

IX. Contact Dermatitis

A. An allergic eczema resulting from hypersensitivity to a substance that has come in contact with the skin.

B. Treatment includes removal of the antigen from contact with the skin, colloid baths and lotions to soothe the skin and dry the weeping lesions and antihistamines to control itching.

X. Acne

A. A skin disorder characterized by papules and pustules occurring at puberty.

B. No specific treatment.

XI. Psoriasis

A. A chronic and recurring disorder characterized by papules and adherent silvery scales that produce pinpoint bleeding when removed.

B. There is no known cure, but coal tar and mercury remedies used in conjunction with cortisone can keep the condition under control.

XII. Fungal Infections (Mycoses)

A. Examples are epidermophytosis (athlete's foot), tinea of the scalp (ringworm) or face (barber's itch) and moniliasis (thrush). All produce some itching and breakdown of the skin.

B. Fungistatic drugs such as griseofulvin are most helpful in the control of fungal infections.

XIII. Cancer of the Skin

A. Almost all cases can be treated successfully if they are caught early.

B. Causes are unknown but hereditary factors and environmental influences such as chronic irritation can increase susceptibility to skin cancer.

C. Treatment consists of surgical removal or radiation therapy.

D. Types include:
  1. Basal cell epithelioma.
  2. Squamous cell epithelioma.
  3. Melanocarcinoma.

XIV. Burns

A. Caused by exposure to heat, electrical agents, strong chemicals or radiation.

B. Classified as first degree, second degree or third degree.

C. Emergency treatment:
  1. All burns should be considered potentially dangerous.
  2. Salves or ointments should not be used without a physician's order.
  3. Immersion in ice water or cold compresses applied to the burn help relieve and reduce edema.
  4. Dangers are shock, infection and fluid loss.
  5. Nurse should anticipate the needs of the physician and have necessary equipment and medications prepared.

D. Treating the wound.
  1. New methods of treatment have reduced the mortality rate for severe burns. Most recent hazard is *Pseudomonas aeruginosa.*
  2. Infection remains the major cause of death in burned patients.
  3. Topical applications include:
     a. Silver nitrate 0.5 per cent soaks. Reaches only surface microorganisms and also produces loss of chlorides.
     b. Sulfamylon acetate cream 10 per cent. Has deeper penetrating effect but stings when applied and can also produce metabolic acidosis or allergic reaction in some patients.
     c. Combination of a sulfa drug and a silver salt is a newer compound now being tried.
  4. Two general methods of treating burn wounds: open and closed. There is no one "best" way to

treat a burn; patient must be treated on an individual basis.

    a. Open method (wound is cleansed and then left uncovered).

    b. Closed method (wound is cleansed and then covered with an occlusive dressing).

E. Record of intake and output essential for aiding physician in restoring and maintaining a normal fluid and electrolyte balance. Also important for determination of kidney damage that can occur in severe burns.

F. Diet—usually high protein with supplements of vitamins and minerals.

G. Emotional aspects must be considered because the patient may have permanent physical handicaps or cosmetic difficulties.

H. Complications of burns.

    1. Infection due to improper handling of burned area or equipment used for patient, or greatly lowered resistance of patient.

    2. Contractures as a result of improper positioning and inadequate exercise.

14

distal higher than proximal
hand & elbow & shoulder

Nursing Care of Patients With Disorders of the Musculoskeletal System

Bryant's Traction
Back Care - Slip hand
under

INTRODUCTION

The special branch of medical science concerned with the <u>preservation</u> and <u>restoration of the functions of the skeletal system</u> is called *orthopedics.* We cannot confine orthopedic nursing to patients with diseases and deformities of bones and joints, however, because the basic principles of orthopedic nursing are applicable to the nursing care of all patients, and most especially to those confined to bed. Whatever the diagnosis may be, attention to the musculoskeletal functions of the patient is essential to his general well-being and continued activity.

The three main functions of the musculoskeletal system are *motion, support* and *protection.* Of these three, the preservation of <u>motion is probably the most important</u> consideration as far as the

practical nurse is concerned. It is the <u>long bones of the limbs which give the body support and provide motion</u> by <u>acting as levers</u> to which the muscles are attached. <u>Joint motion is a result of the shortening and stretching of opposing sets of muscles.</u> For example, when the <u>flexor</u> muscles of the leg <u>contract</u> and shorten, the <u>opposing extensors must relax</u> and lengthen. Disuse or undue strain on these muscles can lead to permanent disabilities and loss of motion.

If we follow the development of bones within a person from conception to old age we can see that the bony tissues of the infant differ greatly from those of the adult. That is because all bone cells do not follow the same pattern of development from the embryonic stage to full maturity. There are <u>two distinct groups of bone cells</u>. Some

211

of them are designed so that they are immediately transformed into mature cells. The normal newborn infant will have this type of firm bone cells in his skull and shoulder bones. In the second group, the bone cells form cartilage first and then are gradually replaced by mature bone cells as the person grows older. Thus, the bones of an infant are really mostly cartilage. Ossification, or replacement of cartilage by more solid bony tissue, is not completed throughout the body until 20 to 25 years of age.

Because the bony structures of infants and young children are softer and more pliable, there is less danger of their breaking bones during the time of life when they are learning to walk and run and are therefore more likely to have frequent falls. If a fracture does occur, however, it will heal more rapidly in a very young person because growth is still taking place within the bone.

On the other hand, the bones of elderly persons are brittle and less compact, breaking easily. In addition, they do not heal readily when a fracture is sustained because the physiological exchange of minerals has decreased with advancing age, making the process of repair much slower.

In studying the process of bone development and repair, it must be remembered that bone is a living tissue, with a complex system of canals through which blood and lymph vessels pass. This system allows for the adequate transportation of nutrients to the bone cells and removal of wastes. There is also a continuous depositing of, storing and removing from the bony tissues certain minerals which are essential to the normal functioning of bones.

Muscles compose one third to one half of the body's entire bulk. In this chapter, we will be concerned only with the skeletal muscles which are instrumental in moving the various parts of the body. Involuntary muscles and cardiac muscle tissues will be discussed in appropriate chapters.

DIAGNOSTIC TESTS

X-ray Films. X-ray is the diagnostic aid most often used by the orthopedic surgeon. Through the use of roentgen rays, which are capable of penetrating structures less dense than bone, thereby presenting an outline of bony structures in the body, the physician is able to discover abnormal changes in the contour, size and density of bones.

Cultures. Samples of infected bone tissues are sometimes taken for the purpose of growing cultures in the laboratory. These cultures make it possible for the physician to determine the specific organism causing the infection and the appropriate drug to be used in the treatment of the infection.

Biopsy. In the case of bone tumors, the surgical removal of samples of the cells within the growth (biopsy) is an important diagnostic aid in determining the type of tumor present.

GENERAL NURSING CARE

Lifting and Turning the Patient. There are special skills necessary for the proper care of a patient with musculoskeletal disorders, particularly in regard to moving the patient and changing his linens.

First, the nurse must use good body mechanics herself so that she can safely and correctly use her strength to the greatest advantage. An awkward posture or failure to use the correct methods of lifting and moving the patient will often cause him unnecessary discomfort and apprehension about being moved and will also lead to painful muscle strain for the nurse.

Secondly, all movements must be gentle and firm. When moving or turning the patient, there should be sufficient help from adequately trained personnel. Each person involved, including the patient, should understand exactly what is going to be done and the steps to take in accomplishing the move. If the patient can help without

pt do as able ē danger to affected limb

danger to the diseased joint or limb, he should be encouraged to do so. If he is not able to help, the nurse explains the procedure to him and asks him to cooperate by relaxing completely during the procedure. Many times the patient is afraid that moving and turning will cause him pain. It is then necessary to help him understand the reasons for frequent changing of the position and gain his confidence and cooperation so that he will not make the task more difficult by resisting all efforts to turn him.

Nurses are sometimes tempted to allow their patient the privilege of assuming any position and remaining in that position as long as he appears comfortable. They reason that it seems unkind and unnecessary to force the patient to move about when he is apparently resting and does not wish to be disturbed. This is actually not a kindness and could be considered as nothing short of neglect when we know the terrible consequences of poor body posture.

The nurse might also take the time to find a reason for the patient's assuming certain postures in bed. It is possible that the patient is curled up in a fetal position because he is trying to keep warm. Older patients and those with poor circulation instinctively huddle their shoulders and tuck their limbs close to their bodies when they are chilly. It is also possible that the patient is flexing his knees, hips and back because he is attempting to relieve pain in his abdomen or lower legs. These possibilities should always be considered, and they should make the nurse even more aware of her responsibility in performing sensible and practical nursing measures for the comfort of her patient.

Orthopedic Bed Making. When a patient has traction applied to an upper or lower limb, or when he is in a large body cast, it is not always convenient to arrange the bed linens in the conventional manner. Some institutions in which there are large orthopedic units provide specially made linens which have been designed so that bed making and changing of linen is much easier for the nurse and less disturbing to the orthopedically handicapped patient. If there is such linen available, the practical nurse should seek specific instructions in its use.

In institutions in which there is no such linen available, the practical nurse must improvise with the materials she has at hand. This requires some ingenuity and imagination, but it can be done. For example, two draw sheets may be used for the foundation of the bed in lieu of one large bottom sheet. This would be useful in instances in which the patient's lower limb is in a traction apparatus which uses a frame resting on the mattress rather than suspended from an overhead frame. Obviously there will be a good bit of disturbance of the frame and the traction if the large bottom sheet must be changed each time it becomes soiled. When two draw sheets are used, however, only the draw sheet under the patient's body need by changed and the frame will not be disturbed at all. Top covers may be folded so that the limb in traction is not covered. If extra warmth is needed for the affected limb, it can be covered with a small baby blanket.

One important point to remember in changing the linen is avoidance of pulling sheets from under the patient and causing friction against the skin. The patient confined to bed for a long period of time must have his skin preserved at all costs. He must be gently turned on and off the sheets being changed; sheets are never pulled from under him.

Prevention of Deformities. The nurse must constantly bear in mind her responsibilities in the prevention of deformities for all of her patients. Maintenance of good body position, preservation of muscle tone and continued joint motion are no less important for the patient with a stroke or the burned patient than they are for the patient with an orthopedic disorder. No matter what the diagnosis, the patient confined to bed over a prolonged period of time will need proper positioning of the joints and adequate exercising of the limbs in order to prevent irreparable damage and deformities. Nursing measures that prevent deformities and helplessness are initiated and consistently carried out by the nursing staff. To wait for a physician's order for care that is the nurse's responsibility is tantamount to negligence on the part of the nurse.

The deformities most commonly associated with poor positioning and lack of exercise are *contractures, loss of muscle tone* and *ankylosis*. The first two are directly concerned with the muscles; ankylosis affects the bones.

CONTRACTURES. When skeletal muscles are not regularly stretched and contracted to their normal limits, they attempt to adapt themselves to this limited use by becoming shorter and less elastic. This "adaptive shortening" is referred to as a contracture. The most frequent contractures occurring in patients confined to bed for long periods of time are "foot drop," knee and hip flexion contractures, "wrist drop" and contractures of the arm (see Fig. 14-1).

LOSS OF MUSCLE TONE. We know that joint motion is a result of the shortening and stretching of opposing muscles. That is, when the flexor muscles of the leg contract and shorten, the opposing extensor muscles must relax and lengthen. Muscle tone is defined as the readiness of the muscles to go to work, to contract and relax as needed. If a muscle is not stimulated to action regularly, or if it is stretched beyond its normal limits for an extended period of time, it will lose its ability to work. An example is "foot drop," in which the calf muscles are shortened and the opposing flexor muscles are stretched so that they lose their "tone."

ANKYLOSIS. Ankylosis is a permanent fixation of a joint and is the result of a disease or injury in which the tissues of the joint are replaced by a bony overgrowth which completely obliterates the joint. Sometimes this process cannot be prevented, as, for example, in some types of arthritis. In these cases, the physician braces the joint in the position that will be most useful to the patient, even though there

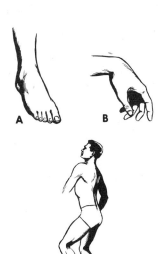

Figure 14–1. *A,* Foot drop resulting from improper support of the feet while patient is confined to bed. A simple footboard could easily prevent this deformity. *B,* Wrist drop resulting from improper support of the hand. *C,* Flexion contracture of knee and hip force this patient to walk on tiptoe on the affected side. If both legs are involved, walking is impossible.

is no motion in the joint. Imagine your wrist locked in a position in which the palm and fingers are dangling at right angles to the lower arm. Now imagine your wrist locked in a position in which the wrist is slightly flexed. If you had your choice of positions, you would choose the one in which your wrist was slightly flexed, because this would allow you to perform many of your daily activities. The term used for these positions of choice is "positions of optimum use" or "positions of maximum function." In her daily care of patients who have their joints braced in positions of this kind, the practical nurse must use care that the limb is in the position established by the physician.

Nursing Care in Prevention of Deformities. We have stated that good body position and exercises are necessary for prevention of the type of deformities defined above. It is important, therefore, that the nurse fully understand her role in the prevention of such deformities.

Good body position for the patient simply means good posture for the patient confined to the bed or wheelchair. The nurse can judge whether her patient has good posture in bed by observing him to see if his position conforms to the following rules:

1. The back is straight with the normal curves of the spine unexaggerated.

2. The legs are *slightly flexed* to relieve the strain on the lumbar spine, the abdomen and the legs.

3. The ribs are elevated and the rib cage supported so that constriction is prevented.

4. The legs are supported so that the weight of one does not fall on the other.

5. Excessive ankle extension is prevented.[11]

Figure 14-2 illustrates the correct positioning and support of the patient according to the above rules. Since any position is tiring if maintained too long, it is also necessary for the nurse to assist the patient in changing his position at least every two hours.

Even though it is well understood by the nurse that changing the body positions from supine to side to prone will prevent decubitus ulcers, circulatory stasis and respiratory and urinary complications, she may not fully appreciate the fact that *changing of the body's position will not guarantee freedom from orthopedic deformities. It is also necessary to change joint positions.* Figure 14-3 illustrates this very important point. In order to prevent ankylosis of the joints and contractures of the muscles, the nurse must remember to flex and extend the limbs alternately when she changes the patient's position.

Another important point in the prevention of orthopedic deformities is the matter of exercise. Physical therapists tell us that all joints should be put through their full range of motion at least once daily, preferably more often. If the patient is not able to do the exercises, the nurse or physical therapist must carry out *passive exercises* – help for him. If the patient is able to perform the exercises under the guidance of the nurse or physical therapist, the term used is *active exercises.* on own

The responsibility of the practical nurse in regard to these exercises lies in her obligation to familiarize herself with the exercises necessary for each individual patient and to carry out these exercises as ordered. She will find that in some cases it will not be possible to exercise all of the joints because of traction to a limb or a cast covering certain parts of the body. In other instances, the more complicated exercises will require the attention of the physical therapist. The ideal time for the administration of passive exercises to the limbs so that each joint is put through its full range of motion is during the morning bath. They take so little time, and they could easily be made a part of the routine morning care.

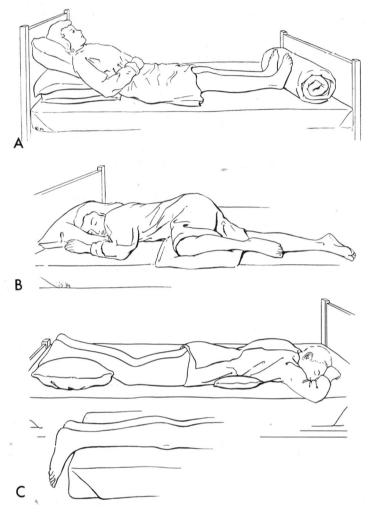

Figure 14–2. *A,* Patient lying on back. Blanket roll or footboard and pillows may be used to keep feet in correct position. Note support of patient's back with pillows. *B,* Patient lying on side. Pillow is placed under knee to maintain good alignment of back. *C,* Patient lying in prone position. Small pillow is placed under abdomen and under lower legs. Alternate position of feet may be used to maintain correct position of feet. (A and B, from Todd and Freeman: *Health Care of the Family.* C, from Montag and Swenson: *Fundamentals in Nursing Care,* 3rd Ed., W. B. Saunders Co., Philadelphia.)

Emotional Aspects of Orthopedic Disorders. Unfortunately, many orthopedic conditions require prolonged periods of confinement to bed, or, at best, immobilization of a part of the body and restricted physical activities. This leads to frustration and a feeling of hopelessness and despair on the part of the patient so confined. When the patient is young and unaccustomed to dependence on others for his personal care, he may react with anger and bitterness toward his plight. If the patient is a wage-earner or an active member of the family, and one upon whom others are dependent, he has the additional burden of financial and social problems.

Immobilization and some degree of helplessness can greatly affect a patient's personality. Some never cease to rebel against the situation, while others

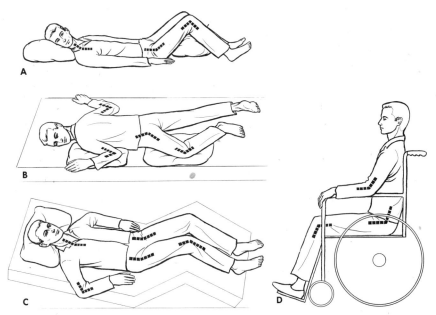

Figure 14–3. In these illustrations, the patient's body position has been changed four times, and yet the positions of the joints at the knees, hips, elbows and neck have been changed very little or not at all.

become "institutionalized" and do not wish to return to their former lives and responsibilities. The nurse must understand that the long convalescent period filled with tedious hours of waiting for the bone to heal and the surrounding tissues to mend is a very difficult time for the patient. She will need much tact and patience as well as a lively imagination to help him spend his time happily and busily. Occupational therapy is available in most institutions and should be used to the fullest for the orthopedic patient. Suggestions offered in Chapter 8 of this text may be of help to the practical nurse in her efforts to provide suitable recreation for the orthopedically handicapped.

NURSING CARE OF THE PATIENT IN A CAST

Casts are used for the purpose of immobilizing a certain part of the body so that it is firmly supported and completely at rest in a specific position.

Types of Casts. Leg and arm casts may cover all or part of the limb. These are called long-leg or short-leg casts, depending on how much of the leg they cover. A walking cast is a leg cast with extra material added to the sole for weight bearing. This is most often a metal bar ("walking iron") covered with rubber. A spica cast covers the trunk of the body and one or both extremities. There are long-leg and short-leg spicas, which cover one or both legs, and shoulder spicas which include the trunk and one arm.

The material most commonly used for casts is plaster of paris. This material is used because it is cheap, durable, fairly easy to apply, and readily available. Plaster of paris is gypsum from which the water has been removed. Strips of crinoline are impregnated with this plaster and are available in various widths. When they are to be used, these strips are soaked in water and applied wet. When the material dries, there is a firm shell of plaster molded to the exact shape of the part of the body to which it has been applied.

Preparation for Application of a Cast. The mattress and pillows of the patient with a cast should be protected with a waterproof material until the cast is completely dry. Most orthopedic surgeons prefer a firm cotton mattress with steel or wooden slats underneath to prevent sagging of the mattress, resulting in improper support of the cast.

Before a cast is applied, the patient's skin is thoroughly cleaned with soap and water, and any breaks in the skin are reported to the doctor if he is not aware of them. Shaving is not done unless surgery is to be performed before application of the cast. In this case, a special orthopedic surgical preparation according to the hospital procedure is necessary.

In emergencies, a thorough explanation of what is going to be done is not always possible. In all other cases, however, it is best if the patient is prepared for the type of cast that will be applied, the precautions that must be taken while the cast is drying and any special devices that may be put on his bed to help him turn and move about in the bed. An example is the trapeze bar attached to an overhead frame which allows the patient to lift himself and turn without strain on the affected part.

Care of the Fresh Plaster Cast. The newly applied cast is usually not dry for a period of time, most often 48 hours, depending on the type of cast. While the plaster is damp, its shape can be changed by careless handling or improper support. It follows, therefore, that extreme care must be used in moving the patient or the cast during this time.

When transferring the patient from the stretcher to the bed, there must be enough help available so that the patient is not "tumbled" into bed. Pillows for support should be placed on the bed before moving the patient onto them. For large casts, pillows are used to support the curves of the cast so that there will be no cracking or flattening of the cast by the weight of the body (see Fig. 14-4).

The patient in a body cast or spica is more comfortable if pillows are not put under the head and shoulders, because they push the chest and abdomen against the front of the cast, causing an uncomfortable crushing sensation and dyspnea.

While a cast is still damp, it should not be grasped by the fingers in the process of lifting or moving it. An effort should be made to use only the palms of the hands or the flat surface of the extended fingers. The reason for this is apparent when we realize that fingertips can sink into the damp plaster and make impressions through the thickness of the cast, thus pressing mounds of plaster against the tissues under the cast. These can harden and will in time lead to pressure sores.

Drying the Cast. The speed with which a plaster cast will dry is directly

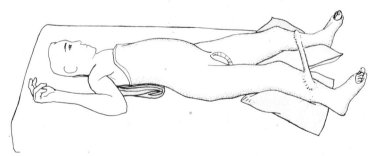

Figure 14–4. Proper support of cast so that weight of body does not flatten curves in cast. (From Wiebe: *Orthopedics in Nursing,* W. B. Saunders Co., Philadelphia.)

affected by (1) the humidity of the atmosphere around the cast and (2) circulation of air around the cast.

Thick body casts sometimes take several days to dry out completely. Others, such as the thin casts for club-foot or long-leg casts, may dry within a few hours. A cast dryer, similar in principle to a hair dryer, may be used to speed up the evaporation of moisture from the cast. The advantage of using the dryer is the increased circulation of air around the cast, NOT the application of heat. The use of heat is dangerous because it may easily lead to burns under the cast. It is also possible that heat exhaustion and excessive loss of body fluids from perspiration will occur. A dryer should not be used without a written order.

Frequent turning of the patient helps the cast dry evenly and prevents prolonged pressure and flattening of one side of the cast. The patient should always be turned onto his "good side," i.e., with the fractured limb uppermost, while the cast is drying.

Bed cradles are not advisable, as they trap the moisture and increase the humidity around the cast. The patient in a cast may experience chilling from the dampness. He should be covered adequately with blankets, but the cast must remain uncovered until it is thoroughly dry.

It is not possible to determine whether a cast is dry simply by feeling its surface; therefore, it should be handled very carefully for the first few days or until the physician states specifically that the cast is dry. A dry cast is white, has a shiny surface and will resound when tapped. A wet cast is grayish and dull in appearance and will give a dull thud when tapped.

Complications to Be Watched for. Gangrene and/or paralysis can result from swelling under the cast or pressure on an area that is not properly supported. It is the responsibility of the nurse to make frequent and intelligent observations of her patient and

to report any unusual events promptly and accurately. The following statements will serve as a guide for the nurse caring for the patient in a cast.

1. *Listen to the patient's complaints.* If he complains of numbness, a tingling sensation or sharp localized pain due to pressure of the cast, report it immediately. Do not attempt to judge whether his complaints are justifiable. A dull throbbing pain can sometimes be relieved by elevating the limb. If not, this should also be reported.

2. *Observe the fingers or toes protruding from a cast for signs of impaired circulation.* These signs include a bluish-gray discoloration of the skin, coldness to the touch or slow return of color to the skin after pressure by a finger.

3. *A sudden, unexplained elevation of temperature or unusual odor may indicate infection.* Either of these signs should be brought to the attention of the nurse in charge or the physician.

4. *Check frequently to see if the cast is properly supported or if there is undue pressure on any one part of the body.*

Daily Care. After the cast is thoroughly dry and the initial swelling under the cast has subsided, the practical nurse must concern herself with the cleanliness of the patient and the cast. The problems involved will vary according to the type of cast and the area it covers. All parts of the body not included in the cast should be bathed daily, using care not to wet the cast with bath water. The skin around the edges of the cast should receive special attention, including massage with alcohol or lotion and close observation for signs of pressure or breaks in the skin. The edges of plaster casts tend to crumble, with bits of plaster dropping down inside the cast and causing the patient discomfort and skin irritation. This can be avoided by covering the rims of the cast with stockinette or tape.

Wetting a cast will cause it to disintegrate rapidly. After it has been thoroughly dried, a cast can be painted with shellac or varnish, which allows for cleaning of the surface and removal of stains without damage to the cast.

The patient in a long-leg cast or a spica can very easily soil the cast when attempting to use the bedpan. The problem of protecting the cast is even more difficult when the patient is a very young child who is not yet toilet trained, or an older patient who is incontinent. To avoid soiling, the perineal area of the cast can be covered with a waterproof material, such as the waxed paper or plastic wrapping used to keep refrigerated foods airtight. The material should be applied so that it covers the outside edge of the cast and extends down inside the cast for a few inches. This covering may be changed as often as necessary and also gives the added advantage of allowing for thorough cleaning of the buttocks and perineal area without danger of wetting the cast with bath water.

When a bedpan is used by the patient in a spica, there is the possibility of a backward flow of urine under the cast unless the head of the bed is slightly elevated. Since the patient cannot bend at the hips to sit up on the pan, the head of the bed should be elevated on shock blocks or some other device and the lumbar area of the cast supported to prevent cracking it.

Itching is a common complaint of the patient in a cast. Patients must be instructed not to use sharp objects such as pencils or rulers to scratch under the cast. These can, of course, tear the skin, leaving an open break for the entrance of bacteria. A coat hanger, bent so there is a safe round edge to use for scratching, will help the patient who is determined to scratch. This can be suggested, but may be done only with the approval of the physician.

When a cast is removed, the underlying skin is usually dry and scaly. Cleaning of these areas should be done under the direction of the physician, since the type of care to be given will depend on whether or not another cast is to be applied. In any case, over-enthusiastic scrubbing of the area must be avoided so as to prevent damage to the deeper layers of skin.

NURSING CARE OF THE PATIENT IN TRACTION

Types and Uses of Traction. Traction is the application of a mechanical *pull* to a part of the body for the purpose of extending and holding that part in a certain position. Through a system of ropes and pulleys, weights are attached to a fixed point below the area of injury or disease. The apparatus is rigged so that the weights on one end and the weight on the patient's body on the other will pull the affected part in opposite directions, thus straightening and holding that part in the desired position. There are several ways of accomplishing this. The two general types of traction are *skeletal* and *skin traction.* In skeletal traction, the surgeon inserts pins, wires or tongs directly through the bone at a point distal to the fracture, so that the force of pull from the weights is exerted directly on the bone. With skin traction, a bandage such as moleskin or ace-adherent is applied to the limb below the site of fracture and the pull is exerted on the limb in this manner. For cervical traction, either method may be used. Crutchfield tongs are inserted directly into the skull for skeletal traction, or a cloth head halter may be applied for skin traction (Fig. 14-5).

The most common types of traction apparatus used are Bryant's traction for small children, Russell traction and the Thomas splint with Pearson attachment (see Fig. 14-6).

Traction is used in the treatment of fractures and contracture deformities and to relieve the muscle spasm of severe back pain.

Most traction patients must lie on their backs with a limited amount of turning on either side. This is not an excuse for neglect of the patient's back. He must still be kept clean and com-

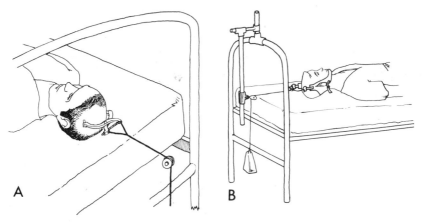

Figure 14–5. *A,* Skeletal traction of the cervical vertebrae, using tongs. *B,* Halter traction, applying straight pull on the cervical vertebrae. (From Wiebe: *Orthopedics in Nursing,* W. B. Saunders Co., Philadelphia.)

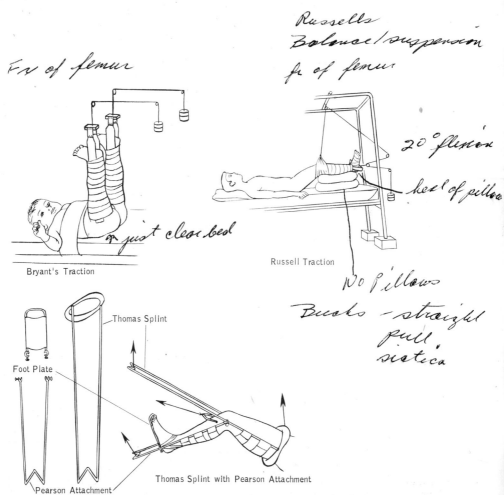

Fx of femur

Russells Balance / suspension fr of femur

20° flexion

heel of pillow

No Pillows

Bucks - straight pull. sistica

Bryant's Traction

Russell Traction

just clear bed

Thomas Splint

Foot Plate

Pearson Attachment

Thomas Splint with Pearson Attachment

Figure 14–6. Various types of traction. (From Wiebe: *Orthopedics in Nursing,* W. B. Saunders Co., Philadelphia.)

fortable and free of pressure sores. Special back care, particularly in the sacral region where pressure is greatest, must be given every hour. This includes a gentle massaging of the area with lotion, use of a rubber ring at intervals to relocate the area of pressure and careful attention to keeping the bottom sheet clean, dry and free of wrinkles.

The bottom sheets are always changed *starting with the unaffected side.* This decreases the number of times the affected side is disturbed. To provide adequate covering of the patient, two sets of top linen may be used if specially made fracture linen is not available. One set covers the upper half of the body and the other set covers the lower half and the unaffected limb. A small cotton baby blanket may be used to cover the limb in traction.

If the physician will not permit turning the patient far enough to allow for adequate back care, the patient may use a trapeze bar to lift himself so that back care can be given and the bottom sheet changed or tightened. The patient should be instructed to lift himself straight up so that the amount of pull exerted on the limb in traction will not be altered. This same maneuver can be used when the patient is placed on a bedpan (see Fig. 14-7). A small, child-size bedpan should be used and the lower back supported by a small pillow or folded blanket.

Frequent observations of both the patient and the traction apparatus should include the following:

1. *Be sure the weights are hanging free.* If the weights are resting on or against any support such as the foot of the bed or the floor, the purpose of the traction is lost. Be careful not to bump against the weights when walking around the foot of the bed. This can be painful to the patient and may cause damage to the diseased bone. It is not necessary to lift the weights when pulling the patient up in bed. The amount of pull on the limb will remain the same as long as the weights are hanging free.

2. *Check the position of the patient, making sure his body weight is counteracting the pull of the weights.* Should the patient slip down in bed so that his feet are resting against the footboard, there will be a loss of force exerted on the limb. *not foot plate against bed*

3. Observe all bony prominences for signs of impaired circulation and tissue necrosis.

4. Observe the patient's posture in bed and position of joints for proper alignment.

CARE OF THE PATIENT ON A FRAME

There are times when the nursing care of a patient with an orthopedic

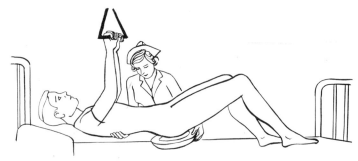

Figure 14–7. Patient lifts body straight up by pushing down with one or both feet and pulling up on trapeze. Small of back is supported by nurse's hand. After patient is on bedpan, a folded towel may be used to support the lumbar curve of spine. (From Wiebe: *Orthopedics in Nursing,* W. B. Saunders Co., Philadelphia.)

condition is extremely difficult if the patient is lying on a conventional hospital bed. To solve the nursing problems brought about by these conditions, there are specially designed frames or orthopedic beds available. The Stryker frame and Foster bed are examples of these frames. They are used (1) to facilitate the nursing care and frequent turning of patients who are helpless, (2) to aid in immobilizing the spine as a means of treating spinal fractures and other diseases of the spine and (3) to provide a means of keeping clean and dry those patients who cannot be moved for placement of a bedpan or those who are incontinent.

There are several modifications of the frames, but the basic structure consists of two metal frames covered with a heavy duck or canvas material. One of the frames is designed so that there is a perineal opening under the buttocks, and this frame is used when the patient is lying on his back. The second frame is covered so that it matches its

mate and is used when the patient is lying in a prone position. The position of the patient may be alternated from back to abdomen by using alternate frames. In the prone position, the head of the patient is supported with a strap across the forehead so that the face is uncovered, allowing for eating, reading or any other simple recreational activity. In addition to the frames, there are detachable supports for the arms, and a footboard attachment for proper positioning of the patient's feet.

Since turning the patient is a comparatively easy procedure when these frames are used, many complications caused by the patient's lying in one position too long can be avoided. It must be remembered, however, that these patients are *more likely to develop decubitus ulcers* than those in a conventional bed unless they are turned at least every two hours.

Turning the Patient. The practical nurse caring for a patient on a frame must seek instruction in the use of

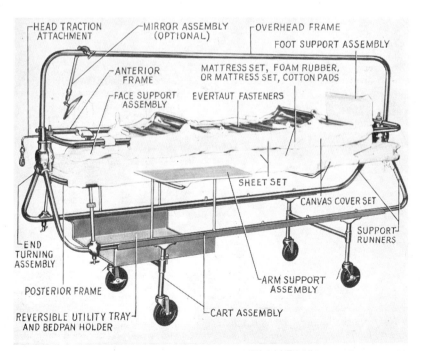

Figure 14–8. The Stryker turning frame. (Courtesy of the Orthopedic Frame Company, Kalamazoo, Michigan.)

these frames before accepting any responsibility for such a task. Unless the patient is turned quickly and smoothly and is adequately strapped onto the frame, there is danger of injury to the patient and disturbance of the body alignment desired by the physician. It is strongly recommended that the practical nurse observe and assist with the use of the frame before attempting to care for the patient on a frame (see Fig. 14-9).

Daily Care. When bathing the patient on a frame, the usual procedure for a bed bath must be altered. The anterior portion of the patient's body is washed while the patient is lying on

Bathe one side turn bed other frame other side bathe

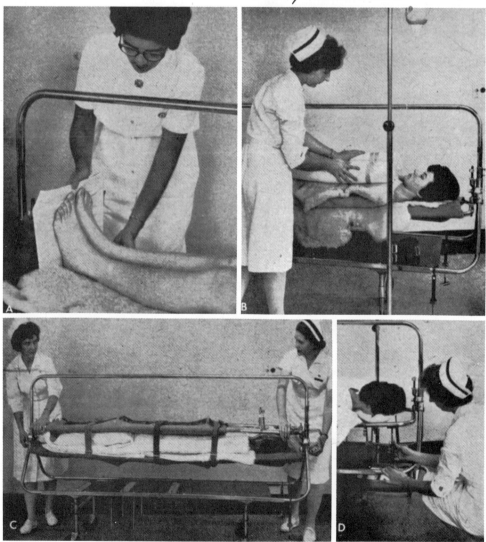

Figure 14–9. A, Foot support, taken from the posterior frame, is used to prevent foot drop. B, Rolls of foam rubber and pillow supports prevent pressure on patient's chest and upper abdomen. C, The anterior frame is securely strapped and screwed into position prior to turning the patient. Nurses stand at head and at foot of frame to execute the turn. D, The turn accomplished, the posterior frame is removed and the arm boards and the utility board are positioned. (From Dalton: American Journal of Nursing, February, 1964.)

the posterior frame. He is then turned onto the matching frame while the remaining portions of the body are bathed.

There should be adequate support of the buttocks over the perineal opening of the frame while the patient is on his back, or there will be a disturbance of alignment of the spine and added pressure on the sacral region. When the patient wishes to use the bedpan, the perineal or buttock strap is removed and the pan is placed on the rack beneath the opening. A piece of waterproof material may be tucked up under the buttocks and the other end placed in the bedpan to direct the flow of urine into the bedpan. Before replacing the supporting strap under the buttocks, the perineum and buttocks are thoroughly cleaned, dried and powdered.

The CircOlectric Bed

The CircOlectric bed (see Fig. 14-10) is an electrically operated frame similar in principle to the Stryker frame, except that the patient is turned head-over-heels rather than from side to side. Although this procedure may be somewhat frightening to both patient and nurse who are unfamiliar with the operation of the apparatus, the bed is relatively simple to operate and has several advantages.

The bed can be rotated so that the patient is in a prone position, a supine position or a sitting position. If the patient is able to do so and is confident about the operation of the bed, he can manipulate it himself using the hand controls. Use of the CircOlectric bed is not limited to patients in traction. It can also be utilized for burned patients to facilitate turning and applications of medication and for patients with neck injuries.[12]

CRUTCH WALKING

Introduction. For the convalescent patient or one who may always need support while walking, crutches can mean the difference between freedom to move about and confinement to one location. Before attempting to walk with crutches, one should have sufficient instruction in their use and manipulation so that they can be handled safely and effectively. The ease with which some persons apparently handle themselves on crutches is the result of patience and hard work to learn the proper use of crutches.

The type of crutch to be used will depend on the amount of disability or paralysis present and the patient's ability to bear weight and keep his balance on his feet. If the crutches are too short or too long, they can create problems of lifting and moving about for the patient. In regard to this, one must bear in mind that the muscles of the arms, shoulders, back and chest are all used in the manipulation of crutches. Since this is true, many physical therapists start the patient on special exercises to strengthen these muscles several weeks before the patient begins to use the crutches.

Gaits. The patient usually learns at least two gaits if he is to be using the crutches for an extended period of time. Usually he learns one for rapid movement and one for walking in crowded conditions or close quarters.

The gaits described in Fig. 14-11 are those most often used. The term "point" indicates the number of points of contact with the ground. A three-point gait, for example, uses two crutches and one foot; a four-point gait uses both feet and two crutches.

FRACTURES

Definition. A fracture is a break or interruption in the continuity of a bone. The amount of injury to the neighboring tissues varies according to the type of fracture, but at the site of injury there is always some degree of tissue destruction, interference with

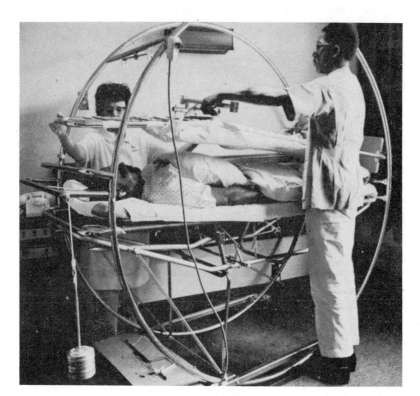

A

Figure 14-10. *A,* Attendant helps place the anterior frame of CircOlectric bed over this patient. Pillows have been placed on his abdomen to provide comfort and to assure that the patient is safely positioned between the anterior and posterior frames. Properly aligning the body and keeping the patient's arms along his sides are points to keep in mind in preparing the patient. (From Hrobsky: American Journal of Nursing, December, 1971.)

the blood supply and disturbance of muscle activity in that area.

Types of Fractures. *Complete fracture* is the breaking of a bone into two parts with complete separation of the two broken ends. An *incomplete fracture* is the breaking of a bone into two parts, but the two fragments are not completely separated.

A *comminuted* fracture is one in which the bone is broken and shattered into more than two fragments.

A *closed (simple) fracture* is one in which there is no break in the skin.

An *open (compound) fracture* is one

c̄ or s̄ protuberance
in which there is a break in the skin through which the fragments of broken bone protrude.

A *greenstick fracture,* commonly found in children, is one in which the bone is partially bent and partially broken. Other types of fracture may be classified according to their appearance on x-ray (see Fig. 14-12).

Treatment. The primary aim in the treatment of fractures is the establishment of a sturdy union between the broken ends of bone so that the bone can be restored to its former state of continuity. The healing and repair of a

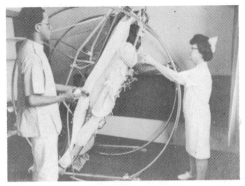

B

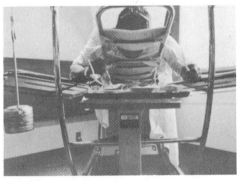

C

B, Attendant uses controls to rotate patient to prone position. *C,* Patient can assume sitting position by using controls himself. (From Hrobsky: Bedside Nurse, December, 1971.)

fracture begins immediately after the bone is broken and goes through four stages:

(1) Blood oozing from the torn blood vessels in the area of the fracture clots and begins to form a hematoma between the two broken ends of bone.

(2) Other tissue cells enter the clot and granulation tissue is formed. This tissue is interlaced with capillaries, and it gradually becomes firm and forms a bridge between the two ends of broken bone.

(3) Young bone cells enter the area and form a tissue called "woven bone." At this stage, the ends of the broken bone are beginning to "knit" together.

(4) The immature bone cells are gradually replaced by mature bone cells and the tissue takes on the characteristics of typical bone structure.

It is hoped that a thorough understanding of these stages of healing in the process of bone repair will make the nurse more aware of the need for gentle handling of a fractured bone while it is in the process of healing.

To facilitate the process of repair and insure proper healing of the bone without deformity or loss of function, the surgeon must bring the two broken ends together in proper alignment and then immobilize the affected part until healing is complete. The procedure for

Text continued on page 231

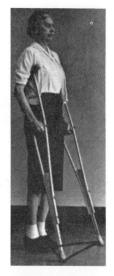

Figure 14-11. Left, the tripod position. All gaits begin from this stance. Below, the four-point alternate gait, the slowest and safest crutch gait. It offers maximum balance and support because there are always three points of contact with the ground. The right crutch is brought forward, then the left foot. The left crutch comes forward and then the right foot. *(Continued on opposite page.)*

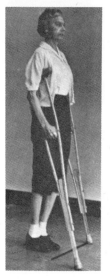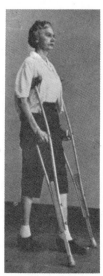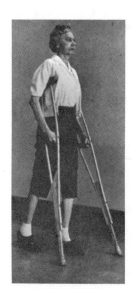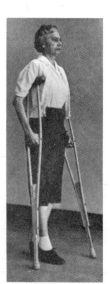

Figure 14–11 *continued.* This three-point gait, used by patients who can bear a little weight on their injured leg or foot, begins from the tripod position. Both crutches and the affected leg are brought forward at the same time. The patient must then rest lightly on the crutches while she moves forward the unaffected limb.

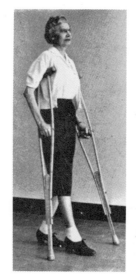
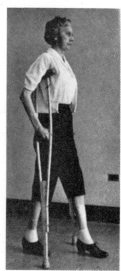

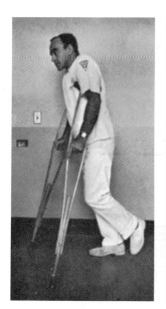
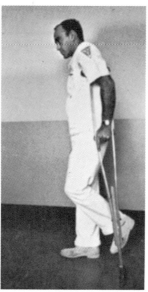

Figure 14–11 *continued.* This three-point is used by patients who cannot bear any weight on the affected leg or foot. It begins from the tripod position. Then both crutches are brought forward, and the uninjured leg is swung through the crutches. The affected leg is kept off the ground. *(Continued on next page.)*

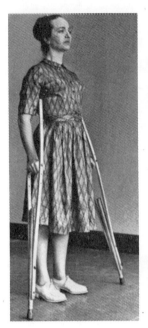
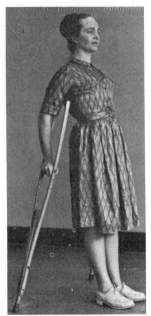

Figure 14–11 *continued.* The swing-through gait is used mainly by paraplegics and severe arthritics who have good balance and muscle power in the arms and hands. From the tripod position, both crutches are brought forward. The patient bears down on the handpieces, lifts the body, and swings it through crutches into a reversed tripod position. To maintain balance in this gait, pelvis moves first, then shoulders and head.

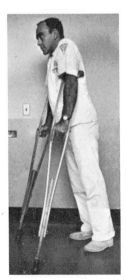
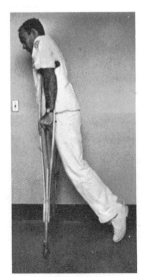
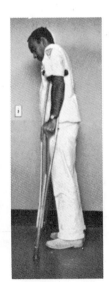

Figure 14–11 *continued.* The swing-to gait is slower than the swing-through gait. From the tripod position, the patient places both crutches forward and then swings his body ahead into a tripod position. The crutches and feet must never be even or patient loses stability. In the drag-to gait, the feet are slid along the ground and not raised. (From: *The Modern Medical Encyclopedia,* Vol. 3, Western Publishing Co., Ind., Racine, Wisconsin.)

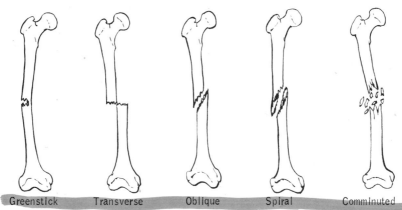

| Greenstick | Transverse | Oblique | Spiral | Comminuted |

Figure 14–12. Types of fractures classified according to their appearance on x-ray. (From Wiebe: *Orthopedics in Nursing*, W. B. Saunders Co., Philadelphia.)

bringing the two fragments of bone into proper alignment is called *reduction of the fracture* (see Fig. 14-13).

There are three methods of reducing a fracture: (1) closed reduction, (2) open reduction and (3) internal fixation.

Closed reduction is done by manual manipulation of the bone without making a surgical incision into the skin. A general anesthetic may be given before the fracture is reduced.

An *open reduction* is done after a surgical incision is made through the skin and down to the bone at the site of the fracture. In cases of open (compound) fractures, or comminuted fractures, an open reduction is always necessary so that adequate cleansing of the area and removal of bone fragments can be done.

When a fracture cannot be properly reduced by either open or closed reduction and it is impossible to guarantee adequate union of the bone fragments, the physician must perform a procedure called *internal fixation* of the bone. This means that pins, nails, screws or metal plates must be used to stabilize the position of the two broken ends. This type of operation is particularly useful in the treatment of fractures in elderly patients whose bones are brittle and will not heal properly (see Fig. 14-14).

In elderly patients who have suffered a fracture of the head of the femur, the surgeon may choose to take out the broken head fragments and replace it with a prosthesis. This device is designed so that it has a ball to replace the head of the femur and is shaped so that it can be fitted into or onto the shaft of the femur in such a way that the patient can bear weight on it. Although a prosthesis is not as good as a normal hip joint, many patients who have such a prosthesis are able to walk again and use the limb effectively.[19]

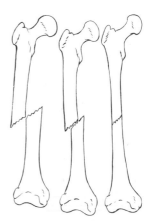

Figure 14–13. Reduction of a fractured bone. A gradual pull is exerted on the distal (lower) fragment of the bone until it is in alignment with the proximal fragment. (From Wiebe: *Orthopedics in Nursing*, W. B. Saunders Co., Philadelphia.)

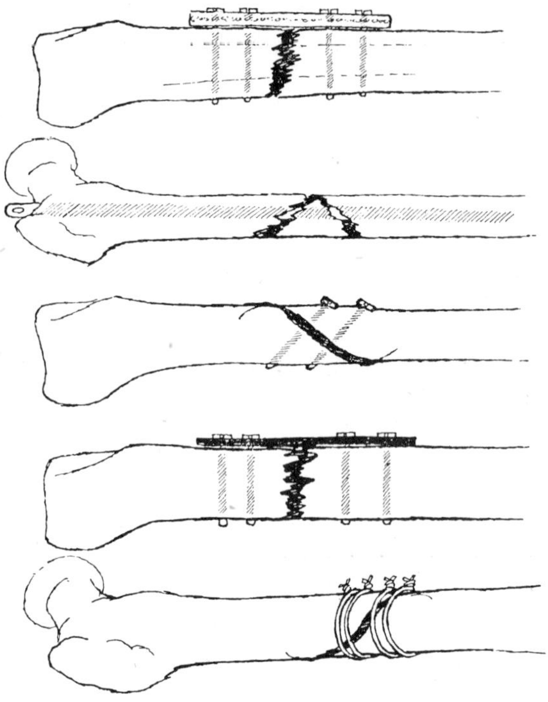

Figure 14–14. Illustrations of various methods of internal fixation, using plates, pins, nails or screws to hold fragments of bone in place. (From Wiebe: *Orthopedics in Nursing*, W. B. Saunders Co., Philadelphia.)

NURSING CARE. The emergency treatment and nursing care of fractures consist of preventing shock and hemorrhage and the immediate immobilization of the part to avoid unnecessary damage to the soft tissues adjacent to the fracture. For the emergency care of a possible fracture, the reader is referred to Chapter 23.

After an x-ray picture of the injured part has been made and the type of fracture and extent of damage established, the physician will decide which method to use in reducing the fracture and providing immobilization. There is always some degree of pain with a fracture because of muscle spasm, but after proper reduction, this pain should be relieved. A constant, unrelenting pain in the area may indicate nonunion and improper reduction and should be reported to the physician.

Since an open fracture is very easily infected, the nurse must use extreme care in changing the dressings and caring for the wound. Any rise in temperature, foul odor or purulent discharge should be reported immediately.

The nursing care of the patient in traction or a cast has been discussed earlier in this chapter.

AMPUTATION

Definition. An amputation is the surgical removal of a limb or part of a limb. It is a very serious operation and brings about many emotional, physical and sometimes financial problems for the patient and his family.

INDICATIONS FOR AMPUTATION. Severe physical trauma, malignancy and gangrene are the most common indications for an amputation. When the surgeon removes a limb, he cuts away only the damaged tissue and always tries to leave enough of a stump so that a prosthesis (artificial limb) may be properly fitted. For some patients, two or more surgical procedures may be necessary before the stump is in

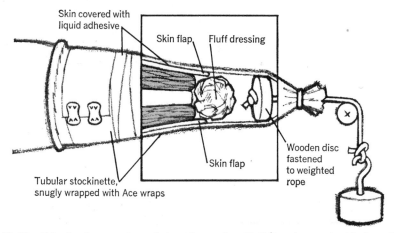

Skin covered with liquid adhesive

Skin flap

Fluff dressing

Skin flap

Tubular stockinette, snugly wrapped with Ace wraps

Wooden disc fastened to weighted rope

Figure 14–15. Prior to closure, stump is kept in traction. Fluff dressing soaked in Betadine covers open end of stump; tubular stockinette is held in place with liquid adhesive, Ace wrap. (From Kirkpatrick: American Journal of Nursing, May, 1968.)

condition to receive a prosthesis. During the time before complete closure of the wound the stump is kept in traction (see Fig. 14-15). This is done to prevent flexion contracture in the remaining part of the limb.

Preoperative Nursing Care. Unless the amputation is an emergency procedure following severe trauma, the physician will tell the patient that removal of the limb is necessary and assist him in plans for rehabilitation, including fitting and use of the prosthesis. Additional plans for rehabilitation of the patient give him something to look forward to. This will be a very difficult time for the patient as he awaits a surgical procedure that will undoubtedly leave him handicapped. He will need sympathetic understanding and a great deal of encouragement from the nursing staff to help him over this period of adjustment.

Physical preparation of the surgical area includes shaving and thorough cleaning of the affected limb. If the surgeon wishes additional preparation with special antiseptics and wrapping of the part in sterile towels, he will give a written order to that effect.

Postoperative Nursing Care. Immediately after surgery, the stump is elevated on a pillow. There will be

some oozing of blood and serum, so the pillow should be protected with some waterproof material. The drainage must be watched carefully and any large or sudden increase in amount or change in its color to a bright red, indicating fresh bleeding, must be reported immediately. Since sudden hemorrhage may occur with any amputation, a large tourniquet must be kept at the bedside at all times during the postoperative period. In order to prevent hip flexion contractures while the amputee is confined to bed, he should be encouraged to lie on his abdomen as much as possible, especially when he is sleeping. The nurse must also be careful to support the limb and hip (if it is not in traction) with a blanket roll or pillow so that external rotation and abduction of the limb are avoided.

Exercises are usually begun soon after the amputation, so that the patient may begin to strengthen the muscles he will use most while wearing an artificial limb. When a lower limb has been removed, the patient must learn how to balance himself on one leg, how to stoop and bend over without losing his balance and how to use his back muscles to maintain good posture while wearing an artificial limb. The use of crutches and fitting and applying an artificial limb are best supervised by a physical therapist.

Sensations referred to as "phantom sensations" or "ghost pains" in the limb which has been removed are not unusual. The patient may insist that he has pain in his toes or cramps in his foot after his foot or leg has been removed. These sensations are very real and are not the result of superstition or an overactive imagination. The patient actually experiences these sensations because the nerves which formerly led to the foot or lower leg are still functioning and therefore carrying impulses to the brain. The nerve ending in the stump may be compared to a "live" electric wire; that is, the wire may have been shortened, but it still carries electrical charges. The nerves may have been shortened, but they are still in the remainder of the limb and their endings are sensitive and capable of transmitting impulses. Early ambulation and early weight bearing on the stump are often helpful in reducing phantom sensations. It is sometimes necessary for the surgeon to reopen the stump and remove more nerve tissue, but this is not always successful, as there are still some nerve endings left, and they can continue to transmit sensations of discomfort.

Emotional Aspects and Rehabilitation. Unless there are complicating factors that will prevent early ambulation, most surgeons agree that the most important factor in successful rehabilitation of the amputee is early ambulation so that the patient can see for himself that he can eventually become independent once again. The elderly and chronically ill can benefit from a positive yet realistic approach to their problems. The nurse must, of course, avoid giving false hopes or unreal assurances that everything is going to be all right. It is insulting to the patient to tell him that he will be "just like new again" when he obviously can't be restored to his former state of health. On the other hand, tears and a long face won't do much toward giving him courage to face his problems and work toward a solution. By helping her patient find short-range goals that can be accomplished without great difficulty and that indicate progress toward independence, the nurse can be of real help to the amputee. For example, she can guide him toward devising ways in which he can meet his own personal needs, such as bathing and shaving. Later, he can be encouraged to sit up, exercise his other limbs and assist with changing his dressing. Finally, she can set for him the goal of wearing a prosthesis successfully and walking without assistance.

SPRAIN

A sprain involves the stretching of the ligaments around a joint so that there is a rupture of the fibers. This leads to an inflammation and some small hemorrhages in the area. The result is pain, bruising and swelling with loss of function. Sprain is treated with rest, support of the joint and ligaments with an elastic bandage, elevation of the part to reduce the swelling and local applications of heat and cold.

DISLOCATION

Definition. A dislocation involves stretching and tearing of the ligaments around a joint with complete separation of the bones which make up the joint. Dislocation occurs most frequently at the shoulder joint, knee joint and the jaw. The symptoms are severe pain aggravated by motion of the joint, muscle spasm and an abnormal appearance of the joint.

Treatment. As soon as possible, a dislocated joint must be reduced, that is, returned to its normal position. If reduction is delayed, certain pathologic changes will take place within the joint, making reduction and future normal motion of the joint very difficult to

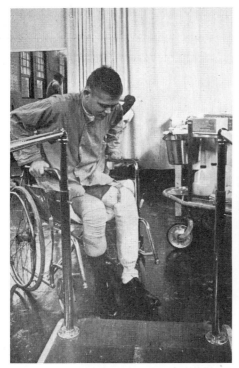
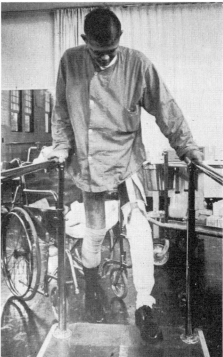
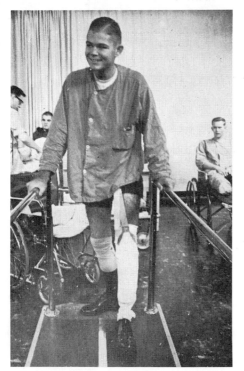

Figure 14–16. A young Marine wheels to parallel bars, gingerly puts his weight on temporary prosthesis and takes his first step. (From Kirkpatrick: American Journal of Nursing, May, 1968.)

accomplish. After reduction, the joint is immobilized by a bandage or cast.

OSTEOMYELITIS

Definition. Osteomyelitis is a bacterial infection of the bone. The causative organism is most often *Staphylococcus aureus,* which enters the blood stream from a distant focus of infection, such as a boil or furuncle, or from an open wound, as in an open (compound) fracture. It occurs most often in children under the age of 15, and is usually found in the tibia or fibula.

Symptoms. Osteomyelitis has a sudden onset with severe pain and marked tenderness at the site, high fever with chills, swelling of adjacent soft parts, headache and malaise.

Diagnosis. Diagnosis is made on the basis of (1) laboratory findings indicating an acute infection, e.g., high sedimentation rate and white cell count, (2) x-rays, which may show bone destruction 7 to 10 days after onset of the disease, (3) history of injury to the part, open fracture, boils, furuncles or other infections and (4) biopsy, in which the bone sample exhibits signs of necrosis.

Treatment and Nursing Care. The earlier the condition is diagnosed and treatment is begun, the better the prognosis. General treatment and nursing care are aimed at improving and maintaining the physical condition of the patient through adequate fluid, mineral and vitamin intake. Specific treatment includes elimination of the infection through the use of antibiotics and immobilization and absolute rest of the affected limb. In some unusually stubborn infections, this treatment is not adequate, and surgical incision for drainage of the abscess and removal of dead bone and debris from the site of infection is necessary.

The problem of keeping a formerly active and alert child quiet and content during the weeks of immobilization of the affected bone is a challenge to the nursing team. The parents should be informed of the purpose of the immobilization so that they may cooperate with the physician and nurses in their efforts to limit the child's activities. Attractive meals and menus that are planned with consideration for the child's preferences will help to maintain adequate nutrition during the time he cannot be active and will not have much appetite or interest in food. It is also important that the child be protected from other infections during the acute and convalescent phases of the disease. After dismissal from the hospital, both the child and the parents should be cautioned against his participation in strenuous games and activities which may lead to injury of the affected limb.

ARTHRITIS

Definition. The term "arthritis" is used to cover all inflammatory diseases of the joints. Actually, research has shown there are approximately 100 different types of arthritis, but all are capable of producing disability, and most are generally treated in the same manner. For classification of arthritis and rheumatism, see Table 14-1.

Etiology. The exact cause of arthritis is not yet known; however, there are some definitely established predisposing factors. These include:
1. Infection, the most common being with streptococcus, staphylococcus and gonococcus.
2. Trauma, overweight and/or poor posture.
3. Prolonged physical stress and strain (see Fig. 14-17).
4. Emotional disturbances.
5. Metabolic disorders (gout).
6. Heredity.

Symptoms. In most cases, the onset of arthritis is slow and gradual

TABLE 14-1. CLASSIFICATION OF ARTHRITIS AND RHEUMATISM*

I. Polyarthritis of unknown etiology
    A. Rheumatoid arthritis
    B. Juvenile rheumatoid arthritis (Still's disease)

II. "Connective tissue" disorders
    A. Systemic lupus erythematosus
    B. Polyarteritis nodosa
    C. Scleroderma
    D. Polymyositis and dermatomyositis

III. Rheumatic fever

IV. Degenerative joint disease
    Primary/secondary osteoarthritis, osteoarthrosis

V. Nonarticular rheumatism
    A. Myositis
    B. Tenosynovitis

VI. Associated with known infectious agents

VII. Traumatic or neurogenic disorders

VIII. Allergy and drug reactions

IX. Miscellaneous and associated diseases

*From Marmor, et al.: American Journal of Nursing, July, 1967. Reprinted with permission.

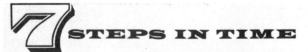

7 STEPS IN TIME

Case histories of women crippled by arthritis usually show long hours of hard work, in the home or outside, with little rest or relaxation.

With this in mind doctors urge women to take steps to prevent arthritis. They have special advice for housewives and mothers:

1	Relax your housekeeping standards a bit
2	Don't do all your ironing in one batch Rest at the half way mark
3	Do your major house cleaning by installments; rest a day between bouts
4	Take it easier with the children.
5	Keep rested, relaxed and well nourished, but not overweight
6	Protect yourself against cold and dampness and get sunshine when possible
7	Avoid strain, fatigue and worry and you will lessen your chances of suffering from arthritis

Figure 14-17. Steps to prevent arthritis in women. (From a pamphlet published by the Arthritis and Rheumatism Foundation, 10 Columbus Circle, New York.)

with weight loss, malaise and pain in the joints. In the less common acute form of arthritis, the symptoms occur more rapidly and are extreme in nature, with a high temperature, severe joint pain, elevated white cell count and prostration of the patient.

Rheumatoid Arthritis

Introduction. The most crippling and one of the most common types of arthritis is rheumatoid arthritis. It is a disease of connective tissue and may affect not only the joints, but the nerves, tendons, muscles and blood vessels as well. Rheumatoid arthritis is second only to heart disease as a cause of permanent disability.

According to the handbook for patients, "Home Care in Arthritis," issued by the Arthritis and Rheumatism Foundation, the progressive changes that occur as a result of rheumatoid arthritis are as follows:

As the disease progresses, structures in and around joints become thickened and shortened, with consequent limitation of motion. Pain itself becomes a very important factor in the limitation of joint motion. In good health there is a happy balance between the opposing sets of muscles, but in rheumatoid arthritis there develops an imbalance, which gradually bends fingers, arms, legs, and even the spine, making it difficult to keep full motion in a joint. One finds it increasingly difficult to straighten out his fingers, or perhaps his knee. Muscles become tight in an effort to protect a joint from the pain resulting from motion to the joint. All these changes tend to limit motion.*

Treatment and Nursing Care. Because rheumatoid arthritis can be such a crippling disease if left untreated, treatment is aimed at relief of discomfort, prevention of deformity, rehabilitation of the patient and physical and emotional support.

RELIEF OF PAIN. The relief of joint pain in arthritis is most often achieved

*See Student Reading No. 1.

by use of the salicylates. These include aspirin, Empirin and sodium salicylate. The amount prescribed is quite large and averages about 12 tablets of 5 grains each per day, or a total of 60 grains daily. These drugs are preferred for most patients because they are relatively safe and inexpensive, and they tend to retard the inflammatory process in the joints as well as provide relief from pain. The nurse should be aware, however, that these drugs can produce side effects such as gastrointestinal irritation and bleeding, ringing in the ears, hearing loss and hyperpnea. Codeine and other narcotics for relief of pain are used with great caution because of the danger of addiction, which can be a real threat when it is necessary to control pain in a chronic disease.

Other drugs used in the treatment of arthritis include *antimalarial compounds* such as chloroquine phosphate and gold sodium thiosulfate, the *corticosteroids* such as prednisone and hydrocortisone and the *phenylbutazones* such as Butazolidin and Tandearil. It should be emphasized that no drug will cure arthritis and that those available for relief of symptoms can produce serious and sometimes irreversible side effects. This is especially true of the phenylbutazones, which are highly toxic. For this reason, they are prescribed with caution and on an individual basis. The effectiveness of these various drugs is extremely difficult to evaluate because arthritis tends to subside and then flare up again for no apparent reason, and if a patient is taking a drug at the time his symptoms subside, he may readily, and perhaps falsely, conclude that the drug was the cause of the remission. Another factor is the hope of the patient that the drug will work. Studies have shown that, as a group, arthritics respond more favorably to placebo medications than other patients. This probably is one reason that fraudulent cures and quackery are so successful in their appeal to many victims of arthritis.

Application of heat is often recommended for temporary relief of pain and reduction of joint stiffness and swelling. Some patients receive hot soaks and paraffin baths on an outpatient basis at a clinic or receive deep heat through short-wave diathermy under the supervision of a physical therapist. The patient also may obtain some relief at home by submerging the painful joint in a tub or pan of water heated to about 100° F. Or, if the joint cannot be submerged with ease, the patient may apply hot towels for 10-minute periods several times a day.

PREVENTION OF DEFORMITY. A regimen of *rest and exercise* is recommended for the arthritic patient. It is important to realize that neither alone will do the job of preventing deformities. To guard against fixation of the joints, contractures or atrophy of the muscles, prescribed exercises are necessary. Because motion can cause pain, both the nurse and the patient must realize the danger of allowing a joint to remain in one position for long periods of time. The exercises should be carried out slowly and carefully and strictly according to the directions of the physician or physical therapist. Overstretching of the muscles and tendons or overuse of the joint can be more

TABLE 14–2. GENERAL EXERCISES*

Back Lying

_____ Times	Hands together, bring arms overhead—elbows as close to ears as possible—stretch but stop at point of pain.
_____ Times	Hands together—make big circles—*OUT UP AND OVER.* May use stick or wand.
_____ Times	Shoulders and elbows at right angles—roll arms forward and backward.
_____ Times	Elbows at right angles—roll forearms so that palms face you and face away from you.
_____ Times	Bring alternate knees to chest. (You should keep other knee and hip bent about 45 degrees if comfortable.)
_____ Times	Straight leg raising with other knee bent at 45 to 90 degrees if comfortable.
_____ Times	Ankle circling—both directions.
_____ Times	Roll legs in and then out.
_____ Times	One at a time, spread legs apart, then bring back to the midline.

Face Lying

_____ Times	Arms at sides—raise arms up, bring shoulder blades together.
_____ Times	Arms at sides—raise head and shoulders.
_____ Times	Bend alternate knees.
_____ Times	Pinch buttocks together.
_____ Times	Raise legs alternately from hips—keep knees straight.

Sitting or Lying

_____ Times	Make fist.
_____ Times	Straighten fingers completely—assist with other hand if necessary.
_____ Times	Keeping hand flat, bring each finger toward thumb (use powder or finger paints if helpful).
_____ Times	Oppose each finger and thumb (ball of digits).

*From Marmor, et al.: American Journal of Nursing, July, 1967. Reprinted with permission.

harmful than helpful. Exercises do not necessarily need to hurt to be effective in maintaining motion.

Rest is also an essential part of the arthritic patient's treatment. It reduces inflammation and relieves some of the emotional strain, tension, fatigue and worry that are frequently associated with an exacerbation of the patient's symptoms.

Good positioning of the body is essential at all times, whether the patient is lying, sitting or standing. Earlier in this chapter, we discussed the various methods of changing body positions as well as maintaining proper joint positions. These must be diligently applied when caring for an arthritic patient, particularly one who is confined to bed for a period of time. When the ambulatory patient is resting, he should understand and follow the principles of good posture in a bed or chair.

ORTHOPEDIC DEVICES. In the early stages of rheumatoid arthritis, severe muscle spasms and accompanying pain can rapidly lead to serious deformities, particularly of the upper and lower extremities. There are specially designed splints and braces that hold the joint in a position of maximum

function and provide rest. These corrective devices are also designed in such a way that they can increase joint function and relieve pain.

When arthritic changes involve the joints of the feet, there are special orthopedic shoes that the patient can wear to prevent deformities. These shoes can also redistribute weight-bearing stresses on the foot so that pain and injury to the joints are lessened.

Self-Help Devices. The patient with arthritis frequently is at a loss to know where to get help in adjusting to a new way of living with his crippling disease. He may not realize that there are ways in which he might possibly continue to carry out many of the simple tasks of daily living, so he gives up in despair and becomes more dependent on others for his care. His family grows impatient with him because he doesn't seem to want to help himself, and he withdraws from the society of others.

The nurse or physical therapist who works with the patient and his family to develop ways for the patient to help himself is performing an invaluable service to all concerned. Figure 14-18 shows a variety of devices that can be

Figure 14–18. Self-help devices. Whether homemade or storebought, they can change the arthritic's world to one of freedom and independence.

(1) Slotted woodblocks can be bought. An inverted, slotted shoe box could substitute. *(2)* Drive two long rust-proof nails up through cutting board with points extending about 2 inches above surface. Nails hold food in place while patient peels, cuts or trims. *(3)* Attach a coat hook, large cup hook or curved piece of splinting material to a long wooden dowel. It helps reach hanging clothes, adjusting bed covers, or removing a robe. *(4)* A long-handled shoe horn and elastic laces that don't have to be tied add to independence. *(5)* Ordinary sponge becomes a back scrubber when attached to lightweight wooden coathanger. *(6)* For stocking aid, cut two rectangular shapes from a bleach bottle, smooth corners and edges, and tape them to form double thickness. Attach a garter to each end of long piece of twill or trach tape, then attach tape, just above garters, to each side of one end of plastic. To use, gather stocking onto plastic, fastening garters to top of stocking. Holding tape, drop stocking-covered plastic to floor, insert foot into plastic scoop and pull tape upward, drawing stocking onto leg. *(7)* To help patient raise and lower himself independently, add height to his chair and bed by placing stable woodblocks under legs. *(8)* Two jar openers eliminate need to grip or twist wrist when removing lids. *Left:* handle type opener grips any size lid. *Right:* rough-surfaced discs on top of and beneath jar provide traction. Patient presses down and turns lid with the flat, strong part of the hand. *(9)* Large thermal mugs protect hands from excessive heat and cold and eliminate need to grip tightly. *(10)* To eliminate weight bearing on fisted hands, here's a trapeze for bed transferring. Enlarge and soften bar with crutch grips or foam rubber. *(11)* Large-handled buttonhook aids independence. *(12)* Twill tape loops attached to washcloth or towel enable patient to reach almost any part of body. *(13)* A rectangular piece of splinting material rolled into a cylinder enlarges or extends slender handles. Warm end of cylinder, then cut slits for insertion of handle. *(14)* A file handle or lightweight wooden coathanger extends or enlarges comb and brush handles. *(15)* Faucet handle extensions can be made from plywood. (From: Nursing, October, 1972.)

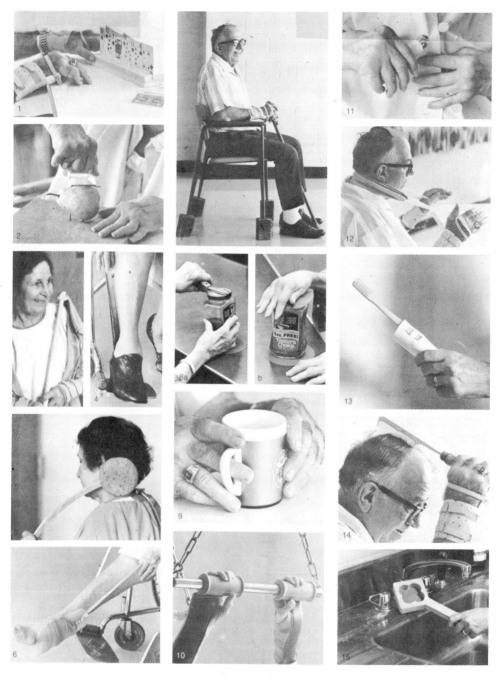

Figure 14–18.

See opposite page for legend.

of great help to the person crippled with arthritis. An imaginative and creative person could probably add many more. The concerned nurse constantly looks for ways to help her patient gain independence and some control of his life.

SURGERY. In recent years there has been an increased use of surgical procedures in the treatment of arthritis. Formerly, surgery was a kind of "last ditch" measure to be used when all other measures had failed and the patient was severely handicapped with serious deformities. It is now considered feasible in some cases to use surgical intervention as a means of preventing such deformities, relieving pain and arresting the progress of the disease.[15]

The type of surgery done will depend on the joint involved and the specific kind of deformity present. For example, if the synovium of the joint is diseased, a synovectomy (removal of the synovium and repair of the tendons) is done. If the muscles and tendons are involved, causing a tightness of the extensor mechanism, these muscles and tendons will also require surgical correction. Total hip replacement is discussed under treatment of osteoarthritis.

DIET. There is no special diet that will cure or relieve arthritis, in spite of many fraudulent claims to the contrary. The patient should eat an average, well-balanced diet with no excess or limitations in amount or types of foods. Obesity can contribute to additional stress on the weight-bearing joints and aggravate the arthritic condition. This should be explained to the patient who has a tendency to be overweight so he can be properly motivated and encouraged to lose weight and continue to keep his weight within normal limits.

EMOTIONAL FACTORS. It is now believed that joint diseases such as rheumatoid arthritis are definitely related in some way to personality and emotional factors. Obviously, any disease that hampers physical activity and produces pain, that often results in an unattractive appearance and that can greatly alter one's everyday life will bring about some unpleasant emotional response in its victims. Whether the emotional upheaval is the cause of the disease or vice versa is a matter of speculation.

There is evidence that response to treatment of arthritis can vary greatly in individuals even though they may have the same amount of joint involvement and are receiving the same treatment. The patients who respond poorly are usually suffering from some emotional problems stemming from feelings of insecurity and lack of confidence in themselves. Those who respond more favorably to treatment are for the most part well-adjusted persons who think well of themselves and believe themselves to be accepted by society. One must realize, of course, that the individual's state of mind can be a result of the successful treatment rather than a cause or contributing factor. There is no doubt, however, that psychological and emotional factors do play an important role in the etiology and progress of arthritic changes in the joints. There are many instances in which emotional traumas resulting from unpleasant and uncontrollable events in a person's life have led to the development of arthritis, or to a flare-up of symptoms in a person who has a chronic form of the disease.

It is important, then, for the nurse to recognize the relationship between the patient's emotional state and his physical symptoms. She must strive to help the patient achieve serenity and peace of mind; and she should always avoid creating, by her words or actions, a situation in which she could add further to the patient's emotional problems and feelings of insecurity.[25]

Education of the Patient. As in all

chronic diseases, the arthritic patient's understanding of his illness and his ability to cooperate with the physician in the treatment of his illness will go a long way toward the success of the treatment. The Arthritis and Rheumatism Foundation issues several excellent booklets for the express purpose of helping the patient and his family understand arthritis. These publications are sold for 10 cents and 15 cents and may be obtained from the local chapter of the Foundation or by writing to the Foundation at 10 Columbus Circle, New York 10019. *ADDRESS*

Osteoarthritis

Definition. Another common type of arthritis is osteoarthritis. In this type of arthritis there is a gradual "wearing out" or degeneration of the joint rather than an acute inflammatory type of process. Osteoarthritis is one of the less serious types of arthritis and rarely leads to crippling. Most persons suffering from this disease are over 40 years of age, and have only mild pain and stiffness of the joints.

The joints of the fingers are often affected, particularly in women. These fingers then take on the characteristic appearance commonly associated with this type of arthritis (see Fig. 14-19).

Treatment and Nursing Care. Since this type of arthritis is basically a process of degeneration, little can be done to reverse the disease process itself. However, much can be done to

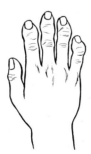

Figure 14–19. Joint deformities commonly associated with osteoarthritis.

eliminate the obesity, poor posture or physical strain which may have predisposed the joints to the disease. The joints should also be protected from injury by accidental falls or twisting of the joints. The application of mild heat gives some relief when the discomfort becomes severe. Exercises as prescribed by the physician or physical therapist also keep the joints active and help maintain good muscle tone. The physician may order salicylates for the relief of pain, and in some cases of poor posture or orthopedic disability he may prescribe certain orthopedic appliances. For the rare cases of severe disability, joint debridement may be necessary.

TOTAL HIP REPLACEMENT. Surgical replacement of the entire hip joint damaged by the degenerative processes of osteoarthritis is a relatively new procedure. There are two different surgical procedures that may be used by the surgeon, the difference between the two being the type of material from which the artificial joint is made. The McKee-Farrar prosthesis is made of a metal called Vitallium. The femoral head of the Charnley prosthesis is made of stainless steel and the cup which fits over the femoral head is made of plastic. Both types are cemented into place with an acrylic cement (see Fig. 14-20).

During the preoperative period, the patient is given instructions in use of the walker and crutches. He may also be taught some basic exercises which strengthen the muscles of the hip and leg. In the immediate postoperative period, proper positioning of the patient and frequent turning to prevent complications are extremely important. A cast or Thomas splint with slings may be applied to immobilize the joint and hold the leg and hip in optimum position for healing. If no splint or cast has been applied, extreme care must be exercised in turning the patient. *At no time* is he allowed to lie on the affected side until there are written orders that

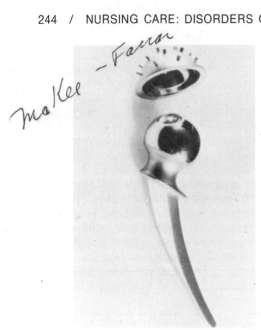
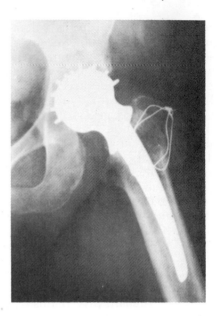
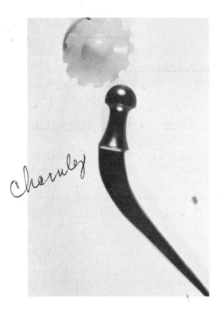
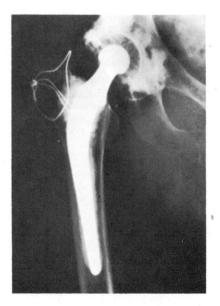

Figure 14–20. Prostheses used in two types of surgical procedure for total hip replacement. The McKee-Farrar procedure involves the replacement of both the femoral head and acetabulum by a metal prosthesis (above: left and right). The Charnley prosthesis (below: left and right) involves total prosthetic replacement of the hip joint. Its components are metal and plastic. (From: Journal of Practical Nursing, August, 1971.)

he may do so. Pillows are placed between the legs to keep them separated and avoid internal rotation and adduction of the hip joint.

The nurse caring for a patient who has had a total hip replacement must use great care in handling and positioning the hip joint during the immediate postoperative period. If she does not know exactly what can and cannot be done in moving, positioning and allowing weight bearing on the joint, she has an obligation to seek information from the physician or nurse in charge. The reward for conscientious nursing care will be the satisfaction of seeing a formerly crippled and pain-ridden patient walk again without fear of pain.

A relatively recent development is that of the total knee replacement. Information relating to nursing care can be found in the article by Shoemaker.[21]

COLLAGEN DISEASES

The collagen diseases affect connective tissue. Although each collagen disease presents a distinct clinical picture, all affect various organs, cause inflammation of the connective tissue and deposit fiber-like material in the ground substance of the tissue. It is not surprising that one or more organs can be involved in a collagen disease since some type of connective tissue can be found in all organs of the body.

The cause of collagen disease is not clearly understood, but they are believed to be related in some way to an autoimmune reaction. This means that the patient develops antibodies that are specific against his own body tissues.

Diseases that are included in the collagen group are scleroderma, systemic lupus erythematosus, polyarteritis and arthritis. Scleroderma involves the skin, joints and blood vessels. It is often confused in its early stage with arthritis and Reynaud's disease because of the symptoms it presents. The skin gradually loses its elasticity and

pigmentation and becomes hardened and mummy-like. Bodily motion is greatly restricted by the fixation of the skin and underlying tissues and involvement of the muscles and soft tissues of the joints. Systemic lupus erythematosus involves skin, blood vessels and serous and synovial membranes. It occurs in both acute and chronic form and is now known to be fairly common, occurring most often in young women.

Treatment for the collagen diseases is limited to the administration of adrenocorticosteroids for the relief of symptoms and measures to keep the patient as healthy as possible under the circumstances. The antimalarial compounds are often successful in relieving the symptoms of lupus erythematosus.

GOUT

Introduction. Gout is not a type of arthritis, but a metabolic disease. It is the result of a defect in the metabolism of purines, which are products of the digestion of proteins. This faulty metabolism results in an accumulation of uric acid in the blood, and eventually there are deposits of sodium urate crystals in the joints, kidneys, cartilage of the ear and sometimes in the heart or other internal organs. Subcutaneous deposits of urea crystals are called tophi, and they appear in about one third of the patients who have gout.

Cause and Incidence. The cause of gout in not known. It is considered a familial disease, and about 95 per cent of its victims are men. Contrary to popular belief, gout is not a rich man's disease resulting from "high living" or overindulgence in expensive and highly seasoned foods. In fact, the disease occurs most often in individuals who are in the middle and low income groups.

Symptoms. Arthritic changes with tenderness, swelling and pain in the joints are characteristic of the acute phase of gout. The joints most often affected are those of the great toe, ankle, instep, knee and elbow. With repeated attacks, there can be permanent damage and deformity of the joint. Renal failure can occur as a result of attacks that produce urea deposits in the kidneys and thereby damage renal cells.

Treatment. Most drugs used in the treatment of gout increase the amount of uric acid excreted in the urine. Probenecid (Benemid) and sulfinpyrazone inhibit the reabsorption of uric acid into the blood at the renal tubule. Allopurinal acts to interfere with the formation of uric acid. Aspirin in *large doses* lowers the serum uric acid level, but, paradoxically, in *small doses* it actually raises the level of uric acid in the blood.[13]

Dietary regulations are not given the emphasis they formerly were before the development of effective drugs. During an acute attack, the patient may be placed on a low-purine, low-fat diet to decrease the production of uric acid. Foods high in purines include brains, kidneys, sweetbreads, liver and other organ meats and their gravies. Sardines and anchovies are also high in purines.

Rest is helpful in reducing the discomfort of gout during an acute attack. A bed cradle to relieve the weight of the bed clothes can also be helpful. Emotional stress and physical trauma should be avoided, since they aggravate the symptoms of gout.

CLINICAL CASE PROBLEMS

1. Mrs. Wilkins, age 38, weight 210 pounds, has been admitted to the hospital with a diagnosis of fracture of the right femur. You have been told that when the patient returns from the cast room, she will have on a hip spica. This cast will cover all the right leg and foot except the toes, and the left leg will be covered down to the knee. The body section of the cast will stop at the waistline. You have been assigned to assist in the care of Mrs. Wilkins when she returns from the cast room.

How will you prepare the bed for the patient's return?

What equipment will you anticipate needing?

How can you support the cast while it is drying?

How is the patient to be transferred from the stretcher to the bed?

What provision can be made for drying the cast?

List the observations you must make while the cast is drying.

If the doctor orders a trapeze bar installed over the patient's bed, how would you plan the procedure for getting Mrs. Wilkins on and off the bedpan?

2. Mr. Moss is a young man, age 33, who has been injured in a fall from a building on which he was working. When you are assigned to the care of this patient, you are told that he has a fracture of the tibia and fibula of the left leg. These fractures were reduced under anesthesia, after which pins were inserted for skeletal traction. The accident occurred three days ago, and now you are assigned to give A.M. care to this patient.

What nursing problems will skeletal traction present?

What special observations must you make?

3. Mrs. Carter, age 50, is a very obese woman who comes to the orthopedic clinic for treatment of arthritis of the knees and ankles. She has great difficulty walking and would use a wheel chair if she could afford one. Her daughter states that the patient is becoming more and more inactive and, though her mother says that she does

not want to become an invalid, that she refuses to move about and do things for herself. Mrs. Carter lives alone and prefers not to live with her daughter because the grandchildren make her nervous. In fact, she prefers to be left alone because she feels that she cannot be of any use to anyone in her condition. Her daughter feels that her mother could find many useful things to do in her neighborhood if she would only try.

What problems can you see in this situation? How could proper instruction help Mrs. Carter in her illness?

What effects could Mrs. Carter's attitude have on her physical condition?

4. Mrs. Lewis, age 52, has been told she has osteoarthritis. She is a very nervous individual and extremely apprehensive about her condition. While you are bathing her one morning, she tells you that she knows she will be helpless and completely useless as a wife and mother within a few months because she has arthritis and she knows what a crippling disease this is. She is very depressed and refuses to help herself during the bath and changing of the bed linen, saying, "I know I will soon be an invalid, and I might just as well get used to having others do everything for me."

How can you help this patient understand the type of arthritis she has and the ways in which she can prevent deformity and crippling?

REFERENCES

1. Adams, J.: "Modern Management of Traumatic Amputation." Nursing '72, Nov., 1972, p. 46.
2. Bailey, J. A.: "Traction, Suspensions and a Ringless Splint." Am. Journ. Nurs., Aug., 1970, p. 1724.
3. Beland, I.: Clinical Nursing: Pathophysiological and Psychosocial Approaches, 2nd edition, New York, The Macmillan Co., 1970.
4. Bennage, B. A., and Cummings, M. E.: "Nursing the Patient Undergoing Total Hip Arthoplasty." Nurs. Clin. N. Amer., Vol. 8, No. 1, 1973, p. 107.
5. Boegli, E. H., and Steele, M. S.: "Scoliosis." Am. Journ. Nurs., Nov., 1968, p. 2399.
6. Brasswell, M. P., et al.: "Helping Patients Adjust to Rheumatoid Arthritis." Nursing '72, Oct., 1972, p. 11.
7. Brunner, et al.: Textbook of Medical-Surgical Nursing, 2nd edition, Philadelphia, J. B. Lippincott Co., 1970.
8. Dalton, A.: "Using a Stryker Frame." Am. Journ. Nurs., Feb., 1964, p. 100.
9. Eyre, M. K.: "Total Hip Replacement." Am. Journ. Nurs., July, 1971, p. 1384.
10. Holley, L.: "The Physical Therapist—Who, What, and How." Am. Journ. Nurs., July, 1970, p. 1521.
11. Harmer, B., and Henderson, V.: Textbook of the Principles and Practice of Nursing, 5th edition, New York, The Macmillan Co., 1960.
12. Hrobsky, A.: "The Patient on a CircOlectric Bed." Am. Journ. Nurs., Dec., 1971, p. 2352.
13. Johnson, E. S. B.: "Understanding Hyperuricemia: Nursing Implications." Nurs. Clin. N. Amer., Vol. 7, No. 2, 1972, p. 399.
14. Kerr, A.: Orthopedic Nursing Procedures. New York, Springer Pub. Co., 1960.
15. "Life-Threatening Scleroderma." Nursing '72, Aug., 1972, p. 23.
16. Marmor, I., Walike, B. C., and Upshaw, M. J.: "Rheumatoid Arthritis—Surgical Intervention." Am. Journ. Nurs., July, 1967, p. 1430.
17. Modern Medical Encyclopedia, Vol. 3. New York, Golden Press, 1965.
18. Molinari, M. G., et al.: "Total Hip Replacement." Journ. Pract. Nurs., Aug., 1971, p. 20.
19. Neufield, A. J.: "Surgical Treatment of Hip Injuries." Am. Journ. Nurs., March, 1965, p. 80.
20. Ranalls, J.: "Crutches and Walkers." Nursing '72, Dec., 1972, p. 21.
21. Shafer, K., et al.: Medical-Surgical Nursing. 5th edition, St. Louis, The C. V. Mosby Co., 1971.
22. Shoemaker, R. R.: "Total Knee Replacement." Nurs. Clin. N. Amer., Vol. 8, No. 1, 1973, p. 117.
23. Smith, D. W., et al.: Care of the Adult Patient, 3rd edition, Philadelphia, J. B. Lippincott Co., 1971.
24. "Traumatic Amputation." Nursing '72, Nov., 1972, p. 40.
25. Walike, B. C., et al.: "Rheumatoid Arthritis." Am. Journ. Nurs., July, 1967, p. 1420.
26. Weibe, A. M.: Orthopedics in Nursing. Philadelphia, W. B. Saunders Co., 1961.

SUGGESTED STUDENT READING

1. Arthritis and Rheumatism Foundation: "Rheumatoid Arthritis," "Home Care in Arthritis," "Osteoarthritis," "Questions and Answers on Arthritis" and "About Gout" (pamphlets).

2. Davis, R. W.: "Surgery for Osteoarthritis of the Hip." Bedside Nurse, May, 1972, p. 24.
3. Eyre, M. K.: "Total Hip Replacement." Am. Journ. Nurs., July, 1971, p. 1384.
4. Foss, G.: "The 'How-to's' of Bed Positioning." Nursing '72, Aug., 1972, p. 14.
5. Holley, L.: "The Physical Therapist—Who, What, and How." Am. Journ. Nurs., July, 1970, p. 1521.
6. Hrobsky, A.: "Small World of the Traction Patient." Bedside Nurse, Dec., 1971, p. 27.
7. Kirkpatrick, S.: "Battle Casualty: Amputee." Am. Journ. Nurs., May, 1968, p. 998.
8. MacGinnis, O.: "Rheumatoid Arthritis—My Tutor." Am. Journ. Nurs., Aug., 1968, p. 1699.
9. Madden, B. W., and Affeldt, J. E.: "To Prevent Helplessness and Deformities." Am. Journ. Nurs., Dec., 1962, p. 59.
10. Molinari, M. G., et al.: "Total Hip Replacement." Journ. Pract. Nurs., Aug., 1971, p. 20.
11. Ranalls, J.: "Crutches and Walkers." Nursing '72, Dec., 1972, p. 21.
12. Scott, M. M.: "Diagnosis of Rheumatoid Arthritis." Bedside Nurse, May, 1971, p. 10.
13. Skinner, G.: "Head Traction and the Stryker Frame." Am. Journ. Nurs., June, 1952, p. 694.
14. Weaver, A. L.: "Management of Rheumatoid Arthritis." Bedside Nurse, May, 1971, p. 14.

NOT HEAT

OUTLINE FOR CHAPTER 14

I. Introduction

A. Orthopedics—concerned with the preservation and restoration of the functions of the skeletal system (motion, support and protection).

II. Diagnostic Tests

A. X-ray films aid in diagnosis of abnormal changes in the contour, size and density of bones.

B. Cultures aid in diagnosing infections of the bone.

C. Biopsy—samplings of cells taken from bone tumors.

III. General Nursing Care

A. Lifting and turning. Nurse must maintain good body posture of the patient.

B. Orthopedic bed making. Make the bed with a minimum of disturbance to the limb in traction and to the skin.

C. Prevention of deformities.
   1. Contractures—adaptive shorten-

ing of the muscles when they are not used and are poorly positioned.
   2. Loss of muscle tone from lack of exercise.
   3. Ankylosis—permanent fixation of a joint.

D. Good body posture of patient, with frequent changes of position.

E. Exercises, active or passive. Each joint should be put through its full range of motion at least once daily.

IV. Care of the Patient in a Cast

A. Cast is used to immobilize a certain part of the body so that it is firmly supported and completely at rest.

B. Preparation for application of a cast includes proper washing of the skin with soap and water and shaving if surgery is to be done.

C. Care of the fresh plaster cast: patient should be handled gently. Wet cast is picked up only with the palms of the hand. Pillows to support the cast to prevent flattening should be waterproofed. Patient must be turned frequently to avoid misshaping the cast.

D. Drying the cast: use of heat is dangerous. Circulating air is best method.

E. Complications: gangrene or paralysis can result from a cast that is too tight. Nurse must check for signs of impaired circulation, numbness or tingling, sudden or unexplained increase in temperature or unusual odor.

F. Daily care.
   1. Use care not to wet cast when patient is bathed or uses bedpan.
   2. Observe condition of skin at edge of cast.

V. Nursing Care of the Patient in Traction

A. Traction extends and holds part of the body in a certain position by mechanical pull. Skeletal traction exerts pull on the bone; skin traction exerts pull on the skin.

B. Nursing care.
   1. Special and diligent back care.
   2. Bed is made so that traction apparatus is disturbed as little as possible.
   3. Weights must be hanging free, and patient positioned so that his body weight is counteracting the pull of the weights. Check bony prominences frequently for signs of impaired circulation.

Patient must be kept in good body alignment.

VI. Care of the Patient on a Frame

A. Stryker frame or Foster bed is used to:
1. Facilitate nursing care and frequent turning.
2. Immobilize the spine as a means of treating fractures and other disorders of the spinal column.
3. Provide a means of keeping clean and dry for those patients who cannot be moved with ease.

VII. CircOlectric bed similar in principle and purpose to Stryker frame.

VIII. Crutch Walking

A. Type of crutch will depend on amount of disability and the patient's ability to bear weight and keep his balance on his feet.
B. Gaits include three-point, four-point, swing-to and swing-through gait.

IX. Fractures

A. A break or interruption in the continuity of a bone.
B. Types.
1. Comminuted—the bone is shattered.
2. Closed (simple)—no break in the skin.
3. Open (compound)—there is a break in the skin through which fragments of broken bone protrude.
4. Greenstick—the bone is partially bent and partially broken.
C. Treatment—to establish a sturdy union between the broken ends of bone.
1. Closed reduction is done by manual manipulation without a surgical incision.
2. Open reduction—a surgical incision is made, and the exposed bone is aligned.
3. Internal fixation—pins, plates or screws are used to stabilize the position of the broken ends of bone.

X. Amputation

A. Surgical removal of a limb or part of a limb because of severe physical trauma, malignancy or gangrene.

B. Preoperative care includes thorough cleaning and shaving of the limb.
C. Postoperative care.
1. Observe for signs of hemorrhage.
2. Encourage patient to lie on his abdomen as much as possible, keeping stump in good alignment to prevent flexion contractures. Exercises are done to keep joints from ankylosing and to prepare limb for fitting of prosthesis.
3. Phantom sensations often can be relieved by pressure on the stump.
D. Emotional aspects and rehabilitation. Early ambulation is important for improving patient's morale and helping him achieve independence. Nurse should have positive, hopeful attitude, provide her patient with short-range goals and avoid giving false hopes.

XI. Sprain

A. Stretching of the ligaments around a joint so that there is rupture of some of the fibers.
B. Treatment: Rest, support of the joint, elevation to relieve edema and local applications of heat and cold.

XII. Dislocation

A. A stretching and tearing of the ligaments around a joint with complete separation of the bones that make up the joint.
B. Treatment: Reduction of dislocation so that joint is returned to its normal position. Immobilization accomplished by bandage or cast.

XIII. Osteomyelitis

A. A bacterial infection of the bone.
B. Symptoms: Sudden onset with severe pain and marked tenderness at site of infection, fever and swelling of adjacent parts.
C. Treatment: rest, antibiotics and measures to improve the general health of the patient. Surgical incision for drainage of abscess and debridement of infected bone if necessary.

XIV. Arthritis

A. Inflammatory diseases of the joints.
B. Exact cause unknown. Predisposing

factors may include trauma, emotional disturbances and metabolic disorders.

C. Symptoms: weight loss, malaise, pain, swelling of the joints and loss of motion.

D. Two main types:
1. Rheumatoid arthritis.
   a. Can cause permanent disability.
   b. Treatment and nursing care aimed at relief of pain, prevention of deformity, rehabilitation of the patient and physical and emotional support.
2. Osteoarthritis.
   a. Gradual wearing out and degeneration of the joint.
   b. Rarely leads to crippling.
   c. Treatment aimed at eliminating factors that may aggravate the condition.

XV. Collagen Diseases

A. A group of little understood diseases that affect various organs, cause inflammation of the connective tissue and deposit fibrous material in the ground substance of such tissue.

B. Includes scleroderma, systemic lupus erythematosus, polyarteritis, and arthritis.

C. Treatment varies but the corticosteroids offer some relief from symptoms in almost all these diseases.

XVI. Gout

A. A metabolic defect in which purines are not completely metabolized, allowing uric acid to accumulate in the blood and sodium urate crystals to be deposited.

B. Cause is unknown.

C. Symptoms include pain and swelling of the joints, especially those of the great toe, ankle, instep and knee. Renal failure can occur as a result of sodium urate crystals in the kidney.

D. Treatment includes administration of colchicine, aspirin or probenecid. Diet should be low in purines and high in aklaline-ash.

E. Early diagnosis and treatment can prevent serious deformities.

15

Nursing Care of Patients With Disorders of the Cardiovascular System

Part One. Nursing Care of Patients With Disorders of the Blood

INTRODUCTION

The blood is actually a tissue. A little more than half of it is liquid and the remainder is composed of cells. These cells carry on some of the most important functions in the body; and since their life span is comparatively short (a red blood cell only lives two or three months), new ones must be manufactured by the bone marrow, lymph nodes and spleen in order to assure the body of a plentiful supply.

The white cells aid in the body's defenses against infection, and the platelets assist in the clotting of blood.

The red cells (erythrocytes) carry on the vital functions of transporting nutrients to all the other tissues of the body, exchanging these nutrients for waste products and then carrying the waste to specific organs for disposal. The erythrocytes contain a pigmented protein called hemoglobin. Without hemoglobin, the red cells would not be red, nor would they be able to transport oxygen, because it is the hemoglobin which absorbs oxygen and carbon dioxide and releases them when they have reached their destinations. We can see, therefore, that a deficiency of hemoglobin as well as a substantial

251

decrease in the number of erythrocytes can lead to serious difficulties for the other cells of the body.

The blood cells are suspended in a liquid. This liquid is called *plasma*. Plasma is a complex fluid containing antibodies, hormones and some nutritive elements and waste products. Plasma also contains *fibrinogen*, a chemical which plays an important part in the clotting of blood. When fibrinogen is removed from plasma through the formation of a clot, the remaining liquid is spoken of as *serum*. Both plasma and cells contain minerals such as calcium, sodium and potassium, the electrolytes so essential to health.

The total volume of blood in the body varies from 4 to 6 quarts in a healthy adult, but it is not always the amount that matters so much as it is the quality of the blood itself. The rapid loss of a quart or more may result in death. However, a gradual loss of blood over a period of time will seriously deplete the number of red cells and lead to a serious anemia.

BLOOD DYSCRASIAS

Definition and Types

A blood dyscrasia is an abnormal or pathologic condition of the blood, especially one that involves some imbalance in its elements. In general, there are two types of blood dyscrasias—those present at birth *(congenital)* and those *acquired* after birth. Most congenital blood dyscrasias are a result of the body's inability to produce blood elements that are primarily concerned with the formation of blood clots. The person who has such a condition maintains most normal physiological functions, but if there is any damage to the blood vessels, he has a tendency to bleed freely because his blood will not clot normally. One of the best known examples of this type of blood dyscrasia that is present at birth is hemophilia.

Blood dyscrasias that are acquired are usually a result of some imbalance between production and destruction of certain blood elements, particularly the red blood cells. Whether production of erythrocytes is decreased or their destruction is increased, there is inevitably a deficiency of these elements. Since erythrocytes are vital to the transportation of oxygen, the body cells, which must have oxygen to carry on the metabolism that is necessary for their existence and functions, will be seriously affected by any deficiency of red blood cells. It can readily be understood, therefore, that a blood dyscrasia can be extremely serious and even fatal if the imbalance between supply and demand is not corrected. The acquired blood dyscrasias include a number of diseases such as the various anemias, the leukemias and hemolytic jaundice.[4]

Drug-induced blood dyscrasias may be the result of any one of three actions: (1) interference with the production of the components of the blood, (2) inhibition of blood cell function and (3) destruction of the blood elements. The anticancer drugs, for example, act to depress the bone marrow which produces blood cells; this action inevitably produces some degree of blood disorder. Some drugs, such as diphenylhydantoin (Dilantin), primidone (Mysoline), barbital derivatives and oral contraceptives may produce anemia by interfering with the absorption and utilization of folic acid, a substance essential to the manufacture of red blood cells.

Although bone marrow depression is an expected action of the anticancer drugs, the same type of situation can develop if a patient has an idiosyncrasy or hypersensitivity to other types of drugs. Chloramphenicol (Chloromycetin—an antibiotic) produces bone marrow depression in about 50 per cent of all patients who receive it. In many cases, the action continues long after the drug is discontinued. Mephenytoin (Mesantoin) and phenylbutazone (Butazolidin) can also cause aplastic anemia in some persons.[3]

Symptoms

Although the congenital and acquired blood dyscrasias vary widely in their specific pathology, they have many symptoms in common. One of these symptoms is fatigue. This is a result of inadequate transportation of oxygen, which must be present for the body cells to transform nutrients into energy. Another symptom is dyspnea, and it too is brought about by inadequate transportation of oxygen. As the body attempts to compensate for the oxygen deficiency, the heart beats faster. This will produce the symptom of increased pulse rate, and the patient may be aware of palpitations of the heart. Another compensatory mechanism is the shifting of blood from the peripheral vessels to the more vital internal organs. The body does this by constricting the peripheral blood vessels so that the flow of blood through them is decreased. This produces the milder symptoms of shock and also impairs proper distribution of body heat so that the patient becomes chilled very easily.

In some dyscrasias, the blood elements necessary for clotting of blood are in short supply. These elements, such as platelets, are obviously essential, and when they are lacking, the patient will suffer from a tendency to bleed and is in danger of hemorrhage from the slightest injury. When blood cells such as white blood cells are lacking in sufficient numbers or behaving abnormally, as in leukemia, the patient has a greatly lowered resistance to infection and has difficulty establishing an immunity to infectious diseases.

Since the blood dyscrasias have many symptoms in common, they will also have certain principles of nursing care in common. In many instances, nursing measures are governed by the patient's symptoms and the needs arising from such symptoms. To avoid repetition, we have presented most of the nursing care under anemia, which is present in almost all blood dyscrasias. The reader should bear in mind that these basic principles of care can be applied to any patient with a blood dyscrasia that presents similar symptoms.

Anemia

Definition and Classification. "Anemia" is a term used to designate an abnormal reduction in the number of red blood cells circulating in the blood. In a healthy person, there is an even balance between the production of new red cells and the disposal of old "worn-out" red cells. When something happens to upset the normal balance, anemia results. Thus, anemia is really a symptom rather than a disease.

There are various types of anemia, but they may be classified into three general groups: (1) anemia from blood loss, (2) anemia resulting from a failure in blood cell production and (3) anemia associated with an excessive destruction of red cells.

Loss of blood leading to anemia may result from severe trauma to the blood vessels and massive hemorrhage, or it may be the result of a more gradual loss of blood, as in a small bleeding peptic ulcer.

The type of anemia caused by a failure in cell production is the result of a deficiency of certain substances necessary for the formation of red blood cells. Examples of this type of anemia are nutritional anemia, in which there is an inadequate intake of foods containing proteins and iron, or pernicious anemia, in which there is faulty absorption of specific nutrients such as vitamin B_{12} and iron.

Anemias associated with excessive destruction of red blood cells are exceedingly rare. They are known as hemolytic anemias ("hemolysis" means the destruction of red blood cells). Some of the hemolytic anemias are inherited, while others are caused by exposure of the erythrocytes to poisonous agents such as chemicals or certain bacterial toxins.

Diagnosis. The diagnosis of anemia is easily established by a red cell count and hemoglobin evaluation. However, the determination of the specific type of anemia present is more difficult and requires a more thorough microscopic examination of the blood because the size and color of the erythrocytes vary in the different types of anemia. For example, the red cells are larger than normal when pernicious anemia is the diagnosis, while in an iron deficiency anemia they are smaller than normal and contain less hemoglobin.

STERNAL PUNCTURE. Since most erythrocytes are manufactured in the red bone marrow there is much information to be gained from an examination of a specimen from the bone marrow. The sternum, being a flat, thin bone and readily accessible for an aspiration biopsy, is usually the site selected for removal of cells from the bone marrow. The procedure is referred to as a *sternal puncture.* It is often used in the diagnosis of several types of blood disease in which impaired production of blood cells is suspected.

SYMPTOMS. The symptoms of anemia are essentially the result of decreased oxygen supply to the tissues. The skin is pale, and the mucous membranes of the mouth and conjunctiva are noticeably lacking in color. The patient may complain of being easily fatigued or "tired all the time." Headache, dizziness, shortness of breath following slight exertion and digestive disturbances are usually present. If the patient is an adult female, there may be menstrual difficulties.

In an acute anemia, the blood pressure falls rapidly, and dyspnea and restlessness appear. Symptoms of shock become apparent, and emergency treatment must be used.

General Treatment and Nursing Care. The treatment of anemia logically begins with determination of its cause. The doctor may order extensive diagnostic tests to aid him in his search for the etiologic factor present. Most physicians feel that treatments which alter the patient's blood picture by increasing the number of erythrocytes or changing their appearance will only confuse the issue. They prefer to order simple hygienic measures to improve the general health of the patient until a definite diagnosis has been made. The nurse may need to explain this to the patient should he complain that nothing is being done to cure him of his disease. Anemia is most often a chronic disease, which means that nursing measures are aimed at conserving the strength of the patient as much as possible over an extended period of time. It also means that these patients will need encouragement and emotional support during their long illness.

REST. It is only in the acute stages of anemia that absolute bed rest will be necessary. If the patient is ambulatory, he should be encouraged to indulge in mild forms of exercise followed by short periods of rest. He must be warned never to exert himself to the point of exhaustion, because of the unnecessary strain this puts on the heart and lungs.

Those who have anemia are suffering from a diminished supply of oxygen to the tissues of the body. When the brain is deprived of a small amount of oxygen, dizziness will occur, and if the supply of oxygen is greatly diminished, as in a severe anemia, a loss of consciousness will occur. Because the patient may easily injure himself during attacks of dizziness or fainting, he should be instructed to lie down when he first begins to feel faint. The best position is flat in bed without a pillow and with the feet slightly elevated. It is often helpful if the ambulatory patient will lie down in this position several times a day to improve the blood flow to the brain, thereby relieving the cause of dizziness.

WARMTH. Other tissues suffer not

only from a decreased supply of oxygen but also from a lack of the warmth which adequate circulation provides. Thus, the anemic patient nearly always feels chilly and suffers from the cold. Caution should be used to avoid drafts when providing adequate ventilation in his room, and extra blankets and warm sleeping clothes will make him more comfortable. Care must also be used in the application of hot water bottles or electric heating pads because of the danger of burning the patient, who has poor circulation and decreased sensitivity to heat.

DIET. The diet is an important part of the treatment of anemia. The patient is encouraged to eat foods which are rich in iron, protein and vitamins B and C because the body uses all of these in the manufacture of new red blood cells. It is not unusual for the anemic patient to have a poor appetite. Factors which contribute to the anorexia are fatigue, weakness and soreness of the tongue and gums. Patients with nutritional anemia usually have very poor eating habits because of ignorance or indifference to the nutritional values of food.

Before attempting to force any kind of diet on the patient, the nurse should try to determine why he does not eat properly. If she will take a few minutes to discuss the diet with the patient, she may find an excellent opportunity to teach him the value of eating a variety of foods and the kinds of food that are rich in the nutrients his condition requires. The nurse might also encourage her patient to eat as much as he can and to learn to rest a little before mealtime so that he will feel more relaxed and ready for his tray when it arrives.

If the tongue and gums are extremely tender and sore, the foods must not be highly seasoned or served too hot. It is also helpful if the foods are of semi-solid consistency so that chewing is kept at a minimum.

SPECIAL MOUTH CARE. Bleeding of the gums may be among the early symptoms of anemia. As the disease progresses, the gums become more tender and bleed quite freely. When this occurs, brushing of the teeth must be discontinued and some form of special mouth care substituted. Crusts of dried blood may form inside the mouth, especially around the teeth. The crusts of blood may be gently removed by cotton applicators dipped in a solution of diluted hydrogen peroxide. Frequent cleansing of the mouth with cotton applicators dipped in a mild mouthwash will also keep down the odor of halitosis and make the patient feel more comfortable. The lips may be lubricated with mineral oil to prevent dryness and cracking.

VITAL SIGNS. The temperature, pulse and respiration should be checked frequently. An increase in the pulse and respiratory rate could indicate an increasing severity of the disease in which the heart and lungs are working harder in their efforts to provide oxygen to the body tissues. The body's resistance to infection is greatly reduced in all blood diseases; therefore, an elevation in the temperature may indicate than an infection is present. Any rise in the temperature of these patients should be reported immediately so that treatment may be begun before the infection becomes widespread.

SPECIAL OBSERVATIONS. It is possible for a patient to lose a small amount of blood continuously from an internal lesion without being aware of what is happening to him. The nursing staff must carefully observe all bodily excretions for signs of bleeding. When this is suspected as a cause of anemia, the stools of the patient should be checked carefully for signs of fresh blood or old blood (tar-colored stools). When the physician suspects intestinal bleeding, he may order a laboratory examination of the gastric contents or stools for occult (hidden) blood. The urine may also show signs of blood. Bright red blood rarely goes unnoticed, but the hazy brown color caused by old blood in the urine may be considered unimportant if the nurse does not realize its significance. The practical nurse should know that any unexplained coloring of body excreta is to be reported immediately.

BLOOD TRANSFUSIONS. The administration of whole blood to replace that which the patient has lost or is unable to produce himself is one of the most common treatments of anemia. The first record we have of such a procedure was in 1818 when an English obstetrician by the name of James Blundell began to treat successfully cases of postpartum hemorrhage with the administration of human blood. He was unaware of blood types and did not fully understand what happened when a reaction to the blood transfusion resulted in serious illness or death. It was not until 1900, when Landsteiner completed his research on blood groups, that an explanation could be given. It was he who determined that there are four main groups of human blood and that these groups cannot be mixed without disturbing the normal action of the red blood cells in the person receiving the transfusion.

Blood Groups. Landsteiner divided human blood into four main groups or "types" and labeled them A, B, AB and O. The reactions of incompatible blood types are a result of an agglutination (clumping together) and destruction of the red cells. The reaction is brought about by a substance on the surface of the red blood cells of the person receiving the blood and is an antigen-antibody reaction. The blood cells of the donor act as *antigens* which stimulate the plasma of the recipient to produce antibodies.

In order to clarify the reactions of incompatible blood types, Figure 15-1 shows what happens when a small sample of diluted blood from one type is mixed with test sera from an incompatible type. This clumping of the red cells can readily be seen, even with a low power microscope.

The Rh Factor. In 1940, Landsteiner and Weiner described yet another means of differentiating human blood. Since much of their work was done using rhesus monkeys, they named the newly discovered factor Rh. This factor is an *agglutinogen*, which means that it is capable of causing a clumping together of red cells. About 85 percent of the population have this factor present in their red cells; they are typed *Rh positive*, and the remaining 15 percent who lack this factor are typed *Rh negative.* As long as Rh positive individuals receive only Rh positive blood in transfusions, no problem will develop, provided they are com-

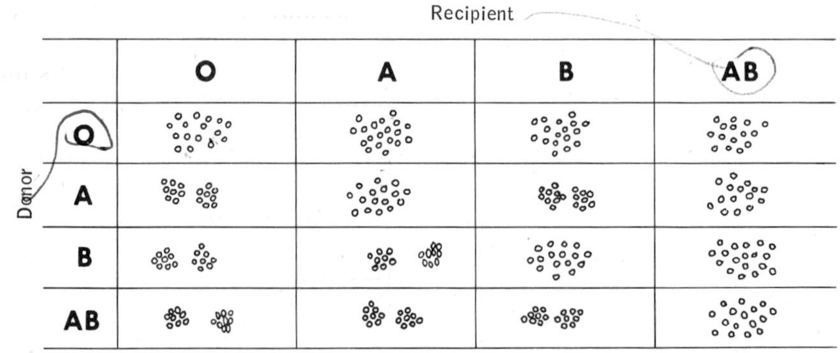

Figure 15–1. Horizontal letters designate blood type of recipient, vertical letters those of the donor. If types are compatible, the red blood cells remain in normal position. If types are incompatible, the red blood cells clump together, producing a reaction in the person receiving the blood.

patible according to other groupings. But if an Rh negative individual should receive Rh positive blood, he will receive the agglutinating factor into his blood and become "sensitized." If he then receives another transfusion of Rh positive blood he will suffer from a serious reaction due to the clumping of the red cells.

Besides transfusions with Rh positive blood, there is another way an Rh negative individual may build up antibodies; that is, during pregnancy in which the plasma of an Rh negative mother is stimulated to build antibodies against the Rh positive fetal blood, which enter her circulatory system and become mixed with her blood. The mother's blood may become sensitized just as it would if she had received a transfusion of Rh positive blood. With subsequent pregnancies, she may build up a high level of antibodies which would affect the fetus in a serious way. The condition which occurs when this happens is called "erythroblastosis fetalis" and may cause the child to be stillborn, or if delivered living, it may present symptoms of a transfusion reaction.

Responsibilities of the Nurse During Transfusion of Whole Blood. Even though the administration of whole blood is now a fairly common procedure, familiarity does not justify an attitude of complacency or indifference on the part of the nurse. Very serious, even fatal reactions can occur during the procedure, and close observation of the patient is always necessary. The following precautions are listed to remind the practical nurse of her responsibilities when caring for a patient receiving a transfusion.

1. Always be certain that the patient is receiving the blood assigned to him. Carefully check the name and blood type written on the label of the container.

2. Check frequently to see that the blood is flowing properly and at the rate prescribed by the physician. If the practical nurse is in doubt as to the proper rate of flow, she should ask the nurse or physician in charge.

3. If chills, rash or other symptoms of a reaction occur during the transfusion, stop the transfusion and notify the physician or nurse in charge immediately.

4. Observe the patient closely during and immediately after the transfusion. Check both temperature and pulse rate for evidence of a transfusion reaction.

5. Inspect the first urine specimen after a blood transfusion for signs of transfusion reaction (hemoglobinuria). The urine will be red or dark brown in color.

IRON THERAPY. We know that iron is one of the substances the bone marrow uses to manufacture normal healthy red blood cells. When the body is lacking in iron, the amount of hemoglobin is decreased in the red cells, making them very small and pale in color. In a simple deficiency anemia, the condition is relieved by administering iron salts. The iron preparation most often used is ferrous sulfate.

Iron salts are irritating to the gastrointestinal tract and should not be given on an empty stomach. There will be fewer gastric upsets if this medication is given in divided doses and immediately after meals. The patient should be warned that the taking of iron salts by mouth produces tarry stools and there is no cause for alarm if he notices this change in the color of his stools. Because iron salts may deposit on the teeth and gums, causing a discoloration, the liquid forms of this medication should be given through a straw. Following administration of each dose, the teeth should be thoroughly cleansed and the mouth rinsed well.

Some patients suffer such severe gastric disturbances from the oral intake of iron salts that the medication must be given by another route. Other patients who are anemic because of gastric or intestinal bleeding cannot take iron by mouth because the irritation aggravates the condition. The drug of choice in these cases is Imferon, an iron preparation which is given into the muscle. These injections must not exceed 2 ml. at each site, and the sites of injection should be rotated to allow for proper absorption and to minimize the hazards of a local inflammation.

Vitamin C is usually given with iron because this vitamin enhances the absorption of iron. Folic acid may also be prescribed, but since body requirements are low, the dosage is usually small.

VITAMIN B_{12} AND LIVER EXTRACT. The glands of the stomach secrete many different substances which help the body absorb and utilize the food which is taken in and digested. There is one specific substance (intrinsic factor) normally secreted by the stomach mucosa that is essential for the proper growth and development of normal red blood cells. In pernicious anemia, the intrinsic factor is missing from the gastric juices so that the iron and protein taken into the stomach cannot be properly absorbed. The result is that the red cell production is decreased and those red cells which are produced are abnormal in structure and function. In order to correct this condition, the physician will order the administration of vitamin B_{12} or liver extract, which contains vitamin B_{12}.

These injections are given daily for the first few weeks and then may be spaced so that they are given weekly. As the patient improves, the injections may be necessary only once a month.

In some ways, the patient with pernicious anemia can be compared to a diabetic. There is no cure for the disease, but the patient can lead a normal life as long as he receives adequate medication and does not indulge in excesses or dissipate his energy. Here, however, the similarity ends. The diabetic cannot neglect his daily doses of insulin or ignore his diet without soon

suffering the consequences. The patient with pernicious anemia may neglect his injections of liver extract or vitamin B_{12} and continue to feel well for weeks or even months. The disease will progress from bad to worse in a gradual manner and eventually lead to serious mental as well as physical deterioration. This neurological damage dulls the patient's awareness of what is happening to him, and thus he may not fully realize that he needs the help of his physician.

In view of these possibilities, the patient and his family must be warned of the dangers involved. They should be made aware of the need for continued treatment for the rest of the patient's life, and informed of the unpleasant outcome they can expect if the injections are neglected. In explaining these things to the patient, the nurse must use tact and patience. The prospect of facing a lifetime of regular injections with the expense and inconvenience this involves is not a pleasant one. With sympathetic understanding and a genuine display of interest in the patient's well-being, the nurse can do much to help him adjust to his illness and the treatments necessary to keep him as well as possible.

Sickle Cell Disease

Definition. Sickle cell disease is a broad term used to include all those hereditary disorders related to the presence of sickle hemoglobin (hemoglobin S) in the red blood cells. In the United States, the most common disorders related to the presence of this specific type of hemoglobin are homozygous sickle cell anemia, sickle cell thalassemia and sickle cell hemoglobin C disease. Of these, homozygous S, or sickle cell anemia, is by far the most common. Sickle cell trait, in which only about 35 per cent of an individual's total hemoglobin is affected, is present in about one out of every 10 to 12 Negroes in this country. Those who

s position & elevate extremeties
edema & shortness of breath

ed skin care
at nails to keep from scratching

No salted nuts or candy because of edema cheek
                                              vitals

Educate Husband on problem
Talks to kids about mental strain about transferring
Promote a good therapeutic environment

have the trait are carriers of the sickle cell gene but as a rule do not have any of the symptoms of sickle cell anemia.

Sickle cell disease is found almost exclusively in Negroes or persons with Negro blood. It is sometimes found in persons whose ancestors were from the Mediterranean region—that is, Greeks, Italians, Spaniards, Frenchmen, Turks and North Africans. Those of Middle Eastern and Indian ancestry may also be affected. In the United States, sickle cell disease afflicts between 30,000 and 50,000 people.[10]

The odds favoring transmission of sickle cell anemia through the genes are very high because nearly 10 per cent of the black population of the U.S. have the trait and are, therefore, carriers. It is for this reason that genetic counseling and adequate screening of the Negro population for early detection of the disease are considered so important in the control of sickle cell anemia. See Fig. 15-2 for illustration of the statistical probabilities of transmission.

Symptoms. As stated earlier, sickle cell trait is not a disease in the true sense of the word. The person with the trait is not anemic and is usually without symptoms unless placed under great physical stress in situations where there is poor oxygenation of the blood; for example, at extremely high altitudes where the percentage of oxygen in the air is decreased.

Sickle cell anemia presents a variety of symptoms which usually appear at the beginning of the second year of life. The disease is rarely fatal. In addition to the anemia that is always present, there may be periodic joint and extremity pain, swelling of the hands and feet, abdominal distention due to liver and spleen involvement, irritability and jaundice.

All of the symptoms are related to the defective hemoglobin, which, when deprived of a sufficient supply of oxygen, forms clumps in the red cells, causing them to assume a sickle shape.

The deformed cells are less easily moved along in the blood stream and cannot pass through small blood vessels as easily as they should. They tend to break apart and pile up against one another, adding to the difficulty of passage through the vessels. The blockage of blood supply further deprives the hemoglobin of its oxygen supply. Thus, a vicious cycle of oxygen deprivation begins, involving clumping of hemoglobin, occlusion of blood vessels and, finally, more oxygen deprivation.

Treatment. There is no cure for sickle cell anemia; treatment is primarily symptomatic and preventive. Upper respiratory infections, poor living conditions and nutritional deficiencies aggravate the condition and precipitate the acute symptoms of thrombosis. The patient is encouraged to drink plenty of fluids to increase the blood volume and remove stagnated cells in the vessels. Acidity promotes sickling, so alkaline foods and liquids are recommended.

The symptoms of severe anemia are treated with blood transfusions and large doses of folic acid and other nutrients essential to the formation of blood elements. Antibiotics are used to combat any secondary infections that may develop. Drugs such as urea and potassium cyanate have been suggested as useful in inhibiting the sickling process, but their effectiveness is still questionable.[5]

Leukemia

Definition. The word "leukemia," when translated literally, means "white blood." Actually, the white blood cells would have to number one million per cubic millimeter before the blood would have a milky white appearance, and although leukemia is characterized by an increase in the number of leukocytes, they rarely rise above 500,000 per cubic millimeter. In addition to the increase in number, the leukocytes of the patient with leukemia are abnormal

The odds[1] for passing sickle cell anemia and trait

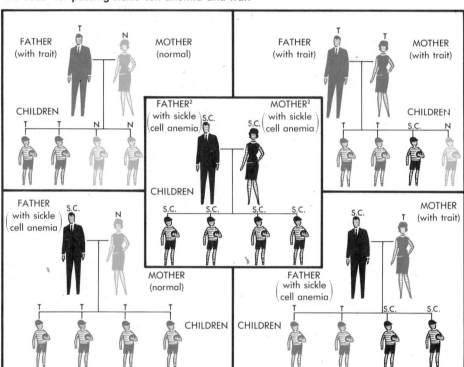

T — Trait
N — Normal
S.C. — Sickle Cell

Figure 15–2. Chart depicting the chances of inheriting sickle cell anemia. (Modified from: Nursing Update, June, 1972.)

---

[1]These are statistical probabilities, but they don't hold true in every case and may vary with the size of the family.

[2]If both partners have sickle cell anemia, they may not be able to produce children.

in appearance and do not function as normal white cells do.

The common lay term for leukemia is "cancer of the blood." The various types of leukemia are classified as progressive malignant diseases because there is a metastatic growth of leukemic cells. These cells can spread from the bone marrow or lymph nodes to the spleen, liver and other highly vascular regions. After they have invaded these organs and surrounding tissues, they destroy the tissues by using the nutritive elements for their own rapid growth. Since the new cells utilize the available amino acids and vitamins at a prodigious rate, the patient with acute leukemia is very likely to suffer from severe debilitation and avitaminosis.[6]

Types. There are various types of leukemia, but they are generally classified as the lymphogenous leukemias and the myelogenous leukemias. This classification is based on the origin of the malignant white blood cells. Lymphogenous leukemias originate in the lymphoid tissues, where they proliferate and spread to other parts of the body. Myelogenous leukemias have their beginnings in the bone marrow.

Another way in which the leukemias can be differentiated is by their rate of progress. Acute leukemia develops rapidly and is more common in younger persons who are going through a rapid stage of development when all body cells are multiplying at an accelerated rate. Chronic leukemia occurs in older persons, usually over 45, who are not in the growth period of their lives.

ACUTE LEUKEMIA. This type of leukemia has an abrupt onset with symptoms of an upper respiratory infection, extreme pallor, ulcerations of the mouth and gums, which also bleed easily, and a high fever. Later there is bleeding from all the body orifices and small hemorrhages under the skin. The disease runs a rapid course and in a short while the patient is critically ill. Death often occurs within weeks or months after the onset of the disease.

CHRONIC LEUKEMIA. As expected

from its name, this type of leukemia progresses more slowly. The onset is insidious, with vague symptoms of fatigue and pallor, a sensation of heaviness in the abdomen, especially in the area of the spleen, and some symptoms of anemia, since there is a decrease in the red cell count and marked reduction of the platelet count. This lowering of the number of platelets accounts for the fact that these patients bleed easily and may have had a history of severe bruising from minor blows years before other symptoms appear.

Later in the disease, there is swelling of the lymph nodes and enlargement of the spleen. Death may result from infection, severe anemia or hemorrhage.

Incidence and Cause. It is estimated that in the United States there are about 14,000 deaths per year resulting from leukemia. The disease most often strikes youngsters under the age of 5 and is the major form of cancer in children aged 2 to 10. There has been an increase in the death rate from leukemia in persons over 45 years of age.[6]

As in other types of cancer, the exact cause of leukemia is not known. There are, however, some factors that are considered to be closely linked with the development of leukemia. Ionizing radiation in relatively large doses is one such factor. Another is certain chemicals that are toxic to bone marrow. The third factor is one that has been the subject of much research in the past few years. This is the theory that tumor viruses are in some way linked to the development of leukemia, but no one has yet been able to isolate a virus that can be identified as the specific cause of leukemia.

Treatment and Nursing Care. There is no known cure for leukemia. Treatment is aimed at: (1) slowing down the growth of the malignant blood cells, (2) maintaining a normal level of red cells, hemoglobin and platelets and (3) providing relief from symptoms which accompany the disease.

The use of chemotherapy as a means

TABLE 15–1. ACUTE TOXICITY OF ACTIVE AGENTS*

	Severity at Therapeutic Dose	Major Toxic Effects
1. Prednisone	±	Hypertension, electrolyte imbalance, osteoporosis
2. Vincristine	+	Peripheral neuropathy
3. 6-Mercaptopurine	++	Marrow depression and nausea and vomiting
4. Methotrexate	+++	Stomatitis and marrow depression
5. Cyclophosphamide	++++	Marrow depression

*From Freireich, E. J., and Frei, E., in Moore, C. V., and Brown, E. B., eds.: Progress in Hematology, Volume IV, 1964. By permission of Grune & Stratton.

of slowing the progress of leukemia and producing a remission of symptoms began in 1942 with the use of nitrogen mustard. Since that time, many drugs have been evaluated, and at this writing, the most effective means of treatment is to use a combination of drugs from a list of the five most promising ones. For the most part, these drugs, when given in combination, have an additive effect; that is, they are more effective in combination than either would be alone. It is also possible to combine a drug with a high toxicity with one that has a low toxicity, thereby increasing the destruction of leukemic cells without causing severe toxic reactions in the patient.

There are five groups of drugs that are used in the treatment of leukemia. Examples of these are presented in Table 15-1 with their major toxic effects.

Blood transfusions are often necessary in order to maintain a near-normal blood picture. Antibiotics may be given to control infections, since the body's defense mechanisms against infection have been impaired by the leukemia.

Of the three aims listed above in the treatment of leukemia, providing relief from symptoms is the most challenging to the nursing staff. Regardless of the type of leukemia present, the nursing care of the leukemia patient is a difficult assignment, one demanding perseverance and ingenuity in solving the many problems this disease presents.

Extreme care must be used in handling these patients because of their tendency to bleed at the slightest injury. Care of the mouth and gums is similar to that described under care of the patient with anemia. If rectal temperatures are necessary, as in the case of a small child or a delirious person, it must be remembered that the mucous membranes are very fragile and injuries are easily sustained.

Protection against infection must be exercised constantly. The skin will require continued observation and special care so that no pressure sores or other breaks in the skin will occur. Pruritus (severe itching) is a very common complaint in some types of leukemia. In these cases, the fingernails should be trimmed to prevent scratching and tearing the skin. Special medications may be ordered to help relieve the itching.

Respiratory difficulty often accompanies leukemia when the lymph nodes of the neck become greatly enlarged. Then proper positioning of the patient for adequate breathing becomes necessary. In severe cases, the physician may order the administration of oxygen.

The patient with leukemia should

remain ambulatory as long as possible because of the pulmonary and circulatory complications which frequently arise from inactivity and confinement to bed. The nurse will then have the added responsibility of providing some mild forms of recreation for her patient so that time will not pass so slowly and his attention will be diverted from his illness.

It is generally believed by authorities that the leukemic patient, even if he is a child, should be told that he has leukemia. Nurses who have worked with leukemic patients have found that deception and trying to avoid direct answers to the patient's questions cause him more frustration and fear than telling him the nature of his illness. This does not mean that one should be brutally frank or morbid in answering the patient's questions. His physician should be the one to tell him his diagnosis. The nurse should encourage the patient to talk about his fears and anxieties when he seems inclined to do so. He will need much emotional and moral support, and his family may not be capable of providing enough of this support for the patient, since they too are going through an emotional upheaval. The nurse must be able to show a hopeful attitude without giving the patient and his family false hopes. She will need to understand the severity of the patient's physical and emotional state without becoming unduly depressed and morose herself.

Hemophilia

Classic hemophilia, which is also known as hemophilia A and factor VIII deficiency, is a relatively rare hereditary disease characterized by a delayed coagulation time which produces a prolonged period of bleeding after injury or surgery. This type of hemophilia almost always occurs in males and is transmitted through the female. Although the female does not have the disease herself, she and all her female descendants can transmit classic hemophilia to their offspring.

There are other types of hemophilia, similar to classic hemophilia, which can affect either sex. In all types, there is a decrease in the amount or the activity of one of the 11 different clotting factors normally present in blood and essential to the formation of clots. Hemophilia A results from a *deficiency* of factor VIII, Hemophilia B, or Christmas disease, is the result of a deficiency of factor IX. In von Willebrand's disease, there is a decrease in the *activity* of factor VIII, even though the factor is present in normal amounts in the plasma. The blood of a hemophiliac forms a clot immediately after injury, but the clot is unstable and does not effectively impede bleeding.

There are varying degrees of severity in the types of hemophilia, depending on the amount of the factor present and the effectiveness of the factor in clot formation. For the mild cases who have 25 to 50 per cent of the deficient factor present in the serum, symptoms may not appear at all until a severe injury or surgery is followed by prolonged bleeding and the hemophilia is thus discovered. In very severe cases in which less than 1 per cent of the factor is present, the affected persons may bleed spontaneously without injury, and severe hemorrhage can develop very quickly whenever an injury does occur.

Symptoms. The most obvious symptom of hemophilia is, of course, bleeding. It is not, however, surface bleeding that causes the most serious complications of hemophilia. Bleeding most often occurs internally with leakage of blood into the joints, the intestinal wall or peritoneal cavity and the deeper tissues of the body. Hemarthrosis, or bleeding into the joints, produces swelling, pain, warmth and limitation of movement similar to that suffered by the patient with rheumatoid arthritis. If the bleeding occurs in the intracranial spaces and thereby increases intracranial pressure, the patient may experience convulsions and brain damage that can be fatal. Other serious complications from internal bleeding in the hemophiliac include obstruction of the airway due to hemorrhage into the neck or pharynx, and intestinal obstruction resulting from bleeding into the intestinal wall or peritoneum.

Treatment and Nursing Care. Within the past few years, there have been made available plasma concentrates which are used to replace the missing factors in the more common types of hemophilia. These factor replacements include those needed to treat von Willebrand's disease, factor VIII deficiency (classic hemophilia) and factor IX deficiency (Christmas disease). The availability of these replacement factors has greatly improved the outlook for hemophilia and helped the hemophiliac live a more normal life.

Hemophilia is a complex disease requiring individual treatment and nursing care based on the needs and priorities of care required by each patient. He should be encouraged to lead an active life insofar as he is able and to avoid situations which predispose him to injury and illness. The parents of a child with hemophilia should avoid over-protecting him, because treating him as an invalid and sheltering him from normal childhood activities deny him the opportunity to develop into a healthy, well-adjusted person. Many persons who have been over-protected in their childhood deliberately indulge in needlessly hazardous activities and take risks that an emotionally healthy person would avoid. Sergis and Hilgartner write of one young man who joined the Merchant Marines without telling anyone he was a hemophiliac, and his brother, who also had hemophilia, chose to race cars in his spare time. Both young men denied their illness and refused to recognize the limitations which it imposed.[8]

Purpura

Definition and Types. The word purpura refers to small hemorrhages in the skin and mucous membranes; they occur as a result of leakage from the capillaries into the tissue spaces of the subcutaneous tissues. If the hemorrhages are small, pinpoint in size, they are called petechiae; the larger ones which resemble bruises are called ecchymoses. Purpura actually is a symptom and may be secondary to a number of diseases including scurvy, liver disease with failure to utilize vitamin K and allergy to certain drugs.

Idiopathic thrombocytopenic purpura is a disease of unknown cause in which the thrombocytes (blood platelets) are destroyed before they reach maturity. It is primarily a disease of young people and is accompanied by enlargement of the spleen.

Treatment of purpura is concerned with curing the primary disease whenever possible and controlling the symptoms. Idiopathic purpura is treated by splenectomy.

CLINICAL CASE PROBLEMS

1. Mrs. Thomas is a young mother who has three small children. She is admitted to the hospital with a severe anemia. Her hemoglobin is 5 gm. and red cell count is also very low. The young mother confides in you that she has never eaten as she should, especially when she was a teen-ager, and with the added strain of having the children to care for at home, she doesn't take the time to cook the meals she knows they should have because she is so tired all the time.

Her husband makes a fairly good salary, but Mrs. Thomas is under the impression that an adequate diet would cost more than they can afford at present.

How can you teach the patient the value of good food and help her with shopping practices which would provide her family with good food that is not expensive?

What could you suggest to help her with the problem of chronic fatigue?

REFERENCES—PART ONE

1. Beland, I.: *Clinical Nursing: Pathophysiological and Psychosocial Approaches,* 2nd edition. New York, The Macmillan Co., 1970.
2. Brunner, L. S. et al.: *Medical-Surgical Nursing,* 2nd edition. Philadelphia, J. B. Lippincott Co., 1970.
3. Eisenhauer, L. A.: "Drug-Induced Blood Dyscrasias." Nurs. Clin. N. Amer., Vol. 7, No. 4, 1972, p. 799.
4. Gurski, B. M.: "Rationale of Nursing Care for Patients with Blood Dyscrasias." Nurs. Clin. N. Amer., Vol. 1, No. 1, 1966, p. 23.
5. Jackson, D. E.: "Sickle Cell Disease: Meeting a Need." Nurs. Clin. N. Amer., Vol. 7, No. 4, 1972, p. 727.
6. Lunceford, J. L.: "Leukemia." Nurs. Clin. N. Amer., Vol. 2, No. 4, 1967, p. 635.
7. Patterson, P. C.: "Hemophilia: The New Look." Nurs. Clin. N. Amer., Vol. 7, No. 4, 1972, p. 777.
8. Sergis, E., and Hilgartner, M. W.: "Hemophilia." Am. Journ. Nurs., Nov., 1972, p. 2011.
9. Shafer, K. N., et al.: *Medical-Surgical Nursing,* 5th edition. St. Louis, The C. V. Mosby Co., 1971.
10. "Sickle Cell Disease Is Not a Textbook Curiosity." Nursing Update, June, 1972, p. 1.
11. Smith, D., Germain, C., and Gips, C.: *Care of the Adult Patient.* Philadelphia, J. B. Lippincott Co., 1971.
12. Vaz, D. D.: "The Common Anemias: Nursing Approaches." Nurs. Clin. N. Amer., Vol. 7, No. 4, 1972, p. 711.

SUGGESTED STUDENT READING

1. Jackson, D. E.: "Sickle Cell Disease: Meeting a Need." Nurs. Clin. N. Amer., Vol. 7, No. 4, 1972, p. 727.
2. Patterson, P. C.: "Hemophilia: The New Look." Nurs. Clin. N. Amer., Vol. 7, No. 4, 1972, p. 777.
3. Sergis, E., and Hilgartner, M. W.: "Hemophilia." Am. Journ. Nurs., Nov., 1972, p. 2011.
4. Shafer, K. N., et al.: "Sickle Cell Disease Is Not a Textbook Curiosity." Nursing Update, June, 1972, p. 1.

OUTLINE FOR CHAPTER 15

Part One   Disorders of the Blood

I. Introduction

A. Blood is a tissue composed half of cells and half of liquid.

B. Blood cells transport essential nutrients and oxygen for proper utilization of these nutrients and remove wastes. Blood is also essential to the body's protective devices.

II. Blood Dyscrasias (Abnormal Conditions of the Blood, Congenital or Acquired)

A. Symptoms common to all blood dyscrasias include fatigue, dyspnea, increased pulse rate and heart beat and sensitivity to cold.

B. Anemia.
1. An abnormal reduction in the number of circulating red blood cells from blood loss, from failure in blood cell production or from excessive destruction of red blood cells.
2. Diagnosis of anemia established by red cell count and hemoglobin evaluation. Determination of exact type of anemia much more complex.
3. General treatment and nursing care:
   a. Rest.
   b. Provision of warmth.
   c. Special mouth care.
   d. Observation of vital signs and checking for hidden blood loss.
   e. Blood transfusions.
   f. Iron therapy, vitamin B_{12} and liver extract.

C. Sickle Cell Disease—a broad term including all hereditary disorders related to the presence of hemoglobin S in the red blood cells.
1. Sickle cell anemia the most common type of sickle cell disease.
2. Genetic counseling and adequate screening of the Negro population for early detection are essential to control and prevention.
3. Symptoms usually appear at the beginning of the second year of life. Joint pain, swelling of the hands and feet, abdominal distention and jaundice are usually present in addition to the anemia.
4. Treatment is essentially symptomatic and preventive. The disease is rarely fatal, but there is no cure for it.
   a. Folic acid prescribed along

with vitamins and other nutrients essential to the production of red blood cells.
   b. Maintenance of general
health and improvement of
living conditions necessary
for prevention of crises and
complications.
   c. Fluids are forced and al-
kaline-ash foods encour-
aged.
   d. Drug therapy not yet established.
D. Leukemia.
   1. A progressive malignancy of the
white blood cells.
   2. Types: lymphogenous (originating in the lymphoid tissue) and
myelogenous (originating in the
bone marrow). Also, acute and
chronic.
   3. Incidence and cause. Occurs
most often in youngsters under
the age of five years. Death rate
from leukemia is increasing.
Factors associated with its development include ionizing radiation, certain chemicals and
viruses.
   4. Treatment and nursing care.
      a. Treatment to slow down
growth of malignant cells
and maintain a normal level
of red cells and hemoglobin.
      b. Nursing care: relieve symp-
toms and help prevent complications, especially those

of infection and hemor-
rhage.
   c. Patient should be told of his
diagnosis.
   d. Chemotherapy involving a
combination of antileu-
kemic drugs.
E. Hemophilia—characterized by prolonged coagulation time.
   1. Three general types: Classic hemophilia, or hemophilia A;
Christmas disease, or hemophilia B; and von Willebrand's disease.
   2. Symptoms of hemophilia primarily related to internal hemorrhage involving the joints, muscles, intestinal wall, peritoneal
and cranial cavities.
   3. The development of replacement factors has improved the
outlook for hemophiliacs.
   4. Over-protective attitudes toward
the child with hemophilia
should be avoided, and he
should be encouraged to live as
normal a life as possible within
the limitations imposed by his
disease.
F. Purpura.
   1. Small hemorrhages in the skin
and mucous membranes.
   2. Symptomatic of primary diseases such as scurvy, liver disease and allergy to certain drugs.
   3. Treatment aimed at control of
primary disorder.

Part Two.   Nursing Care of Patients With Disorders of the Heart

INTRODUCTION

Heart disease is still the major cause
of death in the United States. Circulatory diseases, which include heart
disease, account for a large percentage
of the chronic illnesses that disable to
some degree another large segment of
the population of this country.
   While these facts may be somewhat

sobering, they should not be interpreted to mean that all heart diseases
are either fatal or totally disabling.
There are many different types of heart
disease, and although any disease
which involves the heart is a serious
affair, many heart conditions are relatively minor and can be cured. Even in
the case of these which cannot be
cured, the knowledge that one has a

heart disease may actually prolong his life if he follows his doctor's orders and lives sensibly.

DIAGNOSTIC TESTS AND EXAMINATIONS

Diagnosis of heart disorders can be made using a wide variety of techniques and tests that are now available to the physician; basically, however, most diagnoses are made with relatively simple tools. Of these techniques and tools, the physician most often relies on a thorough physical examination, a detailed and accurate history and a careful evaluation of the patient's symptoms. Special diagnostic procedures may include the electrocardiogram, multiple-view x-ray films and cardiac catheterization.

Electrocardiogram

An electrocardiogram is a means of studying the heart muscle activity by observing the effects of electric current flowing from the heart. Electric current means the rate of movement of electrical charges through a conductor, just as water current refers to the rate of flow of water molecules through a pipe or other conductor.

Activity of the heart muscle generates negative charges of electricity. To take an electrocardiogram, the operator of an electrocardiograph machine places electrodes on various parts of the patient's body. These electrodes pick up the electric impulses, which are then magnified 3000 times or more and conducted through wires (leads) to a very sensitive needle attached to a graph (see Fig. 15-3). As the impulses cause the needle to vibrate, a recording of the movement is made on a moving paper at the front of the electrocardiograph machine. The tracing made on the paper is called an electrocardiogram. Information obtained by the electrocardiographic tracings includes rhythm of the heart beat, site of the

Figure 15–3. (From Sanderson, ed.: *The Cardiac Patient.* W. B. Saunders Co., Philadelphia.)

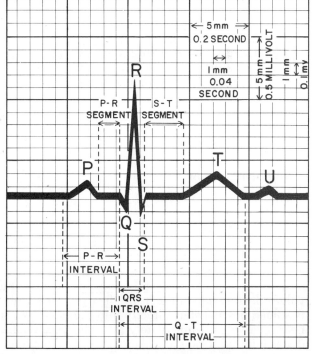

heart's pacemaker, size of the ventricles and abnormal currents passing through the heart muscle.

The electrocardiogram is used to diagnose heart disorders that interfere with proper contraction and relaxation of the heart muscle. It cannot always detect potential heart disease or other disorders of the cardiovascular system.

Preparation of the patient for an electrocardiogram should include some brief explanation of the way in which the machine works. It is natural for the patient to have some fear of a machine that is obviously concerned with electricity. If he understands that the machine transmits electricity from his body and in no way conducts electricity toward him, he will be less apprehensive and more cooperative.

Heart Catheterization

In this procedure, a small, flexible catheter is introduced into a vein of the right arm. The catheter is gently passed into the vena cava, right atrium, right ventricle and on to the pulmonary artery. By using a special manometer, the physician can measure the pressure of the blood in any of these large vessels and chambers of the heart. Samplings of blood are withdrawn from the vessels and chambers for the purpose of determining the oxygen content of the blood as it passes through each of these. The cardiac catheterization is especially useful in diagnosing congenital heart disease.

Angiocardiogram

injected as above

This is a special type of x-ray examination using an opaque dye to aid in visualizing the heart and large blood vessels leading to and from the heart. The dye is injected through a catheter such as is used for cardiac catheterization. In the event the examination involves the left side of the heart, the dye is sometimes injected directly into the heart chambers. Immediately after the dye is injected, x-rays are taken in rapid sequence. This type of examination is done for congenital heart diseases or other structural defects of the heart, its valves or the large blood vessels.

Radioactive Isotopes

Within recent years there has been an increasing interest in the use of radioactive isotopes for the diagnosis of heart disease. For example, structural defects within the heart itself and abnormal routing of the blood to or from the great vessels can be diagnosed by the use of a Geiger counter over the heart to locate radioactive material injected or inhaled into the circulatory system. Radioactive iodine can be used to determine the cardiac output and thereby determine the heart's ability to function as a pump.

Other information that can be obtained through radioactive isotopes include estimation of blood loss and determination of the life span of individual red blood cells.

GENERAL NURSING CARE OF THE CARDIAC PATIENT

The basic principles underlying the nursing care of the patient with heart disease remain essentially the same, even though the diagnosis and treatments may be more specific in each case. In order to avoid repetition in this area, the general nursing care is discussed first. Additional nursing responsibilities involved in specific types of heart disease are included under each disease later in the chapter.

Rest

After the physician has made a definite diagnosis, he decides the amount of rest demanded by the condition of the patient's heart. He may order the patient on complete bed rest, or he may allow some limited activity. In less acute types of heart disease, the patient may be ambulatory.

It is of extreme importance that every one on the nursing team understand exactly what is meant by *absolute or complete bed rest*. When either of these is ordered, the physician does not want the patient to exert himself any more than is absolutely necessary. The nurse may need to interpret the doctor's orders to the patient, explaining the need for absolute rest and enlisting his cooperation. It is very difficult for a person who has always been active suddenly to find himself in a position of total dependence on others even for his most basic needs. The fact that he may feel well enough to exert himself does not alter the situation. *As long as the patient is on absolute bed rest, everything involving the slightest physical effort must be done for him.* He must be fed, bathed, dressed and his position changed by those in attendance. When turning the patient and changing his position, sudden movements and rough handling must be avoided. He should be instructed not to sit up suddenly or turn too quickly.

The clothing of the patient on bed rest should be designed to allow for changing with a minimum of effort. The hospital gown is ideal, but if the patient insists on wearing something different, a gown or pajama coat which does not have to be pulled over the head is best.

It is often a helpless and lonely feeling to be confined to bed for days at a time. The patient on bed rest will need reassurance that his nurse is never very far away. He must never be left without having a call bell at his fingertips, and the nurses on duty should make a special effort to answer his light immediately. A delay in getting to his room may result in undue anxiety or excitement for the patient.

We have spoken of physical rest, but the patient's emotional serenity and peace of mind are equally important. His room should be quiet, neat and orderly, and away from confusion and centers of activity such as the elevator or nurses' station and utility room. The number of visitors is usually decided by the physician or nurse in charge. If the practical nurse notices that a particular visitor leaves the patient agitated and unable to rest after a visit, she must report this to the nurse in charge. It is obvious that the patient must also be protected from any startling news or other occasions of emotional excitement.

The attitude of the nurse caring for him will greatly affect the patient's acceptance of bed rest. If she performs every task willingly and with a genuine desire to be helpful, the patient will be more inclined to relax and cooperate. If, on the other hand, he is made to feel that he is a burden to the nursing staff, causing them a great inconvenience every time he asks for a glass of water or to have his position changed, he will soon start doing things for himself rather than ask for help. *attitude of nurse willing to help - heal better*

Positioning and Exercises. It is the responsibility of the physician to decide when a cardiac patient may get out of bed, sit in a chair, ambulate or exert himself in any way. There are, however, certain implications for nursing care that are derived from the nurse's knowledge of the structure and function of the heart and circulatory system and the particular type of heart disease a patient may have.

Enlargement of the ventricles with improper contraction and ejection of blood from these heart chambers can be aggravated by restriction of the left chest wall. In order to avoid this condition and provide more space for contraction and relaxation of the ventricles, it is best to have the patient lie on his right side or in the supine position. Cardiac output will be impeded less in either of these positions than when the patient is lying on his left side.

If a patient is experiencing respiratory distress, it is best to elevate the head of the bed. This measure allows greater freedom for the diaphragm, since abdominal organs are pulled downward by gravity. Thus, the abdominal organs will not crowd upward toward the thoracic cavity.

It has been noted that children with congenital heart disease often assume a squatting position when they are tired or short of breath. The explanation for this observation is that squatting is an instinctive protective measure taken by the child who suffers from improper pumping action of the heart or valvular deficiency which interferes with proper circulation of blood through the body. The position limits the amount of blood flowing through the legs and thereby decreases the workload of the heart. The adult patient who has a low cardiac output can benefit from sitting up in a chair with his legs dependent or from the nurse rotating tourniquets on his legs. Both of these measures reduce the workload of the heart; however, it is essential that the physician give permission before the nurse carries out either measure.

One must always remain alert to the possibility of sluggish blood flow and clot formation in a patient who is inactive. It is especially important to be alert to this danger in a patient whose heart muscle is damaged and cannot function properly as a pump or whose heart valves cannot ensure adequate circulation of blood through the heart chambers. Bed rest may relieve the workload of the heart, but inactivity is not without its hazards. Mild exercises such as contraction and relaxation of the leg muscles while lying in bed or sitting are helpful in returning pooled blood from the lower extremities and decreasing the possibility of clot formation. Elastic stockings or bandages can also be used to exert pressure on the deep veins and thus facilitate venous return. It is important that the nurse know whether the patient can benefit from full venous return or if he would fare better with a pooling of the blood in the legs and less work for the heart.

Cardiac arrythmias (irregular muscular contractions of the heart) can lead to improper circulation of blood to the brain. Improper circulation, in turn, can lead to signs of poor oxygenation of the brain tissues, such as, for example, light-headedness, mental confusion and extreme drowsiness. These symptoms indicate a need for administration of additional oxygen and for restriction of physical activities that place a burden on the heart. The fact that the patient can feel the irregular rhythm as a fluttering or pounding sensation in his chest contributes to his anxiety. He should be encouraged to rest or sleep as much as possible, and every effort should be made to reassure him so that his anxiety and the effect it has on the heart rate can be reduced. The patient's confidence in the nurse who knows what is to be done and why, and who carries out her duties competently, can greatly reduce his anxiety and the work demanded of his heart.[29]

Diet and Fluids

There are three factors to consider in the diet and fluid intake of the cardiac patient: (1) the amount of food allowed for each meal, (2) the types of food to avoid and (3) the restriction of sodium intake and limiting of fluids when edema is present.

We know that digestion of food requires an increased amount of blood flow to the stomach, which in turn places an extra burden on the heart to supply that blood. It is also true that a full stomach may interfere with the lowering of the diaphragm and complete expansion of the lungs. In view of these facts, it is evident that patients with heart disease should be fed several small meals of easily digested foods rather than three large meals a day. In the acute stages of the disease, the diet may be limited to liquids and semisolid foods to prevent overtaxation of the heart.

In addition to providing small, digestible meals, the diet is also planned so that highly seasoned foods and stimulants such as tea and coffee are avoided, as are all gas-forming foods which may lead to abdominal distention. Most physicians will request that extremely hot and cold foods and liquids be eliminated from the diet, especially cold drinks and iced foods, because of the constriction of blood vessels brought about by cold.

In the presence of edema, sodium is restricted in the diet because of its ability to hold fluid within the tissues. The seasoning of foods with salt substitutes and other condiments may be allowed by the physician to make the diet more palatable. The limitation of fluids by mouth depends on the type of disease present and the wishes of the physician in charge. In some cases, the nurse may find that fluids are limited to as little as 1000 or 1500 ml. within a 24-hour period. In this case, *completely accurate* records must be kept and the intake of liquids scheduled so that the patient does not have to wait an unreasonable length of time before he may have something to relieve his thirst.

Care of the Skin

The fact that the patient must not exert himself and should remain immobile presents quite a problem in the proper care of the skin and prevention of pressure sores. When edema is present, the problem is even more difficult because edematous tissue breaks down more readily than normal tissue. Frequent turning of the patient must be done with adequate help so that the patient does not feel the need to exert himself in an effort to help. As stated before, sudden movements and rough handling are to be avoided. The area of the sacral bone must be given special attention, especially when the patient is in orthopneic position, because of the tendency for edema to localize at the lower spine. Care of the back may be accomplished fairly easily with the patient sitting up and leaning across the overbed table padded with pillows.

Medications

Drugs useful in the treatment of the patient with heart disease consist mainly of three types: (1) those which decrease the rate and improve the strength of the contractions of the heart muscle so that it beats more normally, (2) those which relieve edema and (3) those which provide relief from pain. Other more specific medications are discussed later in this chapter under their related diseases.

The drug used most often to slow and strengthen the heart beat is *digitalis.* This drug is classified as a heart tonic; that is, it improves the muscular contractions of the heart, making it more effective as a pump. There are several different forms of digitalis, and there are preparations which may be given by intramuscular injection as well as by mouth. In the administration of any of these preparations, the pulse should be counted just before each dose is given. It is a generally accepted rule in all institutions that the medication is withheld if the pulse is below 60 per minute, and the doctor is informed of the situation.

Another drug used to control the heart beat is *quinidine.* This drug is a heart depressant. It stops the convulsive twitching of the heart muscle (fibrillation) and improves the rhythm of the heart beat. By depressing the heart's contractions, quinidine allows for a more complete relaxation of the heart muscle between contractions so that the chambers may completely fill with blood. Since it is a heart depressant, the pulse should also be counted before quinidine is administered.

Edema of the tissues may be relieved by the administration of drugs which increase the urinary output. These drugs are called *diuretics.* Diuretics can be classified according to their physiological action. One type increases the rate of glomerular filtration and thereby increases urinary output. A second type affects the osmotic pressure in the tubules of the kidney and prevents reabsorption of fluid back into the blood stream so that these fluids remain in the tubules and are excreted as urine. A third group of diuretics inhibit the secretion of antidiuretic hormone (ADH). As a result of this deficiency of ADH, water is not reabsorbed into the blood stream, and it is excreted in large amounts as dilute urine.[12]

Most physicians wish to have the patient receiving a diuretic weighed daily in order to estimate the amount of fluid lost from the tissues. When weighing a patient daily, the nurse should schedule the procedure so that the patient is weighed at the same time each day (preferably in the morning before breakfast), on the same scales and with the same amount of clothing. In addition to daily weighing, the physician will most likely request that an accurate record be kept of the patient's intake and output of fluids. The procedure for measuring and recording intake and output varies in each hospital. The important point to be emphasized is that everyone who is in any way responsible for the care of the patient must carry out this procedure conscientiously.

Severe pain is most often associated with heart disease of an acute nature, such as myocardial infarction. The drugs used most often are morphine sulfate and Demerol. As the acute phase and severe pain subside, these drugs may be replaced with milder sedatives which promote relaxation and freedom from anxiety. Much of the patient's pain may be due to his nervousness and anxiety, and so the nurse can do much to help relieve his pain by providing complete physical and mental rest for him. In the scheduling of necessary procedures such as turning the patient, skin care, etc., she should use common sense so that the patient is not disturbed any more often than necessary, and most especially she should realize that medications which induce sleep and relieve pain are not given as a substitute for good nursing care.

Rehabilitation of the Patient

The amount and type of activities permitted the patient during convalescence and after discharge from the hospital are governed by the response of the heart to treatment and the amount of residual damage to the heart itself. The physician will impress on the patient the importance of following his orders so that future attacks can be avoided. The patient with a chronic heart disease must adjust his life so that no extra demands are placed on the circulatory system. Members of the health team, including the dietitian, social worker and public health nurse, may all play an important part in teaching the patient how to live with his illness.

Prevention of Heart Disease

As a recognized member of the nursing team, the practical nurse has a responsibility in the education of the public regarding the prevention of heart disease. A few of the "facts of life" in regard to the heart diseases are presented below.

1. Obesity does not directly cause heart disease, but it does place an unnecessary strain on the heart, making it more susceptible to heart disease.

2. A diet that is habitually high in calories, total fats, saturated fats, cholesterol, refined carbohydrates and salt presents a major risk in the development of coronary heart disease.

3. Cigarette smoking increases the proneness to coronary heart disease from two- to six-fold, depending on the number of cigarettes smoked.

4. Elevated blood pressure (that is, a diastolic pressure in the range of 90 to 94 mm. Hg) is closely associated with coronary heart disease.

5. Atherosclerotic heart diseases are closely associated with diabetes mellitus.[31]

6. Exercise does not damage the heart; in fact, light to moderate exercise is a good protective device, provided it

is done regularly. Sudden bursts of strenuous exercise by a person who is not accustomed to exercise can be damaging to the heart.

7. Periodic physical examinations for children will facilitate early detection of congenital heart diseases that are not severe enough to present serious symptoms.

8. There is a definite relationship between streptococcal infections of the throat and rheumatic heart disease. The nurse must encourage early treatment of sore throats and other infections that could be streptococcal in origin.

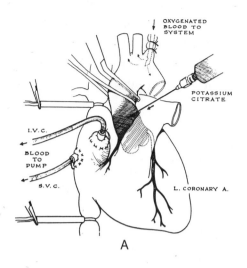

A

SURGERY OF THE HEART

Introduction

Until the 1950's, there was little that could be done in the way of surgical procedures involving the heart itself, because prolonged interruption of circulation meant certain death for the patient. But with the advent of the heart-lung machine and hypothermia techniques, surgeons could repair or replace damaged valves and correct many congenital heart defects.

The heart-lung machine, which has many variations in design and appearance, functions as artificial heart (pump) and lungs (oxygenator). For this reason, it is sometimes called a pump-oxygenator. Since all of this is done outside the patient's body, the procedure is called extracorporeal circulation. The surgeon inserts large tubes in the venae cavae and reroutes the unoxygenated venous blood through the heart-lung machine (see Fig. 15-4). There the blood is exposed to an atmosphere of oxygen in which an exchange of gases takes place— carbon dioxide is released and oxygen is taken up—and the oxygenated blood is returned to the patient via the femoral artery. The blood also may be cooled so that the patient's body temperature is lowered (hypothermia),

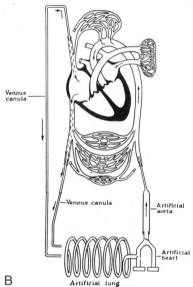

B

Figure 15–4. *A,* Schema of intrathoracic cannulation for extracorporeal maintenance of circulation. Systemic venous return is diverted to oxygenator by intracaval catheters. Although blood return is pictured returning from oxygenator entering aortic arch by way of the subclavian artery, the current mode of returning oxygenated blood is by extrathoracic cannulation of the femoral artery. The diagram also demonstrates the first method of elective cardiac arrest by injection of 4.5 mEq. of diluted potassium citrate into the aortic root. *B,* Diagram of artificial maintenance of circulation. Extrathoracic cannulation: Blood is sucked out of venae cavae into oxygenator and is pumped through a side-branch (femoral artery) back into the aorta. Flow in aorta is reversed. All tissues are perfused with blood coming from the aorta. (From Quinn: Journal of Practical Nursing, November, 1965.)

thereby reducing the body's metabolic needs during surgery.

Extracorporeal circulation and hypothermia permit the cardiac surgeon adequate time to open the heart, visually inspect its internal structures and perform the necessary surgery. Congenital heart defects such as abnormal openings in the septum can be repaired fairly easily. Others that involve more than one defect and require extensive repair of the heart and one or more of the great vessels are less successful and present more of a risk to the patient.

An artificial valve such as the one shown in Figure 15-5 can be inserted as a replacement for a diseased valve that has been damaged in rheumatic heart disease or other acquired heart disorders.

Preoperative Care

Prior to surgery, the patient undergoes a series of diagnostic tests and examinations such as those presented in the previous pages of this chapter. These tests are done to determine as far as possible the exact nature of the heart's structural defects. With this information, the surgeon plans the type of surgical procedure he will perform to correct the condition. If the procedure seems relatively simple, he will so inform the patient and his family. If the defect involves a very high risk, the patient and his family must make the decision as to whether or not the surgery is to be done. The physician or some other qualified person also will instruct the patient, explaining what he can expect to be done, the kind of equipment to be used during and after surgery and the expected results of the surgical procedure. Most authorities agree that the patient should not be told so much as to confuse him and cause undue worry, nor so little that he is apprehensive and frightened when he awakens from anesthesia and finds himself in the midst of complicated machinery. The information given is tailored to each patient's individual

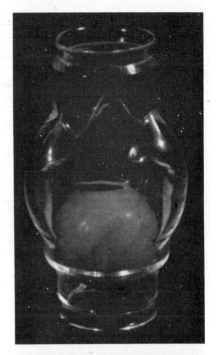

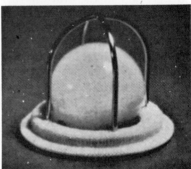

Figure 15–5. Hufnagel (top) and Starr-Edwards cardiac valves operate on the ball-valve principle: a ball regulates an opening by suction and by its own weight. Sound is produced by the forceful back-and-forth movement of the ball as it strikes its stationary cage. (From Slatin: American Journal of Nursing, June, 1967.)

needs, level of intelligence and apparent desire to know what is in store for him.

During the operative procedure, the surgical personnel must function as a team. Each person must be thoroughly trained in his duties. Figure 15-6 shows the many persons and types of equipment involved in open-heart surgery.

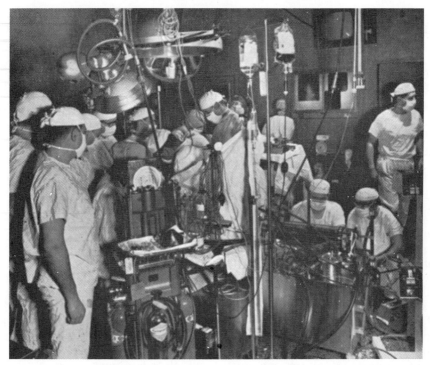

Figure 15–6. The scene in the operating room during open-heart surgery in which an artificial valve was inserted to replace a leaking aortic valve. The artificial heart-lung machine is seen in the lower right hand corner. The full "team" consists of 14 people: four surgeons, two scrub nurses, two circulating nurses, two anesthesiologists, two technicians operating the artificial heart-lung machine, one nurse operating the monitoring and recording equipment, and one cardiologist.

The electrocardiogram, arterial and venous blood pressure, and blood pressures in various chambers of the heart are recorded and visible on the large monitor screen in the upper right hand corner.

Although the maze of wires and tubing seen in this picture seems to have achieved almost nightmarish proportions, when each member of the team carries out his assigned task there is no confusion and the whole operation proceeds with quiet efficiency. (From Rogoz and Holswade: Journal of Practical Nursing, April, 1966.)

Postoperative Care

During the entire postoperative period, intelligent observation is the primary concern of the nurse. The patient is kept in an intensive care unit, where specially trained personnel and monitoring equipment are in constant attendance. After the first 48 hours, the surgeon will assess the patient's condition and decide whether he can be transferred to a general surgical unit. The patient will continue to need nursing care of the most detailed kind. His vital signs must be taken and recorded at regular intervals. His intake and output must be measured and recorded at least every eight hours, and his fluid intake may be restricted for a period of time. Thoracotomy tubes for drainage and proper re-expansion of the lungs will need special attention (see Chapter 16 for details). He may be given oxygen by tent or nasal prongs.

Until the surgeon allows the patient out of bed, it is necessary to encourage gentle daily exercises of the arms and legs. These are necessary to improve circulation and to maintain full range of motion in the joints, especially that of the left shoulder, which the patient hesitates to move and uses as a protective splint to avoid motion in the operative area. The amount of physical activity is very gradually increased and is governed by the type of surgery done and the patient's reaction to surgery.

CONGESTIVE HEART FAILURE

Definition

Congestive heart failure is actually a complication of other cardiac conditions rather than a disease in itself; in fact, it is the chief complication in 70 per cent of all patients who have heart disease. When the heart loses its efficiency as a pump, the result is congestion within the heart chambers. This may develop gradually over a period of years or it may appear suddenly, following an acute disease of the heart or kidneys.

It is usually the left side of the heart that fails first in congestive failure, but eventually both sides will be affected. To understand the mechanism involved in congestive failure, one must have some knowledge of the circulation of blood through a normal, well-functioning heart. Normally, the ventricles contract while the atria relax, so that with each contraction of the ventricle, blood is poured into the atrium on each side of the heart. The ventricles then relax and receive a new supply of blood. In congestive failure, the contractions of the ventricles are weak; thus, they cannot empty, and so become engorged with blood. When the left ventricle fails, there will be a damming up of blood in the left atrium and the pulmonary veins. If the right ventricle fails, there will be a damming up of blood in the right atrium and the vena cava.

Symptoms

The symptoms of congestive failure can readily be understood by analyzing the steps mentioned above. The key word is *congestion*. We know how our progress is slowed down when we approach a congested area of traffic while driving an automobile. So it is with the circulation of blood when congestion is present. The sluggish flow of blood through the pulmonary vessels produces dyspnea, cough and sometimes hemoptysis (the spitting of blood). If the situation continues unchecked, the serum from the blood inside the pulmonary vessels empties into the air sacs of the lung and begins to fill the lower branches of the bronchial tree. When this happens, the patient is said to have *pulmonary edema.*

Congestion of the venae cavae leads to a dependent type of edema, which means that the lower parts of the body are edematous. There is also an accumulation of fluids in the liver and abdominal organs. Congestion of the kidneys may lead to impaired kidney function, which only aggravates the condition of edema. Inadequate circulation of fresh blood to the brain may cause mental confusion and irritability which sometimes progresses to delirium or loss of consciousness.

Treatment and Nursing Care

Medical treatment and nursing care for the patient with congestive heart failure are aimed at three goals: reducing the body's oxygen needs, eliminating edematous fluid from the body and increasing the output of the heart. These are accomplished through rest, proper diet and the administration of oxygen, diuretics, and drugs which increase heart muscle tone, particularly digitalis preparations.

Rest. In providing rest for the patient with congestive failure, the nurse must remember the hazard of the formation of an embolus when the circulation is so sluggish. The doctor may order passive exercises of the lower extremities and flexion of the legs several times a day to speed up the blood flow and discourage the development of clots. If these exercises are ordered, it is important to explain to the patient that they are passive exercises to be done by the nurse and require no effort on his part.

The patient with mild congestive failure may be ambulatory or may be sent home with instructions to perform only light work. These patients usually must receive help and guidance from the public health nurse, social worker, visiting nurse or other individuals and agencies concerned with the welfare of cardiac patients.

Those patients who are confined to bed with acute congestive failure should have side rails on their beds because of the mental confusion and disorientation which frequently accompanies this condition.

Diet. While the patient is in the hospital, he has no responsibilities in the preparation of his meals of (restriction of sodium from his diet) When he is discharged from the hospital, however, he or a member of his family must have some instruction in the preparation of meals and planning of menus within the limitations of a low-sodium diet. Although the dietitian is usually responsible for this instruction, repetition and further explanation by the nursing staff will help to impress on the patient the importance of this phase of his treatment. The physician may or may not allow substitutes for table salt. The nurse might explain to the patient and his family that there is no need for purchasing expensive foods specially prepared for low-sodium diets as long as the person preparing the food at home understands the proper way to modify the family's regular meals so that the patient's food has a low-sodium content. Seasonings such as garlic, onions, lemon juice, vinegar, and other herbs are acceptable on the low-sodium diet and help to make the food more palatable. The patient should be cautioned to read the labels on all cereals and processed foods because some of these have sodium added for preservation. He must also be warned that many patent medicines, cough syrups and dentifrices contain sodium. And finally, though this is obvious to those who know the correct term for baking soda, sodium bicarbonate is not allowed the patient on a low-sodium diet.

Medications. Drugs used in the treatment of congestive failure are most often (diuretics and digitalis) These have been discussed earlier under general treatment and nursing care. However, it may be well to remind the reader that many persons with chronic congestive failure must continue to take digitalis daily for the rest of their lives. *Apical & Radial pulse*

Practical nurses may hear the doctor use the term "digitalized" in reference to the patient. This means that the patient has been given the drug several times a day while in the hospital until it has had the desired effect. After the patient is "digitalized," he must continue to take a maintenance dose of the medication every day so as to sustain the desired effect as long as necessary. The patient should have impressed on him the importance of faithfully continuing his medication once he has been discharged from the hospital, even though he may feel that his condition has improved to the point that he does not need it any more.

Pulmonary Edema *LCHF*

The accumulation of fluid within the lung tissues can occur very suddenly following rapid failure of the left side of the heart or as a result of an abrupt increase in the workload of the heart. This acute condition can be fatal in a very short period of time if not relieved by emergency measures. The patient with chronic congestive heart failure involving the left side of the heart can also suffer from pulmonary edema, and though the symptoms are less dramatic in the chronic form, they are no less uncomfortable or frightening for the patient.

Symptoms. In *acute pulmonary edema,* the patient experiences a sudden, frightening dyspnea. He cannot lie down flat in the bed because such a position only increases the edema in his lungs and aggravates his shortness of breath. He may complain of a heaviness or pressure in his chest rather than a sharp pain. He often becomes slightly cyanotic, and he perspires profusely. His respiration is rapid, and each time he breathes, a moist, rattling sound can be heard some distance away from him. The congestion in his lungs produces a persistent hacking cough, and the sputum brought up is thick at first, becoming thin, frothy and blood-tinged. The pulse rate increases, and the venous pressure becomes so great that the jugular veins become distended and are easily observed. The patient becomes more and more apprehensive and begins to struggle for air, breathing more rapidly (hyperventilating) and thereby further aggravating the situation. Unless the condition is relieved, the heart weakens and begins to beat irregularly, and the patient eventually loses consciousness. Finally, death occurs as the heart and lungs fail.[19]

Treatment and Nursing Care. If the nurse is the first to observe a patient in acute pulmonary edema, she must realize that an emergency situation exists and that without proper treatment, the patient may literally "drown" in his own secretions. She should place the patient in orthopneic position, so that he can breathe as well as possible, and summon help immediately. She also must strive to reassure the patient and keep him as calm as possible. Oxygen is administered, and the patient is given a sedative such as morphine sulfate to relieve anxiety, induce rest and repress the respiratory reflexes. If the patient is not already receiving digitalis, some fast-acting form of this drug is given to slow and strengthen the heart beat.

Because of the congested state of the pulmonary blood vessels, some measures must be taken to reduce the venous return of blood to the heart. One way in which this can be accomplished is by rotating tourniquets on the extremities (see Fig. 15-7). Note that the tourniquets are changed promptly every 15 minutes. This is necessary so that circulation to the extremities is not seriously impaired and blood clots do not form in the veins.

In addition to the preceding measures, the patient may be given a rapid-acting diuretic to speed up the elimination of body fluids and thereby reduce fluid volume in the blood vessels and tissue spaces. Of course, a very accurate record must be kept of the patient's intake and output. Weight is usually checked daily, and the patient's diet restricted in fluids and sodium.

DISEASES OF THE CORONARY ARTERIES

Definition

The heart is actually a muscle and as such must have its own supply of

TABLE 15–2. DOSAGE AND TIME OF ACTION OF DIGITALIS PREPARATIONS*

Preparation	Route	Onset of action	Peak effect	Total digitalizing dose	Daily oral maintenance dose
Digitalis leaf	Oral	2-5 hr.	8-24 hr.	1.5 Gm.	0.1 Gm.
Digitoxin	Oral	2-4 hr.	8-12 hr.	1.5 mg.	0.15 mg.
Gitalin	Oral	2-4 hr.	8-10 hr.	5 mg.	0.5 mg.
Lanatoside C	Oral	varies	6 hr.	5-10 mg.	0.5-1.5 mg.
Deslanoside	I.V.	10-30 min.	2-3 hr.	1.6 mg.	
Digoxin	Oral	1-3 hr.	6 hr.	2.5 mg.	0.375 mg.
"	I.V.	10-30 min.	2-3 hr.	1.5 mg.	

*From "Drugs Used in the Care of the Cardiac Patient," Nurs. Clin. N. Amer., Vol. 4, No. 4, 1969, p. 646.

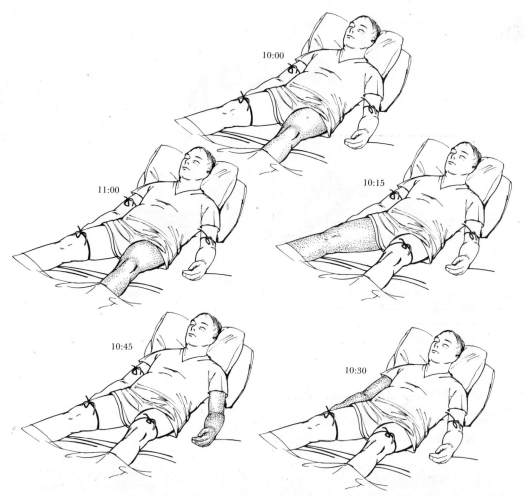

Figure 15–7. Rotation of tourniquets at 15-minute intervals.

blood to nourish it and remove waste products. The blood vessels which supply blood to the heart muscle *(myocardium)* are called the coronary vessels. They were given this name because the main trunks of these vessels encircle the top of the heart like a crown and send their branches downward into the heart muscle (see Fig. 15-8). The coronary arteries are especially important because any disease involving these vessels will ultimately result in a decrease in the efficiency of the heart.

The coronary arteries may be affected by a hardening and loss of elasticity of their walls *(arteriosclerosis)* or deposits of material inside the vessel *(atherosclerosis)*. In either case, the condition causes a narrowing of the lumen of the vessel and predisposes it to a complete blockage of blood flow through the artery.

Types of Coronary Disease

There are two main types of disease processes which may affect the coronary arteries once they have become narrowed. The first is a sudden occluding or closing of the artery by a blood clot. This clot may be formed within the artery at the site of the occlusion *(thrombus)* or may be one which has

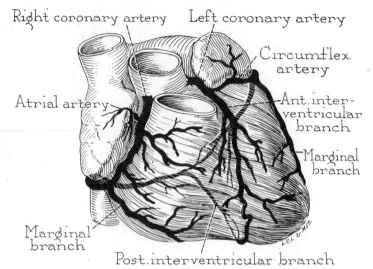

Figure 15–8. The heart, showing the coronary arteries, which encircle the top of the heart and send branches down into the muscle tissue of the heart. (From King and Showers: *Human Anatomy and Physiology*, 6th Ed., W. B. Saunders Co., Philadelphia.)

entered the blood stream at a distant point and been carried along until it reached a vessel too small to allow its passage *(embolus)*. The sudden blocking of a coronary vessel may be referred to as a *myocardial infarction, coronary occlusion* or *coronary attack*.

In the second type of coronary artery disease, the arteries become hardened or filled with layers of deposits over a period of time so that the openings inside these tubular structures gradually become more and more narrow until they are eventually closed. This disease process leads to a condition called *angina pectoris*.

Acute Myocardial Infarction. An *infarction* is an area of necrotic tissue caused by an obstruction to the flow of blood to that area (see Fig. 15-9). Myocardial means "pertaining to the heart muscle." Thus, in a myocardial infarction, there is an area of necrosis in the heart muscle. The prognosis of the patient who suffers an acute myocardial infarction depends to a great extent on the size of the artery plugged by a clot and the amount of heart tissue that artery had formerly supplied with blood. If a large area of the heart is

affected, instant death may occur. Smaller areas may heal if treated promptly and effectively.

SYMPTOMS. The clinical picture presented by the patient with an acute myocardial infarction is one that most lay people recognize as a "heart attack." There is a sudden, severe pain in the chest, usually described as crushing or burning. Sometimes the pain is mistaken as a symptom of acute indigestion. The patient also shows symptoms of shock with pallor, profuse sweating, anxiety and often nausea and vomiting.

Although the above symptoms are usually present in an acute myocardial infarction, they are not always so severe, and in some cases the patients have described their pain as mild. The severity of the symptoms will depend on the size of the area of infarction.

Whenever there is necrotic tissue anywhere in the body, the white cell count increases and the sedimentation rate is elevated. Within 24 hours of an acute attack, the temperature of the patient with myocardial infarction rises and leukocytosis appears.

The use of enzyme studies in the

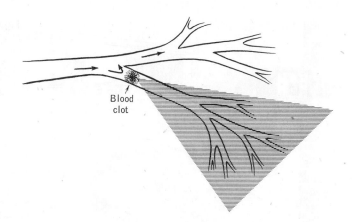

Figure 15–9. Shaded area represents region of infarct resulting from obstruction to the flow of blood through vessel plugged by clot.

Blood clot

diagnosis of myocardial infarction has greatly increased the accuracy with which a diagnosis of this condition can be made. Enzyme studies are described in more detail in Chapter 5 of this text. The specific enzymes whose levels are significant in the detection of myo-

cardial infarction are shown in Fig. 15-10.

TREATMENT AND NURSING CARE

Immediate Care. An acute myocardial infarction is an emergency case and requires immediate treatment to

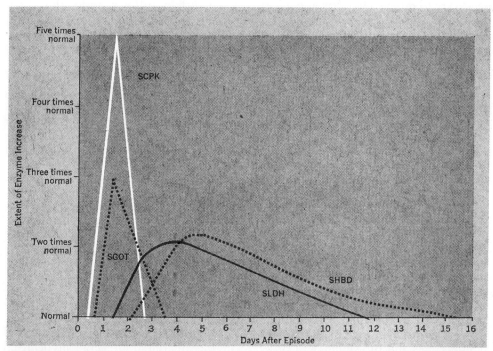

Figure 15–10. Typical changes in serum enzyme levels following myocardial infarction. Early rapid rise of both the serum creatine phosphokinase (SCPK) and serum glutamic oxaloacetic transaminase (SGOT) within first 2 days of infarction contrasts with later rise of lactic dehydrogenase (SLDH) and serum hydroxy butyrate dehydrogenase. SHBD elevation persists 10 to 20 days, thus offering the most persistent evidence of infarction. (From Coodley: American Journal of Nursing, February, 1968.)

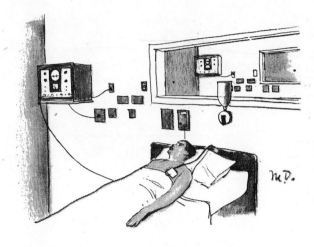

Figure 15–11. Some of the special equipment used in a coronary care unit to provide constant surveillance of coronary patients and immediate treatment of those who go into cardiac arrest, failure or shock, or who show significant arrythmias. Each patient is connected to an electrocardiographic monitor with a pacemaker attachment in place for immediate activation. The monitors have an emergency alarm signal that goes off when the rate or quality of the beats changes. The ECG and pulse rate are constantly displayed on oscilloscopes at the bedside and at the nurses' station. Equipment needed for defibrillation, heart reactivation, cardiopulmonary resuscitation and emergency drug therapy is available. (From Hazletine: American Journal of Nursing, November, 1964.)

combat shock and prevent further circulatory collapse. Pain is relieved by morphine sulfate or Demerol. The first dose is often given directly into the vein by the physician. Oxygen may be necessary to relieve cyanosis and assist the heart in its efforts to circulate oxygenated blood through the body. The patient often feels panic and expresses a sensation of approaching death. This pessimistic attitude may persist for several days after the attack. The nurse must do all that she can to convey a feeling of calm reassurance to the patient and convince him that the situation is in hand and his only concern is to relax and let the medications take effect.

Rest. Most patients who have suffered a myocardial infarction are placed on bed rest for at least one month or more to allow the heart to rest and healing to take place. The principles and practices mentioned earlier in this chapter in regard to providing rest for the cardiac patient are extremely important in the care of the patient with an acute myocardial infarction.

Sometimes the physician will order exercises of the legs to prevent the formation of a thrombus in the veins. These exercises may be done by the nurse (passive) or by the patient (active), depending on the desires of the physician. It is also important in the prevention of phlebothrombosis to avoid pressure on the back of the leg under the knee. This means that the knee rest or pillows under the knees should be used only for brief periods of time and alternated with an exercise in which the patient presses his feet against the footboard or foot of the bed.

Another common complication of acute myocardial infarction is "frozen shoulder." This is a term used to describe limited motion of the shoulder and arm. It is caused by the patient's attempt to relieve the pain in his chest by keeping his left arm immobile against his chest. To avoid this complication, massage and exercises under the doctor's orders may be done. It is also helpful if the nurse will place a pillow between the arm and chest wall to support the arm and relieve the tension of the muscles.

Medications. In addition to the digitalis mentioned under general treatment of heart diseases, there is one group of drugs that is specifically used in the treatment of acute myocardial infarction. These are the *anticoagulants,* so called because they impair the clotting mechanism of the blood. These drugs are usually ordered by the physician daily as "stat" doses only after he has received a laboratory report on the patient's current prothrombin level (see Chapter 5).

PREVENTION OF ACUTE MYOCARDIAL INFARCTION. The high incidence rate of coronary heart disease in men between the ages of 40 and 60 years has prompted Dr. Robert McMillon of Winston-Salem, North Carolina, to write "A Coronary Decalogue." Some of these rules may seem a bit flippant to include in a textbook, but they are all based on sound principles and are presented with the sincere conviction that they offer an excellent guide for those who wish to avoid an acute attack of coronary heart disease.

1. Thou shalt not try to be a champion athlete after 50.
2. Thou shalt not struggle to be a perfectionist.
3. Thou shalt not fill up thy stomach with food nor engage in exercise after eating.
4. Thou shalt consider losing thy temper a luxury to be indulged in sparingly.
5. Thou shalt avoid worry—the government will probably take care of you.
6. Thou shalt keep thy alcoholic intake below the point where it may delude thee into thinking thou art a better man than thou ever were.
7. Thou shalt not smoke tobacco if possible.
8. Thou shalt take regular vacations.
9. Thou shalt avoid cold weather.
10. After a certain age thou shalt not take unto thyself a young wife, nor even a reasonable facsimile.*

Angina Pectoris. The term "angina pectoris" literally means a severe cramplike pain in the chest; however, it is used universally to designate a serious cardiac disorder resulting from a decreased blood supply to the heart muscle. It is caused by a narrowing of the arteries due to arteriosclerosis or atherosclerosis.

Angina pectoris is similar to myo-

---

*Reprinted from the *Atlanta Constitution*, Thursday, February 7, 1963.

cardial infarction in that it results from an inadequate oxygen supply to the myocardium. The difference is that myocardial infarction is a result of a rather sudden blockage of a coronary artery, whereas angina pectoris is a more gradual process in which the coronary vessels cannot bring sufficient blood supply (or oxygen) to the myocardium because they are occluded by atherosclerotic plaque and their walls have lost their elasticity.

The attacks of pain in angina pectoris vary in each patient, so that an activity that precipitates an attack one day may have no effect on the patient the next day. Generally, however, there are some factors that can be considered relevant to an attack. These include sudden physical exertion, especially in the morning, cold air, eating a very heavy meal and emotional upsets.[11]

SYMPTOMS. The type of pain or discomfort may vary in individuals, but in most cases it is described as a dull pain or tightness under the sternum. It may or may not radiate down one or both arms. Sometimes the patient experiences dyspnea, and there may be pallor or flushing of the face and profuse perspiration.

In general, it is felt that the patient with chronic but unchanging angina pectoris is not in serious trouble, and his condition is not critical. However, if his condition becomes worse very suddenly, he most likely will suffer from serious damage to the heart muscle.

TREATMENT AND NURSING CARE. The treatment of angina pectoris is mostly symptomatic, with emphasis on eliminating those factors which are known to precipitate an attack in the individual patient. With guidance from his physician, the patient may soon learn to correlate certain activities with an attack and thereby learn to avoid them whenever possible.

Medications. The most specific type of medications used for angina pectoris are the *vasodilators*, that is, those drugs which expand the blood vessels, allowing for a more rapid flow of blood. The drug of choice is usually nitroglycerine in tablets, administered under the tongue. This drug acts almost immediately and often produces a feeling of warmth, flushing of the face or throbbing in the head. When these patients are hospitalized, it is not unusual for the physician to write an order granting permission for the patient to keep nitroglycerine tablets at his bedside to be taken as needed.

Effects of Cold. We know that cold has a direct effect on the blood vessels, causing them to contract. The patient with angina pectoris is already suffering from a narrowing of the arteries; thus, he must avoid exposure to cold, which will further aggravate the condition. He should be instructed to wear warm clothing and stay indoors when the weather is extremely cold. In the summer months, some patients have suffered attacks when they entered an air-conditioned building after being out in the hot sun.

DISORDERS OF THE HEART'S CONDUCTION SYSTEM

Introduction

One can hardly read a newspaper or magazine today without becoming aware of the great strides being taken in the field of electronics, and the ways in which this advancing research can be of benefit to the health and welfare of mankind. The comparatively new transistors have now been found to be useful in initiating electrical impulses in the hearts of persons suffering from disorders of the heart's electrical conduction system. Although the surgical procedure involved in inserting an artificial pacemaker cannot be termed simple, it probably will become more and more common in the years to come.

We know that the normal heart is capable of generating tiny electrical impulses that can be picked up, amplified and recorded by an electrocardiograph. These impulses are essential to normal contraction of the heart's ventricles and atria. The impulses originate in the sino-atrial (S.A.) node and the atrioventricular (A.V.) node. These are neuromuscular structures. One, the S.A. node, is located in the wall of the right atrium between the openings for the inferior and superior venae cavae. It stimulates contraction of the atria. The A.V. node is located in the septum between the atria and transmits impulses via the bundle of His and the Purkinje fibers to the ventricles, causing them to contract (see Fig. 15-12).

When the heart's electrical conduction system fails, the normal contractions of the heart that are necessary to its pumping action also fail. It is not possible to relieve this condition by implanting the electrodes of an artificial packmaker directly into the heart muscle. These electrodes are attached to the very small pacemaker batteries which are pre-set to stimulate ventricular contractions at a rate of 70 per minute. Pacing may be accomplished temporarily, as in the case of complete heart block following myocardial infarction, or permanently, when the heart's conduction system is irreparably damaged. Temporary pacing is accomplished by transvenous insertion of an electrode catheter through the basilic and jugular vein to the right ventricle (see Fig. 15-13). Permanent pacing involves implantation of the electrodes and the pacemaker within the body (see Fig. 15-14).

Indications for Use of the Pacemaker

There are four general disorders that may respond to the artificial pacemaker. They are: (1) Stokes-Adams disease, a condition characterized by disturbances in the rhythm of ventricular contractions. The arrhythmia inter-

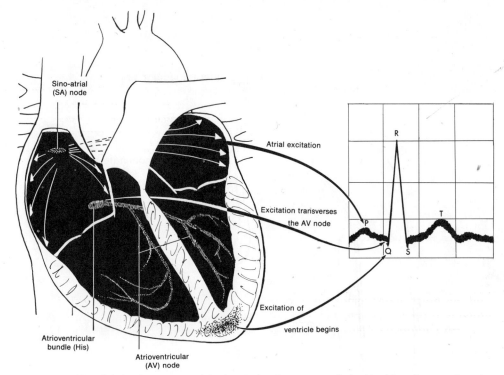

Sino-atrial
(SA) node

Atrial excitation

Excitation transverses
the AV node

Excitation of

ventricle begins

Atrioventricular
bundle (His)

Atrioventricular
(AV) node

Figure 15–12. Conducting system of the heart showing source of electrical impulses produced on electrocardiogram. (After Jacob and Francone: *Structure and Function in Man*, 2nd Ed., W. B. Saunders Co., Philadelphia.)

feres with normal flow of blood to the brain and produces symptoms of dizziness, unconsciousness, convulsions or death. (2) Carotid sinus syndrome, a disorder involving the carotid sinus, which works by reflex action to ensure a steady flow of blood to the brain and other parts of the body. When the carotid sinus does not function normally, the patient suffers from attacks of fainting, lowered blood pressure or convulsions. Such an attack can be precipitated by slight pressure on the carotid sinus, as from turning the head quickly or wearing a tight collar. (3) Surgical injury to the heart's conduction system during corrective cardiac surgery. (4) Arteriosclerosis with atrioventricular block in some elderly patients.[14]

Nursing Care

During the preoperative period, the nurse cooperates with the physician and other members of the medical team in diagnostic tests and other procedures that will be useful in determining the patient's readiness for surgery. She must be especially observant of the patient's vital signs, and if any attacks of fainting or dizziness occur, they should be reported accurately. During such an attack, the patient's pulse should be taken and recorded. The nurse also should chart the duration of the attack and any aftereffects noted.

Instruction of the patient and physical preparation for surgery are approximately the same as for any major surgery. The physician will explain the artificial pacemaker and the expected outcome of the surgical procedure. The patient also should be informed of the type of equipment and special apparatus that will be used postoperatively. This includes thoracic tubes and drainage bottles, intravenous tubes, oxygen and possibly gastric suction.

After the patient recovers from surgery, he will be able to return home

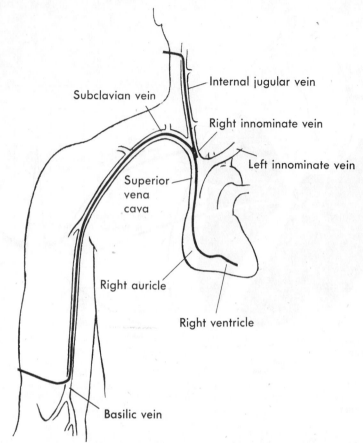

Figure 15–13. Temporary transvenous pacing catheter may be inserted via several routes: shown here are jugular and basilic vein insertion sites. The catheter is guided into the right ventricle using fluoroscopy or by watching the EKG for a characteristic wave form. (From Andreoli et al.: *Comprehensive Cardiac Care*, The C. V. Mosby Co., St. Louis. Reprinted in American Journal of Nursing, April 1969.)

within one to two weeks. The artificial pacemaker should cause him no discomfort and should not hamper the movement of his chest or arm. Many of these patients will be able to indulge in activities that formerly were restricted because of the danger of precipitating an attack. They can lead normal lives again without the constant fear of a serious or even fatal attack.

INFLAMMATORY DISEASES OF THE HEART

Definition

The tissues of the heart are subject to the same inflammatory conditions that may affect other parts of the body. The inflammation may be present in the inner lining (*endocarditis*), the heart muscle (*myocarditis*) or the sac surrounding the heart (*pericarditis*). The process may also involve the valves between the heart chambers or those located at the base of the major vessels leading from the heart.

Bacterial infection of the heart can result from an acute infection elsewhere in the body, such as those caused by staphylococci, pneumococci and gonococci. However, the most common occurrence is inflammation of the heart as a complication of rheumatic fever.

Unfortunately, rheumatic heart dis-

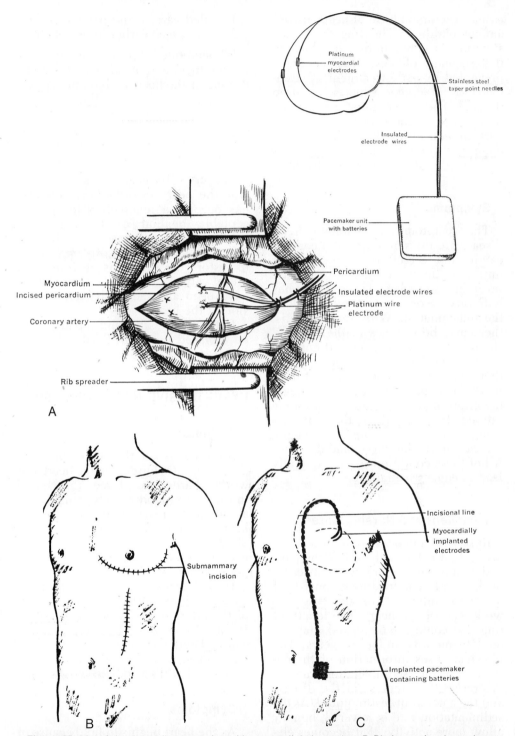

Figure 15–14. *A,* Implantable pacemaker with myocardial electrodes. *B,* Platinum wire electrodes are implanted usually in the left ventricular wall. *C,* Outward appearance of patient with abdominally implanted pacemaker. Position of implanted pacemaker and electrodes is shown at right. (From Heller: American Journal of Nursing, April, 1964.)

ease is a common form of heart disease among children. The tragedy of the situation is compounded by the fact that so many of these cases could be prevented by early treatment of streptococcal infections, especially "strep throat." The nurse must realize the importance of these facts and do her part in educating the public to the danger of allowing cases of tonsillitis and sore throat to continue untreated.

Symptoms

The symptoms of rheumatic heart disease are the symptoms of a complication and therefore do not appear until after the acute stage of rheumatic fever has subsided. These symptoms will vary according to the location of the inflammation. With a myocarditis, there may be changes in the rate and rhythm of the heart beat and enlargement of the heart. In an endocarditis, there may be characteristic heart murmurs, hematuria, small red areas over the entire body (petechiae) and undue fatigue. In pericarditis, there are the symptoms of pain in the heart region, increase in the heart rate and dyspnea. All of these conditions may eventually lead to congestive failure.

Treatment and Nursing Care

Rest. Inflammatory conditions are primarily treated with rest of the part, and so it is with inflammatory diseases of the heart. The treatment consists of measures intended to decrease the work load of the heart. The length of time for confinement to bed may extend to months and even years. The physician uses information of the patient's current sedimentation rate to determine the progress of the disease and the amount of rest required. As the sedimentation rate is lowered, he may allow more activity; if it becomes elevated, he will order the patient back to bed. ↓ sed rate up

↑ sed rate BR

Detailed care of the patient on bed rest is discussed earlier in this chapter.

Medications. Specific medications for the treatment of inflammatory conditions of the heart include the antibiotics, particularly penicillin, which is given in massive doses and often by a continuous intravenous drip. If the causative organism is resistant to penicillin, other antibiotics may be given.

Surgery. In recent years surgery inside the heart, or open heart surgery, has become a relatively safe and acceptable method of treating some forms of heart disease. A technique referred to as *commissurotomy* is used to restore the functions of a diseased mitral valve, or other valves which may have been affected by bacterial invasion of the heart.

If the valve is beyond repair, it can be replaced by an artificial valve (see the preceding discussion).

HYPERTENSIVE HEART DISEASE

Definition

An increase in the blood pressure places an extra burden on the heart as it works harder to force the blood through the blood vessels. This brings about an increase in the size of the heart and impaired function as a result of fatigue of the heart muscle. The term used to describe this condition is "hypertensive heart disease."

Hypertension may result from chronic kidney infections or diseases of the arteries such as arteriosclerosis. It may also occur without any apparent cause, having no known relationship with any other disease. This second type is called *essential hypertension.*

Symptoms

As the heart begins to fail because of fatigue from its attempts to compensate for hypertension, the patient develops dyspnea, undue fatigue, edema of the extremities and eventually cyanosis. Congestive failure develops rapidly if the hypertension is not relieved.

Treatment and Nursing Care

Treatment is aimed at relief of the underlying cause, when this can be determined, and measures to decrease the work load of the heart. The patient with hypertensive heart disease will need intelligent nursing care based on the needs of the individual patient. Physical and emotional rest are of great importance. The patient must learn to use moderation in everything he does, avoiding excesses in eating, drinking, smoking, exercise and emotional excitement.

Medications. Drugs used in the treatment of hypertensive heart disease include those that lower the blood pressure in addition to medications that improve the strength and character of the heart beat. The hypotensive drugs (those that lower the blood pressure) include reserpine (Serpasil) and hydralazine (Apresoline).

CONGENITAL HEART DISEASE

Definition

The word "congenital" means "born with" or "present at birth." Thus, a congenital heart disease is actually a defect in the structure of the heart which has resulted from improper growth and development of the infant's heart or a major blood vessel. There may be one or more defects present, and they constitute abnormal openings or obstructions which impair the circulation of blood (see Fig. 15-15).

The exact cause of the improper development of the heart in a fetus is not fully understood, although a virus infection in the mother (especially German measles) during the first three months of pregnancy is believed to be a causative factor.

Types

There are many different types of congenital heart disease, depending on the number and kind of structural defects present and the symptoms resulting from the impaired circulation. The term "blue baby" is often used to describe any infant who has cyanosis as a result of a congenital heart defect, but it is more correctly used to describe a condition known as "tetralogy of Fallot."

This condition was given the name "tetraology" because there are four defects present, and Fallot is added because that was the name of the French physician who first described the condition.

The four defects that make up this group are:*

1. *Ventricular septal defect:* In the wall (septum) between the two ventricles, there is an abnormal opening, causing unoxygenated blood in the right ventricle to mix with oxygenated blood in the left ventricle.

2. *Overriding aorta:* Instead of rising solely from the left ventricle, the aorta straddles both ventricles, rising from a joint just over the septal defect. Thus it receives both oxygenated and unoxygenated blood and sends this poorly oxygenated mixture through the body.

3. *Pulmonary stenosis:* There is a narrowing in the pulmonary valve, which obstructs the flow of blood through the pulmonary artery to the lungs.

4. *Enlarged right ventricle:* Owing to the strain of pumping blood through the narrowed pulmonary valve, the right ventricle overworks, becomes enlarged and is not able to function effectively.

The main result of this combination of defects is that the blood and the body tissues do not get enough oxygen.

---

*From the booklet "If Your Child Has a Congenital Heart Defect," published by the American Heart Association.

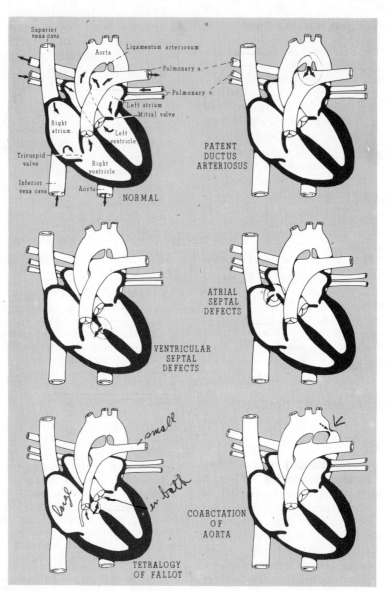

Figure 15–15. Congenital defects of the heart. (From Jacob and Francone: *Structure and Function in Man,* 2nd Ed. W. B. Saunders Co., Philadelphia.)

TABLE 15–3. GENERAL SIGNS AND SYMPTOMS OF CONGENITAL
HEART ABNORMALITIES*

Infants	Children
1. Dyspnea	1. Dyspnea
2. Difficulty with feeding	2. Poor physical development
3. Stridor or choking spells	3. Decreased exercise tolerance
4. Pulse rate over 200	4. Recurrent respiratory infections
5. Recurrent respiratory infections	5. Heart murmur and thrill
6. Failure to gain weight	6. Cyanosis
7. Heart murmurs	7. Squatting
8. Cyanosis	8. Clubbing of fingers and toes
9. Cerebrovascular accidents	9. Elevated blood pressure
10. Anoxic attacks	

*From Congenital Heart Abnormalities. Teaching Reference. Ross Clinical Education Aid, No. 7, Ross Laboratories, Columbus, Ohio.

Since blood which is low in oxygen is a bluish red, this gives the skin a blue tinge. However, certain other defects also cause cyanosis.

Symptoms.

See Table 15-3.

Treatment and Nursing Care

Recent advances in the techniques of open heart surgery have provided methods of successfully treating some but not all types of congenital heart defects. In these surgical procedures, attempts are made to correct the defect so that the circulation of the blood is established to a state as near to normal as possible. In order to accomplish this, the surgeon may repair the defect by enlarging or tying off sections of the major vessels, rerouting the blood through the use of grafts and suturing together openings in the septum.

Medical treatment with drugs may be of more benefit than surgery for some types of heart defects. In cases in which the defect cannot or need not be repaired by surgery, the patient may be

kept under continuous medical supervision for observation of his progress and administration of medications to relieve his symptoms.

CLINICAL CASE PROBLEMS

1. Mr. Wilkins is admitted to the hospital with a diagnosis of myocardial infarction. He is obviously very apprehensive the first few days he is in the hospital and apparently is afraid that he is going to die.

After he begins to recover from his heart attack, Mr. Wilkins does not wish to stay in bed as the doctor ordered, and he demands iced coffee with his meals.

How can you help relieve the patient's anxiety when he is first admitted to the hospital?

What could you say to help Mr. Wilkins understand the need for absolute bed rest until his physician gives permission for him to be up?

Why is it not permissible for Mr. Wilkins to have any iced drinks or foods?

TABLE 15–4. CLASSIFICATION OF HEART DISEASE

Type	Cause	Specific Treatments
Congestive heart failure	Complication of another primary heart disease or renal failure. Ventricles fail to empty properly, leading to congestion of all tissues served by the venae cavae and pulmonary veins.	Rest to relieve stress and strain on the heart. Diuretics and restriction of sodium intake to relieve edema. Drugs which increase the cardiac output by improving the muscular contractions of the heart.
Coronary heart diseases	1. Arteriosclerosis, causing a narrowing of the blood vessels which serve the heart muscle. This results in a decreased supply of oxygen to the heart muscle. 2. Acute coronary occlusion. A sudden blocking of a coronary vessel by a blood clot. This leads to myocardial infarction, with death of the area being deprived of its blood supply.	Vasodilator drugs. Limited activities to avoid overexertion and added strain on the heart. Avoiding sudden exposure to cold. Analgesics for relief of pain. Treatment of shock. Rest. Anticoagulant drugs such as Dicumarol and Coumadin. Oxygen for dyspnea and cyanosis.
Inflammatory diseases of the heart	1. Most often rheumatic fever following a streptococcal infection of the throat. 2. Sometimes following acute infections such as diphtheria and typhoid fever.	Absolute bed rest. Antibiotics to treat the infection. Treatment of anemia, which is usually present. Surgery to restore proper functioning of the heart valves.
Hypertensive heart disease	Hypertension: essential, in which the cause is unknown, or secondary, following chronic kidney disease or a disease of the aorta.	Drugs which lower the blood pressure. Treatment of the primary condition. Sympathectomy to block the nerve impulses to the blood vessels.
Congenital heart disease	Unknown. May be due to viral infections, especially German measles, during the first three months of pregnancy.	Surgery for types amenable to this type of treatment.

REFERENCES—PART TWO

1. Aagard, G. N.: "Treatment of Hypertension." Am. Journ. Nurs., April, 1973, p. 620.
2. American Heart Association: *If Your Child Has a Congenital Heart Defect.* New York, 1960.
3. Beland, I. L.: *Clinical Nursing: Pathophysiological and Psychosocial Approaches,* 2nd edition. New York, The Macmillan Co., 1970.
4. Brunner, L. A., et al.: *Medical-Surgical Nursing,* 2nd edition. Philadelphia, J. B. Lippincott Co., 1970.
5. Cogen, R.: "Cardiac Catheterization: Preparing the Adult." Am. Journ. Nurs., Man., 1973, p. 77.
6. "Drugs Used in the Care of the Cardiac Patient." Nurs. Clin. N. Amer., Vol. 4, No. 4, 1969, p. 645.
7. Forde, T. P.: "Electrocardiography," in *The Cardiac Patient,* ed. R. G. Sanderson. Philadelphia, W. B. Saunders Co., 1972.

8. Germaine, C. P.: "Exercise Makes the Heart Grow Stronger." Am. Journ. Nurs., Dec., 1972, p. 2169.
9. Goldman, M. J.: "Medical Aspects," in *The Cardiac Patient*, ed. R. G. Sanderson. Philadelphia, W. B. Saunders Co., 1972.
10. Grellman, A.: "Diuretics." Am. Journ. Nurs., Jan., 1965, p. 84.
11. Griep, A. H., and Sister DePaul: "Angina Pectoris." Am. Journ. Nurs., June, 1965, p. 72.
12. Guyton, A. C.: *Textbook of Medical Physiology*, 4th edition. Philadelphia, W. B. Saunders Co., 1971.
13. Hanchett, E. S., and Johnson, R. A.: "Early Signs of Congestive Heart Failure." Am. Journ. Nurs., July, 1968, p. 1456.
14. Heller, A. H.: "Nursing the Patient with an Artificial Pacemaker." Am. Journ. Nurs., April, 1964, p. 87.
15. Hunn, V. K.: "Cardiac Pacemakers." Am. Journ. Nurs., April, 1969, p. 749.
16. "How to Read an E.C.G." RN, Jan., 1973, p. 35.
17. Kos, B. A.: "The Nurse's Role in Rehabilitation of the Myocardial Infarction Patient." Nurs. Clin. N. Amer., Vol. 4, No. 4, 1969, p. 593.
18. Lamberton, M. M.: "Cardiac Catheterization: Anticipatory Care." Am. Journ. Nurs., Sept., 1971, p. 1718.
19. Larsen, E. L.: "The Patient with Acute Pulmonary Edema." Am. Journ. Nurs., May, 1968, p. 1019.
20. Olwin, J. H., and Keppel, J. L.: "Anticoagulant Therapy." Am. Journ. Nurs., May, 1964, p. 107.
21. "Pacemaker." Nursing Update, Aug., 1972.
22. Piterak, E. F.: "Open-ended Care for the Open Heart Patient." Am. Journ. Nurs., July, 1967, p. 1452.
23. Quinn, C. A.: "LPN: Heart-Lung Technician." Journ. Pract. Nurs., Nov., 1965, p. 30.
24. Ritchie, M.: "Heart Failure—the Geriatric Patient." Nurs. Clin. N. Amer., Vol. 3, No. 4, 1968, p. 663.
25. Rogoz, B.: "Nursing Care of the Cardiac Surgery Patient." Nurs. Clin. N. Amer., Vol. 4, No. 4, 1969, p. 631.
26. Sanderson, R. G.: "Surgical Aspects," in *The Cardiac Patient*, ed. R. G. Sanderson. Philadelphia, W. B. Saunders Co., 1972.
27. Schneider, W. J., and Boyce, B. A.: "Complications of Diuretic Therapy." Am. Journ. Nurs., Sept., 1968, p. 1903.
28. Shields, H. E.: "Cardiac Anatomy and Physiology." Nurs. Clin. N. Amer., Vol. 4, No. 4, 1969, p. 563.
29. Smith, A. M., et al.: "Serum Enzymes." Am. Mourn. Nurs., Feb., 1972, p. 277.
30. Smith, B. C.: "Congestive Heart Failure." Am. Journ. Nurs., Feb., 1969, p. 278.
31. Stamler, J., et al.: "Coronary Proneness and Approaches to Preventing Heart Attacks." Am. Journ. Nurs., Aug., 1966, p. 1788.

SUGGESTED STUDENT READING

1. Childers, E. D.: "The Nursing Care of Patients with Myocardial Infarction." Journ. Pract. Nurs., Oct., 1969, p. 29.
2. Conway, G. F., and Haverland, M.: "The LPN/LVN in Cardiac Care Unit." Journ. Pract. Nurs., Sept., 1971, p. 2.
3. Deal, J.: "Battery Operated." Bedside Nurse, Nov., 1972, p. 12.
4. Germaine, C. P.: "Exercise Makes the Heart Grow Stronger." Am. Journ. Nurs., Dec., 1972, p. 2169.
5. Gruhl, V. R.: "Some Basic Considerations about Myocardial Infarction." Journ. Pract. Nurs., Oct., 1969, p. 27.
6. Johnson, O. C.: "Low Sodium Diet." Journ. Pract. Nurs., Sept., 1969, p. 19.
7. Rodman, M. J.: "Drugs for Managing High Blood Pressure." RN, May, 1969, p. 73.
8. Rogez, B. D., and Holswade, G. R.: "Care of Patients Having Open-heart Surgery.: Journ. Pract. Nurs., April, 1966, p. 22.
9. "So Your Patient Has a Pacemaker." Nursing Update, Aug., 1972.
10. Yu, P. N.: "Future Trends in Coronary Care." Journ. Pract. Nurs., Oct., 1969, p. 31.

OUTLINE FOR CHAPTER 15

Part Two Disorders of the Heart

I. Introduction

A. Heart diseases are still a major cause of death in the United States, although not all kinds are fatal.

II. Diagnostic Tests and Examinations

A. Electrocardiogram and x-rays.

B. Heart catheterization—determines pressures within heart chambers, takes blood samples for determining oxygen content in various parts of the heart and great vessels.

C. Angiocardiogram—x-ray using dye to visualize the heart and blood vessels.

D. Radioisotopes—aid in diagnosing structural defects of the heart and great vessels. Also can determine the life span of individual red blood cells.

III. General Nursing Care

A. Physical, emotional and mental rest.

B. Diet: serve small, easily digested meals and know types of food to avoid and whether to limit intake of sodium and fluids.

C. Relief of dyspnea and cyanosis—

proper positioning, administration of oxygen.

D. Care of the skin—avoid breakdown of skin during immobility of patient.

E. Medications:
1. To decrease the rate and improve the strength of the contractions of the heart muscle (for example, digitalis).
2. To relieve edema (for example, diuretics).
3. Analgesics (for example, morphine sulfate and Demerol).

F. Rehabilitation—patient can lead a useful, active life within the limitations imposed by his illness.

G. Prevention—adequate exercise and avoidance of obesity, tobacco, emotional strain and other stresses that place an added burden on the heart. Periodic examination of children for early detection of heart disorders.

IV. Surgery of the Heart

A. Introduction.
1. Development of new machinery and techniques has greatly reduced the risk of heart surgery and made open-heart surgery possible.
2. Examples include repair of structural defects and repair or replacement of diseased valves in the heart.

B. Preoperative care includes instruction of the patient and comprehensive tests and examinations to determine the type of surgery needed and the risk to the patient.

C. Immediate postoperative care is given in an intensive care unit. Nursing care includes intelligent observation of vital signs, measuring intake and output, care of thoracotomy tubes and possibly administration of oxygen. Exercise of limbs necessary to avoid circulatory and musculoskeletal complications.

V. Congestive Heart Failure

A. A complication of other cardiac conditions in which the heart loses its efficiency as a pump and the blood flow becomes congested.

B. Symptoms.
1. Left-sided failure produces congestion of the lungs and eventually pulmonary edema.
2. Right-sided failure produces edema of the lower part of the body and impaired circulation to the brain.

C. Pulmonary edema (an accumulation of fluid within the lung tissues).
1. May result from left-sided failure of the heart or an abrupt increase in the workload of the heart. Acute pulmonary edema can be fatal in a short period of time.
2. Symptoms include severe dyspnea and coughing up sputum that may be blood-tinged and frothy.
3. Treatment to relieve symptoms and reduce venous return of blood to the heart includes keeping patient calm, giving him oxygen and a sedative and rotating tourniquets on the extremities. Diuretics aid in elimination of fluids causing pulmonary failure.

VI. Diseases of the Coronary Arteries

A. Coronary arteries provide blood supply to the heart muscle.

B. Main diseases are myocardial infarction and angina pectoris.
1. Myocardial infarction is an area of necrotic tissue in the myocardium resulting from impaired blood supply to the area.
   a. Symptoms — crushing or burning sensation in the chest, pallor, profuse perspiration, anxiety, nausea and vomiting.
   b. Immediate care—relief of pain, oxygen to relieve dyspnea and prevention of shock. Later care—rest and medication.
   c. Prevention—avoidance of predisposing factors such as obesity, high fat diet and smoking. Control of disorders such as rheumatic heart disease and atherosclerosis helps avoid formation of blood clots within the arteries.
2. Angina pectoris is pain in the chest arising from decreased blood supply to the heart muscle, caused by a narrowing or occlusion of these arteries.
   a. Symptoms—a dull pain or

tightness in the chest, profuse perspiration, pallor or flushing of the face and dyspnea.

b. Treatment — vasodilator drugs, especially nitroglycerine, and avoidance of exposure to cold, sudden physical exertion or emotional upsets that may precipitate an attack.

VII. Disorders of the Heart's Conduction System

A. If the sino-atrial node and the atrioventricular node fail to initiate the electrical impulses that stimulate contraction of the heart muscle, an artificial pacemaker can be inserted to stimulate the contractions.

B. Indications for its use include Stokes-Adams disease, carotid sinus syndrome, surgical injury to the heart's conduction system during corrective cardiac surgery, and some cases of arteriosclerosis in elderly persons who are suffering from atrioventricular block.

C. Nursing care—accurate observation of the patient prior to surgery. Reporting of any attacks that occur. Surgeon instructs the patient. Physical preparation same as for any major surgery. Special equipment may include thoracic tubes and drainage bottle, intravenous tubes, oxygen and gastric suction.

VIII. Inflammatory Diseases of the Heart

A. Inflammatory conditions involving the heart muscle (myocarditis), the inner lining (endocarditis), or the sac surrounding the heart (pericarditis).

B. Symptoms vary according to the structure involved.

C. Treatment and nursing care—rest to reduce the workload of the heart, medication to control infection and surgery to repair or replace valves destroyed by the inflammatory process.

IX. Hypertensive Heart Disease

A. High blood pressure places an added burden on the heart and can enlarge the heart and fatigue the heart muscle.

B. Symptoms include dyspnea, fatigue, edema of the extremities and cyanosis. Congestive failure develops rapidly if the condition is not relieved.

C. Treatment aimed at relief of underlying cause and administration of hypotensive drugs to control the blood pressure.

X. Congenital Heart Disease

A. A defect in the structure of the heart that has resulted from improper growth and development during the prenatal period.

B. Exact cause is unknown, but there is a definite relationship between these defects and some viral infections, particularly German measles.

C. Types include a variety of defects in the septum, position of the great vessels and chambers of the heart.

D. Symptoms include dyspnea, cyanosis, increased pulse rate, poor physical development, decreased exercise tolerance and elevated blood pressure.

E. Treatment includes correction by surgery whenever possible. Medications such as digitalis may be given.

Part Three.   Nursing Care of Patients With Disorders of the Peripheral Vascular System

INTRODUCTION

The peripheral blood vessels are those veins and arteries which are situated a distance from the heart. Diseases of the peripheral blood vessels are most often chronic in nature, affecting persons of the older age group and associated with other diseases of the cardiovascular system or the kidneys. Diabetics are also particularly susceptible to diseases of the peripheral blood vessels.

The lower extremities, being farthest

TABLE 15-5. CONDITIONS CAUSING REDUCED ARTERIAL SUPPLY*

Disease	Predisposing Factors
Buerger's disease or thromboangiitis obliterans	Unknown; suspect infection or activity of some toxic agent.
Arteriosclerosis (atherosclerosis)	Diabetes, hypertension, disturbances of lipid metabolism, especially cholesterol.
Arterial embolism	Heart disease—atrial fibrillation, vascular lesions, bacterial endocarditis, coronary occlusion, venous thrombosis.
Arteritis	Systemic infections—syphilis, pneumonia, typhus fever, typhoid fever, influenza, septicemia, scarlet fever, cholera.
Constant constriction of peripheral vessels	Pathologic overactivity of sympathetic nervous system.
Spasmodic cyanosis of the fingers	Spondylitis, cervical rib.
Frostbite	Exposure to cold.

*From Fulcher: Nursing Clinics of North America. W. B. Saunders Co. March, 1966.

away from the center of the body's circulatory system, are often subject to diseases of the blood vessels which diminish the supply of blood to these parts. These conditions will be discussed first in this section of the chapter.

Since the blood vessels leading to and from the brain also come under the general heading of peripheral vessels, cerebrovascular diseases are presented after diseases of the extremities in this same section.

CIRCULATORY DISORDERS OF THE EXTREMITIES

General Treatment and Nursing Care

In order for the body to remain in a state of good health, there must be an equal balance between the metabolic needs of the tissues and the supply of nutrition brought by the blood stream to meet those needs. When the supply cannot meet the demands, the cells begin to degenerate from a lack of nutrition. All treatments and nursing care of the patient with a disease of the peripheral blood vessels are aimed at the establishment of good circulation so as to provide adequate nutrition and at prevention of further breakdown of the tissues.

Use of Heat. Whenever there is impaired circulation to the extremities over a period of time, the peripheral nerves begin to degenerate. The patient then has a decreased sensitivity to all stimuli, particularly heat and cold. Since chilling causes constriction of the blood vessels (the very condition we are trying to combat), these patients must be provided with extra warmth. Their decreased sensitivity to heat rules out the practice of applying local heat in the form of hot water bottles or electric heating pads, because the patient may be burned without his realizing it. In addition, local heat increases

TABLE 15-6. CONDITIONS CAUSING DECREASED VENOUS FLOW*

Disease	Predisposing Factors
Varicose veins	Familial defects of valves, pregnancy, abdominal tumors, ascites.
Phlebothrombosis (noninflammatory clot formation)	Heart disease, obesity, varicosities, trauma, surgery, debility, polycythemia, certain anemias.
Thrombophlebitis (inflammatory clot formation)	Local injury to endothelium by stretching or trauma, chemical irritation, infection, esp. pneumonia, influenza, typhoid fever. Prolonged bed rest during infections.

*From Fulcher: Nursing Clinics of North America, W. B. Saunders Co., March, 1966.

the metabolic activity of the area to which it is applied and further upsets the balance of supply and demand mentioned previously.

The best means of preventing chilling and providing comfort for the patient is to raise the temperature of his environment and dress him in extra warm clothing made of flannel and wool. These will provide an even distribution of heat to the body. It is not unusual for these patients to develop the habit of huddling close to radiators, heaters or open fires in an effort to keep warm. They must be warned that this is a dangerous practice that can easily lead to severe burns and damage to the tissues of the lower extremities.

Instructions to the Patient. So much can be done to prevent complications from diseases of the peripheral vascular system by properly educating the patient and his family in the special care of the lower extremities, that it might well be considered one of the most important aspects of treatment and nursing care. Many special clinics in the larger medical centers have specially printed cards or booklets to distribute to their patients. The following, taken from A. F. Brown's *Medical Nursing,* is an example of the points to be emphasized when instructing these patients.

INFORMATION FOR PATIENTS OF THE
PERIPHERAL VASCULAR CLINIC

1. Keep warm.
2. Do not use tobacco in any form.
3. Take great care that the foot is not injured. Avoid crowded places.
4. Wear wide-toed shoes which cause no pressure and have adequate support for the arches.
5. Do not wear circular garters.
6. Do not sit with the knees crossed.
7. If the weight of the bedclothes is uncomfortable, use a pillow to hold the bedclothes off the feet.
8. Soak the feet in a basin of warm soapy water for five minutes every day. Dry thoroughly, especially between the toes, by mopping, not rubbing.
9. Do not apply any medicine to the feet without directions.
10. If the feet are dry and scaly, rub with lanolin, olive oil, castor oil, or cold cream.
11. If the feet are moist, use talcum powder.
12. Before filing nails, soak feet in warm (not hot) water for five minutes to soften nails. File straight across. Do not use a razor blade or knife.
13. Proper first aid treatment is important. Consult your physician immediately for any redness, blistering, pain, or swelling.
14. Do not attempt to treat corns or calluses. Ask your physician what should be done.
15. Drink an abundance of water, at least the equivalent of 20 glasses of water in each 24-hour period.

Rest and Exercise. Exercises of a special type may be ordered by the physician in an effort to improve circulation in the lower extremities, because much of the movement of blood through the deeper veins in the lower leg depends on muscular activity. These exercises have several contraindications, however, and are to be done only on the specific orders of the physician. Periods of rest are alternated with the exercises to prevent fatigue and to allow the body time for healing and repair.

There are times when the physician advises complete rest of the affected limb, and the patient is confined to bed. When this occurs, the skin must receive particular attention to prevent pressure and breakdown of the tissues. Special notice must be given the heels, and weight relieved by extending the heels over the end of the mattress or placing a pillow under the lower leg. A bed cradle over the legs or footboard with pillows may be used to bear the weight of the top covers.

In using any of these measures to prevent pressure on the heels, it must be remembered that relocating the pressure to another part of the lower leg may also cause difficulties. It is important, therefore, that these patients change position frequently to avoid pressure in any one area for too long. It is also true that sitting or lying in one position over a long period of time decreases the flow of blood and further aggravates the static condition of the circulation.

Ulcers. The starvation of any tissue will inevitably lead to degeneration and death of the tissue cells. An ulcer, or open sore, develops on the skin and erodes the underlying tissues, accompanied by suppuration and drainage of purulent material. Ulcers are quite common in peripheral vascular diseases. Treatment of this condition consists of measures to aid in draining the purulent material and removal of dead tissues so that healing can take place.

Wet compresses, Furacin dressings, surgical debridement of necrotic tissue and irrigation may all be necessary to heal these ulcers. Because of the impaired circulation, they heal very slowly and may require special skin grafting to replace the tissue lost by necrosis.

There are special pressure bandages or paste "boots" which are used in treating ulcers of the lower extremities. These "boots" are applied so that they cover the entire lower leg and have a threefold purpose: (1) they exert an even pressure on the blood vessels, thereby eliminating local areas of congestion, (2) they give support to the veins near the surface of the limb and (3) they protect the ulcer from injury and infection from outside sources.

As stated before, these ulcers heal very slowly. The reason for this is that the body's mechanisms against inflammation and infection cannot function as they should when the supply of blood to an area is decreased. The patient often becomes discouraged and depressed by the lack of progress in healing and will require encouragement and constant reassurance from the nursing staff.

Appliances for Support and Comfort. Even, well-distributed support of the vessels near the surface of the body will help in the return of the venous blood from the legs. To provide this type of support, the physician may recommend that the patient wear an elastic bandage or fitted elastic stockings. Because of their comfort and east of application, the stockings are more satisfactory than elastic bandages for an ambulatory patient. When these stockings are worn daily, the following rules should be observed:

1. The hose should be applied early in the morning before arising from the bed. The blood vessels are less congested after a night's rest.

2. Stockings must be held up with supporters rather than with garters. Circular garters are forbidden.

3. Never roll the tops of the hose and "knot" them as a means of holding them up.

4. Two pairs are necessary to allow for daily washing and drying of the hose.

Diet. Obesity adds an extra burden of weight and pressure on the peripheral blood vessels and further aggravates congestion of these vessels. Overweight patients must be made aware of the dangers involved in being overweight and encouraged to follow the diet recommended by the physician.

The increased intake of fluids to the equivalent of 20 glasses within a 24-hour period mentioned previously is based on the belief that the removal of waste products from the blood is improved in this manner. Many physicians also agree that the intake of such large amounts of liquids will make the blood less thick and therefore more easily circulated through the vessels.

Drugs. Medications used in the treatment of peripheral vascular diseases are of two main types: vasodilators, which enlarge the size of the blood vessels, and anticoagulants, which impair the clotting ability of the blood.

Nicotine, which is found in tobacco, has the effect of producing spasmodic narrowing of the peripheral arteries. It is obviously very dangerous for a patient to continue smoking when the peripheral arteries are affected by disease. The patient may experience some difficulty in giving up smoking if he has developed the habit, but the warning that to continue to smoke may result in gangrene and eventual loss of a limb may help him to adjust.

Arteriosclerosis of the Extremities

Definition. Sclerosis means a gradual hardening. In arteriosclerosis, the walls of the arteries become hardened over a period of years and eventually lose their elasticity. This brings about a narrowing of these vessels and a decreased flow of blood. It also produces an increase in the blood pressure because of the extra force needed to push the blood through the smaller openings. Arteriosclerosis of the lower extremities is more common than that of the upper extremities, and, being farther from the heart, the lower extremities are more likely to suffer from poor circulation. Diabetics frequently have arteriosclerosis of the lower extremities, which is why amputations are so common in persons who have diabetes.

Symptoms. In the early stages of the disease, the lower extremities feel cold to the touch, and the patient complains of being unable to keep his feet warm. He may also experience tingling and numbness in the lower legs. Later, there develop fatigue and weakness of the muscles of the affected limb, and the patient may tell of leg cramps at night which are relieved by rubbing or lowering the leg over the side of the bed. In the last stages, ulcers may appear, or there may be a dry gangrene which first involves the toes and then progresses up the extremity if left untreated.

Treatment and Nursing Care. Arteriosclerosis itself cannot be cured at present. Treatment is therefore aimed at relieving the symptoms and improving and maintaining adequate circulation to the extremities so that gangrene or ulcers will not develop. It is also important to avoid any breaks in the skin which may lead to an infection. Once an extremity becomes gangrenous, little can be done beyond surgical amputation of the limb.

EXERCISE. Active exercising of a muscle will improve the circulation of blood to that muscle. The physician may order the patient with arteriosclerosis of the extremities to take regular exercises. He will encourage him to walk whenever possible, play golf, ride a bicycle or perform some similar form of exercise as consistently and regularly as he would take a medication.

WARMTH. Warm clothing and adequately heated rooms are helpful in maintaining continued dilatation of the blood vessels. The reasons for avoiding extremes in temperatures are discussed under General Nursing Care, earlier in this chapter.

PREVENTION OF INJURY TO THE EXTREMITIES. Arteriosclerosis of the extremities is most common in older persons, and since persons in this age group are frequently in danger of injury from falls because of poor eyesight or decreased muscular coordination, they must be protected from all safety hazards. They should also be instructed carefully in the proper care of the feet and nails mentioned under General Nursing Care. Their shoes should fit snugly enough to prevent blistering, but not so tightly that they impair circulation to the toes. Darned socks or hosiery and stockings that are too loose or too tight must also be avoided.

PHYSIOTHERAPY. Special exercises (for example, Buerger's exercises), sitz baths and whirlpool baths are all of value in maintaining a good flow of blood to the lower extremities.

Buerger's Disease

Definition. Buerger's disease, also called thromboangiitis obliterans, is an inflammatory disease of the medium-sized vessels, particularly the arteries of the legs. It is characterized by the formation of clots within the arteries, a sharp spasmodic pain in the area and eventual destruction (obliteration) of these vessels.

The exact cause of Buerger's disease is not known, but the most outstanding predisposing factor is thought to be excessive smoking over a period of years.

Treatment. Aside from elimination of smoking and other factors that lead to constriction of blood vessels, treat-

ment is primarily symptomatic, as in cases of arteriosclerosis of the extremities (see the preceding discussion).

Buerger-Allen Exercises. These specific exercises are prescribed to improve circulation to the lower extremities. The patient is taught to do these exercises at home several times a day. He is also instructed in proper care of his feet and legs to avoid aggravation of his condition (see "Instructions to the Patient," earlier in this chapter, for details). The Buerger-Allen exercises are as follows:

1. Lie down in a supine position and elevate the lower extremities at an angle of 45 to 90 degrees. Support them in this position until the skin of the extremities turns dead white.

2. Lower the feet and legs so that they are below the level of the rest of the body, being careful that there is no pressure on the back of the knees.

3. When redness appears in the lower extremities, place them flat on the bed for 3 to 5 minutes.

Thrombophlebitis

Definition. A *thrombus* is a blood clot which forms inside a blood vessel and remains attached to the side of the vessel wall. This clot may continue to enlarge until it eventually closes off the flow of blood through the vessel. *Phlebitis* is an inflammation of a vein. Thus, *thrombophlebitis* is an inflammation of a vein resulting from circulatory stasis caused by a blood clot in the vessel.

In thrombophlebitis, there is local inflammation of the vein, and since there is decreased circulation to the area served by the vein, there is also a local inflammation of the tissues adjacent to the vein.

Aside from the local problems presented by impaired circulation, there is also danger that the clot may break away from the wall of the vessel and be carried along in the blood stream until it reaches a vessel too small for it to pass through. This results in an area of

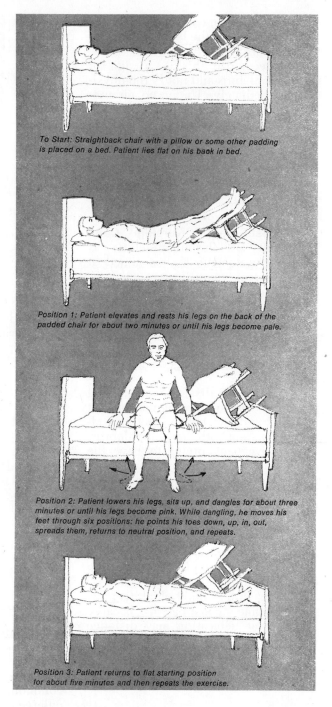

To Start: Straightback chair with a pillow or some other padding is placed on a bed. Patient lies flat on his back in bed.

Position 1: Patient elevates and rests his legs on the back of the padded chair for about two minutes or until his legs become pale.

Position 2: Patient lowers his legs, sits up, and dangles for about three minutes or until his legs become pink. While dangling, he moves his feet through six positions: he points his toes down, up, in, out, spreads them, returns to neutral position, and repeats.

Position 3: Patient returns to flat starting position for about five minutes and then repeats the exercise.

Figure 15–16. Exercises for chronic peripheral arterial disease. (Adapted from Coralt, N. K., *Bed Exercises for Convalescent Patients,* 1968. Courtesy Charles C Thomas, Publisher, Springfield, Illinois.)

infarct as described earlier in this chapter.

Many cases of thrombophlebitis are associated with postoperative of postpartum confinement to bed. That is the reason early ambulation is so important in the care of these patients.

Symptoms. Thrombophlebitis may or may not be accompanied by pain in the affected area. However, whenever a patient complains of severe pain in the calf of the leg that is aggravated by flexion of the foot, the nurse should recognize this as a sign of thrombophlebitis and notify the physician immediately. Under no circumstances should the leg be massaged, because this could easily dislodge the thrombus and produce an embolism.

In addition to the pain in the leg or thigh along the course of the affected vein, the patient may also have an elevated temperature and increased pulse rate.

Treatment and Nursing Care. Treatment of thrombophlebitis is mostly symptomatic and is aimed at prevention of complications such as embolism, local cellulitis or ulceration of the area.

Anticoagulants such as heparin, Dicumarol and Coumadin are given to inhibit the clotting of the blood and thereby prevent enlargement of the thrombus.

There is some disagreement among physicians as to the amount of rest required and the type of activity allowed a patient with thrombophlebitis. Some physicians prefer to have the affected part elevated, while others do not. Whatever the choice of the physician, the nurse must fully understand his wishes and carry out his orders conscientiously.

Warmth in the form of compresses, heating pads set on "low" and extra blankets are all helpful in increasing the blood supply to the area.

Patients with thrombophlebitis must not become constipated, because straining at defecation may dislodge the thrombus. A seizure of coughing may have the same effect. Thus the patient must also be protected from respiratory infections.

Varicose Veins

Varicose veins are veins which have become greatly enlarged and distorted in shape. When blood is returned from the lower extremities, it is kept flowing

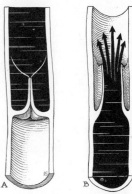

Figure 15–17. The valves of a vein. *A*, Valve is closed and the cusps are filled with blood, thus preventing a backward flow. *B*, Valve is open and blood ascends, passing through the valve. (From King and Showers: *Human Anatomy and Physiology*, 6th Ed., W. B. Saunders Co., Philadelphia.)

in one direction by a system of cup-shaped valves (see Fig. 15-17). These valves open to allow the upward passage of blood and then close to prevent a backward flow toward the feet. If these valves fail to function properly, the vein fills with blood and becomes enlarged and tortuous.

The valves may lose their ability to function properly through injury or disease. In some cases, however, it is believed that weakness of valves in the veins is inherited by some persons, thus making them more susceptible to varicose veins.

Symptoms. In the early stages of development, varicose veins may present mild symptoms of fatigue and a feeling of heaviness in the legs or swelling of the ankles after prolonged standing. Later there may be a dull or sharp pain in the legs. Sometimes the patient complains of cramps in the legs after going to bed at night. Itching along the course of the vein is also very common. As varicose veins continue to enlarge, there are repeated inflammations locally which lead to the formation of ulcers. These are usually found on the lower leg or ankle.

Treatment and Nursing Care. Medical management of varicose veins consists of: (1) support of the veins by the application of fitted elastic bandages, (2) removal of causative factors, such as obesity or prolonged standing or sitting in one position and (3) a prescribed regimen of rest and exercises.

Another form of treatment is the injection of a sclerosing agent into the varicose vein. The solution hardens the vein, obstructing the flow of blood through it and thereby preventing further engorgement. This method is only a temporary measure, however, and does not cure the condition.

Surgical treatment of varicose veins may be necessary when the more conservative methods fail to relieve the symptoms. The surgery may involve a (simple ligation) in which the large saphenous vein is tied off at the upper end (at the thigh). A more common procedure and one that offers more satisfactory results is a "vein stripping." In this procedure, the entire vein is actually pulled out of the subcutaneous tissue. An instrument is inserted in the upper part of the vein through an incision in the thigh. The vein is tied to the instrument, and as the instrument is passed along the course of the vein and pulled out through a lower incision, the vein is "turned inside out," so to speak, and removed. The surgeon then applies even pressure along the course of the vein to control bleeding. After the vein has been removed, the larger, more deeply imbedded veins take over the task of draining blood from the part of the leg formerly served by the surgically removed vein.

After this surgery, the patient is usually out of bed at least once during the first postoperative day so that good circulation is maintained in the lower legs. The dressings and elastic bandages must be checked frequently for signs of hemorrhage. While the patient is in the bed, the limb is elevated on pillows to facilitate the flow of blood through the veins. *only if elevated entire leg*

DISEASES OF THE CEREBRAL VESSELS

Arteriosclerosis of the Cerebral Vessels

Definition. Arteriosclerosis of the cerebral vessels is a hardening of the arteries serving the brain. The condition occurs most often after 50 years of age and increases in frequency with the advancing years.

Symptoms. The symptoms presented are a direct result of a gradual starvation of brain tissue due to a decreased blood supply. These patients manifest signs of mental deterioration with a slowing down of the mental processes and a decrease in intelligence. They often show emotional changes as well, such as being very easily upset and prone to crying and pouting as if they were children once again.

Treatment and Nursing Care. Very little can be done for these patients, because arteriosclerosis is a disease of degeneration in which there is little hope of stopping or reversing the process. The nursing care mainly involves acceptance of the patient as he is and providing a quiet and restful environment so as to avoid any emotional or physical excitement which would aggravate his condition.

Cerebrovascular Accident (Stroke, Apoplexy)

Introduction. Research has shown that by the time we reach the age of 30, one fourth of us will have sufficient hardening of the cerebral arteries to provide the setting for a stroke at any time. By the time we reach 70 years of age, the percentage increases to 80. Stroke is a common disease, more common than many of us realize, for autopsy studies have shown that nearly half the people who die from other causes have had minor strokes without ever having been aware of them. Since stroke is a disease of middle-aged and older persons, we can expect the incidence of this disease to increase as the lifespan increases.

Cause. A cerebrovascular accident may occur as a result of (1) cerebral thrombosis (blood clot forms in the cerebral vessel), (2) cerebral hemorrhage (vessel ruptures and leaks blood into brain tissue) or (3) atherosclerosis of the arteries of the neck and head. Any one of these conditions can lead to an interruption in the flow of blood to the brain tissues, thereby producing ischemia (local anemia) and destruction of the brain cells that formerly were served by the affected blood vessels. High blood pressure, endocarditis and other heart disorders and atherosclerosis are predisposing factors in the gradual blockage of the flow of blood or in a sudden "blow-out" of an artery.

Symptoms. The symptoms of stroke are varied. They depend on the condition causing the stroke and the size and location of the area of brain tissue affected by the vascular accident (see Fig. 15-18).

The patient may have some warning that an attack is coming on, even though he does not know exactly what is wrong. He may feel dizzy, have a headache or lose consciousness for a moment. When a large area of the brain is affected, death may be instantaneous. The most common after-effects of a stroke are disturbances of speech and paralysis on one side of the body.

Fortunately, the cerebral arteries are capable of enlarging and eventually taking over the work of the damaged arteries. This means that there is a possibility that the patient may ultimately regain use of the affected parts of his body. In some cases, there may be slight residual effects such as weakness on one side and a slight limp or dragging of the lower limb.

Treatment and Nursing Care. Emergency treatment consists of loosening all constricting clothing, especially around the neck, and turning the victim's head to one side to prevent obstruction of the air passages. No attempts should be made to move the person until an ambulance has arrived. Never attempt to arouse a person who is unconscious from a stroke.

After the patient has been admitted to the hospital, the vital signs are taken and recorded every hour for the first 24

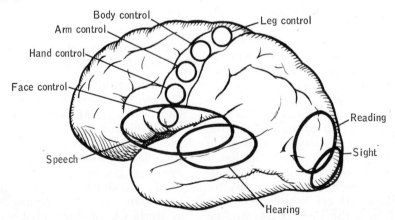

Figure 15–18. Control zones of the cerebral cortex. Nerve cells that control physical and mental activities are located in specific centers or zones of the cerebral cortex, the largest part of the human brain. The left side of the cerebral cortex with its control zones is diagrammed here. If the normal flow of blood to one of these zones is stopped, the activity controlled by the zone will be impaired. (Modified from Stokes, American Heart Association, 1958.)

hours. Observations are made as to the patient's apparent state of consciousness and ability to move his leg or arm, and whether or not he can speak.

During the acute phase of this illness, attention must be paid to maintenance of an airway. This includes positioning of the patient for maximum respiration and suctioning whenever necessary to prevent obstruction of the trachea with mucus or saliva. As long as the patient is unconscious or unable to respond, the head is kept turned to the side to facilitate drainage of mucus and saliva from the mouth.

Fluids may be given by vein until it is definitely established whether or not the stroke victim can swallow. For those who absolutely cannot handle liquids in the mouth, tube feeding may be necessary. If at all possible, the patient should be placed in an upright position, at least a 45° angle, during the tube feeding. The formula should be diluted with water, usually half and half, so that diarrhea is avoided and the patient's fluid intake is adequately maintained. Vomiting and diarrhea can also be prevented by administering the formula slowly. The inconvenience to the patient and the added burden to the nurses brought about by vomiting and frequent watery stools should be sufficient reason for proper administration of tube feedings. Unfortunately, this procedure often is handled in a haphazard way.

Positioning the patient who has had a stroke is of extreme importance. A stroke involves only the *control* centers of muscular activity. It does not affect the muscles themselves. It has been said that in the past, stroke patients have been rendered "tender, loving neglect" because doctors have placed these patients on bed rest, and nurses have proceeded to do everything possible for the patient rather than encourage him to learn to help himself. We must remember that one of the main goals of nursing is to help restore those who are ill to a state of health. The stroke patient cannot move or position himself at first. He must depend

on the nursing staff to keep his musculoskeletal system in good working order until he is able to use it once again.

The body is positioned so that the joints remain movable and the muscles maintain their tone. The patient's position is changed every hour from back to side to prone and then to the back, and so on. While the patient is on his back, the affected arm is raised above his head and the hand tucked under the pillow. This helps prevent "frozen shoulder" so common in these patients (see Fig. 15-19).

In addition to proper positioning, the joints are put through their full range of motion at least once a day. This may easily be done as the daily bath is given. Other exercises for the stroke patient are given only on the order of the doctor in charge and are usually done under the supervision of a physiotherapist. If such a person is not available, however, the booklet, "Strike Back at Stroke," published by the U.S. Government Printing Office, contains excellent, well illustrated directions for these exercises recommended for the stroke patient.

There are many other little things the nurse can do to encourage her patient and strengthen his muscles as well as his will to help himself. Instead of feeding the patient every item on his tray, the nurse can let him hold bread or other "finger foods," suggesting that he feed himself these while she handles the more difficult foods. Strange as it may seem, solids and semisolids are easier for the patient to get down without strangling than water and juices are. Chewing will be very slow for the patient at first; he must not be hurried or allowed to chew to the point of exhaustion.

Combing and brushing the hair is good exercise for the arm and shoulder, as are brushing the teeth and washing the face. The patient may not be able to carry all of these procedures through to completion at first, but with encouragement, he can gradually improve until he is able to perform much of his own

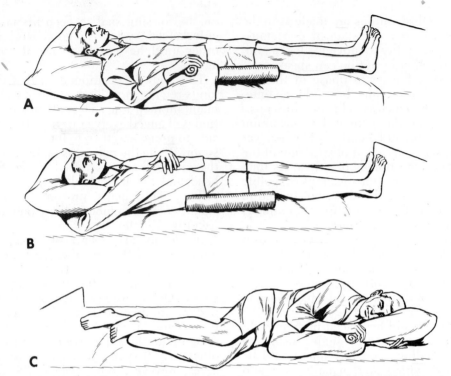

Figure 15–19. *A*, A pillow is placed next to the body on the weak side. The weak arm is placed on the pillow. Make sure that the elbow points away from the body and that the lower arm and hand are placed alongside the body and about 12 inches away from it. A rolled napkin or small towel is placed under the weak hand to keep the fingers open. Note trochanter roll along affected side to keep hip from rotating. *B*, The affected arm is tucked under the pillow with hand flattened to prevent curling of fingers. *C*, In this side-lying position, a pillow is used to support the weak arm. Another pillow is used to support the weak leg. (From *Strike Back at Stroke*, U.S. Government Printing Office, Washington, D.C.)

personal toilet himself. This is a tremendous morale booster to one who might have formerly considered himself totally helpless.

There will be many moments of despair and depression for the stroke patient as he struggles to regain control of his muscles. He will need calm reassurance and sincere words of encouragement—not an artificially gay and hopeful kind of encouragement, but a serious understanding from his nurse that he does indeed have many problems, and her solemn, warm-hearted promise that she will do everything within her power to help him overcome those problems.

SURGICAL TREATMENT OF STROKE. Until recent years, there was no surgical treatment for a cerebrovascular accident. Now, however, it has been found that about one third of all strokes can be traced to obstruction of any one of the four arteries in the neck which supply blood to the brain. These arteries are readily accessible, so that the surgeon may open the artery and remove the obstruction. He then sutures the vessel wall or sews a Dacron patch over the incision, leaving the vessel larger than before. If a long section of the artery is blocked, the surgeon may reroute the blood through a Dacron tube grafted onto the affected vessel (see Fig. 15-20).

These new surgical procedures are also used as means of preventing many major strokes. When the patient experiences warnings such as spells of dizziness or numbness of the limbs, the doctor may suspect "little strokes" and order special x-rays of the arteries serving the brain. If the tests show an

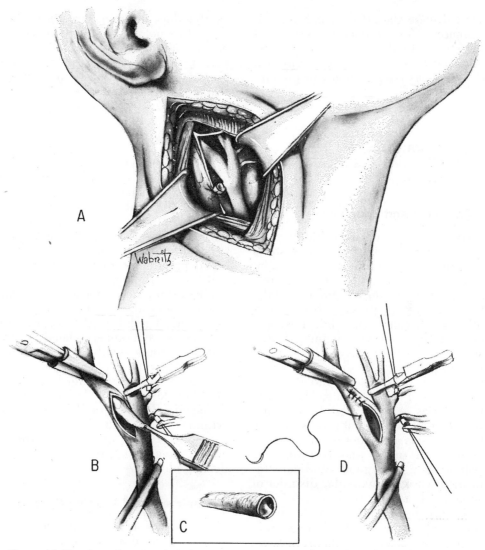

Figure 15–20. Steps in removal of atherosclerotic plaque. *A,* Carotid artery bifurcation is surgically exposed. *B,* Vessel is incised and plaque freed. *C,* Darkened area in vessel lumen is plaque's diaphragm, which further blocks artery. *D,* Vessel is sutured after removal of plaque. (From Long: American Journal of Nursing, September, 1966.)

obstruction, surgical intervention will prevent further development of the obstruction and an eventual cerebrovascular accident.

Prevention. There are measures that can be taken to prevent stroke other than the surgical procedures presented above. Now that more is known about the cause of stroke, we are able to eliminate or at least keep under control some of the conditions that predispose an individual to a cerebrovascular accident.

Control of hypertension is one such factor. Another is adequate treatment of rheumatic heart disease and coronary artery disease, both of which can produce blood clots in the heart that eventually break loose and find their way into the cerebral vessels, thus causing a stroke. Individuals with diabetes, cardiac arrhythmia, atherosclerosis, hypertension and rheumatic heart disease should have periodic examinations for evidence of an impending stroke. In this way, measures can be taken to avoid emotional, physical or infectious stresses that can precipitate a stroke.[12]

HYPERTENSION AND HYPERTENSIVE VASCULAR DISEASE

Definition and Etiology

Hypertension, or high blood pressure, is said to exist when the systolic pressure is consistently above 150 mm. of mercury or when the diastolic pressure exceeds 90 mm. of mercury. Of the two, the diastolic pressure is more significant because it indicates the amount of pressure being exerted against the vessel walls while the heart is in its phase of relaxation, and there is no added pressure of blood being forced out of the left ventricle and into the arteries. A high diastolic pressure reading that is constant means that the blood vessels are under relentless pressure at all times, and therefore the patient is a very good candidate for heart disease or a vascular disorder of some kind.

Systolic hypertension may be due to increased cardiac output of blood, as in hyperthyroidism, or to loss of elasticity in the larger arteries, as in arteriosclerosis. Diastolic hypertension is a result of a narrowing of the small arterioles that control the flow of blood out of the larger arteries.

The exact cause of most cases of hypertension is unknown. The disease may be secondary to another disease or it may be primary in origin (essential hypertension). About 95 per cent of the cases of hypertension are of no known cause and are diagnosed as primary or essential hypertension.

Malignant hypertension is characterized by severe and rapidly accelerated high blood pressure that eventually produces fibrinoid necrosis of the eye,

heart, kidney or brain. If medical treatment does not control the disorder, the patient cannot be expected to live more than two years after onset of severe symptoms. Cause of death may be uremia, heart attack or stroke.

Symptoms

The patient may not have any symptoms at all until years after the onset of the disease. Usually, it is only through routine physical examinations or a screening clinic that the disease is discovered. Essential hypertension tends to be labile and intermittent; that is, the blood pressure level can vary widely and is not constant from day to day.

When symptoms appear, they usually include headache, fatigue, nervousness and irritability. As the disease progresses, symptoms related to the specific organs involved become apparent. Thus the patient may have eye changes with retinal hemorrhage, signs of kidney failure as the kidney cells are damaged, dyspnea and cardiac arrhythmias as a result of heart involvement and fainting spells and giddiness as the oxygen supply to the brain is decreased.

Treatment and Nursing Care

Prevention of the complications presented in the preceding discussion is one of the principal aims of treatment of hypertension. Unless the basic disorder causing secondary hypertension can be eliminated, there is no possible cure for this condition. The patient should avoid obesity and emotional stresses and tensions, limit his intake of sodium and strive for moderation in everything he does.

Drugs used to control hypertension vary from mild diuretics and other antihypertensive drugs to the potent group called ganglion blocking drugs. Many of these medications have side-effects or produce adverse reactions, some mild and some severe, of which the nurse should be aware.

Mild cases of hypertension may respond to the diuretics such as Diuril or Hydrodiuril coupled with a regimen of diet therapy and moderation in living habits. Since the diuretics remove potassium and sodium from the body fluids, the patient receiving one of these drugs should be watched for muscle weakness, cramping and other signs of potassium and sodium deficiency. In most instances, citrus fruits and bananas are added to the diet to provide the needed increased potassium intake. Hyperglycemia may also develop as an adverse effect of the oral diuretics, in which case the patient begins to experience symptoms of diabetes mellitus.

The rauwolfia compounds are often used in combination with other drugs to control hypertension. For example, reserpine, which also acts as a tranquilizer, may be given with a diuretic and also with Apresoline. The combination of drugs is chosen on the basis of the individual patient and his response to the drug therapy prescribed. Rauwolfia preparations may cause peptic ulcer in the patient who is susceptible to this condition. Reserpine sometimes produces depression in certain patients. Apresoline (hydralazine) may cause tachycardia and increased output, which are potentially dangerous to a patient with coronary disease.

Guanethidine sulfate (Ismelin) is a potent antihypertensive drug which has its greatest effect when the patient is standing. Thus, the patient may be lightheaded and even suffer a blackout when he stands up from a sitting position. Patients receiving the drug must be cautioned against strenuous exercise, which can bring about severe hypotension. Another side effect of guanethidine is diarrhea. The dosage of the drug must be tailored according to patient response and ability to tolerate the side effects.

Teaching the Patient

Earlier it was stated that the patient with essential hypertension should try to live a life of moderation and follow the regimen of mental and physical rest, mild exercise, medication and diet as set forth by his physician. This attempt, of course, is easier talked about than done, and there may be many factors which can influence the patient's ability to carry out the prescribed measures. Hypertension, like diabetes mellitus, cannot be cured, but it can be controlled. For this reason, teaching the patient is of primary importance in the management of this disease.

Studies have shown that hypertensive patients have a variety of reasons for not continuing their antihypertensive therapy. Some, for example, discontinue their medications because their symptoms subside and they do not feel the need to take the drugs any longer. Others take more or less of the prescribed dose, depending on whether they feel worse or better on a particular day. Many become discouraged because of the cost of the drugs, lack of family support or annoying side effects that they had not expected the drugs to produce.

It is fairly well established that the patient who knows about his disease, why he needs to follow the instructions given to him and what kinds of benefits can be expected from the regimen he is asked to follow is more likely to cooperate and less likely to require frequent readmissions to the hospital.

Education of the patient should begin with an understanding of his personality, his cultural background, his family life and social life and his feelings about his illness and its effect on his life style. He should be encouraged to talk about himself and his feelings in a relaxed, unhurried atmosphere. The nurse who listens carefully may discover that the patient has many misconceptions about hypertension and his responsibility for control of the disease. He may, for example, think that nervousness and tension are the same as high blood pressure. He may feel that his inability to remain calm under tension is caused by a deficiency within himself and his personality. He may feel guilty about his obesity and the apparent lack of self control that keeps him from adhering to his diet. If his blood pressure varies widely, he may think the variation is due to the incompetence of those checking his blood pressure, and he loses faith in their ability to help him.

These are the kinds of things the nurse should know about if she is to help the patient learn about his disease. If she allows him to talk to her, express his feelings and ask questions freely, she has an excellent opportunity to help him learn what he needs to know to keep his disease under control.

CLINICAL CASE PROBLEMS

1. Mrs. Wolffe is an acquaintance of yours who works at a check-out counter in a grocery store. She has recently complained to you about pain in her legs and the development of unsightly varicose veins. She is about 50 pounds overweight and has tried several times to lose weight on a "crash" diet, but has never been successful. She tells you that her mother also had varicose veins, and so she supposes that the condition is inherited and that nothing can be done about it.

What advice can you give this person?

What treatment is used in the care of varicose veins?

2. You have been assigned to the task of teaching a patient in a peripheral vascular clinic. The patient is suffering from arteriosclerosis of the extremities and has had this condition for several years. You have been told that this is the patient's second visit to the clinic, and he needs instruction in the prevention of complications and in daily care of the feet and legs.

What instructions would you give this patient?

How can you help him understand the importance of following these instructions?

REFERENCES—PART THREE

1. Berni, R.: "Stroke Patient Rehabilitation: A New Approach." Journ. Pract. Nurs., June, 1972, p. 18.
2. Brown, A. F.: *Medical Nursing*, 3rd edition. Philadelphia, W. B. Saunders Co., 1957.
3. Brunner, et al.: *Textbook of Medical-Surgical Nursing*, 2nd edition. Philadelphia, J. B. Lippincott Co., 1970.
4. Fulcher, A. J.: "The Nurse and the Patient with Peripheral Vascular Disease." Nurs. Clin. N. Amer., Vol. 1, No. 1, 1966, p. 47.
5. Goode, M.: "The Patient with a Cerebral Vascular Accident." Nursing Outlook, March, 1966, p. 60.
6. Griffith, E. W., and Madero, R.: "Primary Hypertension—Patients' Learning Needs." Am. Journ. Nurs., April, 1973, p. 624.
7. "Helping the Stroke Patient Come Back." Nursing Update, April, 1971.
8. Jackson, B. S.: "Chronic Peripheral Arterial Disease." Am. Journ. Nurs., May, 1972, p. 928.
9. Shafer, K. et al.: *Medical-Surgical Nursing*, 5th edition. St. Louis, The C. V. Mosby Co., 1971.
10. "Stroke Patients in Camp." Am. Journ. Nurs., July, 1969.
11. Ullman, M.: "Disorders of Body Image after Stroke." Am. Journ. Nurs., Oct., 1964, p. 89.
12. White, P. D.: "Strokes—Prevention, Diagnosis and Patient Care." Journ. Pract. Nurs., Oct., 1965, p. 24.
13. Wilson, S.: "Chronic Leg Ulcers: Nursing Management." Am. Journ. Nurs., Jan., 1967, p. 96.

SUGGESTED STUDENT READING

1. Berni, R.: "Stroke Patient Rehabilitation: A New Approach." Journ. Pract. Nurs., June, 1972, p. 18.
2. Davis, R. W.: "Communication with the Stroke Victim." Bedside Nurse, Dec., 1970, p. 24.
3. "Helping the Stroke Patient Come Back." Nursing Update, April, 1971.
4. "Stroke Patients in Camp." Am. Journ. Nurs., July, 1969.
5. Wakerlin, G. E.: "Strokes: The Hopeful Side." Journ. Pract. Nurs., Nov., 1963, p. 22.
6. White, P. D.: "Strokes—Prevention, Diagnosis and Patient Care." Journ. Pract. Nurs., Oct., 1965, p. 24.
7. Wilson, S.: "Chronic Leg Ulcers: Nursing Management." Am. Journ. Nurs., Jan., 1967, p. 96.

OUTLINE FOR CHAPTER 15

Part Three   Disorders of the Peripheral Vascular System

I.   Introduction

A.   Peripheral blood vessels (situated at a distance from the heart) include the cerebral blood vessels as well as those of the extremities.

II.   Circulatory Disorders of the Extremities

A.   General treatment and nursing care.
  1.   Provide extra warmth. Extreme heat may cause burns or increase the metabolic needs of an area already suffering from poor circulation.
  2.   Instruction to the patient is essential to prevention of injury and avoidance of factors that may predispose the patient to complications.
  3.   Ulcers, a result of tissue death due to impaired blood supply, heal slowly and can be very discouraging to the patient.
  4.   Appliances for support and comfort include elasticized stockings and paste "boots."
  5.   Low-calorie diet may be necessary to avoid obesity, which aggravates the condition. Fluid intake should be increased.
  6.   Drugs include vasodilators and anticoagulants.
  7.   Tobacco must be avoided.
B.   Arteriosclerosis of the extremities.
  1.   Hardening and loss of elasticity in the walls of the arteries supplying the extremities.
  2.   Symptoms — extremities feel cold to the touch. Patient may experience numbness and tingling, fatigue, weakness of the muscles and leg cramps at night. Ulcers will develop, and there may be dry gangrene.
  3.   Treatment and nursing care.
    a.   Treatment is aimed at relief of symptoms and improving and maintaining adequate circulation. No cure.
    b.   Active exercise is helpful in improving blood supply to muscles.

c.   Warmth can help maintain continued dilation of the blood vessels.
d.   Extremities must be protected from injury.
e.   Physiotherapy may include special exercises, warm baths and whirlpool baths to improve circulation.

C.   Buerger's disease.
  1.   An inflammatory disease of the medium-sized blood vessels, particularly the arteries of the legs. Definitely related to excessive smoking over several years.
  2.   Symptoms include severe pain due to clots in the blood vessels and interruption of blood flow.
  3.   Treatment is primarily symptomatic.
  4.   Buerger-Allen exercises maintain adequate circulation to the lower extremities.

D.   Thrombophlebitis.
  1.   An inflammation of a vein resulting from a blood clot in the vessel.
  2.   Symptoms may or may not include pain in the affected area. Patient also may have fever and increased pulse rate.
  3.   Treatment aimed at prevention of complications such as embolism, local cellulitis or ulceration.
    a.   Anticoagulant drugs such as heparin, Dicumarol and Coumadin may be given.
    b.   Physician will prescribe amount of activity he desires patient to have.
    c.   Patient should avoid physical strain until clot is dissolved.

E.   Varicose veins.
  1.   Veins that have become greatly enlarged and distorted in shape.
  2.   Caused by impaired flow of venous blood. Often due to deficient valves in veins.
  3.   Symptoms include fatigue and feeling of heaviness in legs, cramps and itching along course of vessel. Ulcers may form after repeated inflammations.
  4.   Treatment and nursing care: support of the veins by elasticized stockings or bandages, removal of causative factors and

a prescribed regimen of rest and exercise. Surgical correction in severe cases.

III. Diseases of the Cerebral Vessels

A. Arteriosclerosis of the cerebral vessels.
1. Hardening of the arteries serving the brain.
2. Symptoms—patients manifest signs of mental deterioration with a slowing down of mental processes and emotional changes.
3. Treatment and nursing care concerned with accepting the patient as he is and helping him live fully within the limitations imposed by his illness.

B. Cerebrovascular accident (stroke, apoplexy).
1. Caused by sudden interruption of the flow of blood to the brain. Cells served by the affected vessel eventually lose function.
2. May be caused by:
    a. Cerebral thrombosis.
    b. Cerebral hemorrhage.
    c. Atherosclerosis of the neck and head.
3. Predisposing factors may be hypertension, endocarditis and atherosclerosis.
4. Symptoms vary according to the portion of the brain that is affected. Stroke may cause some slight residual paralysis or death. Most common aftereffects are speech disturbances and paralysis on one side of the body.
5. Treatment and nursing care. Primary goal is prevention of complications so that patient can return to useful and active life. Surgical treatment is effective if done early enough—if diagnostic tests or patient's "small strokes" indicate a gradual obstruction of the arteries in the neck. Little can be done surgically once a stroke has occurred.

IV. Hypertension and Hypertensive Vascular Disease

A. Consistent systolic pressure above 150 mm. of mercury or consistent diastolic pressure above 90 mm.
B. Systolic hypertension may be due to increased cardiac output or loss of elasticity of arterial walls.
C. Diastolic hypertension the result of a narrowing of the arterials.
D. Essential hypertension—no known cause.
E. Symptoms mild at first—later depend on organs involved.
F. Treatment and nursing care—aimed at control of the disease through rest, diet, drugs.
G. Instruction of patient essential to successful management of hypertension.

16

Nursing Care of Patients with Diseases of the Respiratory System

VOCABULARY

Atelectasis
Expiration
Inspiration
Intercostal
Mediastinum
Prophylaxis

INTRODUCTION

The respiratory system is chiefly composed of a system of hollow tubes through which we breathe. These tubes are constructed so that they resemble a tree; therefore the term "bronchial tree" is frequently used to describe the respiratory tract. The trunk of the tree is the trachea, the branches the bronchi and the twigs, or smaller branches, the bronchioles. As a breath of air travels down the bronchial tree, it eventually ends its journey in tiny little air sacs called alveoli. These minute sacs comprise most of the tissues of the lungs. It is in the alveoli that the exchange of carbon dioxide and oxygen takes place.

Each lung is covered with a membranous sac called the pleura. There are two layers of the pleura and between these layers there is a fluid which acts as a lubricant to prevent friction when the lung expands and deflates. The pleural sac which encloses each lung is

an airtight compartment. The pressure within the pleural cavity is less than that of the outside atmosphere. Thus, if the pleura is penetrated from the outside, air will rush in and collapse the lung.

While the outer surface of the lungs and bronchial tree are normally protected from contamination by outside sources, the inner lining of the respiratory tract is constantly exposed to dust, germs, and other foreign materials in the air. In defense against these substances, the mucous membranes contain tiny hairlike projections called cilia. These tiny projections trap and help to remove small foreign particles which are inhaled. The membrane also secretes a watery substance that helps prevent infection by cleansing foreign substances from the respiratory tract. If an inflammation does occur, these secretions are automatically increased in an effort to wash away bacteria and other debris. That is why watery eyes, running nose and cough are common to all upper respiratory infections.

Respiration is a very vital function of the body, and yet we are usually unaware of performing this function. It is only when we experience difficulty in breathing that we realize how important normal respiration is to our comfort and well-being.

Diseases of the respiratory system are the most common affliction of mankind. The common cold and other undifferentiated respiratory infections account for more absenteeism from work than any other illness. It is fortunate that most of these illnesses are not of a serious nature. However, there is always the danger of a serious infection and permanent disability, or even death, as a result of complications from a seemingly minor upper respiratory disease.

GENERAL NURSING CARE

There are many symptoms common to all types of respiratory diseases. These symptoms include coughing, increased flow of secretions from the nasal and bronchial mucosa, varying degrees of respiratory difficulty and some elevation of temperature. The nursing care necessary for relief of these symptoms will be discussed first in this chapter. Specific diseases of the respiratory system and the special treatments and nursing care required are discussed after the general nursing care.

Coughing. The act of coughing may be stimulated by any foreign substance in the respiratory tract. A cough may be dry, harsh and *nonproductive*, in which case the patient is unable to produce any sputum, or the cough may be deep, moist and *productive* of moderate to large amounts of sputum. When a cough is productive, the patient should be instructed to take deep breaths and cough up the sputum. Sputum should be expectorated, never swallowed. If coughing is painful to the patient, the nurse may support his chest with the palms of her hands during the seizure of coughing, or the chest may be supported with a binder or elastic bandage.

A nonproductive cough is very irritating to the mucous membranes and exhausting for the patient. Non-narcotic cough mixtures should be given to suppress nonproductive coughing. Any person with a chronic cough should seek medical advice because this is frequently an early symptom of chronic respiratory disease.

There are several different types of cough medicines. Some decrease secretions within the bronchial tract, while others actually increase the flow of these secretions, making them more easily coughed up and expectorated. The latter type are referred to as *expectorant* cough mixtures. Other preparations contain special drugs (for example, codeine) which depress the cough reflex and lessen the desire to cough. These are called *sedative* cough mixtures. Cough preparations are administered in very small amounts at a time and are not followed by water.

Increased Secretions. Since the majority of respiratory diseases are caused by infectious organisms that can easily be transmitted by way of the nasal and bronchial secretions, the nurse must protect herself and others from contamination. It is far better to teach the patient the proper care of these secretions than to try to avoid contact by wearing a mask when in his presence. The patient is usually not offended if he is tactfully told to place a folded tissue over his nose and mouth while coughing and sneezing and to turn his head away from the nurse whenever close contact is necessary, as during a bed bath or other procedure.

Care must be used in handling all nasal secretions and sputum. Disposable tissues should be used and discarded in a small paper bag pinned to the bedside or made readily accessible to the ambulatory patient. A used tissue should never be put in the pocket of one's clothing. If a patient has such a copious amount of sputum that tissues are not practical, he should be given a waxed sputum cup and instructed in its use.

In bacterial infections and chronic respiratory diseases, the sputum is often foul-smelling and leaves a disagreeable taste in the mouth. Frequent oral hygiene is important for patients with this condition, especially before meals, when the taste or odor of the sputum may directly affect the appetite.

Aspiration of the trachea (tracheal suctioning), whether through tubes or through the nose and mouth, is frequently required to remove secretions in the trachea which interfere with adequate oxygen intake. Tracheal suctioning, though a relatively common procedure, is not without its hazards. The removal of secretions may be essential for adequate respiration, but in the process of removing secretions by suction, oxygen—the very substance the patient needs to relieve his distress —is also removed. This accompanying removal of oxygen during suctioning can result in cardiac arrythmias such as tachycardia and bradycardia and may eventually lead to cardiac arrest.

There are some basic guidelines that should be helpful to the nurse in avoiding the serious consequences of oxygen removal by suctioning. (1) Administer oxygen in high concentrations immediately before suctioning the trachea. It is suggested that 100 per cent oxygen be used for five minutes before each suctioning session.[20] This procedure should also be performed immediately after each suctioning attempt. (2) Suctioning periods should be as brief as possible, preferably no more than 10 to 12 seconds. (3) Suctioning pressure should be no higher than necessary to remove secretions. (4) Additional oxygen should be given be-

tween suctioning attempts. (5) If tachycardia develops, continue only if suctioning is absolutely necessary to clear the airway. If bradycardia develops, suctioning should be discontinued and oxygen administered.[9]

Respiratory Distress. There are few persons living today who have not experienced the discomforts of a common cold. The annoyance of trying to breathe in spite of nasal congestion and the discomfort of being awakened in the night with an irritating cough are familiar to all of us. The patient with a severe respiratory disease experiences these discomforts to an even greater degree. He may become physically exhausted and actually suffer from lack of oxygen because of partial obstruction of the air passages or impaired function of the lungs.

The position which best facilitates breathing is the semi-Fowler's or high Fowler's position. The shoulders and back should be supported with a pillow to allow for full expansion of the lungs and to assist in keeping the chin off the chest. The diaphragm and the intercostal muscles are responsible for the mechanical expansion of the thoracic cavity which allows the lungs to inflate with air (see Fig. 16-1). Proper positioning of the patient will allow these muscles to function at their best.

When the deficiency of oxygen is severe, the physician orders administration of concentrated oxygen by mask, catheter or tent to relieve the anoxia.

The air the patient breathes should be kept moist to prevent further irritation of the mucous membranes by drying and to assist in the removal of secretions from the bronchial tree. Whether the air is warm or cool will depend on the wishes of the physician in charge. If warm, moist air is ordered, a vaporizer is set up in the patient's room or a croup tent is arranged. Warmth provides for relaxation of the bronchioles, thus allowing for improved inspiration of air into the lungs.

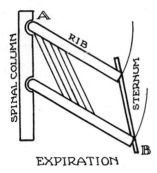 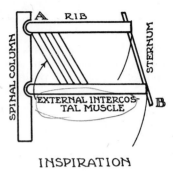

EXPIRATION   INSPIRATION

Figure 16–1. Schematic drawing showing action of first five ribs, sternum, and external intercostal muscles. All act to increase the diameter of the chest during inspiration of air into lungs. (From King and Showers: *Human Anatomy and Physiology,* 6th Ed., W. B. Saunders Co., Philadelphia.)

In the treatment of children with croup, a *croupette* which provides a fine mist of cool, moist air has been proven to be very beneficial. The droplets provided by the croupette are so small they can reach into the smaller bronchioles that the larger droplets of steam cannot reach. The cool air is also considered to be more advantageous than warm air when the patient is suffering from a high fever.

Rest. Whenever an inflammation is present, the affected part must be allowed to rest so that the body can repair the damaged tissues. In a respiratory illness, this same principle is applied. Since any undue exertion places an immediate burden on the respiratory system, bed rest is an important part of the treatment of respiratory diseases. Even minor infections require rest in bed if complications are to be avoided and the infection overcome in a short period of time. The nurse should explain the reasons for the needed rest and anticipate the needs of the patient so that he may be spared undue activity.

Diet. While the inflammation is acute, the diet should consist of high-caloric, high-vitamin liquids. Milk and milk products are especially important because of the need for protein in the repair and rebuilding of damaged tissues.

Later, as the patient progresses, the diet is changed to include soft foods, and eventually a regular diet is resumed. During the convalescent period, the patient will still have need for additional vitamins and proteins while his resistance to infection is low.

Medications. In addition to the expectorant and sedative cough mixtures mentioned earlier, there are several other medications used in the treatment of respiratory diseases. Antipyretics, or drugs which lower the temperature, may be necessary when the fever becomes dangerously high. Aspirin and Pyrilgin are examples of antipyretics. Aspirin has the added advantage of relieving the headache and other general aches and pains frequently associated with respiratory infections.

Antihistamines, which help to dry up secretions of the nasal and bronchial mucosa, are quite often used. These drugs should be taken only on the order of a physician, however, because they often produce undesirable side effects.

Antispasmodics, such as aminophylline, Adrenalin and ephedrine sulfate serve to decrease the muscular contractions of the bronchioles. They are particularly useful in the treatment of asthma.

Antibiotics are useful primarily in bacterial infections. In most viral infections, they are ineffective.

Inhalation Therapy. The inhalation of certain drugs such as bronchodilators and liquefying agents can be of benefit to patients who have difficulty with proper ventilation of the lungs. The drugs are in solution, which can be reduced to a fine spray that is inhaled easily and carried to the lower portions of the respiratory tract. The methods by which inhalation therapy may be carried out include (1) by a hand operated nebulizer, (2) through a nebulizer attached to compressed air or oxygen apparatus and (3) with an intermittent positive-pressure breathing machine.

Drugs administered by inhalation therapy usually are antibiotics, bronchodilators, liquefying agents and diluents. Bronchodilators enlarge the lumen to alleviate spasm of the bronchial tubes and to facilitate breathing for adequate ventilation of the lungs. Examples of bronchodilators are isoproterenol (Isuprel) and epinephrine hydrochloride (Vaponefrin). The liquefying agents and diluents help to thin bronchial secretions and make them more liquid and less tenacious so that they are more easily coughed up and expectorated. These liquefying agents include sodium ethasulfate (Tergemist), distilled water and tyloxapol (Alevaire).

Intermittent   Positive-Pressure Breathing Therapy. The patient with a chronic lung disorder such as emphysema, bronchiectasis or asthma may have partial obstruction of the air passages or damaged lung tissue or both. Every breath he takes is a great effort, and often the breath he has struggled for provides him with less oxygen than he actually needs. The intermittent positive-pressure breathing (IPPB) machine, such as the Bennet respirator, provides for increased inspiration of air into the lungs by introducing air or a mixture of oxygen and air under positive pressure. The machine can be cycled to a respiratory rate set and controlled by the patient. Each time he takes a breath, the machine provides a kind of "boost" that makes inspiration easier. In this way, IPPB helps overcome bronchial resistance to the inward flow of air, allows for more uniform distribution of oxygen to the alveoli, aids in the removal of carbon dioxide and makes coughing easier and more effective in removing secretions that have accumulated deep in the respiratory tree.

Some patients can leave the hospital and visit a local pulmonary clinic on a regular basis for the purpose of receiving IPPB therapy. Others may purchase a machine for their own use at home. Every patient who has IPPB therapy should be instructed in the way in which the machine works and the results that are expected.

There are two main types of respirators: those that provide controlled ventilation and those that give assisted ventilation. They may be used to: (1) provide patient-controlled pressure-breathing assistance for patients who are conscious and able to breathe spontaneously, (2) provide respiratory control for patients who cannot breathe, (3) relieve or overcome insufficient respiration, (4) deliver deep into the bronchial tree medications such as antibiotic and bronchodilator aerosols or liquefying agents that make the mucus less tenacious and easier to cough up and (5) provide a form of deep breathing exercise that "stretches" the respiratory muscles and improves their elastic tone and the circulation of the lungs. In both types of respirators, there are usually controls for the administration of oxygen.

There are at least 50 models and designs of respirators in existence, but the three most commonly used are the Bird, the Bennett and the Engstrom respirators.

Nursing   Responsibilities. Those concerned with the care of patients having controlled or assisted ventilation must have a thorough understanding of the physiology of respiration and the use of respirators. Although the respirators may vary in design and purpose, there are some principles of nursing care applicable to all patients using respirators.

1. The patient who breathes spontaneously usually will breathe through a mouthpiece when assisted ventilation is used. He should be told to purse his lips around the mouthpiece but not to clench his teeth or obstruct the tube with his tongue. He must not breathe through his nose, and if this is difficult at first, he may use a nose clip.

2. He should be given a brief, simple explanation of the purpose of the ventilation and what he can expect from it. The pressure from the respirator helps him inflate his lungs as he inhales. His breathing triggers the machine, and so he can control to some extent the amount of air flowing into his lungs. He should be told to pause after each exhalation.

3. If a mask is used, it should be well fitted so there is no leakage of air.

4. Provide the patient with a quiet, relaxing atmosphere.

5. Check the dials frequently for accidental changes in the readings.

6. Watch for a drop in blood pressure or symptoms of respiratory alkalosis in patients having prolonged controlled ventilation.

7. Pay attention to the skin, state of nutrition and need for suctioning in patients who are paralyzed or comatose.

Breathing Exercises. The mechanics of breathing can become increasingly less efficient as chronic respiratory disease progresses. The patient suffers a loss of lung elasticity, a flattened diaphragm and fixation of the rib cage as he becomes more and more dependent on the muscles of his upper chest and neck for breathing. The purpose of breathing exercises is to help correct this situation by strengthening the abdominal muscles so that they can push upward against the diaphragm and assist in the expiration of air from the lungs. These exercises also help

overcome rigidity of the thorax so that the lungs can inflate and deflate more easily. Patients who follow the exercises prescribed for them often find that they can lead more active and useful lives than formerly because their exertional dyspnea is less severe. This means that they can make better use of all the muscles of their body and are less likely to develop complications that accompany immobility. They also are better able to cough up secretions that would otherwise remain in the lower bronchi and serve as a growth medium for bacteria or as a cause of atelectasis. The psychological value of being able to indulge in ordinary activities that once left the patient breathless cannot be estimated.

Figure 16-2 shows some of the breathing exercises that may be prescribed for a patient with chronic obstructive lung disease.

Postural Drainage. The term postural drainage refers to positioning the patient so that his thorax is lower than the rest of his body. In this way, the force of gravity and ciliary activity of the small bronchial airways will move secretions to the main bronchi and trachea. Once the secretions have reached this point, the patient should be able to remove them by coughing.

The exact position in which the patient should be placed depends on the area of the lung to be drained (see Fig. 16-3). The nurse who assists a patient with postural drainage should obtain specific directions from the physician or physiotherapist so that she can position the patient properly. The physician also may wish to have the nurse use certain tapping, clapping and vibrating techniques during postural drainage. These measures are carried out for the purpose of dislodging mucus plugs so that they can be coughed up more easily. They must be done with precision, preferably by a physiotherapist, but only by someone who has received adequate instruction in the proper technique. Improper

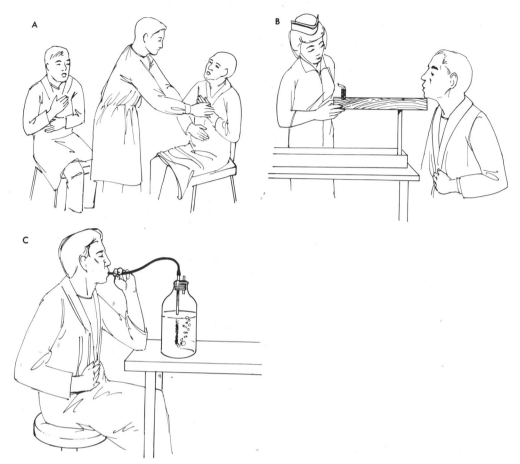

Figure 16–2. Breathing exercises help to improve the patient's respiratory function. *A,* The physical therapist teaches patients abdominal breathing. Placing one hand on his chest and the other on his abdomen helps the patient to recognize when he is doing the exercise correctly. During abdominal breathing the movement of the abdomen is felt with each breath, whereas the chest remains quiet. *B,* Blowing out a candle at various distances. This exercise can be performed also without the chin rest by holding or placing the candle at various distances. *C,* A blow bottle like this one can be prepared easily for use at home or in the hospital. The long glass tube extends below the water and is connected to rubber tubing, through which the patient blows. By taking deep breaths and exhaling, the patient causes the water to bubble vigorously.

clapping and vibrating can cause much discomfort to the patient and accomplish little more than upsetting him to the point that he refuses the treatment.[13]

Because there is likely to be some gagging during coughing episodes that take place during postural drainage, it is best to carry out the procedure <u>before meals, when the stomach is relatively empty and vomiting is less likely.</u> If the patient is to have postural drainage only <u>once a day,</u> it should be done in the <u>morning when he awakens.</u> At this time, secretions that have accumulated during the night's sleep can be removed. <u>After postural drainage is completed, the nurse must be sure to assist the patient with <u>proper oral hygiene, including tooth brushing and a refreshing mouth wash.</u> This will help overcome the foul taste left in the mouth by the sputum.

Irrigations. In order to help the patient eliminate thick, tenacious mucus from the throat and nasal passages, the

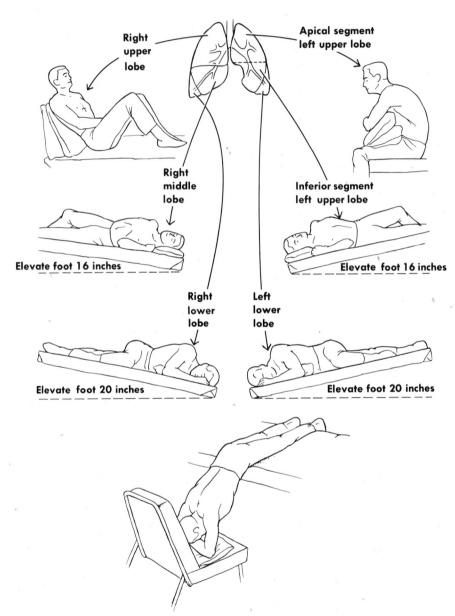

Figure 16-3. Postural drainage requires that the patient assume various positions to facilitate the flow of secretions from various portions of the lung into the bronchi, trachea, and throat so that they can be raised and expectorated more easily. Drawing shows the correct position to drain various portions of the lung. At the bottom of the drawing is illustrated a frequently ordered and less specific position, in which the patient lies across the bed, with his arms resting on a pillow on a chair. (From Shafer et al.: *Medical-Surgical Nursing,* 4th Ed., The C. V. Mosby Co., St. Louis.)

doctor may order gargles and nasal irrigations. Warm salt water (one teaspoonful of salt to a pint of water) is very good as a gargle. It helps remove the mucus and soothes the throat. When nasal irrigations are done, the patient must sit upright, and care must be taken never to use force. To do so may wash the infection up into the sinuses or frighten the patient into aspirating the solution into the trachea. The tip of the irrigating tube is inserted so as to allow space for the return flow of the solution.

OXYGEN THERAPY

Purposes of Oxygen Therapy

The air we breathe contains about 20 per cent oxygen. Under normal circumstances, this percentage is quite adequate, but when there is an obstruction of the intake of air or impaired circulation of the oxygen to the body tissues by way of the blood stream, the percentage of oxygen intake must be increased. The condition brought about by insufficient amounts of oxygen in the body is called *hypoxia.* The symptoms accompanying hypoxia are a result of damage to cells due to a lack of the oxygen so vital to their existence.

Tissues vary in their oxygen requirements. The cerebral cells, for example, receive 20 per cent of the body's oxygen supply and can live for only a few minutes if their supply of oxygen is cut off. Other cells, such as those of the myocardium, can survive as long as 30 to 40 minutes without a fresh supply of oxygen. We can see why it has been said that hypoxia not only stops the machine, but also wrecks the machinery.

The patient who is suffering from hypoxia will complain of headaches and slight visual disturbances, his pulse will become rapid, and his respirations will increase. Restlessness is also present, and cyanosis soon develops if the condition is not relieved. In order to provide the body cells with an adequate supply of oxygen, it may be necessary to administer oxygen by tent, nasal cannula or mask or through a tracheostomy.

Oxygen by Tent. Oxygen tents limit accessibility of the patient for nursing procedures and also provide less accurate oxygen concentrations than other methods. For these reasons, the tent is used less often than other methods of oxygen administration.

Since oxygen is heavier than air, it is possible for a considerable amount to be lost through the mattress unless a rubber sheet is placed over the mattress under the tent area. To make the tent airtight, the sides of the tent are tucked well under the mattress, and the front of the tent is folded inside an extra top sheet or bath blanket across the bed. All holes and tears in the tent must be repaired. When it is necessary to open the side zippers, the nurse should work as quickly as possible and do as much for the patient at one time as is practical so that there is a minimal loss of oxygen. Though speed is important, the patient must not be given the impression that he is being rushed through a procedure for the convenience of the nurse.

Oxygen by Mask. (See Fig. 16-4). If oxygen is administered by mask, care must be taken that the mask fits snugly and follows the contour of the face. It is comforting to the patient to have the mask removed periodically so that his face can be washed gently and powdered to prevent irritation of the skin. Obviously this procedure must be carried out quickly so that the patient does not suffer from a lack of oxygen while the mask is removed.

Oxygen by Nasal Cannula. (See Fig. 16-5). This is the simplest means of administering oxygen. The two-pronged nasal cannula is inserted one-fourth- to one-half-inch into each nostril. This method does not provide sufficient oxygen concentration for a patient with severe dyspnea.

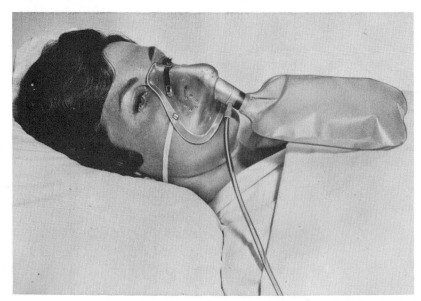

Figure 16–4. Oxygen by mask. (From Secor: *Patient Care in Respiratory Problems*. W. B. Saunders Co., Philadelphia.)

Oxygen by Nasal Catheter. This is the most efficient means of administering oxygen without a tracheostomy.[17] There are several types of nasal catheters available. They are inserted through the nostril and held in place by adhesive tape or a small disk designed to prevent aspiration of the catheter into the bronchial tree. These catheters require periodic changing, and special attention must be given to the nasal mucosa, which may become irritated by the tube and the dryness produced by the flow of oxygen. Another hazard

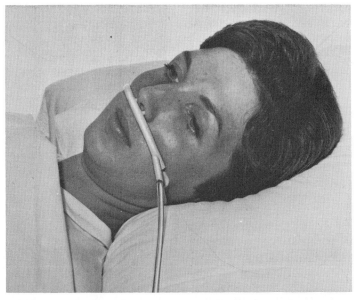

Figure 16–5. Oxygen by nasal cannula. (From Secor: *Patient Care in Respiratory Problems*. W. B. Saunders Co., Philadelphia.)

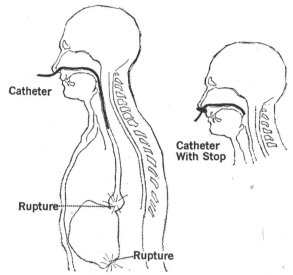

Figure 16–6. A stop placed 12.5 cm. from the catheter tip insures safe insertion in the oropharynx of any adult patient and prevents the catheter from extending into the patient's esophagus. (From Burgess: American Journal of Nursing, December, 1965.)

measure nose to ear lobe

of the nasal catheter is the possibility of rupturing the stomach by inadvertently passing the catheter into the esophagus. This possibility can be avoided by placing a stop on the catheter (see Fig. 16-6).

Precautions to be Taken When Oxygen is Used

Oxygen is NOT EXPLOSIVE. IT DOES SUPPORT COMBUSTION, which means that any spark or flame can cause a major fire in a very short time. The precautions necessary for the prevention of such a catastrophe are usually very clearly stated in every hospital policy book or procedure manual. These precautions include:

1. NO SMOKING signs posted in the area where oxygen is being administered.

2. Use of cotton blankets rather than wool blankets on the patient's bed.

3. Substituting a hand bell for the electric call bell.

4. Discontinuing the flow of oxygen while any electric equipment such as an EKG machine or suction machine is being used at the bedside.

Other precautions include attention to factors that can interfere with the flow of oxygen from the tank to the patient. These may include kinks in the tubing, loose connections and faulty humidifying apparatus. If there is some question whether the oxygen is flowing properly, listen for the hissing sound of air passing into the catheter, mask or tent. To determine whether the tubing is open and oxygen is passing through it, hold your finger over the end of the tube momentarily and then release it. You should hear a "pfft" sound as the oxygen escapes through the end of the tube. Remember that it is not unusual to find that a patient who is supposedly receiving oxygen therapy is actually getting less oxygen than he would under normal circumstances. The physician decides when the patient is to receive oxygen and by what method and in what concentration, but it is the nurse who must see to it that the patient receives what he orders.

Hazards of Oxygen Therapy

Paradoxically, the very oxygen that is needed to sustain life can be toxic. In very high concentrations, given over a period of time, oxygen can actually depress respiration and cause the patient to become cyanotic and comatose. After about 48 hours of administering oxygen in high concentrations and under positive pressure, the lungs fail to expand properly. This is especially true when pure oxygen is being given via a cuffed tracheostomy tube.

The nurse is responsible for seeing to it that oxygen is administered in the concentration ordered by the physician. She must also encourage her patient to take deep breaths periodically if he is able to do so. If the patient complains of discomfort under the sternum or has a cough or very shallow respiration, these symptoms should be reported to the physician in charge, since they may indicate oxygen toxication.

TRACHEOSTOMY

Definition

Tracheostomy is surgical incision into the trachea for the purpose of inserting a tube through which the patient breathes (see Fig. 16-7). It is done when there is complete obstruction of the trachea above the point of the incision and may be an emergency measure, or it may be done in anticipation of obstruction from edema or a growing malignant tumor.

The tracheostomy set consists of three parts: (1) the outer cannula, which is hollow and must never be removed by the practical nurse, (2) the inner cannula, which is also hollow and fits inside the outer cannula (this inner tube may be removed for cleaning) and (3) the obturator, a cone-tipped object which is used during the insertion of the tubes and is shaped to fit into the tubes. The obturator may be inserted to obstruct the inner cannula when the patient is learning to breathe normally again.

Nursing Care of the Patient With a Tracheostomy

The nurse must always remember that the patient with a tracheostomy

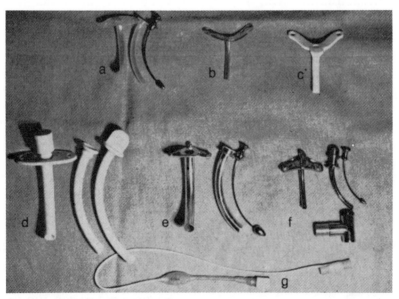

Figure 16–7. A variety of uncuffed tracheostomy tubes are shown above. Non-metal tubes made of nylon (a), polyvinyl chloride (b), and Silastic (c and d) often do not require an inner cannula because crusts do not tend to form. Also available are the traditional metal tubes: Jackson silver (e) and silver with a Morch adaptor on the inner cannula and a T-fitting for a ventilator (f). A cuff (g) can be attached to these tubes for a patient on a ventilator. (From White, H.A.: American Journal of Nursing, January, 1972.)

cannot speak or make any vocal sounds as long as the tracheostomy is open, because the air he inhales and exhales does not pass through the vocal cords. If he is conscious and able to move, he should be given a call bell whenever it is necessary to leave him alone so that he will have a way to summon help quickly. If he is able to write, he should be provided with a pad of paper and pencil or a magic slate so that he can communicate his needs to the nurse. If he is not able to move, he must not be left alone for any reason, as there is danger of a mucus plug obstructing the tracheostomy tube and causing asphyxiation and possible death.

The cleaning and care of the tracheostomy tube and special nursing care of the patient demand constant attention. The practical nurse who is not familiar with this special care should gain experience through observation and assisting with the care of the tracheostomy before she attempts to accept such a responsibility. In some institutions, she may be allowed to take on more responsibility than the information given here will prepare her for. In this case, it is recommended that the practical nurse request additional information and instruction from the physician or nurse in charge. It must be remembered that *the patient with a new tracheostomy incision is always in danger of asphyxiation.*

The special considerations in the nursing care of a tracheostomy patient are as follows:

1. The outer tube is held in place by a woven cotton tape which encircles the neck and ties at the back. This tape must never be cut or untied by the practical nurse because of the possibility that the patient may cough the outer cannula out of the incision.

2. An extra tracheostomy set should be kept in the patient's room at all times.

3. All equipment for cleaning and care of the tracheostomy should be kept at the bedside.

4. When we inhale under normal conditions, the air is warmed and moistened as it passes through the nose and throat. The patient with a tracheostomy does not breathe normally; thus, the air he breathes must be warmed and moistened artificially. A small vaporizer at the bedside will usually accomplish this.

5. Secretions must be removed as soon as they appear at the opening of the tracheostomy tube to prevent their aspiration back into the tube. Great care must be used in wiping or suctioning these secretions so as to avoid trauma to the surgical wound (see Fig. 16-8).

6. Gauze dressings around the tracheostomy opening must be bound with tape so that loose strings will not be aspirated into the tube. Many hospitals have special dressings to be used around a tracheostomy to avoid this hazard.

7. The inner and outer cannulae are often made of very soft metal and may easily be bent by careless handling or improper cleaning methods. The inner cannula should be removed and cleaned on the inside with a pipe cleaner.

8. Until he becomes accustomed to breathing through the tube, and because he cannot speak, the patient may be very apprehensive and easily upset by fits of coughing. He will need continued reassurance and competent, well-informed nurses in attendance.

The Cuffed Tracheostomy Tube. This is a specially designed tracheostomy tube that is used when a patient in acute respiratory failure must receive assisted ventilation with a positive pressure respirator (respirators are discussed later in this chapter). The tracheal end of the tracheostomy tube is encircled by a small balloon. When this balloon is inflated, it fills the space between the tracheostomy tube and the trachea, thereby providing a seal and preventing the escape of air around the tube. When positive pressure is administered, the air passes through the

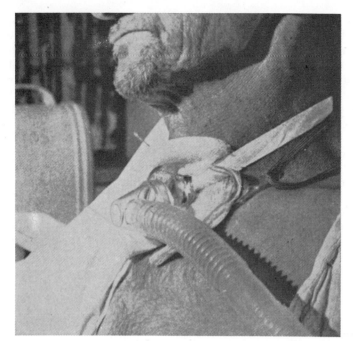

Figure 16–8. High humidity tracheal collar moisturizes oxygen to protect tracheal mucosa from drying and forming crusts. (From White, H.A.: American Journal of Nursing, January, 1972.)

tracheostomy tube *only,* thus providing sufficient pressure to inflate the lungs. The cuffed tracheostomy tube also reduces the chance of aspiration of mucus and fluids in those patients whose protective reflexes in the larynx and trachea are impaired.

Since the lumen of the tube is the only source of air for the patient, he must be watched closely for signs of obstruction of the tube. If the lumen is not suctioned frequently and kept open, the patient will suffocate. To avoid depression of the surface blood vessels in the tracheal wall and resultant necrosis, the cuff must be inflated just enough to seal the trachea without causing extreme pressure against the

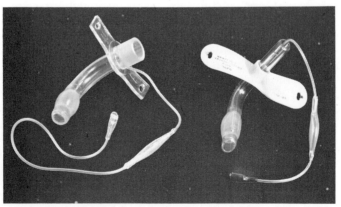

Figure 16–9. Tracheostomy tubes with fixed cuffs. (From Secor: *Patient Care in Respiratory Problems.* W. B. Saunders Co., Philadelphia.)

tracheal wall. A complaint from the patient that he has a sensation of tightness or choking must be reported immediately, as this may indicate overinflation of the cuff.

DIAGNOSTIC TESTS

Chest X-ray

The most common diagnostic aid used for respiratory illnesses is, of course, the chest x-ray. The physician will usually order films taken from the front, back and side of the chest (anterior, posterior and lateral), to obtain views of the lungs from several angles. No special preparation is necessary for a chest x-ray.

Respiratory Function Tests

These tests are done to evaluate functioning capacity of the lungs and to determine specific pulmonary disorders that produce dyspnea. A test for vital capacity measures the greatest amount of air that an individual can exhale after he has inhaled as much air as he can. A tidal volume test measures the amount of air inspired and expired during a normal breath. Expiratory reserve volume is the maximal volume of air expired while a person is resting. Residual volume is the amount of air that is left remaining in the lungs after a person has exhaled as much air as he can. The total lung capacity is the amount of air contained in the lungs after a person has inhaled as much air as he is able.

Sputum Analysis

Laboratory tests of sputum are frequently done in cases of respiratory disease. These tests include stained smears for pathogenic microorganisms or malignant cells and gross examination for color, consistency and general characteristics of the sputum specimen.

The nurse should explain the procedure to the patient, emphasizing the need for coughing up sputum from the lower respiratory tract. If the patient is not instructed properly, he may cough in a shallow and ineffective manner so that he expectorates only saliva. The sputum cup should be kept covered when the patient is not using it, as it may be unpleasant for him and those who enter his room. If a specimen is collected for culture, the container should have a tight-fitting lid so that the spread of the infectious agents in the sputum can be avoided. The best time for collection of the specimen is in the morning upon awakening.

Bronchogram

This is an x-ray of the bronchial tree. The x-ray films are taken after a radiopaque oil has been introduced into the trachea. The patient lies down and is tilted in various positions so the oil will be distributed over the bronchial tree. The oil is a special type that will not damage the mucosa of the respiratory tract, and even though postural drainage may be ordered to remove some of the oil after the test, the remaining oil will not damage the lungs or bronchi.

Bronchoscopy

A bronchoscope is a special instrument designed to be inserted into the bronchi for the purpose of visualizing the inside of the trachea and bronchi (bronchoscopy). The instrument is also used to remove foreign bodies from the respiratory tract or to obtain a biopsy for further study.

For both a bronchogram and a bronchoscopy, the patient's throat is anesthetized so that the gag reflex is no longer present. He is not given any food or liquids for at least 2 hours after either of these examinations because, in the absence of the gag reflex, he is likely to aspirate the material into his trachea.

THE COMMON COLD

Definition

The common cold is an inflammation of the upper respiratory tract. It is caused by a virus. There are so many different strains of viruses which can produce the symptoms of a common cold that immunity is difficult, if not impossible, to establish. Avoiding exposure to those who have a "cold" and maintaining a state of good health and high resistance are the only ways one can avoid catching a cold.

Symptoms

The common cold usually starts with a mild sore throat or a hot, dry sensation in the nose and back of the throat. Within hours after the onset, the nose becomes congested with increased secretions, the eyes begin to water and sneezing and an irritating nonproductive cough appear. There is usually no elevation of temperature, or, if a fever does develop, it is of a low-grade type.

Treatment and Nursing Care

The main purpose of treating a cold is the prevention of complications from a bacterial infection. While the mucous membranes are irritated and inflamed, they are much more susceptible to invasion by bacteria. The patient should stay indoors, preferably in bed, and away from others. Fluids, especially citrus fruit juices, are given in large amounts to keep the temperature down and to help the body remove wastes. Vitamin C in the citrus fruits helps in the repair of inflamed tissues. The patient should avoid chilling and exposure to drafts or sudden changes in temperature. Aspirin are helpful in relieving the aches and pains of a cold and eliminate the headache usually present.

Nose drops of normal saline, or those containing a mild decongestant such as ephedrine, help in the removal of nasal secretions.

ACUTE BRONCHITIS

Definition

This is an acute inflammation of the bronchi. The differentiation between bronchitis, tracheobronchitis, tonsillitis and laryngitis is somewhat difficult and not always necessary, since these upper respiratory infections are generally treated in the same way.

Symptoms

Bronchitis presents approximately the same symptoms as the common cold at the outset. The cough is usually more persistent and later becomes productive of purulent sputum in fairly large amounts. The temperature is usually elevated in bronchitis, and in children it can become high enough to produce febrile convulsions.

Treatment and Nursing Care

The coughing and dyspnea which accompany bronchitis are best relieved by the inhalation of moist air. A vaporizer in the room will increase the general humidity and relieve some of the coughing and dyspnea. For small children in a crib, a croup tent can be improvised by placing a cotton blanket or sheet over the top and sides of the crib and adjusting the flow of steam under this covering. Extreme care must be used with all types of vaporizers in the home or the hospital. They must be placed so that the child cannot reach the vaporizer or its nozzle, and the steam must be directed away from the patient. Adult patients or others in the room may easily turn over a vaporizer which is not placed out of the way.

The patient with chronic bronchitis usually has a persistent cough and copious amounts of sputum, especially upon arising in the morning. Postural drainage is helpful in removing sputum from the lower parts of the respiratory tract. These patients should avoid exposure to cold, damp weather and dust or smog, which will further irritate the bronchi. They should maintain a sensible schedule of rest and good nutrition so that their resistance to bacterial infections is kept high.

PNEUMONIA

Definition

Pneumonia is an extensive inflammation of lung tissues. There are two general types of pneumonia: (1) bacterial pneumonia, which is most often caused by pneumococci and (2) primary atypical pneumonia, or viral pneumonia. This second type of pneumonia is caused by a virus or a combination of several different organisms (mixed infection).

Symptoms

A bacterial pneumonia usually begins abruptly with severe chills and elevated temperature. The onset of atypical pneumonia is usually much more gradual. The patient complains of a severe stabbing pain in the chest or side, which is aggravated by coughing or taking a deep breath. The sputum is frothy and white at first and then changes to a characteristic rust color. Cyanosis is not uncommon, and the skin is moist and hot. "Fever blisters" (herpes simplex) frequently are present around the nose and lips. Patients with pneumonia appear exhausted and usually do not wish to be disturbed for even the most essential of nursing care. Delirium is not an uncommon occurrence in pneumonia and demands constant attendance by the nursing staff so that the patient will not injure himself.

Treatment and Nursing Care

The aims of treatment of pneumonia include: (1) conservation of the patient's strength and energy, (2) relief of symptoms and (3) control of the infection.

The patient is placed on absolute bed rest with medications and nursing care scheduled so that he is disturbed as little as possible. Fluids are forced to combat dehydration and help the body in eliminating wastes. Special attention to the mouth is necessary because the patient usually breathes through his mouth, which produces drying and cracking of the lips and inside of the mouth.

The patient is kept warm and away from drafts. Bedclothes, dampened by perspiration, should be changed as often as necessary to keep the patient dry and comfortable. The patient must be protected from chilling during the bed bath and change of linens.

Since pneumonia is an infectious disease and easily transmitted by droplet infection, the patient is isolated and extreme care is taken with nasal secretions and sputum.

Abdominal distention frequently accompanies pneumonia. The measures used to relieve this condition include rectal tubes and low enemas as ordered by the physician.

The vital signs of the patient must be observed closely and checked frequently. Any change in the pulse rate, falling blood pressure or difficult respiration must be reported immediately. Other signs of danger to be reported include increasing cyanosis, restlessness or delirium.

Complications following pneumonia are not uncommon, especially if the patient does not exercise caution during the convalescent period. Pneumonia is a dangerous disease. It is very exhausting and depletes the body's reserve of energy, thus lowering the resistance to infections. Empyema is a common complication of pneumonia (see the discussion following). Congestive heart failure may also occur as a complication of pneumonia.

BRONCHIECTASIS

Definition

Bronchiectasis is a chronic disease of the respiratory system characterized by

Bronchiectasis

permanent dilatation of the bronchi. This condition may follow pneumonia and other respiratory infections, or it may be the result of a congenital defect in the alveoli. These small sacs are not as elastic as they should be, and they fill with secretions. Because the bronchioles are enlarged and unable to remove the secretions, the sputum collects and becomes stagnant.

Symptoms

The most outstanding symptom of bronchiectasis is severe attacks of coughing in which the patient brings up large amounts of thick, foul-smelling sputum. The coughing is most noticeable in the morning when the patient first gets out of bed. In addition to the coughing attacks, the patient may complain of fatigue and loss of weight. The majority of individuals with true bronchiectasis begin having symptoms by the time they are 20 years of age. As the disease progresses, they develop clubbing of the fingers, which is characteristic of many chronic respiratory diseases (see Fig. 16-10).

Treatment and Nursing Care

There is, unfortunately, no cure for bronchiectasis other than surgical re-moval of the affected part. If the involved area is so extensive that surgery is not possible, the patient's prognosis is very poor.

Other measures to aid in the removal of mucus plugs from the bronchioles include expectorant drugs, removal by way of a bronchoscope and inhalation or aerosol therapy. Antibiotics may be given during acute attacks to prevent further infection of the lungs. They also help in decreasing the amount of sputum produced.

General measures of good nutrition and adequate rest are necessary to conserve the strength of the patient and prevent the development of complications.

CANCER OF THE LUNG

Introduction

In 1930, the lung cancer death rate for males was 3.6 per 100,000 population; in 1960, the rate had increased to approximately 32.5 per 100,000. Today, while death rates from other forms of cancer are decreasing or remaining stable, lung cancer has become a leading cause of death in white males. Factors that contribute to this increase include increasing air pollution, the increase of cigarette smoking by young

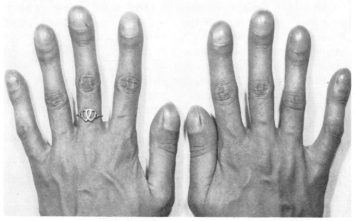

Figure 16-10. Clubbed fingers of patient with chronic respiratory difficulties and cyanosis. (From Brown: *Medical Nursing,* 3rd Ed., W. B. Saunders Co., Philadelphia.)

persons and the increasing numbers of older persons in the population. The condition is found most often in men 40 years of age or older, but the incidence in females is rising.

Symptoms

Most lung tumors begin in the epithelial lining of the bronchi. There are few symptoms at first, usually only a cough and some wheezing. As the tumor grows larger, the patient may have some pain or discomfort in the chest, exertional dyspnea and expectoration of blood-streaked sputum. Diagnosis is confirmed by an x-ray showing a definite mass or by removal of malignant cells during bronchoscopy.

Treatment

The only possible cure for cancer of the lung at this time is by surgical removal. The type of surgery, lobectomy or pneumonectomy, depends on the size and location of the malignant growth. Radiation therapy and chemotherapy may help in some cases to retard growth of the tumor and provide some relief from symptoms.

ASTHMA

Definition

Bronchial asthma is an allergic reaction characterized by swelling of the mucous membranes of the respiratory tract and increased production of secretions within the bronchioles. These conditions produce dyspnea and wheezing because they obstruct the flow of air through the respiratory passages.

Symptoms

Most patients with asthma are free from symptoms between attacks. During an attack, which is usually brought on by exposure to one or more antigens,

the patient has itching and watering of the eyes, cough, and a wheezing type of dyspnea. Respirations may be so difficult that the individual uses all accessory muscles of respiration, such as the chest and abdominal muscles, in an effort to breathe. The patient cannot lie down and may sit up all night struggling for breath during the attack.

Treatment and Nursing Care

The treatment of asthma begins with determination of the substances to which the individual is allergic. Once these allergens have been determined, every effort is made to avoid them. Dust is a very common offender in adults, while foods such as eggs, wheat and milk are common causes of asthmatic attacks in children.

Emotional factors also play an important role in precipitating attacks of asthma. The patient and his family will need help in understanding the relationship between emotional anxiety and attacks of asthma. In some cases, professional counseling for the patient and family can help in removing sources of tension for the patient.

Other factors which may contribute to an attack of asthma are sudden changes in temperature, physical exhaustion, contact with animal dander and overeating.[1] Teaching the patient to look for situations which lead to an attack so that he may avoid them in the future will help in reducing the number of attacks.

Drugs used in the treatment of asthma are given primarily to relieve the symptoms. They do not cure the condition. Bronchodilators such as epinephrine and aminophylline are frequently used in the treatment of asthma. Aerosol therapy with Isuprel also is used. Expectorants such as potassium iodide and ammonium chloride assist the patient in raising sputum by thinning the secretions, thus making them more easily coughed out of the bronchioles.

Sometimes an acute attack of asthma

does not respond to treatment, and the symptoms persist for days. When this happens, the patient is said to have *status asthmaticus.* In this situation, the patient is very seriously ill, and death may occur from excessive strain on the heart. The nursing care includes providing a quiet and restful environment for the patient. All possible sources of dust, pollen and other allergens are removed from the patient's room, and a special air filter may be installed in the window. The patient is placed in Fowler's position to facilitate breathing. Oxygen is usually administered, for these patients often have severe cyanosis. The nurse must anticipate the needs of the patient and do everything possible for him so that he will not exert himself. The patient must be protected from too many visitors and all other sources of emotional excitement.

PLEURISY

Definition

Pleurisy is an inflammation of the pleural membranes surrounding the lungs. In *pleurisy with effusion,* there is also an increase in the amount of serous fluid within the pleural cavity.

Symptoms

The most outstanding symptom of pleurisy is a sharp, stabbing pain in the chest. The pain is aggravated by taking a deep breath. Pleurisy may occur alone or in conjunction with another disease of the respiratory system.

Treatment and Nursing Care

The patient is placed on bed rest and observed carefully for signs of the development of an infection in the respiratory tract. The chest may be supported by strapping with adhesive tape. This offers some relief from the pain.

When pleurisy is accompanied by effusion of serous fluid, the physician may remove this fluid from the thorax for diagnostic tests or relief of symptoms. The procedure for removal of fluid from the pleural cavity is called a *thoracentesis.* It is not uncommon for as much as 500 ml. to be removed at one time during a thoracentesis.

EMPYEMA

Definition

When the fluid within the pleural cavity becomes infected, the exudate becomes thick and purulent, and the patient is said to have empyema. The organisms causing the infection may be the staphylococcus, streptococcus or pneumococcus.

Treatment and Nursing Care

Empyema is treated by eliminating the infection through the use of specific antibiotics and the removal of the excess fluid from the pleural cavity. The physician may order that a sampling of the fluid collected during a thoracentesis be sent to the laboratory and a *sensitivity test* done. This test determines the exact antibiotic which will most effectively destroy the organism causing the infection.

PULMONARY EMPHYSEMA

Definition

This is a chronic respiratory disease that results from a long-standing inflammation of the bronchi as in chronic bronchitis, asthma and bronchiectasis. The small bronchioles at the end of the respiratory tree become plugged with infectious material which prevents normal expansion and contraction of the air sacs (alveoli) of the lung. Air becomes trapped in the alveoli, causing them to become distended, and eventually the alveolar walls thicken and become less elastic. The damaged alveoli then cannot be emptied completely during expiration, and so the lungs remain partially expanded at all times. The patient cannot rid his lungs of stale air to make room for oxygenated air.

One patient who has had emphysema for more than 26 years suggests that a healthy person can get some idea of the effects of emphysema by doing the following: take a deep breath and then exhale only about one third of the air you have breathed in. Continue trying to breathe while retaining the two thirds of that original breath.[10] If you should try this, you would find that it is little wonder that emphysema often is called the "living death."

Cause and Incidence. Although there is no one specific causative factor in all cases of emphysema, many authorities believe that cigarette smoking is the leading cause of chronic bronchitis which eventually leads to emphysema. Other contributing factors include asthma, chronic upper respiratory infections, congenital defects in the respiratory tract and continued irritation of the bronchi by polluted air.[3]

According to the U.S. Public Health Service, emphysema is a major health problem that is second only to heart disease as a cause of disability. It is more widespread than lung cancer and tuberculosis combined, disabling one out of every 14 wage earners over the age of 45.

Symptoms

The first symptom usually is a chronic or recurring cough that often is ignored by the patient. He finds it distressing, but does not consider it serious. As the disease gradually progresses, the individual notices a shortness of breath every time he exerts himself (exertional dyspnea). This can continue for quite a number of months or years, and the patient may not be inconvenienced enough to seek medi-

cal treatment. If he chooses to continue to ignore his symptoms, he eventually finds that breathing is becoming more and more difficult, especially during the expiratory phase. He coughs continuously—a moist, wheezing cough —but he is not able to clear his respiratory tract satisfactorily. He then becomes less and less active; his thorax becomes fixed and assumes a barrel shape, and there are large spaces between the ribs. If x-rays are taken, they will show inflated lungs, a flattened diaphragm and abnormal heart shadows.[17] The appearance of the emphysematous patient is usually quite characteristic, and one can almost diagnose his condition by looking at him. He wears an anxious and strained facial expression. He cannot lie down flat in bed, but sits up on the edge of his bed or chair leaning forward and using his abdominal muscles to exhale. He makes an obvious effort to exhale with each breath and often puffs out his cheeks on expiration. He must speak quickly and in short sentences because he has so little breath.

Complications

The most common complications of emphysema are infection, respiratory acidosis and a heart condition called cor pulmonale. One should bear in mind that cor pulmonale is cardiac failure produced by a lung disease rather than a result of some disorder of the heart itself. It is generally agreed that cor pulmonale occurs because of hypertension within the pulmonary artery. This hypertension places a tremendous burden on the right ventricle because it must work doubly hard to overcome the pressure within the pulmonary artery. Eventually the ventricle enlarges and becomes fatigued. Then the patient has right-sided cardiac failure with symptoms arising from accumulation of fluid in the abdominal cavity, in the peripheral tissues and in the thoracic cavity. The liver becomes enlarged as a result of congestion in the portal circulation. Treatment for cor pulmonale is the same as for other types of cardiac failure; that is, digitalization, use of diuretics and restriction of sodium and fluid intake.

Treatment and Nursing Care

Unfortunately, by the time a patient manifests these severe symptoms, there is nothing that can be done to reverse the pathologic changes responsible for them. There are, however, some therapeutic measures that can help relieve the symptoms. If the disease is detected early, and treatment and rehabilitation plans are carried through, it is possible to help these patients maintain adequate ventilation and continue to lead a fairly comfortable and moderately active life.

Treatment usually consists of administration of medications to prevent infections, bronchial obstruction and chronic inflammation. These drugs include antibiotics, bronchodilators and corticosteroids. Also, the patient must learn to avoid conditions that further aggravate his symptoms. This includes not smoking, avoiding cold air, dust or other irritants that can bring spasm and constriction of the bronchioles, regulation of physical activity so that he does not overexert himself, avoiding emotional upsets and stressful situations that increase breathing difficulties and maintaining adequate nutrition and other measures that will maintain a resistance to infection.

Exercises such as those described earlier in this chapter are of benefit to some patients who do not have severe dyspnea or are not otherwise greatly debilitated. These exercises improve ventilation of the lungs by strengthening the abdominal muscles and other accessory muscles of respiration so that they can be used efficiently in breathing.

Intermittent positive-pressure breathing also can be of benefit in proper ventilation of the lungs and "stretching" of the respiratory muscles so that there can be adequate removal of carbon dioxide from the lungs. This treatment also allows for administration of aerosol drugs which facilitate coughing and bronchial expansion for removal of accumulated secretions.

The patient with emphysema is usually treated at home unless he is suffering from acute respiratory distress. His activities are regulated so that he has frequent periods of rest, and all undue physical exertion is avoided.

Special exercises which increase the contracting ability of the diaphragm and thereby help in deflating the lungs are of some benefit. Abdominal support with elastic bandages or girdles also assists in maintaining good contraction and elevation of the diaphragm.

Aerosol therapy is especially beneficial to the patient with emphysema. There are a variety of medications that may be used to dilate the airways and facilitate the breathing of a patient with chronic obstructive lung diseases such as emphysema.

Isoproterenol (Isuprel) is given by intermittent positive pressure, using a respirator and nebulizer. Patients receiving this drug should be watched closely for signs of cardiac arrythmias and changes in blood pressure. Aminophylline, Tedral (a mixture of theophylline, ephedrine and phenobarbital) and Madrax are administered for the purpose of dilating the bronchi. Expectorants such as potassium iodide and ammonium chloride may also be prescribed. When narcotics or hypnotics are prescribed for these patients, the nurse should be aware of the potential danger posed by these drugs because of their tendency to depress respiration and thereby aggravate the patient's respiratory distress.

PULMONARY TUBERCULOSIS

Definition

Pulmonary tuberculosis is an infectious disease of the lung characterized by lesions within the lung tissue. The lesions may continue to degenerate and become necrotic, or they may heal by fibrosis and calcification. The causative organism is the tubercle bacillus.

Incidence. The widespread use of anti-tuberculotic drugs has brought about some changes in the distribution of tuberculosis in the United States. In the mid-1940's, tuberculosis could be found in almost all communities and in all social and ethnic groups. Today it is primarily found in nonwhite males; nonwhite females rank second, and all persons in the age group of 65 years or older run a close third. Crowded urban areas show a much higher rate than do rural areas.[24]

Diagnosis

Early detection of tuberculosis is of great importance, because the anti-tuberculotic drugs are more effective in the early stages of the disease, the period of disability is much shorter and the complications are fewer.

A tuberculin test such as the Mantoux intradermal test or the Heaf multiple puncture skin test are valuable in ruling out tuberculosis. If the skin test is positive, it indicates a need for further testing by x-ray and a complete physical examination.

X-ray examination of the chest also is useful in detecting tubercular lesions of the lungs. The Public Health Department and other health agencies such as the state Tuberculosis and Health Associations offer free x-ray films from a mobile unit that visits neighborhoods. In this way, cases of tuberculosis can be detected in persons who might not otherwise be tested for lung disease. These x-ray programs have been especially effective in communities known to have a high tuberculosis rate.

Analysis of sputum for the presence of the tubercle bacillus is another diagnostic test that is used. If the bacilli are present, a diagnosis of tuberculosis is very definitely established. Since persons are quite likely to swallow sputum rather than expectorate it, a sample of the stomach contents can be examined for the presence of tubercle bacilli.

Symptoms

The symptoms of tuberculosis include cough, low-grade fever in the afternoon, loss of weight, night sweats and sometimes *hemoptysis* (spitting of blood).

Treatment and Nursing Care

All of the general principles essential to the proper care of a patient with a respiratory disease are applied to the nursing care of a patient with pulmonary tuberculosis. Rest, good nutrition, proper handling of secretions from the respiratory tract and control of coughing are all important aspects to be considered. Of these, rest is probably most important. For the specific procedures and methods of isolation of the patient and destruction of the tubercle bacillus, the student is referred to a text on communicable diseases.

Tuberculosis is more a chronic disease than acute in nature and has a prolonged period of convalescence. Because the patient is confined to an institution or his home for months or even years, some provision must be made for occupational therapy and other diversional activities. The student is referred to Chapter 8 of this text for further information on the care of the chronically ill.

Drugs used in the treatment of tuberculosis are usually given in combination; that is, two drugs are chosen and given simultaneously for maximum effect. The most common drugs used are *streptomycin, para-aminosalicylic acid (PAS)* and *isoniazid (INH)*. These drugs have a specific action against the tubercle bacillus and have greatly facilitated arrest of the disease.

The patient must receive these injections over such an extended period of time that it is extremely important that the sites of injection are rotated faithfully. The patient often becomes discouraged by the number of painful injections necessary, and the nurse must help him understand the need for uninterrupted administration of the medication. When drugs are not administered regularly, the bacilli become resistant, and the drugs are no longer effective.

Surgery is also used in the treatment of tuberculosis. Surgical removal of a diseased lobe of the lung is referred to as a *lobectomy.* A *pneumonectomy* is surgical removal of the entire lung. A *thoracoplasty* is removal of several ribs for the purpose of collapsing the lung. *Artificial pneumothorax* is the injection of air into the pleural cavity for the purpose of collapsing the lung. Both a thoracoplasty and an artificial pneumothorax are done so that the collapsed lung may be in a state of complete rest, thereby aiding in the healing of the tuberculous lesion.

Prevention

Tuberculosis is an infectious disease that is contracted by inhaling the tubercle bacillus. This microorganism is capable of surviving for long periods of time in dark, damp places. It cannot survive more than two hours of direct sunlight and also can be killed by boiling for a full five minutes. Autoclaving is the most efficient method of killing the tubercle bacillus. Ultraviolet light is especially effective in destroying the bacillus in rooms which cannot be reached by direct sunlight.

The best way in which the spread of tuberculosis can be controlled is through adequate detection and treatment of active cases and through education of the public about the disease. Once a person is diagnosed as tubercular, he should be taught the ways in which the disease can be spread and his responsibility in following directions so that he does not contaminate others. He must learn to cover his nose and mouth with a disposable tissue each time he clears his throat, coughs or sneezes. The contaminated tissues should be flushed down a toilet or wrapped in paper and burned. Ordinary face masks are not effective in screening out the tubercle bacillus and should not be relied upon by the nurse as protection from the patient who cannot or will not cover his nose and mouth. There are some specially made masks that are effective barriers against the bacilli, and they should be used when a patient is unable to cooperate.

Strict isolation of the tubercular patient is not considered necessary. When adequate drug therapy is instituted and general safety measures are used, there is no danger of transmission of pulmonary tuberculosis. He and his family should understand, however, exactly how the disease is spread and what precautions they should take when the patient is staying at home. Since small children and infants are particularly susceptible to the disease, special precautions must be taken to protect them from contamination.

There is available a vaccine made from living, attenuated bacilli. It is called BCG (bacille Calmette Guérin) and is capable of offering some protection but cannot be depended upon to provide complete immunity to tuberculosis. The BCG vaccine has the disadvantage of causing a positive reaction to the tuberculin test, and this interferes somewhat with the usefulness of tuberculin testing programs. Public health officials in this country advise the administration of BCG vaccine only to those persons who live in communities that have a very high rate of tuberculosis. In New York City, for example, every child entering the seventh grade is offered the vaccine. In rural areas where the tuberculosis rate is low, the vaccine is not recommended.

If, during the tuberculin testing program, an individual shows a positive reaction within six months after a negative reaction, some authorities recommend that he receive isoniazid as a prophylaxis. The drug is given for one full year. It also may be given as a preventive medication to individuals with silicosis, because they are more susceptible than usual to tuberculosis.

EXTRAPULMONARY TUBERCULOSIS

Definition

It is possible for the tubercle bacillus to attack and damage parts of the body other than the lungs. This is called extrapulmonary tuberculosis. The areas most frequently affected are the bones, meninges, urinary tract and the reproductive system.

Tuberculous meningitis involves infection of the meninges which line the brain and spinal cord. This disease can be fatal unless it is promptly treated with anti-tuberculotic drugs. The symptoms of this disorder are essentially the same as those in other types of meningitis.

Tuberculous infection of the bone is now less common than it formerly was because of better methods of detecting pulmonary tuberculosis and. elimination of contaminated milk as a source of infection. Because of extensive bone destruction in a tubercular infection, there can be serious orthopedic deformities in this disease. Tuberculosis of the spine, called Pott's disease, is now quite rare in the United States. The deformity most commonly seen in Pott's disease is kyphosis, or "hunchback."

NURSING CARE OF THE PATIENT HAVING CHEST SURGERY

Preoperative Care

The preoperative period is somewhat longer when chest surgery is done, because the breathing capacity of the patient will be greatly diminished during the immediate postoperative period and the patient will need to be in the best possible health to withstand the strain. Special exercises may be done under the supervision of a physiotherapist. These exercises are planned so that the chest and shoulder muscles and the muscles of respiration will be able to provide the maximum respiration possible after surgery.

The patient may have extensive diagnostic tests, including a bronchoscopy and sputum examination, immediately before surgery. Postural drainage and expectorant drugs are given to remove as much sputum from the bronchi as possible.

Postoperative Care

When the patient returns from surgery, he will require close observation for signs of respiratory distress. Dyspnea, cyanosis or sudden severe pain in the chest must be reported immediately because these may indicate a collapse of the lung due to a leakage of air into the pleural cavity. The vital signs of the patient are checked frequently and recorded. Oxygen is usually administered for the first few postoperative days.

The position of the patient once he has recovered from the anesthesia will depend on the type of surgery performed and the orders of the surgeon. The patient is turned every 2 hours or more often as ordered. Before attempting to turn the patient, the practical nurse must ascertain whether or not the surgeon wishes to allow the patient to lie on the *unoperative* side. Many surgeons do not allow the patient to lie on the unoperative side because this position diminishes the expansion of the good lung and thereby adds to respiratory distress. There is also danger of infection of the good lung by drainage from the affected lung when the patient lies with the operative side up. When the patient has a tube inserted for drainage from the operative site, lying on the operative side facilitates the flow of drainage. Unless contraindicated, the most comfortable position is semi-Fowler's. After the vital signs have become stable, the head of the bed may be elevated to a 45° angle. In this position, the diaphragm stays down, and there is more room for lung expansion.

Coughing is encouraged during the postoperative period so that secretions will be removed from the bronchial tree and complications thereby avoided. The nurse must realize that coughing is painful for the patient, and he will need support of the chest during a seizure of coughing.

It is not unusual for the patient who has had chest surgery to return from the operating room with a tube inserted through the surgical incision in his chest. This tube provides *closed drainage* of the fluids which accumulate in the pleural cavity during and after surgery.

Special Points in the Care of a Closed Drainage System

1. Remember that the pleural cavity is an airtight compartment. The apparatus for closed drainage must also remain airtight *at all times*.

2. Never raise the drainage bottles from a thoracotomy tube above the level of the surgical incision. It is best to keep the bottles on the floor at all times.

3. Never disconnect the tubing from the bottle. If the tubing becomes disconnected accidentally, pinch the tubing leading to the patient's chest and summon help immediately.

4. Do not allow the tubing to become kinked or obstructed by the weight of the patient.

5. Never pin the tubing to the bedclothes.

6. Do not empty a thoracotomy drainage bottle. The surgeon usually prefers to do this himself. If the bottle becomes filled with fluid, notify the

nurse in charge. The surgeon will want to know immediately if the patient is having that much drainage.

7. Dressings may be reinforced but are never changed by the practical nurse as long as closed drainage is being used.

8. If the patient has two thoracotomy tubes, each one must be connected to its own water-seal drainage bottle. The purpose of the two tubes is to provide drainage of air and fluid from the pleural space (see Fig. 16-11).

9. Check tubing at least once every two hours to be sure that there is no obstruction to the flow of drainage. If the tube is open and unobstructed, the saline in the drainage bottle will rise and fall with each inspiration and expiration. Blood clots that are obstructing the tubing can be removed by gently "milking" the tube in the direction of the bottle.

PNEUMOTHORAX

Definition

The term pneumothorax refers to an accumulation of air or gas in the pleural cavity. Normally the pleural space is an airtight compartment with a negative pressure that allows for expansion of the lungs. If any external or internal chest injury causes a break in the wall of the pleural space, air will rush into the cavity and collapse the lung. This also will cause a shift of the heart and mediastinum toward the unaffected side.

Spontaneous pneumothorax can occur during the course of a pulmonary disease, or it may follow a perforating injury to the external chest wall. *Artificial pneumothorax* is a surgical procedure sometimes used in the treatment of tuberculosis in order to collapse the lung and give it rest.

Symptoms

Spontaneous pneumothorax is characterized by severe dyspnea, a sudden,

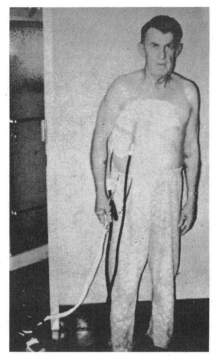

A

TO SUCTION

TO PLEURAL CAVITY

ADHESIVE
MARKER

B

Figure 16–11. *A,* Unwilling but able, patient walks every four hours trailing drainage bottles with rope. Kelly hemostats clamped to pajamas prevent pull on tubes. *B,* Underwater drainage bottles act as one-way valves, permitting air and blood to escape from, but not to return to, pleural cavity. Escaping air causes saline to bubble. Rising fluid level in bottles is marked to indicate amount and rapidity of blood loss. (From Dittbrenner and Herbert: American Journal of Nursing, October, 1967.)

sharp pain in the chest with cessation of normal chest movement on the affected side, and a fall in blood pressure with a weak, rapid pulse.

Treatment and Nursing Care

Spontaneous pneumothorax usually is treated conservatively with bed rest until the lung is reinflated and the administration of oxygen when needed to relieve dyspnea. If the internal lesion causing the leak of air into the pleural cavity eventually seals off and air becomes trapped in the pleural cavity, a thoracentesis may be necessary to remove the air and allow the lung to inflate.

Traumatic pneumothorax may involve more extensive surgery to repair the chest wall and other damaged internal structures. If air continues to leak from a defect in the lung surface or from an outside wound, tubes are inserted and attached to a closed water-seal drainage apparatus. These tubes are removed when the lung expands and the wounds heal. The patient is allowed up and about as soon as lung expansion is complete.

CLINICAL CASE PROBLEMS

1. You are assigned to the care of a 16-year-old girl who has pneumococcal pneumonia. She is receiving oxygen by mask to relieve her dyspnea and cyanosis. The doctor has placed her on absolute bed rest, and though the girl appears exhausted, she does not wish to have others do anything for her. She appears to be delirious at times, and when you check her temperature, you find that it is 104.6° rectally.

What nursing problems do you see in this situation?

How can you help this patient be more comfortable without further exhausting her?

What special observations must you make?

What nursing measures may be used for the high temperature?

2. Mr. Cook, age 45, is admitted to the hospital with the diagnosis of cancer of the lung. The surgeon has scheduled Mr. Cook for a pneumonectomy 10 days after admission. What preoperative care would you expect this patient to receive? When Mr. Cook returns from surgery, he has a thoracotomy tube in place. The surgeon attaches this tube to a water-seal apparatus in the patient's room. You are assigned to assist in the care of this patient on his second postoperative day.

What position would be best and most comfortable for this patient?

What are your responsibilities in regard to the thoracotomy tube and drainage apparatus?

3. Mr. Brown, age 69, is assigned to your care. He has chronic bronchitis with an acute flare-up of symptoms. He also is an arthritic and has great difficulty moving about. One of the treatments ordered for Mr. Brown is postural drainage.

When would you give the patient postural drainage?

What problems will you have with this procedure? How can you overcome them?

Why is postural drainage ordered for this patient?

4. Mr. Warner is a 59-year-old man who has a moderate amount of dyspnea from emphysema. He was admitted to the hospital for a foot infection and, while there, his emphysema was diagnosed. Mr. Warner is not a very agreeable person. He complains about the temperature of his room and the treatment prescribed for his emphysema (which he feels is a very minor thing compared to his foot infection), and he is especialy upset about the restriction on smoking that has been imposed on him by his physician. One day, while

you are applying warm soaks to Mr. Warner's foot, he asks you, "Just what is emphysema, anyway? What will happen if I don't follow my doctor's orders?"

How would you answer Mr. Warner's questions?

How could you motivate him toward taking sensible precautions against aggravating his condition?

What are some of those precautions?

How would you explain intermittent positive-pressure breathing to Mr. Warner?

REFERENCES

1. Beland, I. L.: *Clinical Nursing: Pathophysiological and Psychosocial Approaches,* 2nd edition. New York, The Macmillan Co., 1970.
2. Brunner, E., et al.: *Textbook of Medical-Surgical Nursing,* 2nd edition. Philadelphia, J. B. Lippincott Co., 1970.
3. Burgess, A. M.: "A Comparison of Common Methods of Oxygen Therapy for Bed Patients." Am. Journ. Nurs., Dec., 1965, p. 96.
4. Ciuca, R.: "Cor Pulmonale." Nursing '73, Jan., 1973, p. 10.
5. Conner, S. H., et al.: "Tracheostomy." Am. Journ. Nurs., Jan., 1972, p. 68.
6. Flatter, P. A.: "Hazards of Oxygen Therapy." Am. Journ. Nurs., Jan., 1968, p. 80.
7. Foley, M. F.: "Pulmonary Function Testing." Am. Journ. Nurs., June, 1971, p. 1134.
8. Foss, G.: "Postural Drainage." Am. Journ. Nurs., April, 1973, p. 666.
9. Jacquette, G.: "To Reduce Hazards of Tracheal Suctioning." Am. Journ. Nurs., Dec., 1971, p. 2362.
10. Jones, W. R.: "Living with Emphysema." Nursing Outlook, Sept., 1967, p. 53.
11. Kinney, M.: "Rehabilitation of Patients with C.O.L.D." Am. Journ. Nurs., Dec., 1967, p. 2528.
12. Koonz, F. P.: "Nursing in Tuberculosis." Nurs. Clin. N. Amer., Vol. 3, No. 3, Sept., 1968, p. 403.
13. Kurihara, M.: "Postural Drainage, Clapping and Vibrating." Am. Journ. Nurs., Dec., 1965, p. 76.
14. McCallum, H. P.: "The Nurse and the Respirator." Nurs. Clin. N. Amer., Vol. 1, No. 4, 1966, p. 597.
15. Morgan, C. V., and Orcutt, T. W.: "The Care and Feeding of Chest Tubes." Am. Journ. Nurs., Feb., 1972, p. 305.
16. Nett, L. M., and Petty, T. L.: "Acute Respiratory Failure." Am. Journ. Nurs., Sept., 1967, p. 1847.
17. Secor, Jane: *Patient Care in Respiratory Problems.* Philadelphia, W. B. Saunders Co., 1969.
18. Sedlock, S. A.: "Detection of Chronic Pulmonary Disease." Am. Journ. Nurs., Aug., 1972, p. 1407.
19. Shafer, K. N., et al.: *Medical-Surgical Nursing,* 5th edition. St. Louis, The C. V. Mosby Co., 1971.
20. Shim, C., et al.: "Cardiac Arrythmias Resulting from Tracheal Suctioning." Ann. Internal Med., Vol. 71, 1969, p. 1149.
21. Smith, D. W., et al. *Care of the Adult Patient,* 3rd edition. Philadelphia, J. B. Lippincott Co., 1971.
22. Sovie, M. D., and Israel, J. B.: "Use of the Cuffed Tracheostomy Tube." Am. Journ. Nurs., Sept., 1967, p. 1854.
23. Ungvarski, P.: "Mechanical Stimulation of Coughing." Am. Journ. Nurs., Dec., 1971, p. 2358.
24. Weg, J. G.: "Tuberculosis and the Generation Gap." Am. Journ. Nurs., Mar., 1971, p. 495.
25. White, H. A.: "Tracheostomy, Care with a Cuffed Tube." Am. Journ. Nurs., Jan., 1972, p. 75.

SUGGESTED STUDENT READING

1. Alexander, et al.: "Caring for the Tuberculosis Patient." Journ. Pract. Nurs., Jan., 1971, p. 22.
2. Ciuca, R.: "Cor Pulmonale." Nursing '73, Jan., 1973, p. 10.
3. Fontana, V. J., and Rappaport, I.: "Asthma." Journ. Pract. Nurs., Dec., 1965, p. 24.
4. Gosselin, M.: "Tuberculosis: Why Cling to Isolation Practices." Journ. Pract. Nurs., March, 1972, p. 22.
5. Gurevich, I.: "Some New Concepts in Tracheal Suctioning." RN, Sept., 1972, p. 52.
6. Sweetwood, H.: "Emphysema." Nursing '72, Nov., 1972, p. 8.
7. Tewinkle, M. B.: "Care of the Patient with Chest Surgery." Journ. Pract. Nursing, Feb., 1970, p. 24.
8. "Total Tracheostomy Care for Johnny at Home." Bedside Nurse, June, 1972, p. 14.
9. Tyler, M. L.: "Artificial Airways." Nursing '73, Feb., 1972, p. 22.

OUTLINE FOR CHAPTER 16

I. Introduction

A. Respiratory organs take the form of a tree. Alveoli are small air sacs through which the oxygen and carbon dioxide are exchanged.

B. Diseases of the respiratory tract are the most common afflictions of mankind.

II. General Nursing Care

A. Concerned with <u>relief of symptoms</u> and <u>prevention of complications</u>.

1. Coughing—stimulated by a foreign substance in the respiratory tract. Nonproductive cough —no sputum brought up. Productive cough—varying amounts of sputum brought up.
2. Increased secretions—body attempts to rid itself of irritating and infectious agents. Secretions can spread infection if not handled with care.
3. Respiratory distress. A very disturbing and frightening symptom. Proper positioning can give relief. If distress is severe, the physician may order concentrated oxygen by mask, nasal prongs or catheter. Warm, moist air can provide relief in cases of croup and less severe respiratory disorders.
4. Rest reduces the need for oxygen and prevents exhaustion.
5. Diet should be high-caloric, high-vitamin liquids for patients with acute diseases of the upper respiratory tract. All patients should have a well-balanced diet to provide resistance to infection.
6. Medications.
   a. Expectorant and sedative cough mixtures.
   b. Antipyretics.
   c. Antihistamines to dry up secretions.
   d. Antispasmodics and bronchodilators.
   e. Antibiotics.
7. Irrigations help remove thick mucus from the nose and throat.
8. Inhalation therapy—administration of drugs as a very fine spray that can be inhaled deep into the respiratory tract. Drugs may include antibiotics, bronchodilators and liquefying agents. These drugs combat infection, enlarge the lumen of the air passages and liquefy mucus so that it is thinner and more easily coughed up.
9. Intermittent positive-pressure breathing therapy—use of a respirator to increase the amount of air inhaled into the lungs. This allows for more uniform distribution of air to the alveoli, aids in the removal of carbon dioxide and makes coughing easier and more productive of sputum.
10. Breathing exercises strengthen the abdominal muscles and increase the patient's tolerance to physical exertion.
11. Postural drainage—patient is positioned so that the force of gravity and ciliary action of the bronchioles will move secretions to the main bronchi and trachea so they can be coughed up. Position depends on the area of the lesion in the lung.

III. Oxygen Therapy—Used to Relieve Hypoxia

A. Methods include tent, nasal cannula, nasal catheter and mask. Nasal catheter is the most efficient method.

B. Precautions must be taken to avoid fire hazards.

C. Oxygen can be toxic—symptoms of oxygen intoxication should be reported immediately.

IV. Tracheostomy—Relieves Symptoms of Tracheal Obstruction

A. Tubes may be cuffed or uncuffed. Those with cuffs allow for assisted ventilation by use of respirator.

B. Tracheostomy patient with new incision is always in danger of asphyxiation.

V. Diagnostic Tests

A. Chest x-ray.

B. Respiratory function tests—vital capacity, tidal volume, residual volume and total lung capacity.

C. Sputum analysis for microorganisms, malignant cells, blood, etc.

D. Bronchogram—an x-ray of the bronchial tree using a radiopaque dye.

E. Bronchoscopy—visual examination of the bronchi by utilizing an endoscope.

VI. The Common Cold

A. Caused by many different strains of viruses.

B. There is no cure, but one can increase his resistance to a cold.

C. Purpose of treatment is to prevent complications such as bacterial infection or development of a chronic bronchitis.

VII. Acute Bronchitis

A. An acute inflammation of the bronchi.

B. Symptoms similar to those of the common cold, but usually there is a more persistent cough that is productive of purulent sputum.

C. Treatment includes rest, humidifier and antibiotics. Can develop into chronic bronchitis if not completely relieved and patient continues to be exposed to irritants that inflame the bronchi.

VIII. Pneumonia

A. An extensive inflammation of the lungs.

B. Two general types are bacterial and primary atypical or viral pneumonia.

C. Symptoms include chills, elevated temperature, cough and severe stabbing pain in the chest or side that is aggravated by coughing or taking a deep breath.

D. Treatment and nursing care concerned with conservation of the patient's strength and energy, relief of symptoms and control of infection.

IX. Bronchiectasis

A. A chronic disease of the respiratory system characterized by permanent dilatation of the bronchi.

B. May follow pneumonia or other respiratory infections or result from a congenital defect in the alveoli.

C. Most outstanding symptom is severe attacks of coughing during which the patient brings up large amounts of foul-smelling sputum.

D. Treatment and nursing care are aimed at relief of symptoms. No cure. Postural drainage helps remove stagnant sputum from the lower bronchi.

X. Cancer of the Lung

A. Leading cause of death in white males.

B. Tumors usually begin in epithelial lining of bronchi. Symptoms include coughing and wheezing and, later, pain and bloody sputum.

C. Surgical removal only possible cure. Radiation and chemotherapy may help retard tumor growth.

XI. Asthma

A. An allergic reaction characterized by swelling of the bronchial mucosa and increased production of sputum in the bronchioles, causing wheezing.

B. Symptoms include cough, wheezing, dyspnea and watering of the eyes.

C. Treatment is aimed at removal of the offending allergen and avoidance of emotional upsets or other situations that may precipitate an attack.

XII. Pleurisy

A. An inflammation of the pleural membranes surrounding the lungs. Pleurisy with effusion is accompanied by an increase in serous fluid in the pleural cavity.

B. Symptoms—sharp, stabbing pain in the chest.

C. Treatment includes bed rest and measures to prevent infection. Thoracentesis may be necessary in pleurisy with effusion.

XIII. Empyema

A. The presence of thick and purulent fluid within the pleural cavity.

B. Treated by antibiotics and removal of fluid from the pleural cavity.

XIV. Pulmonary Emphysema

A. A chronic respiratory disease that results from chronic inflammation of the bronchi.

B. The alveoli lose their elasticity and become distended with air. The patient cannot exhale stale air so as to make room for oxygenated air.

C. Symptoms include exertional dyspnea, persistent cough that does not effectively clear the respiratory passages, fixation of the rib cage and a barrel shaped chest.

D. Treatment is aimed at preventing complications and improving ventilation of the lungs. If the disease is detected early, the pathologic changes can be halted and the patient can be rehabilitated to lead a moderately active life. Medications include antibiotics, bronchodilators and the corticosteroids.

XV. Pulmonary Tuberculosis

A. An infectious disease of the lung caused by tubercle bacillus.

B. Characterized by lesions that may continue to degenerate and become necrotic or may heal by fibrosis and calcification.

C. Symptoms include cough, low-grade fever in the afternoon, loss of weight, night sweats and hemoptysis.

D. Diagnostic tests include tuberculin skin tests, x-ray examination, analysis of sputum and examination of gastric contents for tubercle bacilli.

E. Treatment includes rest, good nutrition, proper handling of secretions from the respiratory tract and control of coughing. Specific anti-tuberculotic drugs are streptomycin, para-aminosalicylic acid (PAS) and isoniazid (INH).

F. Surgical treatment may involve removal of part or all of the affected lung.

XVI. Extrapulmonary Tuberculosis

A. Tubercle bacillus infects parts of the body other than the lungs, like the bones, meninges, urinary tract or reproductive system.

B. Tuberculous meningitis is treated with the specific anti-tuberculotic drugs.

C. Involvement of the bone can cause serious orthopedic deformities.

XVII. Nursing Care of the Patient Having Chest Surgery

A. Preoperative care involves diagnostic tests, measures to remove as much mucus from the respiratory tract as possible and special exercises to strengthen the muscles of respiration.

B. Postoperative care involves careful attention to drainage tubes that remove air and fluid from the pleural space. Collapse of the lung is possible.

C. Special points in the care of a closed-drainage apparatus:

    1. Keep the drainage bottle below the level of the chest at all times.

    2. Keep all connections airtight.

    3. Observe the tubes to be sure they remain unobstructed.

    4. Observe thoracotomy bottles to determine amount of drainage. Do not empty these bottles.

XVIII. Pneumothorax

A. Accumulation of air or gas in the pleural cavity.

B. May be spontaneous or artificially induced. In both types the lung is collapsed.

C. Usually treated conservatively unless severe trauma to the thoracic cavity requires surgical repair.

17

Nursing Care of Patients with Diseases of the Digestive System

VOCABULARY

Decompression
Duct
Enzyme
Hemolytic
Sinus

INTRODUCTION

The main portion of the digestive system is actually one long tube which extends from the mouth to the rectum. This tube is known as the *alimentary tract* or *intestinal tract.* For the sake of clarity, the various sections of this tract are considered as organs. Thus, the large bulge just below the esophagus is known as a separate organ, the stomach, even though it is only a continuation of the same tube that forms the esophagus above it and the small intestine below it.

As food enters the alimentary tract by way of the mouth, it immediately begins to undergo physical and chemical changes; that is, it is not only changed in appearance but new substances are formed from the original material. These changes are the first stages of digestion. The food is propelled downward through the alimentary tract by wavelike motions of involuntary muscles within the walls of the alimentary tract. This rhythmic squeezing action is called peristalsis. As the food passes down the digestive tube, it continues to undergo changes until it reaches a liquid state and can then be taken into the blood stream. The transfer of nutrients from the intestines into the blood is referred to as *absorption.* Substances such as cellulose which are not digested and absorbed continue through the tube and are eventually eliminated through the anus. The conversion of the food elements into energy and production of body tissues is called *metabolism.*

The accessory organs of digestion are those organs outside the alimentary tract which are directly concerned with digestion. They include the liver, which manufactures bile, and the gallbladder, which stores the bile until it is needed to help in the digestion of fats. The pancreas is also an accessory organ of digestion. The cells of the pancreas secrete pancreatic juice, which contains six enzymes. These enzymes are special substances necessary for the

345

chemical breakdown of foods. Ducts leading from the liver, gallbladder and pancreas empty their secretions directly into the small intestine, where all digestion is completed (see Fig. 17-1).

In this chapter, the diseases of the digestive tract and diseases of the accessory organs will be considered separately. It must be remembered, however, that the two groups of organs are closely related, and diseases which primarily affect the accessory organs will inevitably affect the function of digestion.

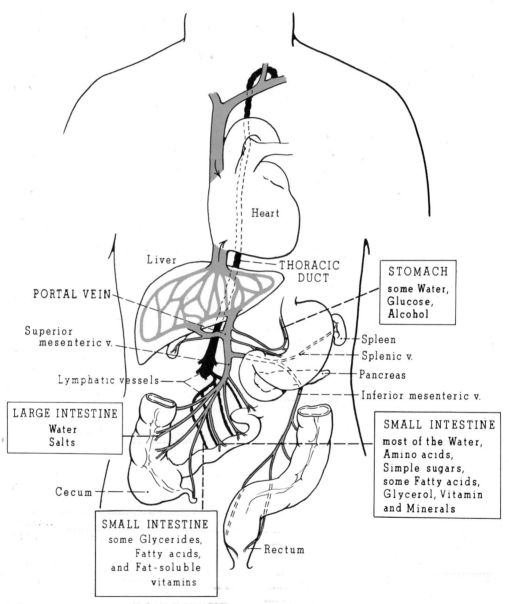

Heart

Liver

THORACIC DUCT

PORTAL VEIN

STOMACH
some Water,
Glucose,
Alcohol

Superior mesenteric v.

Spleen

Splenic v.

Pancreas

Lymphatic vessels

Inferior mesenteric v.

LARGE INTESTINE
Water
Salts

SMALL INTESTINE
most of the Water,
Amino acids,
Simple sugars,
some Fatty acids,
Glycerol, Vitamin
and Minerals

Cecum

SMALL INTESTINE
some Glycerides,
Fatty acids,
and Fat-soluble
vitamins

Rectum

Figure 17–1. Products of digestion are absorbed in the stomach and small and large intestines. (From Jacob and Francone: *Structure and Function in Man*, 2nd Ed., W. B. Saunders Co., Philadelphia.)

Part One. Nursing Care of Patients With Diseases of the Digestive Tract

DIAGNOSTIC TESTS

X ray Examination

Special x-ray examinations of the digestive tract should include a *gastrointestinal series* and a *barium enema.* In a gastrointestinal series, the patient drinks a barium suspension. This substance is radiopaque, and therefore outlines the hollow organs as it passes through them. The filling and emptying of the esophagus, stomach and duodenum may be observed by the radiologist through a fluoroscope. Films of the stomach are taken after the patient drinks the barium and again 6 hours after the fluoroscopy to determine how much barium has passed through the stomach. The gastrointestinal series is useful in diagnosing obstructions, ulcerations and growths within the esophagus, stomach or duodenum.

In preparation for a gastrointestinal series, the patient is not allowed food or fluids for at least 6 to 8 hours before the examination.

The x-ray examination of the lower digestive tract using a radiopaque substance is called a *barium enema.* As the name implies, the barium suspension is instilled through a rectal tube. The barium must be retained by the patient while x-ray films are taken, thus allowing for visualization of the lower bowel. The barium enema is useful in the diagnosis of ulcerations, tumors, obstructions and other abnormalities in the structure of the walls of the lower intestine.

Preparation of the patient for a barium enema usually includes the administration of laxatives and enemas the night before and again on the morning of the examination. The responsibilities of the nurse in preparing a patient for these special x-ray examinations are discussed more fully in Chapter 5.

Gastroscopy and Esophagoscopy

In both of these examinations, the physician is actually able to see the inner lining of the stomach or esophagus. He does this by inserting a special instrument through the mouth and into the esophagus (see Fig. 17-2). The instrument may be passed further down into the stomach if a gastroscopy is done. Foods and liquids are withheld 6 to 8 hours before the examination. The patient is sedated lightly and the procedure explained so that he may be more cooperative during the examination. While there is no actual pain associated with the procedure, it is uncomfortable for the patient.

Proctoscopy and Sigmoidoscopy

These examinations are similar in principle to the gastroscopy. They are done for the purpose of visualizing the inner lining of the anus, rectum and sigmoid colon (see Fig. 17-3).

The patient is prepared for the examination with enemas until the return solution is clear. According to Brown, "By clear returns one means that there is no solid matter in the returns. No more than three enemas should ever be given without consulting the doctor." Other methods of cleansing the lower bowel depend on the individual wishes of the examining physician.

The position of the patient during the examination is usually the knee-chest position unless a special examination table which breaks in the middle is available.

Gastric Analysis

In this test, a tube is passed into the stomach and samples of the gastric contents are withdrawn. The first spec-

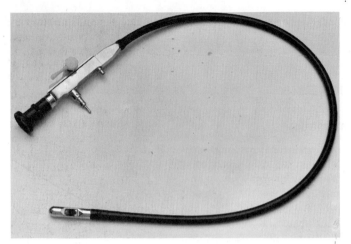

Figure 17-2. Fiber optic gastroscope. (Courtesy American Cystoscope Makers, Inc., Pelham Manor, N.Y.)

imen taken is called the "*first* fasting speci-men." Other specimens are taken after a substance is given to stimulate the flow of gastric juices. The specimens are then taken to the laboratory where they are tested for the amount of hydrochloric acid present.

A *tubeless gastric analysis* may be done when the physician wishes to know whether or not there is any hydrochloric acid in the gastric contents. A tubeless gastric analysis cannot give information on the exact amount of hydrochloric acid present.

As the name implies, there is no need to insert a tube into the stomach for a tubeless gastric analysis. Instead, the patient is given special granules to drink in 240 ml. of water. At prescribed intervals, urine specimens are collected. If hydrochloric acid is present, the urine will be blue; if none is present in the stomach, the urine will remain straw-colored.

Stool Examination

The stool may be examined for: (1) presence of blood, (2) presence of specific bacteria and (3) cysts, ova and parasites.

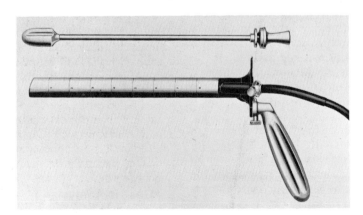

Figure 17-3. Fiber optic proctoscope with obturator. (Courtesy American Cystoscope Makers, Inc., Pelham Manor, N.Y.)

When the stool is examined for occult (hidden) blood, the patient must abstain from red meat for 48 to 70 hours before a specimen is collected. If an examination for amebas is ordered, the specimen must be kept warm and taken to the laboratory immediately after it is collected.

STOMATITIS

Definition and Symptoms

The term stomatitis refers to a generalized inflammation of the mucous membranes of the mouth. It may be caused by certain drugs, trauma from ill-fitting dentures or malocclusion of the teeth, other mechanical irritants in the mouth, nutritional deficiencies, pathogenic organisms and excessive smoking or drinking. Poor oral hygiene can be a major factor in the development of stomatitis.

General symptoms include pain and swelling of the oral mucosa, increased salivation, severe halitosis and sometimes fever. More specific symptoms will depend on the type of inflammation or infection present.

Aphthous Stomatitis

This is commonly called "canker sores" and is characterized by small, white, crater-like ulcers in the mouth. They are quite uncomfortable and frequently interfere with eating because of the discomfort they cause. The exact cause of aphthous stomatitis is unknown, but it is probably a viral infection to which certain individuals are highly susceptible. There is no specific treatment or cure for this disorder.

Vincent's Angina

Another name for this inflammation of the mouth is "trench mouth" because it was quite common during the First World War. It is believed to be caused by a combination of two organisms—a fusiform bacillus and a spirochete. The characteristic lesions are shallow ulcers that are covered with a grayish membrane. These are painful and can interfere with eating. Treatment consists of mouthwashes using sodium perborate and antibiotics.

GASTRITIS

Definition

Gastritis is an inflammation of the mucous membrane lining of the stomach. It may be acute or chronic in nature.

The main causes of acute gastritis are overeating, drinking an excessive amount of alcohol, eating contaminated food or the ingestion of a poisonous drug or chemical.

Chronic gastritis usually follows ingestion of highly spiced food or excessive amounts of alcohol over an extended length of time.

Symptoms

In both acute and chronic gastritis, the main symptoms are nausea, vomiting, pain and tenderness in the stomach region and sometimes diarrhea. The patient with chronic gastritis may also have massive hemorrhage from the stomach.

Treatment and Nursing Care

Acute gastritis is usually of very short duration. Treatment consists of withholding all foods by mouth and administration of drugs which slow down the peristaltic action of the alimentary tract. If severe dehydration occurs, fluids may be given intravenously. The nursing care of a patient having nausea, vomiting and diarrhea is discussed more fully in Chapter 4.

Chronic gastritis is not as easily treated as acute gastritis. Diet therapy is of primary importance in chronic gastritis because the patient frequently admits to indiscretion in his dietary and drinking habits and finds it difficult to change. The diet for these patients is basically a bland diet in which all strong seasonings and roughage are avoided. Frequent small feedings are recommended to prevent overloading of the stomach and unnecessary stimulation of the flow of gastric juices. It is always difficult to change one's eating habits of long standing, and the nurse must use tact and patience in encouraging the patient to follow the prescribed diet faithfully.

Medications which coat the gastric mucosa also help prevent ulceration of the stomach lining. Examples of this type of drug are *bismuth* and *barium*. Since the patient frequently suffers from painful spasmodic contractions of the stomach, antispasmodic drugs are also used.

ULCERATIVE COLITIS

Definition

Ulcerative colitis is an inflammation, with the formation of ulcers in the mucosa of the colon. It is often a chronic disease, and the patient is usually free from symptoms between acute flare-ups.

The exact cause of ulcerative colitis is not known. Acute infections and emotional tension frequently bring about acute attacks.

Symptoms

The chief symptom is diarrhea. The stools are frequent and watery, containing shreds of mucus, blood and pus. Nausea and vomiting, or loss of appetite without actually vomiting, are also common symptoms. The loss of body fluids soon brings about dehydration and malnutrition.

Treatment and Nursing Care

Treatment for this condition is difficult, and the prognosis is poor. Supportive measures, such as blood transfusions, and a diet high in proteins, vitamins and calories must be used. Rest and freedom from anxiety help in the relief of the symptoms. *Antidiarrheic* drugs containing paregoric and kaolin are also of some benefit in the control of the diarrhea.

In caring for the patient with ulcerative colitis, the nurse must bear in mind the importance of the patient's individual personality. These patients are often tense and nervous individuals who are easily offended by the remarks of others. They keep their anxieties well hidden, however, and may give a false impression of serenity and resignation to their illness. Yet these are the very patients who are most in need of small, extra attentions and encouragement.

The stools must be carefully observed and their number and character reported to the nurse in charge or written on the patient's chart. For further information on the nursing care of a patient with diarrhea, see Chapter 4.

APPENDICITIS

Definition

Appendicitis is an inflammation of the vermiform appendix. It is called "vermiform" because it is wormlike, and "appendix" because it is an appendage of the cecum. The appendix is a blind pouch and is therefore easily infected by bacteria passing through the intestinal tract.

Symptoms

Pain in the lower right side, halfway between the umbilicus and the crest of the ileum, is the best known symptom of appendicitis. However, the location of the pain may and often does vary with individuals. An elevated temperature, nausea and vomiting and an increase in the white cell count are also characteristic of appendicitis.

Treatment and Nursing Care

Treatment is surgical removal of the appendix *(appendectomy)*. Before surgery, the patient is allowed nothing by mouth and an ice bag may be placed on the abdomen to slow down localization of the inflammation and thus avoid rupture of the swollen and inflamed appendix. Under no circumstances should laxatives be given when appendicitis is suspected. Hot water bottles to relieve abdominal pain are also forbidden.

The patient is usually allowed out of bed the day after surgery if no complications are present. The convalescent period is most often uneventful, and the patient may return to his former activities within two or three weeks.

PERITONITIS

Definition

The peritoneum is a serous sac that lines the abdominal cavity and encloses the intestines, stomach, liver and spleen and partially encloses the uterus and uterine tubes. Peritonitis is an inflammation of the peritoneum. It usually occurs when one of the organs it encloses ruptures or is perforated so that the organ's contents (including bacteria) are spilled into the abdominal cavity. Examples of common causes of peritonitis are ruptured appendix, perforated duodenal or gastric ulcer, ruptured ectopic (tubal) pregnancy and traumatic rupture of the spleen or liver.

Symptoms

As the peritoneum becomes inflamed, there is local redness and swelling of the membrane with production of serous fluid that becomes more and more purulent as the bacteria multiply. Normal peristaltic action of the intestines slows or ceases altogether, and the symptoms of intestinal obstruction occur. The patient experiences nausea, vomiting, severe abdominal pain and distention, high fever, tachycardia, pallor and other symptoms of shock. Unless the patient is treated promptly and successfully, peritonitis can be fatal.

Treatment and Nursing Care

Antibiotics are given in massive doses to combat infection, fluids and electrolytes are administered to restore a normal balance, and gastric or intestinal suction is instigated to relieve distention. Surgical procedures such as those done to repair a ruptured organ are done as soon as the patient's condition will permit.

Nursing care is primarily concerned with close, intelligent observation of the patient and prompt and accurate reporting of unexpected changes in his condition. He is usually placed in semi-Fowler's position to facilitate breathing, prevent respiratory complications and aid in localizing the purulent material in the lower abdomen or pelvis. His vital signs are noted and recorded every four hours during the critical stage. If he is nauseated and vomits, the characteristics and amount of vomitus are noted. The emesis of fecal material indicates complete intestinal obstruction. If the patient passes flatus or feces rectally, this should be recorded on his chart, as it indicates return of peristalsis. Because of the high fever and toxicity that accompany peritonitis, the patient may be delirious or disoriented, and he must be protected from self-injury. This includes putting side rails on the bed and supervising the patient at all times. High fever and the presence of the gastric tube demand frequent mouth care to protect the lips and prevent halitosis and a foul taste in the mouth. The patient should be turned *very gently* and moved in the bed with care because of the extreme tenderness in his abdominal region.

PEPTIC ULCER

Definition

, A peptic ulcer is an open lesion on the mucosa of the stomach or small intestine. When the ulcer is located in the stomach, it is called a *gastric ulcer* (see Fig. 17-4); if it is located in the upper third of the small intestine, it is called a *duodenal ulcer.*

The ulcerated area is actually the result of digestion of the membranous lining of the stomach or small intestine by the gastric juices secreted by glands in the stomach. The exact reason that an ulcer should develop is not known; however, there are many predisposing factors. They include: (1) a particular type of personality characterized by the expression of constant anxiety and inner tensions, (2) poor eating habits, such as over-indulgence in alcohol, highly seasoned foods or an irregular pattern in mealtimes and (3) an increased secretion of hydrochloric acid in the stomach.

Symptoms

The most common symptom of peptic ulcer is a burning and gnawing pain in the stomach region. This pain is more pronounced when the stomach is empty and is relieved by eating. The attacks of pain are seasonal; that is, they are more likely to occur during the spring and fall than at other times of the year. Other symptoms may include nausea, frequent belching, vomiting (vomitus may contain blood) and tarry stools.

An ulcer that becomes chronic may continue to erode into deeper tissue until it has finally penetrated the stomach wall. This complication is referred to as *perforation.* Other complications include *hemorrhage* and *obstruction.*

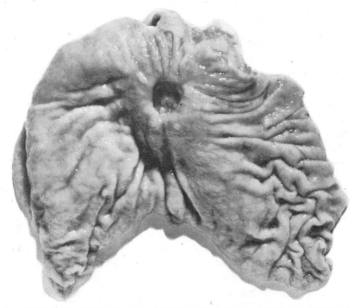

Figure 17–4. Ulcer of the gastric mucosa. Note how deeply the ulcer has penetrated into the stomach wall. (From Bockus: *Gastroenterology,* Vol. 1, 2nd Ed., W. B. Saunders Co., Philadelphia.)

Medical Treatment and Nursing Care

Medical treatment of a peptic ulcer is aimed at relief of the patient's symptoms and removal of the causative factors.

Rest. The patient is placed on bed rest. If hemorrhaging is present, the patient is put on absolute bed rest. His environment must be controlled so that he may have relaxation and freedom from worry.

Diet. There are several dietary regimens useful in the medical management of peptic ulcer. They all are concerned with neutralizing gastric acid, preventing chemical or mechanical irritation of the gastric and intestinal mucosa and gradually progressing from small, frequent feedings to a more normal diet.

The Sippy diet and the Meulengracht diet, named after the physicians who devised them, are the two progressive diets most often used. The administration of milk and cream (90 ml. each) is an initial part of the Sippy diet and is frequently used with other diets. The purpose of giving milk and cream every hour can readily be understood when we realize the need for providing a continued supply of food or liquid in the stomach so that the gastric juices will digest the stomach contents rather than the stomach mucosa. Milk is given because it is a protein which will neutralize the acids of the stomach. Fat is given because it inhibits the flow of gastric juices and also slows down the passage of milk from the stomach.

The physician often orders milk and cream every hour on the hour and an antacid drug every hour on the half hour so that there is no time when the stomach acids are not being rendered neutral. Later on, small, frequent feedings are given so that the stomach is not empty and there is no free hydrochloric acid present for long periods of time. The patient usually is not allowed raw fruits and vegetables or high residue foods that are capable of mechanically irritating the stomach or intestinal mucosa. Spices, meat broths, fried foods, coffee and alcoholic beverages usually are restricted because they stimulate the flow of gastric juices and increase the muscular action of the stomach.

Medications. Specific drugs used in the treatment of a peptic ulcer are as follows:

1. *Antacids,* which neutralize gastric acid. Examples: Amphojel, Gelusil and Maalox.

2. *Antispasmodics,* which reduce muscle spasm and decrease gastric secretions. Examples: atropine, tincture of belladonna and Pro-Banthine.

3. *Sedatives,* which reduce emotional tension. Examples: phenobarbital and the tranquilizers.

Education of the Patient. Before a peptic ulcer can be successfully controlled, the patient must understand how and why he probably developed an ulcer in the first place. Once he has understood the predisposing factors, he must then be helped to avoid them as much as possible. Unless he can cooperate fully with the physician and nurses, there is a strong possibility that he will continue to develop ulcers in spite of medical or even surgical treatment.

Below is a list of some of the important points to be emphasized in teaching a patient with a peptic ulcer.

1. He must learn to regulate the type of foods he eats and the manner in which he eats them. Mealtime should be unhurried, relaxed and spaced at regular intervals.

2. His emotional health, ability to cope with distressing situations and his occupation and home life are all important to his state of physical health. He must learn either to avoid situations of anxiety or to strive to develop a more placid and serene outlook on life.

3. Most patients who have peptic ulcers drink very little water. Since water dilutes the gastric juices and thereby makes them less corrosive, the

patient should develop the habit of taking several swallows of water at least every hour during the day.

4. It is presumed that there is some relationship between the use of tobacco and aggravation of a peptic ulcer. If the patient is unable to discontinue smoking altogether, he might at least use more moderation in his smoking habits.

5. The patient is encouraged to cooperate with his physician and remain under medical supervision for as long as the physician deems advisable. He must report regularly for periodic x-ray examinations of the stomach to determine his progress.

6. There are certain side effects from antacids which should be reported to the physician should they occur. These include constipation or diarrhea, flatulence and signs of edema due to sodium retention. Since drug interactions can occur, the patient should inform the physician about all the drugs he is taking, particularly the amphetamines, sulfonamides, enteric coated tablets and anticoagulants.

7. Unless otherwise ordered, antacids should be taken one hour after meals. If antacid tablets are used in preference to liquid preparations, the tablet must be chewed thoroughly and followed by a full glass of water.

8. Effervescent antacid tablets should be completely dissolved and the bubbles settled before drinking the solution.[5]

Surgical Treatment of a Peptic Ulcer

Indications for Surgery. Surgical treatment becomes necessary when a chronic ulcer fails to respond to medical treatment or when complications such as perforation, obstruction or hemorrhage occur.

Types of Surgical Procedures. In plastic repair of a perforated ulcer, the hole in the stomach is sutured and the area is reinforced with a graft from the peritoneal fold over the stomach.

Subtotal gastrectomy (gastric resection) is removal of a part of the stomach and then joining the remaining portion to the small intestine by anastomosis. Anastomosis is the joining of two hollow organs by suturing the open ends together so that they become one continuous tube.

Total gastrectomy is the surgical removal of all of the stomach. The esophagus is anastomosed to the small intestine.

The vagus (tenth cranial nerve) stimulates the stomach cells to secrete hydrochloric acid. A vagotomy is the cutting of the vagus nerve so that the stomach does not receive impulses from the brain and therefore does not secrete hydrochloric acid. A vagotomy is often done at the same time a gastric resection is performed.

NURSING CARE OF PATIENT HAVING GASTRIC SURGERY

Preoperative Care

The patient who is to have gastric surgery will usually have an x-ray series and other diagnostic tests before the surgery is done. The exception to this rule is an emergency situation in which complications demand immediate surgery and there is not time for an extensive preoperative work-up.

A Levin tube is usually inserted the morning of the operation. This tube is left in place during and after surgery (see gastric decompression below).

The patient will receive routine preparations necessary for all major abdominal surgery. This includes enemas so that the colon is emptied of fecal material. In case the patient has had a barium enema, the nurse should look for and report returns which contain whitish material. This is barium, and it will become hardened if left in the colon, thus presenting the possibility of a fecal impaction later on.

The diet of the patient is restricted to liquids only during the 24 hours before surgery. In case of obstruction, a Levin tube is inserted and gastric suction begun to remove all stomach contents before surgery.

Postoperative Care

When the patient returns to his room and has fully recovered from the anesthesia, he is placed in semi-Fowler's position. This position is more comfortable and facilitates drainage from the stomach when a gastric tube is in place.

Gastric or intestinal decompression is used in almost all types of gastric or intestinal surgery. The type of tube used will depend on the area involved. The Levin tube is used to aspirate or convey liquids to the stomach (see Fig. 17-5). A Miller-Abbott tube and a Cantor tube are used to remove intestinal contents (see Fig. 17-6).

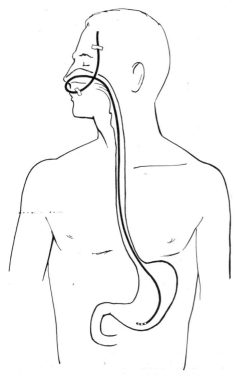

Figure 17–5. A Levin tube in place. The Levin tube is used to aspirate gastric contents or to convey liquids to the stomach.

Gastrointestinal decompression is accomplished by connecting the nasogastric tube to a suction apparatus such as the Gomco electric suction machine. Common indications for gastrointestinal suction include (1) distention following surgery or accompanying intestinal obstruction, (2) withdrawal of specimens of stomach or intestinal contents and (3) removal of stomach or gastrointestinal contents before surgery.

During continuous gastrointestinal decompression by electric suction, the machine should be turned on "low." If the machine is left on "high" continuously, it may cause damage to the gastric mucosa. It is important that the tube be kept open and draining freely. Irrigations, which can be helpful in removing mucus plugs and blood clots, are *not* routinely done; they require a physician's written order. The nurse should know what solution is to be used, how much to use and whether the procedure requires aseptic technique or clean technique.

All drainage obtained via the nasogastric tube should be measured accurately and the amount recorded on the patient's chart for every 24-hour period. Since fluids and electrolytes removed by suction must be replaced, the physician will use the nurse's notes as a guide to fluid replacement. It is also important to record the color and consistency and any unusual odor or other characteristic noted in the fluid in the drainage bottle. Although some bloody drainage is to be expected after gastric surgery, an excessive amount of drainage or bright red blood coming through the tubing must be reported immediately.

The tubing connected to the nasal tube should be long enough to allow for adequate turning of the patient from side to side. The nostril into which the tube is inserted is very tender, and rough handling of the tubing will cause the patient much discomfort. A special clamp which attaches to the bedclothes should be used to pre-

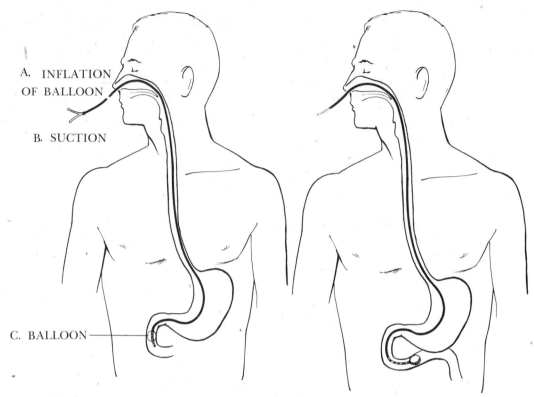

A. INFLATION OF BALLOON

B. SUCTION

C. BALLOON

Figure 17–6. *Left,* A Miller-Abbott tube in place. It is advanced through the intestines to the prescribed point. The Miller-Abbott tube has a double lumen. *A,* Portion of the metal tip leading to the balloon. *B,* Portion of the metal tip leading to the lumen that can be suctioned. *C,* Balloon inflated with air. *Right,* A Cantor tube in place. This intestinal tube ends in a bag that is filled with mercury to help it to pass along the gastrointestinal tract to the point prescribed by the physician. Intestinal tubes are not taped in place until they have advanced fully. The holes for suctioning are behind the balloon.

vent pulling and unnecessary motion of the tube.

After the tubing is removed, the patient is given small amounts of liquids to determine if he can tolerate them. These liquids are gradually increased according to the patient's ability to take them without nausea, vomiting or abdominal distress. If the liquids are well tolerated, the patient then progresses to small, frequent feedings. Within six months, most patients are able to take three regular meals a day as the remaining portion of the stomach stretches to accommodate more and more food. Patients who have had a *total* gastrectomy are usually restricted to small frequent feedings of easily digested semisolids for the rest of their lives. When the patient is to be dismissed from the hospital, the hospital dietitian usually is called to help the patient and his family in the ways and means of planning and preparing his special diets after gastric surgery.

"Dumping" Syndrome

Some patients who have had gastric surgery experience a complication known as the "dumping syndrome." The patient feels weak and faint and may perspire profusely or experience palpitations of the heart. These sensations probably are due to the rapid passage of large amounts of food and liquid through the remaining portion of the stomach (if any) and into the jejunum. This occurs because part or all of the stomach and duodenum have been surgically removed and are no longer present to slow down the progress of the intestinal contents through the upper portion of the gastrointestinal tract. When a patient experiences the dumping syndrome, he is instructed to avoid eating large meals and to drink a minimum of fluids during the meal. He may take the fluids in small amounts later, between meals. If sweet foods and liquids seem to aggravate the condition, and sometimes they do, the patient should try to avoid them. It also may be helpful for the patient to lie down flat in bed for 30 minutes after a meal.

CANCER OF THE STOMACH

Definition

Cancer of the stomach is a malignant growth within the stomach. It is frequently associated with chronic inflammation or ulceration of the stomach mucosa. It is often difficult to distinguish between gastric ulcer and gastric cancer without extensive diagnostic tests.

Symptoms

The symptoms of gastric cancer are very similar to those of a gastric ulcer. Frequently the symptoms are not severe until the malignancy has reached the advanced stages and spread to neighboring tissues.

Treatment and Nursing Care

When gastric cancer has been positively diagnosed, the treatment is surgical removal of all or part of the stomach.

The nursing care of the patient hav-

ing gastric surgery is discussed earlier in this chapter.

CANCER OF THE LARGE INTESTINE

Definition

Malignant growths within the large intestine occur most frequently in persons over 50 years of age and are among the most common diseases affecting this part of the digestive tract. The cause is unknown. Polyps or chronic ulcerations located in the large intestine tend to undergo malignant changes.

Symptoms

As in cancer of the stomach, cancer of the large intestine may present only mild symptoms until it has reached an advanced stage. Any change in a person's bowel habits may be an early sign of cancer of the colon. Either constipation or diarrhea, or alternate attacks of each, are the most common signs. As the growth enlarges, it obstructs the normal passage of fecal material through the colon, and this results in changes in the shape of the stool and loss of blood rectally. If the growth completely obstructs the intestinal tract, the patient experiences the symptoms of an intestinal obstruction.

Treatment and Nursing Care

Cancer of the colon is treated by surgical removal of the affected portion of intestine. There are several different operative procedures which may be carried out. The surgeon's choice will depend on the location of the growth and the extent of the area involved. The purpose of the surgery is to remove the diseased section of the intestine and at the same time provide a means of elimination of fecal material.

INTESTINAL OBSTRUCTION

Definition

Intestinal obstruction is a blocking of the intestinal tract, thereby preventing the normal passage of gastrointestinal contents through the intestine. The condition may occur suddenly or progress gradually over a period of time. Obstruction of the intestines may result from strangulated hernia, cancer, twisting of the bowel *(volvulus)*, telescoping of one part of the bowel into another *(intussusception)* or interference with the passing of nerve impulses to the bowel.

Symptoms

In acute intestinal obstruction, the onset is sudden, with severe pain as a result of increased peristalsis above the point of obstruction. The abdomen becomes distended as the intestinal contents accumulate and fill the intestines. Increased pressure then may constrict blood vessels in the walls of the intestines, resulting in gangrene of the affected portion. Nausea and vomiting are common symptoms of intestinal obstruction. The vomiting is extremely forceful *(projectile)*, and the emesis is often foul in odor because of the back flow of fecal material into the stomach.

In chronic intestinal obstruction, the outstanding symptom is an increasing constipation as the bowel becomes occluded. Nausea and vomiting may be present, and anemia is also frequently present as a result of loss of appetite.

Treatment and Nursing Care

The treatment of intestinal obstruction is immediate surgical correction of the condition. Any one of the surgical procedures listed below under "Types of Surgical Procedures" may be used in the treatment of intestinal obstruction.

The patient with acute intestinal obstruction is very seriously ill. He often has respiratory difficulty because of the pressure of the distended abdomen against the diaphragm. Placing the patient in Fowler's position will help relieve this pressure and also aids in the removal of gas and intestinal contents through the intestinal tube. This tube is inserted before the patient goes to surgery and offers some relief of the symptoms of intestinal obstruction until surgery can be performed.

The postoperative nursing care of the patient with surgery of the large intestine is discussed below.

NURSING CARE OF THE PATIENT WITH SURGERY OF THE LOWER INTESTINAL TRACT

Types of Surgical Procedures

Colectomy. This is simply the removal of the diseased portion of the colon.

Colostomy. In this procedure, an abdominal incision is made and the colon is brought to the outside for the purpose of providing a means of draining fecal material. A colostomy is usually done after a colectomy. The colostomy may be permanent or temporary. If it is a temporary colostomy, the patient must return to surgery later for anastomosis of the open ends.

Abdominoperineal Resection. This is a very extensive surgical procedure in which part of the colon and the entire rectum and anus are removed. Both an abdominal incision and perineal incision are necessary for this procedure. Because of the nature of the surgery, a permanent colostomy is necessary.

Preoperative Care

Before surgery of the large intestine, efforts are made to remove as much fecal material from the colon as possible. To accomplish this, the patient is usually placed on a low-residue diet as

NPO

early as 7 to 10 days before surgery. The last 24 to 72 hours before surgery, his diet is changed to liquids only. Vitamins and minerals may be given to supplement these restricted diets.

In addition to the dietary preparation, laxatives and enemas are administered to cleanse the lower bowel further. Contents of the stomach are removed by inserting a Levin tube and connecting it to a suction apparatus the morning of surgery. If it is necessary to remove the contents of the small intestine, a specially designed tube which passes through the stomach and into the duodenum is inserted. This tube is called a Miller-Abbott tube. It is attached to the suction apparatus and given the same care as a gastric tube. The tube is usually left in place after surgery to remove accumulations of mucus and gas which may cause distention and strain on the sutures.

Postoperative Care

The immediate postoperative care is the same as for other patients having major abdominal surgery. Operations of the large intestine are usually of long duration. The prolonged period of anesthesia and exposure of the body, with loss of essential fluids, leaves the patient particularly susceptible to shock. Therefore, the patient must be watched more closely than usual for signs of shock during the immediate postoperative period.

Difficulty in voiding after surgery is a common problem with these patients. To avoid the retention of urine in the bladder during the postoperative period, a Foley catheter is usually inserted in the operating room. As soon as the patient returns to his room, the catheter is connected to a sterile bedside bottle and an accurate record of his intake and output kept.

The gastric or intestinal tube is connected to an electric suction as soon as the patient is returned to his room. The physician usually does not want the patient to have anything by mouth for the first 48 hours after surgery. Peristalsis usually becomes active after this period of time, and the patient will then be able to take liquids by mouth. The passing of gas, liquids or solids through the rectum is an indication of active peristalsis. In any surgery of the intestine, the surgeon is always concerned with the return of normal peristalsis. It is the nurse's responsibility to observe these patients carefully for evidence of the return of peristalsis and to report such evidence to the doctor.

Special Aspects in the Care of the Patient with a Colostomy

Preoperative Period. The prospect of having an artificial anus in an abdominal opening through which bowel movements will pass is a difficult situation for even the most stalwart person to face. The first thoughts are those of repulsion and absolute despair that an adjustment can ever be made. The nursing staff must recognize the emotional shock for a patient having a colostomy and be prepared to offer adequate moral support. Preparation of the patient during the preoperative period will depend on the physician. He may or may not choose to explain a colostomy fully to the patient before surgery. He will have good reasons for his choice, and the nursing staff must know and respect his wishes in this matter. It is not the responsibility of the nurse to inform the patient of the exact surgical procedure that will be done when he goes to surgery. Her responsibility lies in finding out how much the patient has been told so that she can exercise care in answering any questions he may ask. Some patients do not wish to be told, while others insist on a detailed explanation from the doctor. In other cases, the surgeon does not know himself what procedure will be necessary until after he has opened the abdomen and evaluated the patient's condition.

If the surgeon does tell the patient that a colostomy will be done, he will also explain what a colostomy is, how it works and methods which can be used to control the bowel movements so that the patient's activities are not restricted when he is discharged from the hospital.

There are times, however, when a patient will listen to every word the doctor says and apparently accept the situation calmly. Later, after the initial shock has worn off, he becomes extremely agitated or depressed and begins to display his true emotions. At this time, the nurse must realize why the patient is behaving as he is and strive to help him by answering his questions with intelligence and encouragement.

There are thousands of persons in every walk of life who have colostomies. They are able to continue their regular activities with few restrictions, and most of their associates are not aware that they have a colostomy. It is important that a patient who must adjust to a colostomy knows and understands that such a surgical procedure does not mean invalidism and permanent withdrawal from society.

If there is a person available who has had a successful experience with his own colostomy, arrangements may be made for him to talk with the patient and tell him what he can expect immediately after surgery and during the convalescent period. Information should never be forced on the patient, however. Written material should be made available if he wishes to read about colostomies and how they are cared for, but if he is upset by thinking about his future life with a colostomy, he may not want to discuss the subject with anyone. That is his choice and privilege.

Postoperative Period. Immediately after surgery, the patient with a colostomy will receive the same general care necessary for any patient who has had surgery of the large intestine.

Since the intestinal tract has been thoroughly cleansed before the operation, there will be no fecal material passing through the colostomy for several days. The patient also has a gastric tube in place, and this will remove secretions which might collect in the stomach. Later, as the intestinal tract resumes its normal functions and peristalsis begins, the stomach tube is removed and the patient is allowed liquids by mouth. If these are well tolerated, the diet gradually progresses to a low-residue diet.

Most surgeons wish to have the patient get out of bed the first postoperative day. The gastric tube and retention catheter are clamped off while the patient sits up in a chair at the bedside.

On the third or fourth day after surgery, the surgeon usually irrigates the colostomy for the first time. This is sometimes a difficult experience for the patient, even though he has had some preparation and should have some idea of what to expect. His first glimpse of the colostomy is bound to produce some emotional shock, and his eventual acceptance depends to a great extent on the reactions of those around him who must help him care for his colostomy. He must never be made to feel that the colostomy is an inconvenience to others or that they are repelled by the task of caring for him.

Gradually, the patient is taught to irrigate and care for his own colostomy. As long as there is some drainage through the colostomy, the skin around the artificial anus must be kept clean and protected from irritation by applying ointments or salves as ordered. It may be necessary to change the dressings frequently at first and, if so, Montgomery straps should be used to hold the dressing in place (see Fig. 17-7). Soiled dressings must be wrapped in paper and removed from the patient's room immediately. It is encouraging to the patient if he understands that regular bowel movements will come in time, and frequent changing of the dressings will no longer be necessary.

The restriction of the diet is a vital

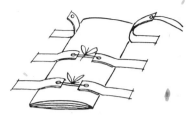

Figure 17–7. Dressing fastened with Montgomery tapes. (From Sutton: *Bedside Nursing Techniques,* 2nd Ed., W. B. Saunders Co., Philadelphia.)

part of controlling the number and consistency of the stools. A low-residue diet is used until the patient learns to control the bowel movements with irrigations. As regularity is established and the patient gains self-confidence, the diet is changed to one that is less strict.

Establishing a regular pattern for evacuation of the bowel takes much time and patience on the part of the patient and the nurses who are teaching him to care for his colostomy. There are several important points to be considered.

1. The colostomy should be irrigated at the same time every day. Later on, the irrigations may be necessary only every two or three days. Some patients adjust very well and have spontaneous evacuations regularly without irrigations.

2. The length of time required for complete evacuation of the bowel varies from 15 minutes to one hour.

3. The amount of solution necessary may vary with individual patients from one pint to several quarts.

4. Irrigations and evacuation seem more normal to the patient if he is sitting on the toilet during the procedure.

5. If the patient is physically able, he should begin irrigating his colostomy soon after surgery and gradually assume responsibility for its care.

6. Foods which are likely to cause diarrhea or lead to the formation of gas should be avoided.

There are various kinds of appliances and colostomy bags available. These are used to collect the intestinal contents until the colostomy is under control. The patient may wish to use such equipment in the early stages of adjustment because it gives him a sense of security. Colostomy bags should not be used indefinitely, however, because they are a source of odor and do not allow the patient complete freedom. The ultimate goal is complete control of the bowel movements so that only a gauze square is needed over the opening to collect mucus that may leak from the colostomy.

The patient who cares for his own colostomy at home needs adequate instruction and careful follow-up to help him solve some colostomy care problems that may arise after he leaves the hospital. Many large institutions employ enterostomal therapists who are trained and experienced in ostomy care and teaching patients. If such a person is not available, however, it becomes the responsibility of the nurse to instruct the patient and assist him in learning to care for his colostomy.

The patient will need to know how to irrigate his colostomy, and he should be familiar with some possible causes of difficulties that he could encounter. Table 17-1 presents some common colostomy care problems, possible causes and relief measures.

ABDOMINAL HERNIA

Definition

The internal organs of the body are contained within their respective cavities by the outside walls of the cavity. In the abdomen, the wall is muscular. If there is a defect in this muscular wall, the contents of the abdominal cavity may protrude through the defect. This protrusion is called a *hernia.* The lay term for hernia is "rupture."

The most common locations for a hernia are in areas where the abdominal wall is normally weaker and more

Table 17–1. COLOSTOMY CARE PROBLEMS

Problem	Possible Cause	Preventive Measures
Exhaustion following irrigation or prolonged return.	Too much water used.	Reduce amount of water or gentle abdominal massage to stimulate bowel activity.
Abdominal cramps during irrigation.	Solution too hot or too cold; too much water or given too rapidly.	Water temperature should be 105° F. Control the flow using clamp. Irrigation can be held no higher than 18 inches above colostomy.
Prolonged instillation.	Partially blocked catheter.	Keep catheter patent.
Breakdown of skin around stoma.	Poor skin care.	Clean skin with soap and water, dry thoroughly and apply tincture of Benzoin or Karaya gum powder to skin. Apply ointment or jelly to stoma if 4 × 4 gauze dressing is applied.
Diarrhea or constipation.	Unbalanced diet, inadequate fluid intake or inconsistency in irrigating times.	Avoid gas-forming foods causing diarrhea. Constipation may be relieved by eating raw fruits and vegetables.

likely to allow protrusion of a segment of intestine. These areas include the center of the abdomen at the site of the umbilicus and the lower abdomen at the points where the inguinal ring and the femoral canal begin. Figure 17-8 shows the most common contributing factors in the development of a hernia.

Hernias are classified as *reducible,* which means the protruding organ can be replaced by pressing on the organ, and *irreducible,* which means that the protruding part of the organ is tightly wedged outside the cavity and cannot be pushed back through the opening. Another name for an irreducible hernia is *incarcerated* hernia. If the protruding part of the organ is not replaced and its blood supply is cut off, the hernia is said to be *strangulated.*

Symptoms

There is a "lump" or local swelling at the site of the hernia. The most common sites are the umbilicus, groin or along a healed abdominal incision.

When pressure on the abdominal wall is removed by lying down, the swelling disappears. Lifting of heavy objects, coughing or any activity which puts a strain on the abdominal muscles may force the organ back through the opening, and the swelling reappears. Pain occurs when the peritoneum becomes irritated or when the hernia is incarcerated or strangulated. The flow of intestinal contents becomes blocked by an incarcerated hernia, and the patient has the symptoms of an intestinal obstruction.

Treatment and Nursing Care

Hernias are best treated by surgery. If surgery is not possible because of age or poor surgical risk, then the patient may be fitted with an appliance called a *truss.* The truss is put on each morning before the patient gets out of bed, because the hernia is more likely to be reduced at that time. A truss simply reinforces the weakened cavity wall and prevents protrusion of the

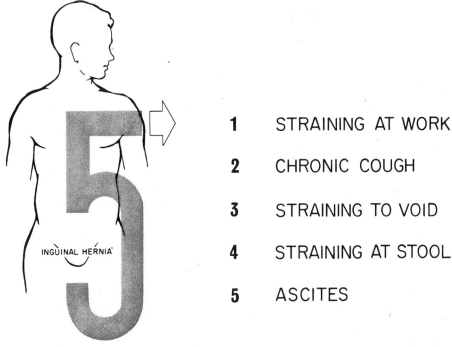

1 STRAINING AT WORK

2 CHRONIC COUGH

3 STRAINING TO VOID

4 STRAINING AT STOOL

5 ASCITES

INGUINAL HERNIA

Figure 17–8. The five major predisposing factors in hernia development. (From LeMaitre and Finnegan: *The Patient in Surgery,* 2nd Ed., W. B. Saunders Co., Philadelphia.)

intestines. It is only a symptomatic measure and does not cure the hernia.

The surgical procedure used in the treatment of a hernia is called a *herniorrhaphy,* which means a surgical repair of a hernia. The defect is closed with sutures. If the area of weakness is very large, a *hernioplasty* is done. In this procedure, some type of strong synthetic material is sewn over the defect to reinforce the area.

During the postoperative period, the patient must be protected from respiratory infections so that coughing does not place a strain on the abdominal wall.

The doctor instructs the patient in the activities he may perform during the convalescent period so that the surgical area will have time to heal completely before any strenuous activities are resumed.

DIVERTICULA

Definition

The term "diverticula" refers to small blind pouches resulting from a protrusion of the mucous membranes of a hollow organ through weakened areas of the organ's muscular wall. Diverticula occur most often in the intestinal tract, especially in the esophagus and colon. When they are present, the patient is said to have *diverticulosis.* If the diverticula become inflamed or infected, the condition is referred to as *diverticulitis.*

Symptoms

A person may have diverticulosis and remain unaware of his condition for quite a while because it often presents no symptoms. Eventually, however, the diverticula may fill with some material passing through the intestinal tract and become inflamed or infected, causing symptoms. If the diverticulitis is in the esophagus, the patient may have difficulty in swallowing, foul breath and emesis of food that was eaten several days prior to the vomiting. Diverticulitis of the intestine produces symptoms of diarrhea or constipation, abdominal pain, fever and rectal bleeding. The condition may be complicated by intestinal obstruction or by peritonitis if the intestinal wall ruptures.

Treatment

The symptoms of the patient will govern to some extent the treatment necessary. Esophageal diverticulitis, if severe, usually is treated by surgical removal of the sacs and repair of the muscular wall. Intestinal diverticulitis often can be managed conservatively with low-residue diet and a lubricating, mild laxative such as mineral oil to control constipation. In some stubborn cases or those likely to be complicated

by obstruction or rupture of the intestine wall, surgical removal of the affected portion of intestine may be necessary.

HEMORRHOIDS

Definition

Hemorrhoids are varicosities of the veins of the rectum. They may be *internal* (inside the sphincter muscles of the anus) or *external* (outside the sphincter muscles) (see Fig. 17-9).

Symptoms

Local pain and itching are the most common symptoms. Bleeding from the rectum at the time of defecation may also be present. External hemorrhoids are less likely to bleed, but they are more evident to the examiner and appear as tumor-like projections around the rectum.

Constipation, prolonged standing or sitting and pregnancy are predisposing causes of hemorrhoids. The habit of sitting on the toilet and straining at the stool for long periods of time is one of

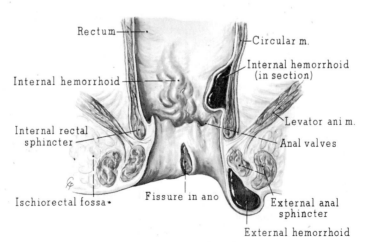

Figure 17–9. Common disorders of the anal canal. (From Jacob and Francone: *Structure and Function in Man*, 2nd Ed., W. B. Saunders Co., Philadelphia.)

the primary factors responsible for many cases of hemorrhoids.

Treatment and Nursing Care

The symptoms of hemorrhoids may be relieved by elimination of constipation, local applications of heat or cold, sitz baths and the use of ointments which contain a local anesthetic. The patient should also be instructed to wash the anal region with warm water and soap after each bowel movement.

The most effective treatment is surgical removal of the hemorrhoids. The procedure is called a *hemorrhoidectomy.*

Most patients experience a good bit of pain after a hemorrhoidectomy. This is relieved by cold applications or warm compresses to the rectum as ordered and the administration of pain-relieving drugs. Mild, wet dressings which are commercially prepared may also be used on the operative area. These dressings have a glycerine base and contain a mild astringent which reduces swelling and relieves pain.

The patient may be more comfortable lying on a rubber ring so that pressure is removed from the rectal area. Sitz baths are also effective in the relief of pain. These are usually ordered twice a day.

After rectal surgery of any kind, there is usually difficulty in voiding because the patient is afraid to completely relax the perineum and the sphincter muscles. Nursing measures to induce voiding should be tried first, and if they are unsuccessful, the patient must be catheterized.

Most patients dread the first bowel movement after a hemorrhoidectomy. There is no doubt that it will cause some pain, and the usual procedure is the administration of mineral oil to soften the stool and thus make defecation less traumatic. A sitz bath after each bowel movement will offer relief and also cleanses the operative area, keeping it free from irritation. The practice of sitting in a tub of warm water may be continued after the patient goes home. During the convalescent period, the patient should avoid roughage in his diet until the operative area has had time to heal completely.

PILONIDAL SINUS (PILONIDAL CYST)

Definition

The word "pilonidal" means "having a nest of hair." A pilonidal sinus is a lesion located in the cleft of the buttocks at the sacrococcygeal region. It is sometimes called a pilonidal cyst, but it is believed to be a subcutaneous canal (sinus) with one or more openings into the skin, rather than a true cyst, or fluid-filled sac. The condition occurs when the stiff hairs in the sacrococcygeal region irritate and eventually penetrate the soft skin in the cleft of the buttocks. Conditions which can lead to development of such a sinus include local injury, improper cleansing of the area and obesity. Persons who have more than the usual amount of body hair are particularly susceptible.

Symptoms and Treatment

A pilonidal sinus may cause no trouble until it becomes infected, and then the patient experiences pain in the area, with swelling and a purulent drainage. When this occurs, the area must be incised surgically and the connecting canals opened and drained. Hairs and necrotic tissue must be removed so the area can heal.

Postoperative care includes changing of dressings and measures to avoid contamination of the wound. A lubricating laxative and oil enema usually are given before the first bowel movement to avoid strain on the sutures. Antibiotics may be given to control infection.

Part Two. Diseases of the Accessory Organs of Digestion

SPECIAL DIAGNOSTIC TESTS

X-ray Examinations

The gallbladder and ducts which carry bile to the small intestine may be visualized by x-ray if a contrast medium of radiopaque dye is used. The dye is given to the patient by mouth or directly into the vein. It is then carried to the liver, where it is secreted with the bile. As the dye travels from the liver to the gallbladder and on through the bile ducts, the hollow structures may be outlined on the x-ray film. Obstructions within the ducts or failure of the gallbladder to fill are thus more easily diagnosed.

Cholecystogram, gallbladder studies or *choleangiogram* are all terms which are used to describe x-ray examinations of the type described above. In the oral method, the patient is given a fat-free meal the evening before the morning of the x-ray examination. After the meal is completed, the dye is given orally in tablet form, and then the patient receives nothing by mouth until after the x-rays are completed. Cleansing enemas and laxatives are usually given to prepare the patient for the test.

The *intravenous* method of administering the dye does not require the administration of laxatives and repeated enemas. This method of giving the dye is usually used for patients who cannot tolerate the dye orally. There is, however, some danger of a serious allergic reaction to the dye given by the intravenous route.

Specific orders for preparation of the patient for gallbladder studies may vary slightly according to the wishes of the radiologist in charge of the examination. The practical nurse is responsible for familiarizing herself with the routine used in the institution in which she works and for carrying out these directions conscientiously.

Bilirubin Test

Bilirubin is a pigment normally found in the blood as a result of the breakdown of hemoglobin and is removed by the liver. The liver secretes the pigment in bile which enters the intestinal tract and gives the stools their characteristic brown color. When the liver is diseased, bilirubin accumulates in the blood stream; thus, a bilirubin test of the blood is a measurement of liver function.

Bromsulphalein Test

Bromsulphalein is a dye that is administered by injection. Under normal circumstances, the liver will remove this dye from the blood stream. The Bromsulphalein test measures the rate at which the liver is able to remove the dye from the blood stream. If the liver is not functioning properly, the dye will remain in the blood longer than it normally would.

Prothrombin Level

This test is sometimes used as a diagnostic test for liver disease because prothrombin is manufactured by the liver. For more details on the prothrombin test, see Chapter 5. Other liver function tests are included in Table 17-2.

JAUNDICE

Definition

Jaundice is actually a group of symptoms rather than a disease. It is only an indication of excessive amounts of bile pigment in the blood stream. When the bile pigment reaches a certain level, it stains the skin a yellowish color, and the patient is said to be jaundiced.

TABLE 17-2. THE NORMAL HEPATOGRAM*

Function	Test	Normal Range
Excretory	Bromsulphalein	With 2 mg./kg. dose, less than 4% retention at 30 min.
	Alkaline phosphatase	2-4 Bodansky units
	Bilirubin	Direct: 0.0-0.2 mg./100 ml.
		Total: 0.2-1.4 mg./100 ml.
	Icterus index	8 units or less
	Urobilinogen	Trace
	Cholesterol	Total: 135-260 mg./100 ml.
		Ester: 95-200 mg./100 ml.
	Cholinesterase	0.7-1.4 pH units/hr.
	Lactic dehydrogenase	Less than 300 units
	Transaminase (SGP-T)	5-35 units
	Serum proteins	Total: 6.5-8.0 Gm./100 ml.
		Albumin: 4.0-5.5 Gm./100 ml.
		Globulin: 2.0-3-0 Gm./100 ml.
		Fibrinogen: 0.2-0.3 Gm./100 ml.
	Prothrombin time	12-15 sec.
	Prothrombin production	Shortening of prothrombin time after dose of vitamin K
Metabolic	Galactose tolerance	Oral: less than 3 Gm. excreted in 4 hr.
		Intravenous: complete removal in 45-60 min.
Detoxication	Hippuric acid	Oral: at least 3 Gm. excreted in 4 hr.
		Intravenous: at least 1 Gm. excreted in 1 hr.
Miscellaneous	Cephalin flocculation	Negative to 2+
	Zinc turbidity	4-8 units
	Thymol turbidity	1-4 units

*From French: Nurses' Guide to Diagnostic Procedures, 2nd edition. Copyright McGraw-Hill, Inc., 1967. Reprinted with permission of McGraw-Hill Book Company.

Types of Jaundice

Jaundice may be divided into three general types based on the underlying cause of the symptoms. The three types are:

1. *Obstructive jaundice,* caused by a plugging of the bile ducts, which in turn causes a back flow of bile. The obstruction may be caused by gallstones or neoplasms in the ducts.

2. *Nonobstructive jaundice,* associated with damage to the cells of the liver. An inflammatory process within the tissues of the liver or nutritional deficiencies may cause this type of jaundice.

3. *Hemolytic jaundice.* Hemolysis means destruction of blood cells. When excessive amounts of red blood cells are destroyed, their pigment is released into the blood stream, and the patient becomes jaundiced. This condition is primarily a disease of the blood.

Nursing Care of a Patient with Jaundice

The other symptoms which accompany jaundice are not always so obvious as the yellowish cast to the skin, but they nevertheless require attention and care from the nurse.

Itching of the skin frequently accompanies jaundice. The itching is of an intense nature and may be very disturbing to the patient. Baths of starch or sodium bicarbonate (baking soda) solutions offer some relief. Mild lotions and frequent changing of the patient's gown and bed linen are also helpful. If the itching is so severe that it disturbs the patient's rest, the nurse should report the situation to the doctor. He may wish to order antihistamine drugs for relief of the itching.

Because the bile is not being secreted into the small intestine, fats eaten by the patient are not properly digested. This leads to *indigestion, loss of* appetite, flatulence and constipation. The patient may be placed on a low-fat diet to avoid these distressing symptoms. A low-fat diet is sometimes difficult for the patient to accept, however, because the foods are not palatable. If the patient understands that fats are directly responsible for many of his digestive discomforts, he may accept the restricted diet more readily. Some imagination in the use of other seasonings besides fat in the preparation of his meals will also help him remain within the limits of his restricted diet.

The stools of a patient with jaundice are lacking in the bile pigment and are therefore very light in color. The urine is very dark because the kidneys have removed some of the pigment from the blood stream and excreted it in the urine. The observations of the nurse in regard to the color of the stools and urine of the patient with jaundice are very important in helping the doctor determine the patient's progress.

Earlier in this chapter, we mentioned the prothrombin level in the diagnosis of diseases of the liver. It was stated that prothrombin was manufactured by the liver; thus, a patient who has jaundice as a result of liver cell damage will also be expected to have a low prothrombin level. Prothrombin plays an important role in the clotting of blood, and so we can expect a patient with a deficiency of prothrombin to hemorrhage easily. This condition demands intelligent observation on the part of the nurse so that she may protect her patient from massive hemorrhage or

severe anemia from loss of blood. Any symptoms which might indicate the loss of blood internally as well as externally must be reported immediately so that treatment may be started.

VIRAL HEPATITIS

Definition

Viral hepatitis is an imflammation of the liver caused by a virus. Hepatitis may be caused by more than one virus. Consequently, a person who has had an attack of viral hepatitis is not immune to the disease if he is exposed to a different virus.

Types of Viral Hepatitis

Viral hepatitis is an infectious disease, which means that it can be transmitted from one person to another. There are two general types of viral hepatitis according to the mode of transmission.

The first type is called *epidemic hepatitis,* or *catarrhal jaundice.* This type is transmitted by the ingestion of foods or liquids contaminated by the virus. There is also a possibility that the virus may enter the body by way of the respiratory tract.

The second type of viral hepatitis is *serum hepatitis.* It gets its name from the serum of human blood which contains the virus. The source of infection may be whole blood or blood derivatives such as pooled plasma, or needles and syringes which contain the blood of persons with the virus in their blood.

Symptoms

The early symptoms of viral hepatitis are very similar to those of an upper respiratory infection. The victim has a low-grade fever, malaise, indigestion and loss of appetite. Later there is local tenderness in the region of the liver and some enlargement of the liver. As the inflamed liver cells cease to function, jaundice becomes evident and the stools become lighter and the urine darker than normal.

Treatment and Nursing Care

Bed rest is necessary until the patient is free of symptoms. After the symptoms subside, the patient may have his physical activities restricted for as long as two or three months so as to avoid permanent damage to the liver. This limiting of activities may be difficult for the patient to understand because he usually feels well and quite able to resume his former activities. He must be encouraged to follow the doctor's orders because of the danger of possible cirrhosis of the liver and other complications if adequate rest is not provided during the long convalescent period.

The patient is isolated during the acute phase of the disease to prevent the spread of the infectious organism (see Chapter 9). Extreme care must be used with all needles and syringes used in treating the patient with hepatitis, as these are dangerous sources of infection. Careless handling of contaminated needles may easily lead to a pricked finger and the entrance of the virus directly into the blood stream.

All articles and equipment containing bodily excretions from the patient also require special handling and disinfection.

The patient's diet is planned to provide an adequate intake of calories and protein. The diet is usually high in protein because protein helps in the repair and rebuilding of body tissues, and high in carbohydrates because these are thought to have a protective effect on the liver cells. Even though nausea is a common occurrence in hepatitis, the patient should eat everything on his tray. His refusal to eat all or part of his meals and extra feedings should be reported so that supplements may be given.

There are no specific drugs used in the treatment of infectious hepatitis other than antibiotics which may sometimes be given to prevent secondary bacterial infections.

CIRRHOSIS OF THE LIVER

Definition

Cirrhosis is a chronic disease characterized by degenerative changes within the structure of the liver cells. The cells are first loaded with fat, and then they begin to degenerate and die. These necrotic cells are then replaced by scar tissue.

The specific cause of cirrhosis of the liver is not known. Although the incidence of cirrhosis is high among known alcoholics, this does not mean that all persons with cirrhosis have a history of excessive drinking. The underlying factor in cirrhosis is a nutritional deficiency, and alcoholics are subject to cirrhosis because they prefer to drink alcohol rather than eat an adequate diet.

Symptoms

In the early stages of cirrhosis, the patient has symptoms similar to those of acute hepatitis. As the disease progresses, the liver cells begin to degenerate, and the blood vessels within the liver also fail to function normally. This results in congestion of the blood vessels which drain the digestive organs and transport the blood to the liver. The next step in the process is an accumulation of fluids within the intestinal tract. The excess fluid produces symptoms of indigestion and diarrhea or constipation.

As the fluid in the intestines continues to accumulate, it may eventually pass through the walls of the intestines and fill the abdominal cavity. This excess fluid within the abdominal cavity is called ascites. The patient's abdomen becomes extremely swollen, and respiratory function may be affected. Ascites is relieved by tapping the abdominal cavity with a large needle and draining off the excess fluids. This procedure of withdrawing fluids from the abdominal cavity is called a *paracentesis.*

The backing up of venous blood may also lead to varicose veins of the esophagus. The varicosities tend to bleed easily and thus cause vomiting of blood. In some cases, massive hemorrhage can occur in this way.

Other symptoms of cirrhosis include edema, jaundice and small hemorrhages under the skin. These hemorrhages are very close to the surface of the skin and have a "spidery" appearance.

Treatment and Nursing Care

There is no known cure for cirrhosis of the liver, and treatment is aimed at relief of the patient's symptoms.

Rest in bed becomes necessary as the disease progresses. The patient with ascites is usually more comfortable with his head and shoulders elevated. This position relieves some of the pressure of the abdomen against the diaphragm and thus facilitates breathing.

There is frequently generalized edema as well as the local collection of fluid within the abdomen. The patient's intake and output are carefully recorded. He is also usually weighed every day to determine the increase or decrease of fluids held in the body. A low-salt diet is given these patients.

Care of the skin is important, not only because of the edema but also because the patient frequently has jaundice with severe itching.

Distended veins and a tendency to bleed are common and predispose the patient to hemorrhage. The nurse must be alert for early symptoms of hemorrhage and report them immediately. Loss of blood through the intestinal tract, no matter how slight it may appear, must be reported to the physician in charge.

The dietary treatment of cirrhosis consists of a high-protein, low-sodium, low-fat diet. Vitamins, especially the vitamin B group, are given in large amounts to supplement the diet.

In the last stages of cirrhosis, some patients undergo mental and emotional changes. The edema may cause increased intracranial pressure and result in irritability and confusion. Depression and despair are also common because the patient realizes that very little can be done to help slow down the disease process and there is nothing which will cure him of the disease. Delirium and coma or convulsions must be watched for and all precautions taken to protect the patient from injury should these appear.

CHOLECYSTITIS

Definition

Cholecystitis is an inflammation of the gallbladder. The cause of cholecystitis is not known, but it is often associated with gallstones. It occurs most frequently in middle-aged women who are overweight.

Symptoms

The symptoms of cholecystitis may be mild or severe, depending on the degree of inflammation present in the gallbladder. In mild cases, the symptoms are those of indigestion and abdominal distention and are most noticeable several hours after eating. There is usually a chronic pain in the upper part of the abdomen on the right side.

In an acute inflammation of the gallbladder, the patient has severe pain in the gallbladder region, nausea and vomiting, and chills and fever. The gallbladder may become filled with pus and will eventually rupture, spilling its contents into the abdominal cavity and leading to a severe peritonitis.

Treatment and Nursing Care

Treatment may vary according to individual cases. The conservative medical treatment consists of measures to improve the general physical condition of the patient and relieve the symptoms until the inflammation has subsided.

Surgical treatment may be resorted to immediately during the acute stage to prevent complications, or the physician may choose to wait and perform surgery after the conservative treatment has had its effect. A *cholecystectomy,* or surgical removal of the gallbladder, is the surgical procedure performed. Nursing care of the patient having a cholecystectomy is presented later in this chapter. If the surgeon wishes to open and drain the contents of the gallbladder, he performs a procedure called a *cholecystostomy.* The nursing care of the patient having this type of surgery is similar to that of the patient having a cholecystectomy.

CHOLELITHIASIS

Definition

Cholelithiasis is the presence of gallstones within the gallbladder or bile ducts. The stones vary in size and may grow to be as large as an orange, but it is usually the smaller stones which cause the most trouble because they are passed into the bile ducts where they become lodged, causing an obstruction in the flow of bile (see Fig. 17-10).

Symptoms

The most outstanding symptom of cholelithiasis is a severe and almost intolerable pain in the region of the gallbladder. Nausea and vomiting are also present, and the patient is frequently drenched in perspiration and near shock because of the pain. A his-

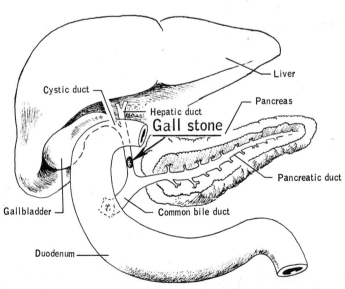

Figure 17–10. Bile is drained from the liver by the hepatic duct and from the gallbladder by the cystic duct. An obstruction due to a gallstone, as pictured above, prevents the flow of bile into the digestive tract. (Modified from Manner: *Elements of Anatomy and Physiology,* W. B. Saunders Co., Philadelphia.)

tory of intolerance to fatty foods over a period of time is a common complaint of patients with gallstones.

Treatment and Nursing Care

The treatment of gallstones is surgical correction of the condition. The specific type of surgical procedure will depend on the location of the stone and the condition of the gallbladder at the time of surgery.

The long names given to surgical procedures involving the gallbladder and ducts may seem very perplexing and difficult to understand, but they are actually only various combinations of prefixes and suffixes.

Cholecystectomy. *Chole* refers to gall, *cyst* means bladder and *ectomy* is the surgical removal of. Thus cholecystectomy means the surgical removal of the gallbladder.

Cholecystostomy. The suffix *ostomy* means cutting into an organ for the purpose of providing drainage. Cholecystostomy is a surgical incision into the gallbladder and the insertion of a drain.

Choledocholithotomy. *Lith* refers to stone, *docho* refers to duct. Thus a choledocholithotomy is a surgical incision into the bile duct for the purpose of removing a stone.

NURSING CARE OF THE PATIENT HAVING SURGERY OF THE GALLBLADDER

Preoperative Care

Unless the surgery is performed for emergency relief of the condition, the patient will have extensive diagnostic tests before the operation is scheduled. These tests help the surgeon determine the location of the difficulty so that he may be prepared for the type of procedure he will need to perform. If jaundice is present, the patient's prothrom-

bin level may be checked to see if he may safely undergo surgery. Vitamin K is given to improve the clotting ability of the blood.

Patients who are having acute pain or abdominal distention often have Levin tubes inserted to remove the gastric and intestinal contents. This tube may be left in place during and after surgery.

Postoperative Care

Because the surgical incision is in the upper section of the abdomen, the patient is placed in semi-Fowler's position after he recovers from anesthesia. Aside from the fact that he will be more comfortable and there will be less strain on the sutures, the patient will also be able to take deep breaths and cough more easily in this position.

One of the most confusing aspects of nursing a patient who has had gallbladder surgery is proper care of the drains or tubes which may be in place when the patient returns from the operating room.

In most cases, the surgery has been performed to relieve an obstruction to the flow of bile through the bile ducts or to provide a means of draining purulent material to the outside. If the patient has had an infection of the gallbladder, the drainage is absorbed by the dressings over the surgical wound. These must be changed often and should be checked quite frequently for signs of fresh bleeding. The drain is left in as long as necessary and is then removed by the surgeon.

When an obstruction of the common bile duct has occurred because of stones or tumors, the surgeon may insert a small tube directly into the common bile duct. This tube is called a *T tube* because it is shaped like the letter T (see Fig. 17-11). This tube must be kept open at all times and is connected to a bedside bottle as soon as the patient returns to his room. The length of time the T tube is left in place depends on the condition of the patient. While

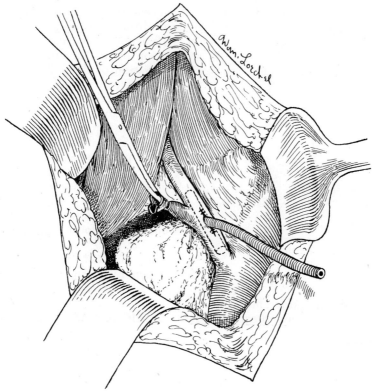

Figure 17–11. Diagrammatic drawing showing the T tube inserted into the common bile duct and sutured in place. The hemostat on the left holds the end of the cystic duct, which has been cut and tied. The gallbladder has been removed. The T tube is brought to the outside and attached to a drainage bottle (From Ferguson and Sholtis: *Eliason's Surgical Nursing,* 11th Ed., J. B. Lippincott Co., Philadelphia.)

the tube is in the common bile duct, there will be no bile going to the duodenum as it normally would.

Precautions must be taken that no tension is put on tubes or drains which have been inserted in the surgical wound (see Fig. 17-12). T tubes are sutured in place, and if they are accidentally pulled out, the patient must be returned to the operating room and the incision reopened to replace the tube. Dressings must be changed with careful handling of the tube or drain. There is usually so much drainage that the dressings must be changed often, and Montgomery straps are best for holding the dressings in place. The sight of so much greenish yellow discharge (bile) on the dressings may

upset the patient unless he is told that this is to be expected.

Since the surgeon will be concerned with whether or not bile is beginning to flow through the duct and on into the duodenum as it normally should, the nurse must carefully observe the color of the patient's stools. A return of the characteristic brown color to the stools is an indication that bile is entering the small intestine. If the obstruction remains in the bile duct, the patient will show signs of jaundice. Light-colored stools, dark urine and the early appearance of a yellowish cast to the skin must be reported as soon as any one of these is noticed by the nurse.

There is no specific diet recommended for the patient who has had

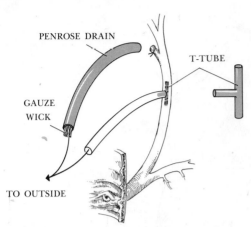

PENROSE DRAIN

T-TUBE

GAUZE
WICK

TO OUTSIDE

Figure 17–12. After cholecystectomy the Penrose drain helps to remove exudate from the area formerly occupied by the gallbladder. The T tube diverts bile to the outside.

surgery of the gallbladder, although he is usually warned to avoid excesses of fatty foods.

PANCREATITIS

Definition

Pancreatitis is an inflammation of the pancreas. It may be acute or chronic in nature and frequently accompanies obstruction of the pancreatic duct due to gallstones or the back flow of bile into the pancreatic duct.

Symptoms

An attack of acute pancreatitis may be mistaken for an attack of acute indigestion. The patient experiences severe pain in the region of the stomach, and nausea and vomiting are usually present. The pain radiates through to the back and may be so severe as to cause the patient to go into shock.

Treatment and Nursing Care

Pancreatitis is usually treated medically. Nitroglycerine under the tongue sometimes relieves the pain, but morphine given intravenously may be

necessary in extreme cases. The patient is allowed nothing by mouth during the acute phase, so as to prevent stimulation of the pancreas and further aggravation of the inflammation. Fluids are given intravenously until the edema of the pancreas and the pancreatic duct has subsided and the digestive juices from the pancreas can once again flow into the duodenum. Most patients with acute pancreatitis recover with this type of treatment.

If the pancreatitis becomes chronic, there is some destruction of the pancreas cells, and the pancreatic duct becomes fibrotic. A diet low in fat and the administration of antispasmodic drugs are helpful in treating chronic pancreatitis. Alcohol is forbidden.

CLINICAL CASE PROBLEMS

1. Mr. Long, age 42, is admitted to the hospital with a diagnosis of bleeding gastric ulcer. He has had the ulcer for more than a year, and even though he has been informed of the type of restricted diet he should follow, he does not always follow it.

Mr. Long is placed on milk and cream every hour on the hour and an antacid medication every hour on the half hour. While you are giving him P.M. care, he becomes nauseated and begins to vomit bright red blood. He also complains of a sharp pain in his upper abdomen. His wife, who is in the room at the time, tells you that he has been vomiting blood at home, and since milk and cream make him nauseated, she thinks you should just omit them and he will be all right. Mr. Long seems resigned to letting his wife do all the talking.

What problems do you see in this situation?

Do you think it is necessary to report his episode of vomiting immediately?

2. Mrs. Knight is a 45-year-old mother of 5 children who has had a

colostomy for treatment of an intestinal obstruction. On her fourth postoperative day, she is assigned to your care. She has received instructions in the care of her colostomy from the nurse in charge, but so far she has refused to take care of it herself.

Mrs. Knight has been told by the surgeon that he may be able to close the colostomy in several months if all goes well. When you enter her room to begin caring for Mrs. Knight, she becomes very upset and tells you that she cannot face the future knowing that she may have to be inconvenienced by the colostomy. She feels that she will be a burden to her family and completely incapacitated by her illness.

How can you help the patient accept her illness?

What can you do to encourage her to take care of herself?

What other problems can you see in this situation?

3. Mr. May is admitted to the hospital with a diagnosis of cirrhosis of the liver. He is 59 years of age and has been hospitalized several times for his condition. He suffers from shortness of breath due to a swollen and enlarged abdomen, is anemic because of minimal but constant esophageal bleeding and appears jaundiced. He has several abrasions on his arms, legs and abdomen from repeatedly scratching to relieve his pruritus. Mr. May is very depressed and will not converse with you when you enter his room with his breakfast tray the first morning you are assigned to his care. He refuses to eat and indicates his attitude by pushing the tray away and turning on his side, face to the wall.

What nursing measures might help relieve some of Mr. May's symptoms?

Why do you think he is mentally depressed?

How would you go about helping him emotionally?

What special observations must you make while caring for Mr. May?

How would you explain a paracentesis to Mr. May if one were ordered for him?

4. Mrs. Luke, age 46, is admitted to the hospital for a cholecystectomy. She is extremely obese and enjoys eating rich, fatty foods even though she knows this will add to her obesity and precipitate attacks of cholecystitis. You are assigned to care for Mrs. Luke when she returns from surgery.

How will you position this patient postoperatively?

If she has a large amount of drainage from the surgical incision, how will you take care of this problem?

When you get this patient out of bed the next day, how are you going to manage the dressings and prevent strain on the sutures?

What other problems might you anticipate?

REFERENCES

1. Amshel, A.: "Hemorrhoidal Problems—Medical and Surgical Treatments." Am. Journ. Nurs., Dec., 1963, p. 87.
2. Barnes, M. R.: "Clean Colons without Enemas." Am. Journ. Nurs., Oct., 1969, p. 2124.
3. Beland, I. L.: Clinical Nursing Pathophysiological and Psychosocial Approaches, 2nd edition. New York, The Macmillan Co., 1970.
4. Brunner, L. S., et al.: Textbook of Medical-Surgical Nursing, 2nd edition. Philadelphia, J. B. Lippincott Co., 1970.
5. Cupit, G. C., et al.: "Antacids." Am. Journ. Nurs., Dec., 1972, p. 2210.
6. DeLuca, J. C.: "The Ulcerative Colitis Personality." Nurs. Clin. N. Amer., Vol. 5, No. 1, 1970, p. 23.
7. Gibbs, G. P., and White, M.: "Stomal Care." Am. Journ. Nurs., Feb., 1972, p. 268.
8. Glenn, F. A.: "Surgical Treatment of Biliary Tract Disease." Am. Journ. Nurs., May, 1964, p. 88.
9. Gutowski, F.: "Ostomy Procedures: Nursing Care Before and After." Am. Journ. Nurs., Feb., 1972, p. 262.
10. Hayter, J.: "Impaired Liver Function and

Related Nursing Care." Am. Journ. Nurs., Nov., 1968, p. 2374.

11. Henderson, L. M.: "Nursing Care in Acute Cholecystitis." Am. Journ. Nurs., 1964, p. 88.
12. "Helping Patients Live with Colostomy." Nursing '72, July, 1972, p. 5.
13. "Hepatitis—When You're Asked About Getting Gamma Globulin." Nursing Update, June, 1971, p. 3.
14. Horowitz, C.: "Profiles in OPD Nursing—A Rectal and Colon Service." Am. Journ. Nurs., Jan., 1971, p. 115.
15. Jackson B. S.: "Ulcerative Colitis." Am. Journ. Nurs., Feb., 1972, p. 258.
16. Murray, C., et al.: "The Patient Has an Ileal Conduit." Am. Journ. Nurs., Aug., 1971, p. 1560.
17. Shafer, K. N., et al.: *Medical-Surgical Nursing*, 5th edition. St. Louis, The C. V. Mosby Co., 1971.
18. Sheridan, B.: "After Hemorrhoidectomy." Am. Journ. Nurs., Dec., 1963, p. 90.
19. Smith, D. W., et al.: *Care of the Adult Patient*, 3rd edition. Philadelphia, J. B. Lippincott Co., 1971.
20. Usher, F., and Matthews, J.: "Surgery: Treatment of Choice for Hernias." Am. Journ. Nurs., Sept., 1964, p. 85.

SUGGESTED STUDENT READING

1. Ahnafield, A.: "Ileostomies and Urinary Ostomies: Preoperative and Postoperative Care." Journ. Pract. Nurs., March, 1972, p. 30.
2. "Cancer of the G.I. Tract—A Symposium." Journ. Pract. Nurs., July, 1969, p. 23.
3. "Care and Management of Ostomies." Bedside Nurse, June, 1970, p. 24.
4. Davis, R. W.: "Nursing Care of the Colostomy Patient." Bedside Nurse, Sept., 1970, p. 21.
5. Harmon, N., and Wayne, P.: "Fiber Optics: Photography in the Stomach." RN, July, 1971, p. 30.
6. "Helping Patients Live with Colostomy." Nursing '72, July, 1972, p. 5.
7. "Hepatitis—When You're Asked About Getting Gamma Globulin." Nursing Update, June, 1971, p. 3.
8. Katona, E. A.: "Learning Colostomy Control." Am. Journ. Nurs., March, 1967, p. 534.
9. Kitzes, G.: "What the Nurse Should Know about Peptic Ulcers." Journ. Pract. Nurs., Jan., 1970, p. 20.
10. Lamberty, K.: "Diet Therapy for Ulcers." Journ. Pract. Nurs., June, 1965, p. 25.
11. Smith, K. R.: "Living with an Ileostomy." Journ. Pract. Nurs., Aug., 1970, p. 27.
12. Welch, G. D.: "The Acceptance of a Colostomy." Journ. Pract. Nurs., June, 1971, p. 36.

OUTLINE FOR CHAPTER 17

I. Introduction

A. Digestive tract is concerned with digestion (physical and chemical changes which foods undergo) and absorption (passage of nutritive elements from the intestines to the blood).

B. Accessory organs of digestion: liver, gallbladder and pancreas.

Part One   Nursing Care of Patients with Diseases of the Digestive Tract

I. Diagnostic Tests

A. X-ray examinations—gastrointestinal series and barium enema.

B. Gastroscopy—direct visualization of the lining of the stomach.

C. Esophagoscopy—direct visualization of the esophageal lining.

D. Proctoscopy—direct visualization of the anus and rectum.

E. Sigmoidoscopy—direct visualization of the inner lining of the sigmoid colon.

F. Gastric analysis—examination and analysis of the contents of the stomach.

G. Stool examination—examination of fecal material for presence of blood, specific bacteria, cysts, ova or parasites.

II. Stomatitis (Inflammation of the Mucous Membranes of the Mouth)

A. May be caused by certain drugs, trauma, nutritional deficiencies or pathogenic microorganisms.

B. Aphthous stomatitis, commonly called "canker sores," is probably a viral infection. No specific cure.

C. Vincent's angina ("trench mouth"). Caused by a combination of a bacillus and spirochete. Treated with sodium perborate mouthwashes and antibiotics.

III. Gastritis (Inflammation of the Mucous Membranes of the Stomach)

A. Main causes—overeating, excessive drinking, contaminated food or ingested poisons.

B. Symptoms—nausea, vomiting and tenderness in the gastric region.

C. Treatment—restriction of foods followed by a bland diet, medications that coat the gastric mucosa and antispasmodics.

IV. Ulcerative Colitis

A. Inflammation with formation of ulcers in the mucosa of the colon.

B. Symptoms—diarrhea, nausea and vomiting or loss of appetite. Dehydration and malnutrition may occur in chronic cases.

C. Treatment—rest, freedom from anxiety and antidiarrheic drugs.

V. Appendicitis

A. Definition—an inflammation of the vermiform appendix.

B. Symptoms—pain the the lower right side, elevated temperature, nausea and vomiting and increase in white cell count.

C. Treatment and nursing care—surgical removal of appendix.

VI. Peritonitis (Inflammation of the Peritoneum)

A. Common causes—ruptured appendix, perforated ulcer and ruptured ectopic pregnancy.

B. Symptoms—vomiting, severe abdominal pain, fever, tachycardia and symptoms of shock.

C. Treatment—massive doses of antibiotics, intravenous fluids and electrolytes and gastrointestinal decompression.

D. Vital signs taken and recorded frequently, patient observed for signs of intestinal obstuction and protected from injury when delirium is present. Semi-Fowler's position helps localize purulent material in pelvis.

VII. Peptic Ulcer

A. Open lesion on the mucosa of the stomach (gastric ulcer) or small intestine (duodenal ulcer).

B. Exact cause unknown. Predisposing factors—anxiety, tension, poor eating habits and increased secretion of hydrochloric acid.

C. Symptoms—gnawing, burning pain in epigastrium (relieved by eating), frequent belching, vomiting and tarry stools.

D. Medical Treatment—rest and bland, non-irritating diet. Medications include antacids, antispasmodics and sedatives.

E. Surgical treatment for chronic ulcers that fail to respond to medical treatment or are complicated by perforation or hemorrhage.

VIII. Nursing Care of Patient Having Gastric Surgery

A. Preoperative care—diagnostic tests, physical preparation of skin, enemas and insertion of Levin tube.

B. Postoperative care—semi-Fowler's position to facilitate drainage of stomach contents. Keep Levin tube open and draining freely. Irrigations if ordered. Mouth care while tube is in place. Observe drainage for color, consistency and amount.

C. "Dumping syndrome"—occurs in some patients who have had part or all of stomach removed. Occurs after eating when large amounts of food pass rapidly into small intestine. May be relieved by eating small meals, avoiding liquids during the meal and lying down after eating.

IX. Cancer of the Stomach

A. Diagnosis difficult as symptoms may be quite similar to those of gastric ulcer.

B. Treatment—surgical removal of all or part of the stomach.

X. Cancer of the Large Intestine

A. Symptoms—constipation or diarrhea (or alternate attacks of each) and rectal bleeding.

B. Treatment—surgical removal of the affected portion.

XI. Intestinal Obstruction (Blocking of the Intestinal Tract)

A. Causes—strangulated hernia, twisting or telescoping of the bowel or interference with conduction of nerve impulses.

B. Symptoms—acute intestinal obstruction characterized by projectile vomiting, nausea and abdominal pain. Chronic type may have less abrupt onset. Symptoms include nausea, vomiting and constipation.

C. Treatment—surgical correction of obstruction and intestinal decompression.

XII. Nursing Care of the Patient with Surgery of the Lower Intestine

A. Types of surgical procedures: colectomy (removal of the diseased portion of colon), colostomy (creation of an artificial anus with bowel opening on the abdominal surface) and abdominoperineal resection (removal of the affected portion of colon, the entire rectum and the anus).

B. Preoperative care—low residue diet, cleansing of lower bowel and intestinal decompression.

C. Postoperative care—observation for signs of shock, care of retention catheter, care of gastrointestinal tube and observation of drainage. Watch for signs of returning peristalsis.

D. Special care of patient with colostomy.

    1. Preoperative period should include adequate explanation of surgical procedure and plans for rehabilitation.

    2. Postoperative care includes instruction of patient in the care of his colostomy.

XIII. Abdominal Hernia (a Protrusion of the Intestines through a Weakened Area in the Abdominal Wall)

A. Most common sites are the umbilical area and beginning of inguinal canal and femoral canal.

B. Reducible hernia—protruding organ can be replaced by pressing on the organ. Incarcerated hernia—cannot be reduced. Strangulated hernia—blood supply to the organ has been obstructed.

C. Surgery most effective means for treating hernia (herniorrhaphy).

XIV. Diverticula

A. Small, blind pouches of mucous membrane that have protruded through a weakened wall of a hollow organ.

B. Symptoms not apparent until inflammation (diverticulitis) or infection occurs. Esophageal diverticulitis may produce difficulty in swallowing, foul breath and emesis. Intestinal diverticulitis produces abdominal pain, fever, diarrhea or constipation and rectal bleeding.

C. Treatment may be surgical removal of affected portion of organ or low-residue diet and lubricating laxatives.

XV. Hemorrhoids (Varicose Veins of the Rectum)

A. Symptoms—local pain, itching and bleeding at time of defecation.

B. Treatment — hemorrhoidectomy. Postoperative care concerned with prevention of infection and relief of pain.

XVI. Pilonidal sinus

A. Subcutaneous canal located in the cleft of the buttocks in the sacrococcygeal area. Produces pain and purulent drainage.

B. Treatment—surgical incision of canal, drainage of purulent material and removal of hairs and necrotic tissue. Antibiotics given to control infection.

Part Two Diseases of the Accessory Organs of Digestion

I. Special Diagnostic Tests

A. Cholecystogram and choleangiogram—x-rays of the biliary tract after injection of a radiopaque dye.

B. Bilirubin test—measurement of pigment normally removed from the blood by the liver.

C. Bromsulphalein test—done to determine the liver's ability to remove a dye from the blood stream.

D. Prothrombin level—the liver manufactures prothrombin.

II. Jaundice (Excessive Amounts of Bile Pigments in the Blood Stream)

A. Three types:

    1. Obstructive jaundice.

    2. Nonobstructive jaundice.

    3. Hemolytic jaundice.

B. Nursing care—frequent bathing to relieve itching, low-fat diet, observation of stools and urine for bile pigments, observation for signs of bleeding.

III. Viral Hepatitis (Inflammation of the Liver)

A. Symptoms—low-grade fever, malaise, indigestion, local tenderness over liver and jaundice.

B. Treatment and nursing care—rest, isolation to prevent spread of infection and high-protein, high-carbohydrate diet.

IV. Cirrhosis of the Liver

A. Specific cause unknown. Underlying factor seems to be prolonged nutritional deficiency.

B. Symptoms—early symptoms similar to those of hepatitis. Later there is congestion of the portal circulation, edema, indigestion and diarrhea. Tendency to bleed. Jaundice and small hemorrhages under the skin.

C. Treatment and nursing care—rest, low-salt, high-protein and vitamin supplements. Paracentesis to relieve ascites. No cure.

V. Cholecystitis

A. Inflammation of the gallbladder. Often associated with gallstones.

B. Symptoms—indigestion, abdominal distention and chronic pain in the upper right abdomen. Severe, acute inflammation produces severe pain, chills, fever, nausea and vomiting.

C. Treatment—surgical removal of gallbladder (cholecystectomy) or incision and drainage of gallbladder (cholecystostomy).

VI. Cholelithiasis (Stones in Gallbladder or Biliary Ducts)

A. Symptoms—severe pain in gallbladder region, nausea, vomiting and history of intolerance to fatty foods.

B. Treatment—exact surgical procedure depends on location of stones.

VII. Nursing Care of the Patient Having Surgery of the Gallbladder

A. Preoperative care—diagnostic tests, care of Levin tube and gastric suction and vitamin K to prevent bleeding.

B. Postoperative care—semi-Fowler's position. Care of tubes, frequent changing of dressings, careful observation of stools for indications of the return of bile to the intestine.

VIII. Pancreatitis (Acute or Chronic Inflammation of the Pancreas)

A. Symptoms—acute attack similar to acute indigestion. Patient has severe pain in the region.

B. Treatment and nursing care—medications to relieve pain, restriction of foods and fluids and intravenous feedings. Chronic pancreatitis treated with antispasmodic drugs and restriction of alcohol and fat.

18

Nursing Care of Patients with Disorders of the Urinary System

VOCABULARY

Contour
Distention
Excreted
Hypercalcemia
Intracranial
Secreted

INTRODUCTION

The urinary system is composed of the kidneys, ureters, urinary bladder and urethra. Their functions are secretion, storage and excretion. The kidneys are two bean-shaped organs which lie on either side of the vertebral column at the level of the last thoracic and first lumbar vertebrae. They are richly supplied with blood from branches of the aorta and vena cava.

The need for an abundant supply of blood to the kidneys becomes apparent when one realizes that nearly one fourth of the body's blood is filtered by the kidneys at one time. Waste products are retained in the kidneys in urine to be excreted, while the remainder of the fluid is returned to the blood. During a 24-hour period, the kidneys handle as much as 200 quarts of liquid, excreting only 1½ to 2 quarts as urine.

The nephron is the functioning unit of the kidney. Each kidney is composed of about one million nephrons, and each nephron can form urine by

itself. Thus, to understand the function of the nephron is to understand the function of the kidney. The basic function of the nephron is to filter a large portion of the blood plasma out of the blood stream and through the glomerular membrane. Unwanted substances such as urea, creatinine, uric acid and other wastes are retained in the tubules, while water and many electrolytes are allowed to re-enter the blood stream. The water and wastes remaining in the tubules are excreted as urine.

The ureters, one from each kidney, convey the urine by peristaltic action from the kidney to the urinary bladder. The bladder serves as a reservoir and holds the urine until its normal distention of 300 cc. to 400 cc., when the urge to urinate compels emptying the bladder. The urine passes from the bladder through the urethra to the outside. The urethra is approximately 1½ inches long in the female and 8 inches in the male.

The kidneys and urinary tract are responsible for maintaining the proper balance of fluids, minerals and organic substances necessary for life. In view of this fact, it is not surprising that a diseased condition of any one system of the body may have a direct effect on the kidneys and urinary tract. Generalized diseases such as arteriosclerosis, other circulatory lesions, infections or disturbances in the metabolic processes may very seriously impair the proper functioning of the kidneys. Similarly, involvement of the heart, lungs or circulatory system can arise from kidney failure.

Diseases, like human beings, will not always conveniently fit into clearly defined categories. The body functions as a whole, and the systems are interdependent. This chapter will be concerned primarily with diseases of the urinary system; however, it should be remembered that the nurse will frequently have need for a good working knowledge of the basic principles of urologic nursing in a wide variety of cases under her care.

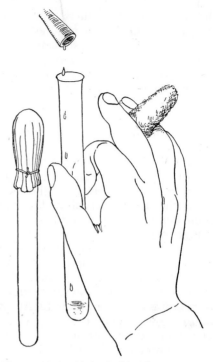

Figure 18–1. Method of holding stopper and tube to collect urine for culture. At left is sterile tube with cotton stopper and paper wrapping. Newer tubes may have cork stoppers. (From Davis and Warren: *Urological Nursing*, 6th Ed., W. B. Saunders Co., Philadelphia.)

DIAGNOSTIC TESTS AND EXAMINATIONS

Urine Culture

A sample of urine is taken by catheter under sterile technique and placed in a sterile culture tube (see Fig. 18-1). After the catheter has been inserted, a small amount of urine should flow through the catheter into the waste basin. This will flush out and partially cleanse the urethra. Approximately 10 cc. of urine should be allowed to drop into the tube, making sure not to let the catheter touch the inside of the tube. The culture tube must be maintained in an upright position so that the urine does not come in contact with the stopper. The tube is then carefully labeled and sent to the laboratory, where cultures are grown under controlled conditions to determine specific types of bacteria present in the urine.

P.S.P. Test

These initials stand for phenolsulfonphthalein, which is a dye administered directly into the vein. The purpose of the test is to estimate the ability of the kidneys to excrete the dye in a given number of hours. Normally, the bright red color will become apparent in the urine within 30 minutes after injection, and after 2 hours have elapsed, more than half the dye should appear in the urine.

Fishberg Concentration Test

This is a relatively simple method for determining the ability of the kidneys to concentrate urine. Normally the kidneys remove a large amount of water from the blood plasma as it passes through the nephron (this is called dilution). Waste products and some water are retained in the tubules, while the remaining water and some minerals are reabsorbed into the plasma. If the renal tubules fail to allow for reabsorption of the water, it remains and is excreted as very dilute urine. If the nephron functions normally, the urine is more concentrated because it contains less water.

In the Fishberg concentration test, the patient is allowed no food or water from after the evening meal the night before the test until after the test, which begins about 10:00 A.M. when the first specimen of urine is collected. An hour later, a second specimen is obtained, and both are properly labeled and sent to the laboratory, where they are tested for specific gravity. A normal specific gravity is between 1.020 and 1.025. A lower specific gravity would mean more dilute urine and would indicate impairment of the kidney's ability to concentrate urine.

X-ray Examinations

Visualization of the urinary tract with x-ray may be achieved by the injection of a contrast medium (one that is opaque to x-ray). The medium used may be given in any one of three ways: (1) directly into the vein (for an intravenous pyelogram), (2) by way of a ureteral catheter (retrograde pyelogram) or (3) through a urethral catheter (cystogram).

The intravenous pyelogram is probably the one used most often, being the simplest and least dangerous method of examining the kidneys, ureters or prostate. It is helpful in diagnosing impairment of kidney function, obstruction, foreign bodies or tumors in the ureters or prostate. The urine should be concentrated in this test so as not to dilute the dye, thus preventing its effectiveness on x-ray film. For this reason, fluids are restricted during preparation of the patient for this test. The retrograde pyelogram must be done during cystoscopy (see the fol-

lowing material) because a catheter is inserted into the ureters and dye injected directly into the ureters.

The cystogram is done to visualize the bladder contour. X-ray films are taken before and after sodium iodide is injected into the bladder through a urethral catheter.

The success of an x-ray examination of the pelvic and abdominal area depends to a great extent on the thoroughness of the preparation. It cannot be stated too often or too strongly that the preparatory procedures done by the nurse must be carried out efficiently and well. Poor preparation leads to unnecessary expense of time and undue taxing of the patient's energy and pocketbook. Methods of cleansing the lower intestinal tract of gas and fecal matter for proper visualization of the urinary tract will vary according to the radiologist's and attending physician's wishes and the individual patient's needs. The nurse must understand the specific orders for catharsis and enemas and carry them out effectively. She must personally supervise the procedures on all patients, male or female.

Blood Analysis

When the filtering plant of the kidney has been affected by disease, there is a slowing down of absorption of wastes from the blood stream. These wastes then begin to accumulate in the blood, upsetting the normal balance in the body. The two most common laboratory tests for these waste products are blood urea nitrogen (BUN) and nonprotein nitrogen (NPN). Both of these must be a "fasting blood" specimen and are drawn in the morning before breakfast. The normal range for these two tests are: BUN, 10 to 20 mg. per 100 ml., NPN, 20 to 40 mg. per 100 ml.

Following all tests requiring restriction of fluids, there will be some dehydration; fluids should be forced during the day unless contraindicated.

Cystoscopy

This is a surgical procedure in which the physician inserts an instrument (the cystoscope) into the bladder through the urethra for the purpose of examining the interior of the bladder.

Patients who are not anesthetized for this procedure should be reassured and encouraged to relax as much as possible during examination. This will decrease the pain and help the examining physician.

Following cystoscopy, the patient may have a general reaction with chills and elevation of temperature. The patient may also have some low back pain and a full sensation with frequent desire to void because of irritation to the mucous membrane. Extensive bleeding or sharp abdominal pain should be reported.

MEASURING THE PATIENT'S LOSS OF FLUIDS

Because the functions of the urinary system are so closely related to the maintenance of the proper fluid balance in the entire body, the loss of fluids from the body is of primary importance in diseases of the urinary system. The physician must depend on the nursing staff for accurate and intelligent observation, measuring and reporting of the patient's output, or loss of fluids. If measurement of the *total urinary output* is required, the nurse must make sure that urine from all points of drainage is measured and the exact amount recorded. For example, urine from a ureterostomy tube and from a urethral catheter should both be included. When *total output* is to be measured, this must include vomitus, watery stools, urine excreted and an estimate of the amount of fluid lost through perspiration.

There are several terms used to describe abnormalities in the flow of urine. These include *retention, suppression* and *residual urine.*

Retention of urine refers to a retaining or holding of urine in the bladder. It may be relieved by inserting a catheter and draining the urine from the bladder. If a catheter is not passed to relieve distention, the bladder will not rupture, but urine will begin to dribble out through the urethra. The retention of urine in the bladder and resulting stretching of the bladder cause severe discomfort to the patient. Nursing measures to induce voiding may be successful, but if they are not, a catheter must be passed. Catheterizations may very easily lead to an infection of the urinary tract and should not be done without a written order from the doctor.

Suppression of urine indicates that the kidneys are unable to produce urine because of some serious malfunction of the kidney cells. There is simply little or no urine being filtered from the blood stream, and if the condition cannot be relieved, uremia (and ultimately death) will follow.

Residual urine is urine retained in the bladder after voiding. When there is poor bladder tone or a partial obstruction of the urethra, the patient may dribble or void only the "overflow," leaving the bladder still unemptied. Residual urine is measured by having the patient void as much urine as possible and then catheterizing him immediately after. Fifteen milliliters is considered a normal amount of residual urine. Any amount over this will become more and more concentrated over a period of time and may lead to an infection or the formation of stones in the bladder.

NURSING CARE OF THE PATIENT WITH A RETENTION CATHETER

A retention catheter is one which is inserted through the urethra into the bladder and left in place so that urine is constantly drained from the bladder. The catheter used most often for this

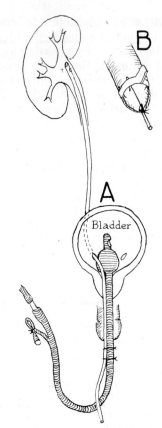

Figure 18–2. *A,* Foley catheter with inflated balloon in place. The balloon may be deflated by releasing tie on small tube or by cutting the small tube if the catheter is the disposable type. The Foley catheter may be used for both male and female patients. *B,* The small tube to left of the Foley catheter is a ureteral catheter, which is passed through the bladder and into the ureter. (From Davis and Warren: *Urological Nursing,* 6th Ed., W. B. Saunders Co., Philadelphia.)

purpose is the Foley catheter, which is specially designed with an inflatable balloon at its tip. The balloon is inflated after the catheter is inserted into the bladder, thereby holding the catheter securely in place so that it is not easily pulled out (see Fig. 18-2).

A retention catheter should always be kept open and draining freely unless there are specific orders to clamp it off. Usually the urine drains by gravity flow, which means that the tube leading from the catheter must lead to a collection bottle which has been placed *below the level of the bladder,* and there must be no looping of the tube below the level of the bottle. A closed container presents fewer possibilities for introducing infectious agents into the urinary tract than does an open container. The amount of drainage in the bottle is measured at least every 8 hours and the amount recorded on the patient's chart. The nurse should report any sandy residue collecting in the tubing or catheter so that they may be changed before there is complete obstruction of the tubing. Sandy residue may be determined by rubbing the tube or catheter between the thumb and fingers. The urinary system is considered to be sterile. For this reason, all tubing and apparatus used in caring for the catheter must be sterile. One must use rigid asepsis when handling the connections for catheter, tubing and drainage bottles (see Fig. 18-3).

The amount, color and content of the urine should be observed closely. Sometimes mucus shreds and bits of tissue or clots may be seen. Various antiseptics, such as pyridium, will cause the urine to be red. Other drugs, dyes and some foods will sometimes change the color and odor of the urine. The presence of what appears to be bright red blood in the catheter should

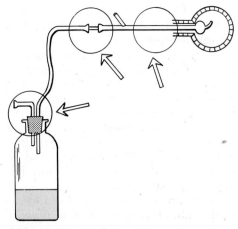

Figure 18–3. Sites at which contamination is most likely to occur.

always be reported immediately, even though the practical nurse may suspect that the coloring is due to something other than blood.

While a catheter is in place, the genitalia and surrounding skin will need extra care. The areas must be kept clean and dry, and creams and powders must be avoided because they tend to cake and further irritate the skin. Soap and water, gently and frequently applied, with thorough rinsing and drying, will do much to prevent odors, irritations and general discomfort of the patient.

If there are clots, mucus plugs or other material obstructing the flow of urine through the catheter, the physician may order irrigations of the catheter. Sometimes it is possible to remove obstructing material by alternately pinching and releasing the tubing as shown in Figure 18-4. The upper hand rapidly squeezes and releases the tube, while the lower hand holds the catheter closed.

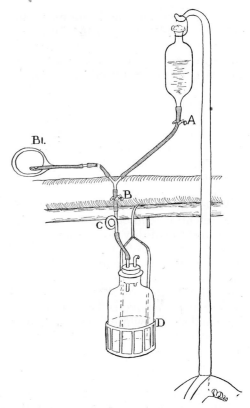

Figure 18–5. Simple apparatus for irrigating bladder through retention catheter. The upper jar is filled with irrigating fluid. Ordinarily clamp A is closed and clamp B is left open so that urine drains freely into bottle D. When irrigation is desired, clamp B is closed and clamp A is opened, thus allowing fluid to run into the bladder (Bl.). After desired amount runs into bladder, clamp A is closed and clamp B is opened. Bottle D rests in a metal frame hung from the bed rail. C is a glass coil used to keep air out of the drainage tube. (From Davis and Warren: *Urological Nursing*, 6th Ed., W. B. Saunders Co., Philadelphia.)

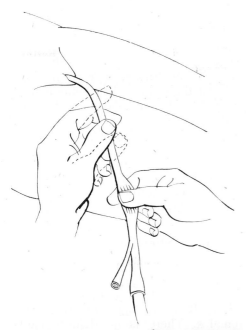

Figure 18–4. Method of "milking" a catheter for the purpose of removing a blood clot or mucus plug obstructing the catheter. (From Sutton: *Bedside Nursing Techniques,* 2nd Ed., W. B. Saunders Co., Philadelphia.)

Constant or intermittent irrigation of the bladder may be necessary to cleanse the bladder and remove clots or other material which may obstruct the catheter. In order to accomplish this, various types of apparatus may be used. The type of equipment will vary according to the wishes of the doctor and the equipment available (see Fig. 18-5). When caring for this type of irrigation, the nurse must have a clear understanding of the type of fluid used for irrigation, any medications or antiseptics to be added to the fluid and the rate of flow desired by the doctor. If measurement of the urinary output is ordered, the amount used for irrigation must be subtracted from the total amount of fluid in the drainage bottle. Care must be taken to avoid contamination of fluids and equipment used for any irrigation, because the irrigating fluid flows directly into the bladder and an infection can easily result.

When the doctor orders removal of the retention catheter, the nurse accepts responsibility for removing the catheter and carefully observing the patient for signs of retention of urine. If a Foley catheter has been inserted, the balloon must, of course, be deflated before it is removed. The catheter is removed slowly while the patient takes a deep breath and lets it out slowly. This will relax the patient and reduce the discomfort. The genital area is washed thoroughly with soap and water and dried. The time of removal of the catheter is recorded, and the patient is observed carefully for signs of difficulty in voiding. A patient with proper fluid intake ought to void within eight hours after removal of a retention catheter. The nurse should report any bleeding, incontinence or dribbling of urine, the last of which may indicate an excessive amount of residual urine.

OTHER MEANS OF ESTABLISHING URINARY FLOW

Aside from the retention catheter mentioned previously, there are several other ways in which a urologist may provide for adequate drainage of urine. The term "retention catheter" or "indwelling catheter" usually refers to a catheter that has been inserted through the urethra. This is the most commonly used method of draining urine. Other means include the following:

Ureteral catheters are very small and of narrow gauge. They are inserted by the urologist directly into the ureters, usually by means of cystoscope. They may be attached to a urethral catheter (see Fig. 18-2).

A *ureterostomy* is a surgical incision into the ureter by way of the abdominal wall. A tube is left in the ureter and permits drainage to the outside.

Nephrostomy and *pyelostomy* tubes are placed directly into the kidney pelvis by way of a surgical wound over the kidney.

Care of these special tubes requires much skill and knowledge and is the responsibility of the physician or registered nurse. A practical nurse must have additional training in urological procedures before attempting to care for a patient who has any one of the previously mentioned tubes inserted.

NEPHRITIS

Definition

Nephritis, sometimes called Bright's disease, refers to a general inflammation and resulting degeneration of the cells of the kidney. The inflammation is not due to an invasion of bacteria and is therefore classified as a *noninfectious* disease. There are two specific diseases classified under the general heading of nephritis. These diseases are glomerulonephritis and nephrosclerosis. Glomerulonephritis may be acute or chronic.

Acute Glomerulonephritis

This condition occurs most frequently in the winter and spring months and is seen primarily in children and young adults. It affects males more often than females. There is no definite cause known; however, it is closely related to and believed to be a complication of an infection by some strains of streptococci. Usually the patient has a history of a recent attack of "strep throat," scarlet fever or chickenpox.

Symptoms. The patient with acute glomerulonephritis usually becomes ill suddenly, with widespread edema, puffiness about the eyes, visual disturbances and marked hypertension. If treatment is not successful, the disease will rapidly progress to uremia and death.

Treatment and Nursing Care. The nurse's first responsibility in the treatment of acute glomerulonephritis is to provide rest for the patient and for the kidney. Absolute bed rest is usually ordered. Though the patient may respond quickly to treatment and, feeling better, wish to become more active, the nurse must explain the need for continued rest and provide an atmosphere for rest. An attitude of willingness to do everything necessary for the patient cheerfully and efficiently will do much to assure the patient of the nurse's sincere interest in him. She should be especially aware of the need for special attention to the diet and fluid intake during the acute phase. The doctor will usually order a sodium restricted diet if edema is present and a limiting of fluids if there is *oliguria* (diminished urine) or *anuria* (absence of urine). The nurse should be sure the patient understands the importance of these factors in the treatment of the disease and do all she can to encourage his cooperation.

Edema that is obvious from external signs may very well be present in the internal organs. For this reason, the blood pressure and pulse must be checked frequently for indications of cerebral edema with increased *intracranial* pressure. Cardiac failure or pulmonary edema may also develop, and the patient must be watched closely for extreme restlessness, increased respiratory difficulty or cyanosis.

Prognosis for acute glomerulonephritis varies, depending upon the extent of permanent damage done to the kidneys or other vital organs.

Chronic Glomerulonephritis

Chronic glomerulonephritis may develop rapidly or progress slowly over a period of years.

Symptoms. There is insidious edema, headache associated with hypertension and dyspnea. The prognosis for this disease is ultimately poor. However, the speed with which it progresses to renal failure and uremia varies with the individual. The exact reason for this is not known. Some patients who develop chronic glomerulonephritis may have acute exacerbations (flare-ups) which subside. Then they may live for several years before damage to the glomeruli of the kidney brings about the uremic state. Others will rapidly pass into uremia and succumb to the disease in a short period of time.

Treatment and Nursing Care. The treatment for chronic glomerulonephritis in the latent stage is primarily *symptomatic* with emphasis on avoiding fatigue and infections, particularly of the upper respiratory tract.

The patient with chronic glomerulonephritis requires much patience and understanding. Often he is aware of the eventual outcome of the disease and may appear stubborn and uncooperative with those who are trying to help him. The nursing care is essentially the same as for acute glomerulonephritis, but is more difficult because of the need for prolonged and constant care and attention to proper rest and diet, with prevention of an infection anywhere in the body. The patient will have periods of irritability and depression. Everything should be done to eliminate undue mental and physical strain on the patient. Obesity must be avoided, and pregnancy is considered extremely dangerous because of the additional work placed on the kidneys during that time. The family will need help in understanding the severity of the disease and adjusting to the fact that the prognosis is poor and death is the eventual outcome.

Nephrosclerosis

Definition. The primary difficulty in this condition is the hardening and narrowing of the small arteries in the kidneys. As the blood supply decreases, the kidney cells degenerate and lose their ability to function. Nephrosclerosis is frequently associated with hardening of the arteries elsewhere in the body.

Symptoms. The symptoms of nephrosclerosis are similar to those of the patient with chronic glomerulonephritis, and the treatment and nursing care are also similar.

PYELONEPHRITIS

Definition

In contrast to the diseases which come under the heading of nephritis, pyelonephritis is an *infection* of the kidney. It is caused by bacterial invasion of the kidney and urinary tract.

Normally the glomeruli of the kidney not only filter the blood passing through them but also destroy the bacteria being carried by the blood. When something happens to interfere with this process, the bacteria may enter and infect the kidney. There are three basic situations which may contribute to the development of a kidney infection: (1) an increase in the number and strength of the bacteria in the blood stream, (2) lowered resistance of the patient to the bacteria and (3) back pressure of urine because of poor drainage from the kidney.

The terminology used in describing the various processes which take place in a kidney infection often confuses those who expect the various steps in the process to represent three distinct diseases. Actually, the classification of infections of the kidney are three stages of the same disease process. *Pyelitis* is an infection of the pelvis of the kidney. *Pyelonephritis* is an inflammation of the kidney pelvis and the kidney cells.

Pyonephrosis is a collection of pus in the kidney pelvis. So we can see that as the infection spreads and pus collects, the diagnosis or name of the disease may change. For the sake of simplifying the discussion of these stages of an infection of the kidney, we will cover the symptoms, treatment and nursing care of the patient with pyelonephritis.

Symptoms

In the acute stage of pyelonephritis, the symptoms include fever, chills, nausea and vomiting and pain in the flank radiating to the thigh and genitalia. The chronic phase is more often insidious, with gradual scarring of the kidney tissues, which results in loss of weight, low-grade fever and weakness. Eventually the urine becomes loaded with bacteria and pus.

Treatment and Nursing Care

Since approximately 90 per cent of the cases of pyelonephritis are associated with an obstruction in the urinary tract, treatment is aimed at removal of the obstruction as well as destruction of the bacteria causing the infection.

Bed rest and forcing fluids are important in the treatment of pyelonephritis. In addition, the nursing care is basically the same as for any severe infection during the acute stage. The urine must be observed closely for amount, changes in color and the presence of pus or a foul odor.

Special diagnostic tests may be done to determine the location of the obstruction if one is suspected.

Specific drugs to destroy the bacteria are usually chosen according to the sensitivity of the causative organism, so that the most effective antibiotic is given. Urinary antiseptics are useful because they are excreted and concentrated in the urine and are capable of inhibiting the growth of bacteria within the urinary system. The sulfonamides, Urotropin and Mandelamine are examples of urinary antiseptics.

The prognosis of the patient depends on the success of the treatment of the active infection before destruction and scarring of the kidney cells can occur. If chronic pyelonephritis develops, the patient may live for years without significant symptoms before renal damage leads to hypertension or uremia.

RENAL FAILURE

Definition

Renal failure or insufficiency means that the kidneys have ceased to function or are only partially functioning as filters. Some substances such as albumin, globulin and red and white cells are not normally passed through the kidneys and into the urine. Their presence in the urine indicates kidney damage and disturbance of kidney function. When renal failure occurs, waste products such as urea salts remain in the blood, and the patient is said to be in a state of uremia. Uremia may occur as an acute condition or develop slowly as a chronic condition.

Acute Uremia. In acute renal failure, the damage is more sudden and rapid in its progress, with injury or total destruction of masses of kidney cells. The causes of acute uremia are usually poisoning from mercury, transfusion reaction or prolonged shock or dehydration. The outlook for acute uremia is better than for chronic uremia; the prognosis depends on the successful restoration of kidney function before permanent damage has been done to the kidney cells.

Chronic Uremia. Chronic uremia is a much slower process, occurring over a period of time. It may present mild symptoms at first, which increase in severity, or the symptoms may be severe at the outset. Prolonged inflammation or damage to the vesicles leads to scarring, and the glomeruli are permanently lost. Hypertension is usually present, and oliguria and anuria are nearly always present. No

SYMPTOMS. Uremia is characterized by depression of consciousness, muscular twitching, impaired vision, convulsions, vomiting, acidosis and dehydration. There is an elevation of nonprotein nitrogen in the blood. There is loss of appetite, and there may or may not be edema.

TREATMENT AND NURSING CARE. Treatment is concerned with decreasing the workload of the kidney and establishing a normal fluid and electrolyte balance. Fluids may be restricted if there is edema and must be spaced at intervals over a 24-hour period.

Nursing care of the patient with uremia presents a real challenge to the nurse. Because the breath is foul and carries odors of urine, diligent mouth care is important. If vomiting is present, there must be a careful measuring and recording of emesis. Fluids may be increased as edema subsides, but if nausea is present, fluids should be given in small amounts at intervals. The skin may itch and be very dry, increasing the irritability of the patient. Sponging the skin with a mild acid solution using two tablespoons of vinegar to one pint of warm water will help to relieve the pruritis. Constipation prevents elimination of wastes through the alimentary tract and must be avoided. Edematous extremities should be elevated on pillows above the level of the heart. Pillows should be protected, since there may be oozing of fluids through pores of the skin. Meticulous care is needed to prevent a breakdown of the skin and resulting pressure sores.

All precautions must be taken to prevent respiratory infections. The nurse must not allow the patient to become chilled, must prevent contact of the patient with others who may have an upper respiratory infection and must turn the patient carefully at least every two hours, avoiding friction of the skin against the sheets.

Observe the patient at all times for twitching or impending convulsions, as they may occur at any time if intracranial pressure increases. Keep equipment at the bedside for prevention of injury to the patient during convulsions. The patient may become extremely irritable and confused; all external stimuli such as noise, bright lights and disturbing visitors should be kept at an absolute minimum.

The family will need help and sympathetic understanding from the nurse during the final stages of chronic uremia. The nurse should avoid assuming a morbid attitude, remembering that the patient may appear comatose, yet still be able to hear what is being said in the room. Attention should be given to the patient's spiritual needs as well as his physical needs. Whatever her personal beliefs may be, the nurse should do all that she can to cooperate with the patient's minister and offer any spiritual and moral support she may be able to give the patient and his family.

DIALYSIS WITH THE ARTIFICIAL KIDNEY

In recent years, medical science has made great strides in development of highly complicated machines and devices designed to assist the human body in its vital functions when trauma or disease have temporarily disrupted these functions. The artificial kidney is one such device that has been developed and is used in large medical centers. It has received much publicity, and since many patients have read or heard of the artificial kidney, the practical nurse should know something of its limitations and the principles on which it operates.

Essentially, the artificial kidney is used to remove from the blood waste products that ordinarily would be filtered by the normal kidney and excreted in the urine. The artificial kidney utilizes the principle of diffusion: solutes in a solution of higher concentration will pass through a semipermeable membrane into a solution of lower concentration. This natural movement

of molecules will continue to take place until the two solutions are of equal concentration. In hemodialysis, the blood of the patient represents the solution of higher concentration. As the blood is circulated through the tubing of the artificial kidney, the impurities pass through the cellophane filter into a "bath" solution containing salt, sugar, sodium bicarbonate and other components of normal plasma. The waste products such as urea are thus removed from the patient's blood (see Fig. 18-6).

At the beginning of each treatment, the artificial kidney is primed with blood that is of the same type as that of the patient. This insures a continuous flow of blood through the tubing. A small pump keeps the blood circulating through the artificial kidney during the treatment, which lasts from 10 to 16 hours, depending on the patient's body size, the amount of renal function that remains and the amount of wastes to be removed.

Artificial kidneys have been used for treatment of patients with acute renal problems since the early 1900's, but it was not until 1960 that those with chronic renal failure could hope to benefit from the artificial kidney. It was at this time that a specialized type of cannula was devised (see Fig. 18-7). The cannula is left in the patient's arm at all times and is replaced only once or twice a year. It eliminates the need for a cutdown each time the patient receives hemodialysis and provides ready access to the patient's blood stream when hemodialysis is indicated.[5]

At the present time, there are many patients whose lives depend on the artificial kidney. These people must return to a chronic dialysis unit in a hospital two or three times a week for an indefinite period. Since their kidneys are functioning very little or not at all, they must depend on the dialysis unit to remove urea and other waste from their blood. They must maintain strict adherence to a low-protein diet to help reduce the amount of waste prod-

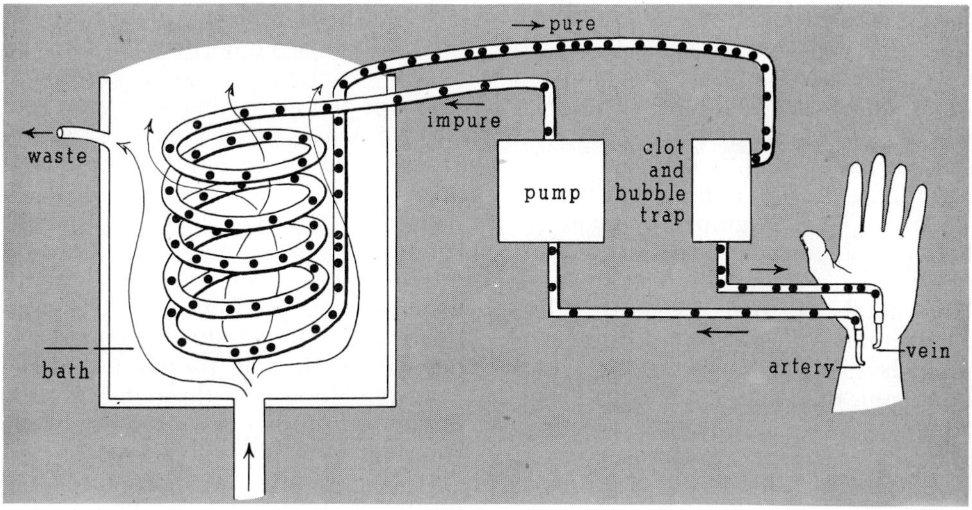

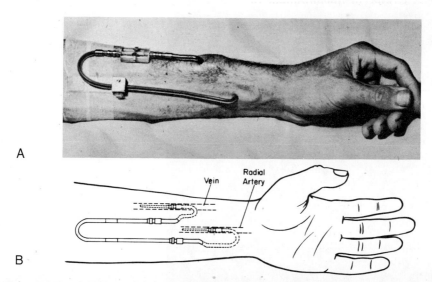

Figure 18–6. Schematic diagram of the artificial kidney. (From Jacob and Francone: *Structure and Function in Man,* 2nd Ed., W. B. Saunders Co., Philadelphia.)

ucts in the blood, and they must limit their sodium intake so that edema and hypertension can be controlled.

One factor that limits the availability of hemodialysis to all patients who can benefit from it is the tremendous cost of the unit. Also, it is difficult or impossible for some individuals to make repeated visits to a clinic. At this writing, there are more persons needing treatment than there are hemodialysis units available for their use. This means that

Figure 18–7. *A,* The cannula, the semipermanent appliance in a patient's arm. The Silastic material is shown coming out of the patient's skin; one side is long and the other side short. The Silastic is connected to the Teflon joint, and the metal rings hold the Teflon inside the Silastic so that the cannula does not come apart. *B,* Schematic drawing showing the two Teflon tips within the vein and artery. The diameter of the beveled tips that are inserted in the vessels ranges from size 13 ($^1/_8$ inch) to size 18 (less than $^1/_{16}$ inch). (From Fellows: Nursing Clinics of North America, December, 1966.)

someone must make the difficult decision as to who will receive the treatment and who will not. There has been some effort to establish a program whereby the hemodialysis unit is installed in the patient's home so that he can utilize the unit at night while he is sleeping. This program has many inherent problems for the patient and his family and may not be feasible for a large number of patients, but it is less costly than a hospital unit and some patients feel that the advantages of a home unit outweigh its disadvantages.

PERITONEAL DIALYSIS

This procedure can be used as an alternative to the use of an artificial kidney. The semipermeable membrane in this case is the peritoneum and the "wash" solution is introduced into the space of the abdominal cavity. There are two phases in peritoneal dialysis— the infusion phase and the withdrawal phase.

In the infusion phase, 2 liters of solution of glucose and electrolytes are introduced into the abdominal cavity via a catheter (see Fig. 18-8). The solution is left in the cavity about one hour, during which time the wastes in the patient's blood pass through the walls of the local blood vessels and into the solution in the abdominal cavity.

During the withdrawal phase, the fluid, which now contains the wastes, is removed by gravity flow. The cycle of infusion, dialysis and withdrawal is

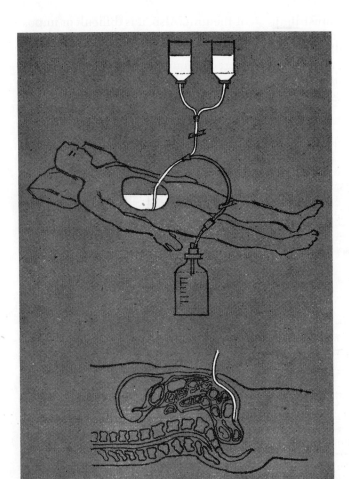

Figure 18–8. Peritoneal dialysis. (From Watkins: American Journal of Nursing, July, 1966.)

repeated until blood tests reveal a near normal level of chemicals in the blood.[13]

The chief disadvantage of peritoneal dialysis is the danger of peritonitis. One also should realize that peritoneal dialysis will not permanently relieve the symptoms of a patient with chronic renal failure. It can be used to remove wastes until a kidney transplant or other procedure is done or until an acute renal condition is corrected, but it is not a cure for renal failure.

CYSTITIS

Definition

Cystitis is an inflammation of the bladder and one of the most common disorders of the urinary tract. It is rarely a primary disease and is often a symptom of some other disturbance in either the urinary tract or the genital tract. Acute cystitis occurs more frequently in females because of the close proximity of the bladder to the genital area and the relative shortness of the female urethra in comparison to the male urethra.

Symptoms

The patient with cystitis is extremely uncomfortable, with frequent and urgent desires to void. There is often a burning sensation at the completion of each act of voiding. Hematuria (blood in the urine) is sometimes present. A general reaction with fever and chills is not characteristic of cystitis and suggests an extension of the infection to the kidneys.

Treatment and Nursing Care

Treatment of cystitis is aimed at removal of the underlying cause and prevention of the spread of the infection beyond the bladder. Urinary antiseptics and, sometimes, antibiotics may be necessary to control the infection. The nursing care consists of simple mea-

sures to relieve the symptoms. Rest is important, and heat in the form of sitz baths, vaginal douches or suprapubic heat will do much to allay the discomfort.

URETHRITIS

Definition

Urethritis is an inflammation of the urethra. It can be caused by many different organisms. Urethritis is one of the most common symptoms of gonorrhea, however, and should be investigated when it is first noticed. In the female, trauma from childbirth and the proximity of the genital organs to the urethra predispose the urethra to infection.

Symptoms

The chief symptoms of urethritis are burning, itching, frequency in voiding and painful urination. A discharge is present and becomes increasingly more purulent if gonorrhea is present. The urinary meatus is swollen and inflamed.

Treatment and Nursing Care

Treatment begins with determination of the causative organism and the administration of specific drugs to combat the infection. The nursing care is similar to that for the patient with cystitis. The nurse should be especially aware of the possibility of a gonorrheal infection until a definite diagnosis has been established and carry out the necessary precautions against spread of the infection to the eyes.

OBSTRUCTIONS OF THE URINARY TRACT

Hydronephrosis

Definition. Whenever the normal flow of urine is obstructed, there follows a backward flow of fluid into the kidney pelvis. If this condition is not relieved by removal of the obstruction, the kidney becomes dilated and continues to fill with fluid. Soon the kidney cells will atrophy until all normal function ceases and the kidney becomes merely a thin, walled cyst. This condition is known as *hydronephrosis*. It can eventually result in complete destruction of the kidney. The condition may be *unilateral* or *bilateral* (one or both kidneys). If it occurs only on one side, the other kidney may enlarge and efficiently carry on the work of two kidneys. This is called *compensatory hypertrophy.*

Symptoms. Severe pain is present only if hydronephrosis develops rapidly. Otherwise, there are no outstanding symptoms, and the patient may develop signs of uremia only after serious damage has occurred.

Treatment and Nursing Care. The primary goal of the treatment is removal of the obstruction so the kidney may drain properly. The ideal situation is drainage of the kidney in the early stages. If the damage is irreparable, the kidney is removed by surgery. The nursing care of the patient with hydronephrosis is concerned with close observation and accurate reporting of urinary output, and of early signs of impending uremia. If nephrectomy is necessary, the nursing care is the same as for any patient with nephrectomy.

Nephroptosis

Definition. The kidney usually lies with its flat surface against the posterior wall of the body and is well padded with fat. If the pad of fat is absent or the *pedicle* of the kidney is longer than usual, the kidney may move backward and forward freely or sag below its normal position when the patient stands. This condition is known as nephroptosis or "floating kidney." It occurs most commonly in middle-aged women who are thin and long waisted.

Symptoms. Nephroptosis may cause no symptoms or disability; however, it has the potential of causing a twisting or kinking of the ureters with resulting hydronephrosis. In some patients, there is pain in the kidney region, aggravated by standing and relieved by lying down and elevating the hips.

Treatment and Nursing Care. Palliative treatment is directed at relief of symptoms by bed rest, weight-gaining techniques and abdominal support with belts or braces. The patient wearing supporting belts or braces should be instructed to apply them on arising in the morning, when the kidney is nearest to its normal position after a night's rest. Surgical fixation of the kidney by suturing it in its normal position (*nephropexy*) is sometimes done when other measures fail. The nursing care after nephropexy is the same as for nephrectomy, though there is less danger of hemorrhage and the patient should have a more rapid recovery. The foot of the bed is sometimes elevated postoperatively to help the kidney maintain a normal position and to avoid strain on the sutures.

Renal Calculi

Definition. For reasons not yet fully determined, some people have a tendency to manufacture stones in the kidney from deposits of crystalline substances normally excreted in the urine. These stones may vary in size from "sand or gravel" to large stones the size of an orange. Some are star-shaped and are called "renal stars." They may be found anywhere in the urinary tract and, if small enough, are flushed out by the urine without any noticeable symptoms. Otherwise, they may obstruct the flow of urine at any point from the kidney to the bladder. These stones are closely associated with urinary tract infections, hyperparathyroidism and its accompanying hypercalcemia, or bone lesions. Men are more often affected than women.

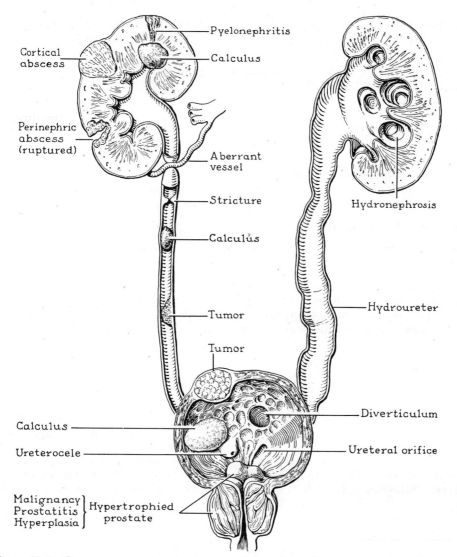

Figure 18-9. Commonly encountered male urogenital problems. (From Brunner et al.: *Textbook of Medical-Surgical Nursing*, J. B. Lippincott Co., Philadelphia.)

Symptoms. Usually there is a dull aching in the lower back with increased production of urine. Blood and pus are found to be present in the urine. If the stone is small and attempts to pass through the ureter, it will often scrape the lining of the ureter and present the dramatic symptoms of *renal colic*. The pain of renal colic is a sudden agonizing pain starting in the flank of the affected side and radiating from there down the ureter to the genitalia and along the inner side of the thigh. These symptoms are frequently accompanied by nausea and vomiting and extreme *diaphoresis*.

Treatment and Nursing Care. The simplest method of treating stones would be by dissolving them or causing them to pass spontaneously; however, though much research is being done, at present there is no way known to accomplish this. When a patient is admitted for kidney stones, most urologists choose to wait a reasonable length of time for the stone to pass spontaneously, as a large percentage do. During this period, the nurse should encourage fluids unless otherwise ordered and strain all urine through cheesecloth or gauze in order to catch the stone should it pass with the urine. If the stone is not passed, a surgical procedure is necessary to remove it. The type of surgery will depend upon the location of the stone.

TUMORS OF THE KIDNEY

Definition

Neoplasms of the kidney are fairly uncommon, actually constituting less than 1 per cent of all malignant tumors of the body. They are, however, nearly always cancerous and are extremely difficult to treat in the later stages. Except for Wilm's tumors (see the material following), they occur mostly in middle life.

Symptoms

The principal symptom of malignant tumors of the kidney is *hematuria* (blood in the urine), which is usually not accompanied by pain in the early stages. There may be an enlargement of the affected kidney. Diagnosis can be made fairly easily by a retrograde pyelogram.

Treatment and Nursing Care

The only treatment that has met with any degree of success is surgical removal of the affected kidney before *metastasis* has occurred. Unfortunately, this is difficult to achieve, because the patient usually does not have symptoms severe enough to send him to the doctor until it is too late. Postoperative radiation is sometimes used to deter further involvement after nephrectomy. The nursing care of the patient is that for patients receiving radiation therapy and postoperative care following nephrectomy.

Wilms' Tumors

Definition. Wilms' tumors of the kidney are thought to be congenital in origin. The average age of onset is three years. Since these tumors are highly malignant and metastasize quickly, the death rate is very high.

Treatment and Nursing Care. Treatment of Wilms' tumor is by nephrectomy. If the tumor is caught early and the kidney removed during the first year of life, the chances of cure are much better.

CARE OF THE PATIENT WHO HAS HAD SURGERY OF THE KIDNEY

Types of Surgery

The two main types of surgical procedures which may be performed on the kidney are *nephrectomy* and *nephrostomy.*

Nephrectomy is the surgical removal of the kidney. Although this is always a serious operation, a person may live with only one kidney. The remaining kidney enlarges and is usually able to carry on the work formerly done by two kidneys.

Nephrostomy is a surgical incision into a kidney for the purpose of providing an artificial means of draining the kidney. This procedure may be done in the treatment of obstructions from large stones or strictures of the ureter or to drain purulent material from an infected kidney.

Nursing Care

In either a nephrectomy or nephrostomy, the surgical incision may be lumbar, transabdominal or thoracic. When the patient returns from surgery, the nurse must check carefully for the location of the surgical wound and the presence of any drains or tubes that may have been inserted during the operation. Attachment of these tubes to drainage bottles or other bedside equipment is the responsibility of the nurse in charge.

Dressings over the surgical wound may be reinforced, but they should not be changed by the nurse unless there are specific written orders to do so. The drainage on these dressings will be blood-tinged at first, but it should gradually become clearer. If bright red blood appears or there is a sudden change in the amount of drainage, the doctor should be notified. Sometimes the drains will have a sterile safety pin attached to the end. This pin must be kept closed at all times and must never be attached to the dressings, the patient's gown or the bedclothes. Extreme care must be taken during the changing of dressings that the drains or tubes are not dislodged or pulled from the surgical incision.

Positioning of the patient depends on the wishes of the surgeon. He may prefer to have the patient lie only on the operative side. The nurse must determine his wishes and follow his orders explicitly in this matter. Turning the patient may be difficult at first because it is usually quite painful for him to move about. The nurse should explain the need for frequent turning and deep breathing so that complications may be prevented.

Hemorrhage is always a danger after surgery of the kidney. It will be remembered that the kidneys have a very rich supply of blood directly from the aorta and vena cava. The vital signs are carefully checked and any indication of shock or hemorrhage reported immediately.

Adequate drainage from the opposite kidney after surgery is of great concern to the physician. Urinary output must be very carefully measured and recorded. Fluids are usually restricted immediately after surgery and then are gradually increased as the remaining kidney compensates for the loss of its partner. If a nephrostomy has been done, fluids are restricted until the affected kidney can recover sufficiently and resume its functions.

TUMORS OF THE BLADDER

Definition

Most tumors of the bladder are malignant, and the prognosis for cure is generally not good. However, superficial tumors, if detected in the early stages, have a more favorable prognosis.

Symptoms

Frequency of urination, *dysuria* (painful or difficult urination) and hematuria are the most common symptoms of bladder tumor. In the later stages, as the tumor becomes larger, there may be an obstruction of the flow of urine.

Treatment and Nursing Care

The treatment for bladder tumor is complete or partial removal of the bladder with transplantation of the ureters to the outside or to the intestinal tract. During the preoperative period, extra care must be taken to observe the patient for hemorrhage from the bladder. Clots or obstruction of the urinary flow or the tumor itself may cause severe bladder spasms and pain. If the patient has a retention catheter in place, care must be taken to maintain open drainage.

CARE OF THE PATIENT HAVING SURGERY OF THE BLADDER AND URETERS

Types of Surgery

Cystectomy is the surgical removal of the bladder. *Ureterostomy* is a surgi-

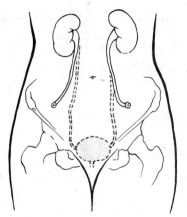

Figure 18–10. Cystectomy and cutaneous ureterostomies. (From *Essentials of Cancer Nursing*, American Cancer Society, Inc.)

cal incision into the ureter for the purpose of diverting the flow of urine. If the bladder is removed, there obviously must be some means of diverting the flow of urine that normally would pass through the ureters and into the bladder. One procedure is a *cutaneous ureterostomy* in which the ureters are transplanted to the skin on the abdomen (see Fig. 18-10). This is a relatively safe procedure, but it is fre-

quently complicated by stricture of the ureter at the point where it joins the skin or fascia.

Another surgical procedure necessitated by cystectomy is ureterosigmoidostomy, in which the ureters are attached to the sigmoid colon, which then acts as a reservoir for the urine (see Fig. 18-11A).

A third procedure involves suturing the ureters to an isolated section of ileum that is connected to an opening in the skin (see Fig. 18-11B). The open ends of intestines where the section of ileum was removed are rejoined by anastomosis. ILEAL CONDUIT

Nursing Care

Nursing care following cystectomy is always difficult because of the danger of hemorrhage and infection. There are also problems involved in devising a satisfactory arrangement for the collection of urine. If ureterostomy tubes have been inserted and brought to the outside, the drainage will keep the dressings wet because urine is constantly dribbling through the ureters from the kidney. The dressings must be

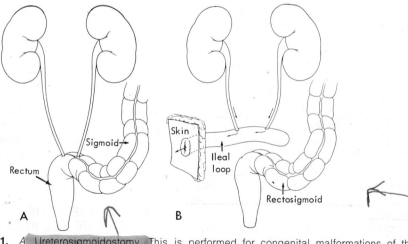

Figure 18–11. *A,* Ureterosigmoidostomy. This is performed for congenital malformations of the bladder and carcinoma of the bladder and pelvic organs. Problems: chronic infection of the urinary tract, reabsorption of urinary electrolytes, and malignancy at the site of ureter implantation. *B,* Ileal conduit. Performed when the bladder (and often the rectum also) has been removed. Problems: patient must wear ileostomy appliance and stricture may develop at the implant site. (From Bloom and Merrill: G. P., *23:*91, 1961.)

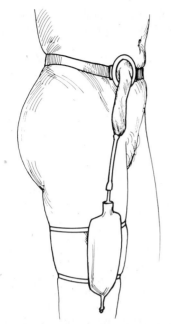

Figure 18–12. A rubber leg urinal draining urine from a ureter implanted into the skin. The end of the bag can be unplugged periodically during the day to allow the urine that has collected to flow out.

changed quite frequently and some waterproof material used to protect the patient's gown and bed linens. The skin around the tubes must also receive special attention to prevent irritation.

There are special cups and appliances available for the collection of urine after a cutaneous ureterostomy or ileal conduit (see Fig. 18-12). These are similar in principle to the colostomy bag, but must be worn constantly because there is no way to control the flow of urine from the kidneys. The patient must have adequate instruction in the daily care of his ureterostomy cup. It is possible for many patients to wear these appliances, resuming their former activities without embarrassment or restriction.

Practical nurses wishing to know more about cutaneous ureterostomies are referred to references at the end of this chapter.

TRAUMATIC INJURIES TO THE KIDNEY AND URETERS

Definition

Accidental injury to the kidneys, ureters, bladder or urethra occurs frequently and should always be considered a possibility whenever there has been trauma to the abdominal cavity or thoracic cage.

Symptoms

The chief symptoms indicating trauma to the kidney are: gross hematuria, pain and tenderness in the renal area and an enlarged mass in the flank.

Treatment and Nursing Care

Since bleeding in the kidney is often self-limiting, most urologists advocate a period of watchful waiting before doing surgery. This is done with the hope that the kidney may be saved. During this time of observation, the nurse must be constantly alert for the early signs of shock and hemorrhage in the patient. Strict bed rest must be enforced, and precautions taken against infections. Nephrectomy may be necessary if there is persistent hemorrhage or an infection developing. Nursing care of the patient with a nephrectomy is discussed in the preceding material.

TRAUMATIC INJURIES TO THE BLADDER

Definition

Any violent blow or crushing injury to the lower abdomen may result in rupture or perforation of the bladder wall with resulting leakage of the urine into the pelvic tissues or peritoneal cavity. This brings about a severe inflammation in these areas.

Symptoms

Early symptoms of bladder injury are painful hematuria, or inability to void, marked tenderness and spasm in the suprapubic area or the development of a large mass in that area.

Treatment and Nursing Care

If the bladder has ruptured or is perforated, treatment consists of a suprapubic cystostomy for the purpose of providing drainage of blood and urine. Care of the patient demands meticulous care and attention to drains and dressings to avoid infection and maintain good drainage. Cold applications may be ordered to the swollen area before surgery and to the operative area following surgery. The nurse should observe the patient carefully for postoperative shock and massive hemorrhage. Any formation of a mass in the suprapubic area before or after surgery, or any change in the vital signs, should be reported immediately.

In addition to physical distress, the patient with bladder injuries is likely to have emotional difficulties in dealing with the problems arising from the sudden loss of his control over the urinary flow and the intimate procedures and treatments necessary. The nurse must be prepared for this and do all she can to encourage and help the patient through this difficult period of adjustment.

Regardless of the diagnosis, patients with urological problems must be approached with an attitude of dignity and composure. Depending on his age, personality, place in the family and community and severity of his illness, the patient's attitude toward these problems will vary. Whatever his reaction to necessary treatments and nursing care, the nurse must remain in control of the situation. By her professional bearing and dignity, she can alleviate much embarrassment, indicating that her primary concern is for the welfare of the patient.

CLINICAL CASE PROBLEMS

1. Mrs. Spence, age 45, is admitted to the medical service with a diagnosis of chronic glomerulonephritis. Her blood pressure is 190 diastolic and 80 systolic, pulse 88 and irregular. She has generalized edema and shortness of breath. Her skin is very dry and shows marked excoriation where she has scratched herself to relieve itching. She has very long, heavily polished fingernails in which she takes great pride.

Mrs. Spence's two children, aged 25 and 23 years, have heard about the artificial kidney and are very anxious to have Mrs. Spence sent to the city 80 miles away for treatment. They ask you if you think they should change doctors and have her transferred.

Mr. Spence travels, and on his visits to his wife, he displays an attitude of indifference and impatience toward her illness. In an effort to show some interest, he usually brings her a box of chocolate candy and salted nuts.

What nursing problems do you find in this situation?

How would you, as a practical nurse, be able to help in the solution of some of these problems?

What special nursing care would you expect this situation to require?

2. Mrs. Downs is a 35-year-old patient who has had a nephrostomy for treatment of hydronephrosis. She returns from surgery with a urethral catheter, a ureteral catheter and a rubber Penrose drain in place.

Explain the purpose of a ureteral catheter.

gravity 5 – 8 cc only in ureteral cath returned by gravity

Type and amt of solution – amt returned STERILE

tissue closes fast

What special care must be taken with the urethral catheter and the drainage apparatus?

What information should you have before irrigating the urethral catheter? *Label which R & L*

What special care will be required by the drain that has been inserted in the operative area? *✓ dry – sterile*

Not in place Call Dr immediately

3. A friend of yours tells you that she has been very uncomfortable during the past week because of frequency of urination and burning when she voids. Last night, she had a severe chill and some elevation of temperature. She has been told that she probably has a very common ailment in women and that if she will drink a lot of fluids, it will probably go away.

What would be your advice to this person?

How would you explain the need for her to follow your advice? *cystitis*

fever & chills often indicate
kidney involvement –
control infection – antibiotics
Dr find cause

REFERENCES

1. Beland, I. L.: *Clinical Nursing: Pathophysical and Psychosocial Approaches,* 2nd edition. New York, The Macmillan Co., 1970.
2. Brand, L., and Komorita, N.: "Adapting to Long-Term Hemodialysis." Am. Journ. Nurs., Aug., 1966, p. 1778.
3. Brunner, L. S., et al.: *Textbook of Medical-Surgical Nursing,* 2nd edition. Philadelphia, J. B. Lippincott Co., 1970.
4. Downing, S.: "The Patient Who Has Peritoneal Dialysis." Am. Journ. Nurs., July, 1966, p. 1572.
5. Fellows, B. J.: "The Role of the Nurse in a Chronic Dialysis Unit." Nurs. Clin. N. Amer., Vol. 1, No. 4, 1966, p. 577.
6. Fellows, G.: "Hemodialysis at Home." Am. Journ. Nurs., Aug., 1966, p. 1775.
7. Isler, C.: "Hemodialysis." RN, Dec., 1970, p. 23.
8. Jacob, S. W., and Francone, C. A.: *Structure and Function in Man,* 2nd edition. Philadelphia, W. B. Saunders Co., 1970.
9. Langford, T. L.: "Nursing Problem: Bacteria and the Indwelling Catheter." Am. Journ. Nurs., Jan., 1972, p. 113.
10. Murray, B. S., et al.: "The Patient Has an Ileal Conduit." Am. Journ. Nurs., Aug., 1971, p. 1560.
11. Shafer, K. N., et al.: *Medical-Surgical Nursing,* 5th edition. St. Louis, The C. V. Mosby Co., 1971.
12. Smith, D., et al.: *Care of the Adult Patient,* 3rd edition. Philadelphia, J. B. Lippincott Co., 1971.
13. Watkins, F. I.: "The Patient Who Has Peritoneal Dialysis." Am. Journ. Nurs., July, 1966, p. 1575.

seperate areas on I & O sheet

SUGGESTED STUDENT READING

1. Davis, J. E.: "Drugs for Urologic Disorders." Am. Journ. Nurs., Aug., 1965, p. 107.
2. Fellows, G.: "Hemodialysis at Home." Am. Journ. Nurs., Aug., 1966, p. 1775.
3. Murray, et al.: "The Patient Has an Ileal Conduit." Am. Journ. Nurs., Aug., 1971, p. 1560.
4. Santora, D.: "Preventing Hospital-Acquired Urinary Infection." Am. Journ. Nurs., April, 1966, p. 790.
5. Schlotter, L.: "Dialysis for Kidney Failure." Journ. Pract. Nurs., Sept., 1970, p. 24.
6. Zielinski, J.: "Terminal Uremia." Journ. Pract. Nurs., Feb., 1965, p. 33.

OUTLINE FOR CHAPTER 18

I. Introduction

A. Urinary system composed of kidneys, ureters, urinary bladder and urethra.

B. Urinary system maintains proper balance of fluids, minerals and organic substances necessary for life.

C. Generalized diseases such as circulatory disorders and metabolic disturbances can affect function of the kidneys.

II. Diagnostic Tests and Examinations

A. Urine culture determines specific microorganisms causing infection.

B. P.S.P. test estimates ability of kidneys to excrete dye.

C. Fishberg concentration test determines kidney's ability to concentrate urine.

D. X-ray examinations visualize the urinary tract through the use of a radiopaque material, which can be given directly into the vein (intravenous pyelogram), by way of a ureteral catheter (retrograde pyelogram) or through a urethral catheter (cystogram).

E. Blood analysis determines the kidney's ability to remove wastes such as urea nitrogen and nonprotein nitrogen from the blood.

F. Cystoscopy is insertion of a cystoscope into the bladder for the purpose of examining the interior surface.

III. Measuring the Patient's Loss of Fluids

A. Nursing staff responsible for accurate measuring and recording of output.

B. Total urinary output measures all urine obtained from all catheters.

C. Total output must include vomitus, watery stools, urine excreted and an estimate of fluid lost through perspiration.

D. Retention of urine means urine is held in the bladder, patient is unable to void.

E. Suppression of urine means kidneys are unable to produce urine.

F. Residual urine remains in the bladder after the patient has voided.

IV. Nursing Care of Patient with Retention Catheter

A. Catheter must be kept open and draining freely.

B. Drainage bottle must be kept lower than bladder.

C. Tubing and container must be handled with care to avoid introducing infection into the bladder. Tubing is changed when sandy residue builds up.

D. Urine amount is measured at intervals. Urine is observed for color, content, peculiar odor or other noticeable characteristics.

E. Genitalia and surrounding skin must receive extra care.

F. Irrigations should be done according to the physician's orders. Nurse must be sure to use correct solution and amount.

G. After removal of retention catheter, patient is watched for ability to void, bleeding, incontinence and dribbling of urine.

V. Other Means of Establishing Urinary Flow

A. Ureteral catheter—inserted directly into the ureter.

B. Ureterostomy—a surgical incision into the ureter to insert catheter or drain.

C. Nephrostomy—surgical incision into kidney for the purpose of drainage.

VI. Nephritis (General Inflammation and Resulting Degeneration of the Renal Cells)

scarlet fever

A. Acute glomerulonephritis—closely related to streptococcal infections.
   1. Symptoms—widespread edema, visual disturbances and marked hypertension.
   2. Treatment—rest, low-sodium diet and observation for signs of increased intracranial pressure, cardiac failure or pulmonary edema.

I = 0

B. Chronic glomerulonephritis—may develop rapidly or over a period of years.
   1. Symptoms—insidious edema, headache associated with hypertension and dyspnea.
   2. Treatment and nursing care—primarily symptomatic with emphasis on avoiding fatigue and infections. No cure.

C. Nephrosclerosis—hardening and narrowing of the small arteries in the kidneys leading to degeneration of renal cells.
   1. Symptoms and treatment similar to those of chronic glomerulonephritis.

VII. Pyelonephritis (Infection of the Kidneys Due to Bacterial Invasion)

A. May develop from:

Pyelonephritis

1. Increase in strength and number of bacteria in the blood stream.
2. Lowered resistance of the patient.
3. Back pressure of urine because of poor drainage from kidney.

B. Symptoms—fever, chills, nausea and vomiting and pain in the flank radiating to the thigh and genitalia. Later symptoms— weight loss, weakness and bacteria and pus cells in the urine.

C. Treatment and nursing care—bed rest, fluids, careful observation of urine for amount, color and odor, urinary antiseptics and antibiotics.

VIII. Renal Failure (Renal Insufficiency)

A. Kidneys fail to function as filters. Indicated by the presence in the urine of albumin, globulin and red and white blood cells.

B. Uremia—the accumulation in the blood stream of waste products such as urea and urea salts.

  1. Acute uremia—sudden and rapid injury or destruction of masses of renal cells. Caused by poisoning from mercury or other heavy metals, transfusion reaction, prolonged shock or dehydration.

  2. Chronic uremia. Caused by prolonged inflammation or damage to renal cells.

    a. Symptoms—depression of consciousness, muscular twitching or convulsions, impaired vision, vomiting, acidosis and dehydration. Elevation of nonprotein nitrogen in the blood.

↑ NPN

    b. Treatment and nursing care—concerned with decreasing workload of kidneys and establishing normal fluid and electrolyte balance. Mouth care, skin care, prevention of respiratory infections, observation of patient for convulsions, delirium and disorientation and provision of nonstimulating environment.

IX. Artificial Kidney

A. Utilizes the principle of dialysis for removal of waste products.

B. Patient's blood is circulated through tubes of cellophane that filter out waste products. Cleansed blood is returned to the patient's body.

C. Development of a specialized type of cannula has made hemodialysis with artificial kidney feasible for patients with chronic renal failure.

X. Peritoneal Dialysis

A. Similar to the artificial kidney, but using the peritoneum as semipermeable membrane. Fluid is injected into the abdominal cavity. Waste products leave blood stream and enter fluid, which is then removed by gravity flow.

B. Chief disadvantage is danger of peritonitis.

XI. Cystitis (Inflammation of the Bladder)

A. Often a symptom of some other disturbance in the urinary tract.

B. Occurs most often in females.

C. Symptoms—frequent urge to urinate, burning sensation during voiding and hematuria; fever and chills in more extensive involvement of urinary tract.

D. Treatment—urinary antiseptics, antibiotics, sitz baths and rest.

XII. Urethritis (Inflammation of the Urethra)

A. Can be caused by many different organisms but often is a symptom of gonorrhea.

B. Symptoms are burning, itching, frequent voiding and painful urination. Purulent discharge may indicate gonorrhea.

C. Treatment involves determination of causative organisms and specific antibiotic to control infection. *c9s*

XIII. Obstructions of the Urinary Tract

A. Hydronephrosis—flow of urine from the kidney obstructed. Kidney becomes dilated and fills with fluid.

1. Symptoms—severe pain occurs only if condition develops rapidly. Otherwise, symptoms are mild and patient may not be aware of condition until uremia develops.
2. Treatment—aimed at removal of obstruction. Patient observed closely for signs of impending uremia, and urinary output noted and recorded. Nephrectomy may be necessary if damage is extensive.

B. Nephroptosis—a sagging of the kidney below its normal position. Condition can lead to kinking of ureter, causing hydronephrosis.
1. Symptoms—sometimes pain in the kidney region that is aggravated by standing.
2. Treatment—bed rest, weight gain, abdominal support with belt or brace and possibly surgical fixation of the kidney by suturing it in its normal position (nephropexy).

XIV. Renal Calculi (Kidney Stones)

A. Exact cause unknown, but closely associated with urinary tract infections, hyperparathyroidism and bone lesions.
B. Symptoms—dull aching pain in lower back with increased urine production. Attempt to pass stone down ureter may cause patient renal colic.
C. Treatment—stone may pass spontaneously, so fluids are encouraged, and urine is strained. Surgical removal necessary for stones which cannot be passed in the urine.

XV. Tumors of the Kidney

A. Neoplasms fairly uncommon but nearly always malignant.
1. Symptoms—hematuria and enlargement of affected kidney.
2. Treatment—surgical removal of affected kidney before metastasis has occurred.
B. Wilms's tumor—a tumor of the kidney thought to be congenital.
1. Average age of onset—three years. Highly malignant and metastasizes rapidly.

2. Treatment—surgical removal as soon as possible.

XVI. Care of the Patient Who Has Had Surgery of the Kidney

A. Two main types of surgery—nephrectomy and nephrostomy.
B. Nursing care.
1. Patient must be checked carefully for catheters and drains and turned carefully to avoid tension on them.
2. Dressings may be reinforced but usually are changed by the surgeon. Some blood-tinged drainage is expected, but bright red drainage must be reported. Most common complication is hemorrhage.
3. Urinary output is measured carefully. Fluids may be restricted.

XVII. Tumors of the Bladder

A. Usually malignant. Prognosis generally not good.
B. Symptoms—frequency of urination, dysuria and hematuria. Possibility of later obstruction to the flow of urine from the bladder.
C. Treatment—surgical removal of part or all of bladder.

XVIII. Care of the Patient Having Surgery of the Bladder and Ureters

A. Cystectomy—surgical removal of the bladder.
B. Ureterostomy—surgical incision into ureter for purpose of providing drainage.
C. Surgical procedures to provide for diversion of flow of urine:
1. Cutaneous ureterostomy—ureters are transplanted to the skin.
2. Ureterosigmoidostomy—ureters are attached to the sigmoid colon.
3. Ileal conduit—a section of ileum connects ureters to abdominal opening.
D. Patient must wear some type of bag or cup for collection of urine. Will require instruction similar to that given a colostomy patient.

XIX. Traumatic Injuries to the Kidney and Ureters

A. Always a possibility when there has been trauma to the abdominal cavity or thoracic cage.

B. Symptoms—gross hematuria, pain and tenderness in renal area and an enlarged mass in the flank.

C. Treatment—watch for signs of shock and hemorrhage. Strict bed rest. Surgery, possibly nephrectomy.

XX. Traumatic Injuries to Bladder

A. Caused by violent or crushing blow to lower abdomen.

B. Symptoms—painful hematuria, inability to void and marked tenderness, spasm or large mass in suprapubic area.

C. Treatment—meticulous care of drains and dressings to avoid infection and to maintain good drainage of urine.

19

Nursing Care of Patients With Disorders of the Endocrine System

calcium from ↓ blood Ca
thyroid & bone breakdown
inhibit bone breakdown

VOCABULARY

Atrophy
Coma
Hypothalamus
Lethargy
Idiopathic
Pruritus

INTRODUCTION

The endocrine system is composed of glands which have no ducts; that is, they pour their secretions directly into the blood stream. These secretions are of great importance to a person's health because they affect the activities of the body tissues; in fact, the nervous system and the endocrine system share the responsibility for controlling *all* activities of every cell in the human body.

The secretions from the endocrine glands are called *hormones*. Hormones are chemical substances capable of stimulating or inhibiting the activities of the cells. They do this by acting as catalysts, which means that they speed up or slow down the chemical changes which take place within the cells and tissues.

The glands of the endocrine system do not always function independently of one another. In some instances, the hormones from one endocrine gland may directly affect the function of other endocrine glands, thus making the study of these glands and their functions very complex and somewhat difficult to understand. There is still much research and scientific investigation to be done before the endocrine glands and the part they play in our health and well-being can be completely understood.

Diseases resulting from an abnormal functioning of the endocrine glands may result from overactivity and increase in secretions from the gland or underactivity and a decrease in production of hormones. The prefixes *hyper-* and *hypo-* are often used to designate the condition present. For example, hyperthyroidism means overactivity of the thyroid gland and an increase in the secretion of its hormone, *thyroxine.* Hypothyroidism is just the opposite—that is, underactivity of the gland and deficiency in the secretion of thyroxine.

TABLE 19–1. FUNCTIONS OF ENDOCRINE GLANDS

Gland	Hormone	Action of Hormone
PITUITARY		
Anterior lobe	Thyrotropic hormone	Stimulates thyroid gland.
	Somatotropic hormone	Stimulates growth.
	Gonadotropic hormones (LH, FSH, LTH)	Affect growth, maturity, and functioning of primary and secondary sex organs.
	Adrenocorticotropic hormone (ACTH)	Stimulates cortex of adrenal glands.
Posterior lobe	Antidiuretic hormone	Decreases production of urine.
	Oxytocic principle *Pitocin*	Stimulates uterine contractions.
THYROID	Thyroxin	Stimulates metabolism (catabolic phase).
PARATHYROID	Parathormone	Regulates blood calcium level. *increase blood ca*
ADRENAL		
Cortex	Hormones divided into three main groups:	
	Glucocorticoids	Tend to increase amount of sugar in blood.
	Mineralocorticoids	Tend to increase amount of blood sodium and decrease amount of potassium in blood.
	Androgens (male hormones)	Govern certain secondary sex characteristics. All corticoids important for defense against stress or injury to body tissues.
Medulla	Epinephrine (Adrenalin); "fight or flight" hormone	Elevates blood pressure. Converts glycogen to glucose when needed by muscles for energy. Increases heartbeat rate. Dilates bronchioles.
OVARIES	Estrone and progesterone	Stimulate development of secondary sex characteristics. Affect repair of endometrium after menstruation
TESTES	Testosterone	Essential for normal functioning of male reproductive organs. Stimulates development of male secondary sex characteristics.
ISLANDS OF LANGERHANS ON PANCREAS	Insulin	Promotes metabolism of carbohydrates.

DISEASES OF THE THYROID GLAND

Introduction

The thyroid gland is located below the pharynx in front of and on either side of the trachea. It secretes *thyroxine* and several other closely related hormones that regulate the rate at which the tissues of the body work. Since thyroxine acts to increase the metabolic activities in most cells of the body, it can, by increasing the nutritive demands of the tissues, affect the heart rate, blood flow, respiration, secretion of gastric juices and muscular functions.

In order to maintain a normal basal metabolic rate, there must be precisely the right amount of thyroxine secreted at all times. The control of the rate of thyroid secretion is a function of the adenohypophysis (anterior lobe of the pituitary gland), which is often called the master gland. The adenohypophysis secretes a hormone called thyrotropin, or thyroid-stimulating hormone (TSH). As is obvious from its name, TSH stimulates the thyroid gland to secrete *its* hormone, thyroxine. This process of one hormone regulating the secretion of another hormone is just one example of the many ways in which the endocrine glands affect one another.

Special Diagnostic Tests

Basal Metabolic Rate. Because thyroxine is so closely related to metabolism, a measurement of the metabolic rate when the body is completely at rest will give information on the functioning of the thyroid gland. This test is used less often than in the past and has been replaced by laboratory tests.

Radioactive Iodine Uptake. The thyroid gland readily absorbs and utilizes the mineral *iodine* in the process of manufacturing thyroxine. To test the activity of the thyroid gland, radioactive iodine is given to the patient by mouth, and after 24 hours, the amount of iodine taken up by the thyroid is measured with a Geiger counter. The overactive thyroid gland will accumulate more iodine than one that is normal or underactive.

Protein-Bound Iodine. This test is another way of measuring iodine content, except that the iodine measured is that which is found in the plasma of the patient's blood. It is called protein-bound iodine because the iodine is chemically bound to proteins in the plasma. Normally there are 4 to 8 μg. (micrograms) of such iodine in the plasma. In hyperthyroid persons, the iodine content is above normal.

Cholesterol Level. Cholesterol is the principal animal sterol, and it is found in many tissues of the body. The concentration of cholesterol in the serum is high when the thyroid is underactive and low when the thyroid is overactive. Although a change in the cholesterol level does not necessarily indicate a disorder of the thyroid gland, determination of the cholesterol level can be used with other diagnostic tests to confirm or rule out thyroid disease. *chol ↑ hypothyroid* *chol ↓ hyperthyroid*

Simple Goiter

Definition. There is often some confusion as to the proper classification of diseases of the thyroid, especially those concerned with enlargement of the gland. A *simple goiter* is only an enlargement of the thyroid, and there is no oversecretion of thyroxine in this condition. The cause of simple goiter has been proven to be a deficiency of iodine in water or food.

Symptoms. As stated before, there are no constitutional symptoms or changes in the metabolic rate of persons with simple goiter. The first sign to be noticed is enlargement of the neck. Later, as the goiter continues to grow, it presses against the esophagus and causes *dysphagia* (difficulty in swallowing). The goiter may also press against the trachea and produce dyspnea.

Treatment and Nursing Care. If goiter is treated early with medications containing iodine, the growth of the gland may be halted, and the enlargement may even disappear eventually. These medications must be given well diluted and administered through a straw because they may stain the teeth. Examples of iodine preparations are *Lugol's solution* and a saturated solution of *potassium iodide* (S.S.K.I.).

A very large goiter which continues to grow and produce local symptoms of pressure, or presents the possibility of the development of malignant disease in the gland, may be removed surgically.

Hyperthyroidism

Definition. Hyperthyroidism is a systemic condition resulting from overactivity of the thyroid gland and overproduction of the hormone thyroxine. This disorder is also known as *Graves' disease, toxic goiter* and *thyrotoxicosis.*

The reason for this increased activity of the gland is not known. In some cases, there has been a history of severe emotional distress or physical strain just before development of the symptoms.

Symptoms. The symptoms produced by the disease are all a result of an increase in metabolism in the body tissues. The patient is extremely nervous, tense and overactive. He seems compelled to indulge in physical activities even though he has an increasing sense of fatigue. He is very sensitive and may laugh or cry at the slightest provocation. His appetite is enormous, and he eats great quantities of food but does not gain weight. The thyroid gland may or may not be greatly enlarged.

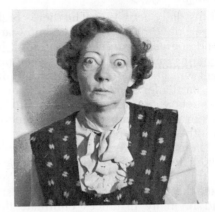

Figure 19–1. Patient with exophthalmic hyperthyroidism. Note protrusion of the eyes and retraction of the superior eyelids. The basal metabolic rate was +40. (Courtesy of Dr. Leonard Posey. From Guyton: *Basic Human Physiology,* W. B. Saunders Co., Philadelphia.)

Another symptom found in about one third of all patients with hyperthyroidism is protrusion of the eyeballs (exophthalmos) (see Fig. 19-1). The exact cause of this condition is not fully understood, but it may be quite severe. It can lead to blindness through stretching of the optic nerve or through ulceration of the cornea due to incomplete closure of the eyes while the patient is sleeping, which lets the epithelial surfaces of the eyes become dry, irritated and eventually infected.

Treatment and Nursing Care. Hyperthyroidism may be treated by conservative medical methods, or it may be treated surgically, depending on the individual case and the response of the disease to conservative measures.

Physical and mental rest are of extreme importance because of the relationship between physical stress or emotional upset and increased activity of the thyroid gland. Rest also helps to conserve the strength of the patient.

The diet of the hyperthyroid patient is based on his metabolic needs. If his metabolic rate is very high, he must eat enough to compensate for this so that he will have sufficient energy to carry

↑ metabolic rate

on his daily activities. The diet is high in carbohydrates, which we know are good sources of quick energy, high in vitamins and high in calories. The patient will need to receive instruction in the particular foods which will meet his dietary requirements and should be encouraged to substitute those foods for others less beneficial to him.

There are several drugs available which temporarily inhibit the release of thyroxine. These drugs greatly reduce the symptoms of hyperthyroidism and in many instances eliminate the need for hospitalization and surgical treatment. Lugol's solution and potassium iodide are both examples of iodine preparations which temporarily inhibit the release of thyroxine. Another drug

called *propylthiouracil* also blocks the release of thyroxine.

In recent years, *radioactive iodine* has been given to reduce the size and activity of the thyroid gland. Those on the nursing staff who must constantly handle the drug need to take radium precautions, but the patient is not exposed to enough radiation to cause concern. Radioactive iodine is excreted in the urine, and the patient must be instructed to dispose of the urine promptly if he is receiving this drug as an out-patient. In the hospital, the nursing staff should use caution in handling the bedpans and urinals and quickly dispose of the urine of all patients receiving radioactive iodine.

The surgical removal of the thyroid gland is called a *thyroidectomy*. If ma-

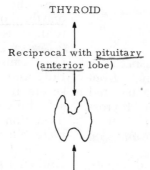

THYROID

Reciprocal with pituitary
(anterior lobe)

Thyroid hormone — stimulates basal metabolic
rate (active principles: thyroxin and triiodothyroxine)

Drug therapy: Used to stimulate basal metabolic
activity and to treat many conditions

For stimulation or substitution:
Thyroid extract, U.S.P.
Refined thyroid, U.S.P
Thyroxin, U.S.P.
Sodium liothyronine, U.S.P. (Cytomel)
Sodium levothyroxine, U.S.P. (Synthroid)

To depress activity of gland:

Strong iodine sol., U.S.P.
Sodium iodide, U.S.P.
Potassium iodide, U.S.P.
Sodium radioiodide sol., U.S.P.
   tracer — 1-100 microcuries
   therapy — 1-100 millicuries
⦁Thiouracil
⬤Propylthiouracil
Methylthiouracil (Methiacil,
   Muracil, Thimecil)
Iothiouracil sodium (Itrumil)
Methimazole, U.S.P. (Tapazole)
Carbimazole

Figure 19-2. Endocrine system in relation to drug therapy. (From Falconer, Norman, Patterson and Gustafson: *The Drug, The Nurse, The Patient,* 5th Ed., W. B. Saunders Co., Philadelphia.)

lignant disease of the gland is diagnosed, the entire gland is removed. In other cases, such as unsightly simple goiter or highly toxic goiters, only a portion of the gland is removed, and the remaining portion continues to secrete thyroxine. Thyroidectomies are not as common as they formerly were because the newer antithyroid drugs have made medical control of hyperthyroidism more successful.

PREOPERATIVE NURSING CARE. The preoperative nursing care of the patient having a thyroidectomy is much less difficult than it was before the antithyroid drugs became available. Most patients who enter the hospital for this type of surgery are much calmer emotionally and less active physically than formerly because they have received medications to stabilize the activity of the gland.

Whereas the practice of "stealing a thyroid" used to be a common occurrence so that the patient would not be unduly upset by surgery, the patients today usually know the exact day and hour of surgery and the type of surgery to be done. The responsibility of the nurse for preparation of the patient who is to have a thyroidectomy is essentially the same as for other types of major surgery. If the patient does appear nervous, tense and apprehensive, his condition should be reported to the physician. These symptoms may indicate improper control of the activities of the thyroid gland and may predispose the patient to the postoperative complication of "thyroid crisis" (see below).

POSTOPERATIVE NURSING CARE. As soon as the patient returns from the operating room, he is placed in *high Fowler's* position to facilitate breathing and reduce swelling of the operative area. The head may be supported with sandbags on either side to relieve tension on the sutures.

Close observation of the patient is an essential part of postoperative care. The vital signs are checked at frequent intervals, and the patient is watched closely for signs of bleeding and swelling of the operative area. Any rise in the temperature, pulse, or respiration rate should be reported when first noticed, since they may indicate a high level of thyroxine in the blood stream. External swelling may cause constriction of the bandage around the neck. Difficulty in swallowing or breathing should also be reported immediately, as they may indicate internal edema and pressure on the esophagus and trachea. In many hospitals, a tracheostomy set is kept at the bedside of the postoperative thyroidectomy patient in case severe respiratory embarrassment develops. Persistent hoarseness or loss of the voice are other symptoms to be reported, as they may indicate damage to the vocal cords.

Tetany and *thyroid crisis* are other complications of a thyroidectomy which may occur. These complications are rare, but when they do occur, the surgeon expects the nurse to be alert for the beginning signs and report her observations immediately.

Tetany is actually a symptom and results from injury to, or accidental removal of, the parathyroid glands. These small glands are located on the posterior surface of the thyroid gland. *Parathormone* is secreted by the parathyroid glands and is important in the regulation of the calcium and phosphorus level in the body tissues. A deficiency of this hormone produces muscle cramps, twitching of the muscles and, in some cases, severe convulsions.

This complication is treated by the administration of calcium intravenously during the emergency stage and subsequent maintenance doses of parathyroid hormone to maintain the proper calcium and phosphorus balance in the body.

Thyroid crisis, sometimes called *thyroid storm,* is another complication to be considered following a thyroidectomy. The condition is caused by a sudden increase in the output of thyroxine *thyroxin Cytomel Synthroid*

due to manipulation of the thyroid as it is being removed. Another cause may be improper reduction of thyroid secretions before surgery (see Preoperative Nursing Care).

The symptoms of thyroid crisis are produced by a sudden and extreme elevation of all body processes. The temperature may rise to 106° or more, the pulse increases to as much as 200 beats per minute, respirations become rapid and the patient exhibits marked apprehension and restlessness. Unless the condition is relieved, the patient quickly passes from delirium to coma to death from heart failure.

Treatment of thyroid crisis must be begun immediately after the first symptoms are noticed. Measures are employed to reduce the temperature, cardiac drugs are given to slow the heart beat, and sedatives, such as one of the barbiturates, are given to reduce restlessness and anxiety.

Hypothyroidism

Definition. Underactivity of the thyroid gland with a deficiency in the production of the hormone thyroxine is called hypothyroidism. The symptoms vary according to the age at which the disease presents itself. In young children, the condition is called *cretinism,* whereas if the disease develops in adulthood, the condition is called *myxedema.*

Symptoms. The child who has a deficiency in thyroxine has retarded physical and mental growth and development. Adults who have myxedema have a decrease in appetite but an increase in weight gain. In both children and adults, there is a tendency to sleep for long periods of time, the speech is slurred and the individual is very sluggish in his mental and physical activities. The skin is dry and scaly, and the patient often complains of increased sensitivity to cold.

Treatment. Hypothyroidism is successfully treated with the administration of thyroid extract. The dosage is gradually increased until a proper level has been reached, and then a delicate balance must be maintained so that the patient does not suffer from either hypothyroidism or hyperthyroidism.

The results of treatment of hypothyroidism are very striking, and most patients show a remarkable abatement of their symptoms. The practical nurse may not see many cases of hypothyroidism in the hospital because treatment usually does not require hospitalization. If the patient is admitted for some other condition of illness and is also being treated for hypothyroidism, some special considerations must be made. As stated previously these patients have very rough and dry skin, and they will need massage with lotions and creams to prevent cracking and peeling of the skin. Provisions for extra warmth must also be made for those patients who have an increased sensitivity to cold as a result of their hypothyroidism.

The nurse must also bear in mind the psychological aspects of hypothyroidism. She must avoid rushing these patients or giving them the impression that she is annoyed and inconvenienced by their sluggishness. Forgetfulness, inability to express themselves vocally and physical inertia are mannerisms which are a direct result of the deficiency in thyroxine, and the nurse must recognize them as unavoidable and embarrassing to the patient as he struggles to overcome his handicap.

DISORDERS OF THE PARATHYROIDS

Introduction

The parathyroid glands, usually four in number, are located on the posterior aspect of the thyroid gland. The parathyroid hormone exerts an important regulating effect on the calcium and phosphorus concentration of body fluids. In general, the parathyroid hor-

normal ↓ phos ↑ Ca

mone depresses the concentration of phosphorus and increases the concentration of calcium in the blood by removing the calcium from the bones so that it circulates in the blood stream.

In order to understand the disorders produced by malfunctioning parathyroid glands, one must be familiar with the metabolism of calcium and phosphorus. Calcium is important to four main functions of the body: bone formation, blood clotting, maintenance of normal cell permeability so that nutrients may enter and waste products may leave, and proper conduction of nerve impulses to and from the muscles. Phosphorus also is essential to bone formation and to the metabolism of carbohydrates and proteins.

Hypoparathyroidism (Tetany)

↓ Ca ↑ phos

Definition. Hypoparathyroidism is a deficiency of the parathyroid hormone. It is sometimes seen following thyroidectomy when too much of the parathyroid tissue is accidentally removed. It can also occur with idiopathic atrophy of the parathyroid glands.

Symptoms. A deficiency of the parathyroid hormone is accompanied by a drop in the level of calcium in the blood and an increase in the phosphorus level. The chief symptom occurring as a result of the lowered calcium level is *tetany.* Muscular twitching and spasms occur because of extreme irritability of the muscular tissue. If the calcium level continues to fall, the patient will suffer from severe convulsions and spasms of the larynx.

Treatment. Acute hypoparathyroidism is treated by oral or parenteral administration of calcium salts. In chronic hypoparathyroidism, treatment is aimed at restoring and maintaining normal calcium levels in the blood. This can be accomplished by injections of parathyroid extract, vitamin D in massive doses to enhance the absorption of calcium by the small intestine

and oral administration of calcium salts.

Hyperparathyroidism (von Recklinghausen's Disease)

↑ blood Ca ↓ phos

Definition. Excessive secretion of the parathyroid hormone is due to an overgrowth of the parathyroid glands. It can also occur in a patient with chronic nephritis. High levels of parathyroid hormone in the blood leads to removal of calcium from the bones (decalcification) and accumulation of this mineral in the blood (hypercalcemia). The calcium is then precipitated in the kidney, where it brings about the formation of kidney stones.

Symptoms. Hyperparathyroidism is characterized by fatigue, muscular weakness, formation of kidney stones and changes in the skeletal system. The bones become tender and painful and are easily fractured or deformed.

Treatment. The condition is treated by surgical removal of the excess glandular tissue so that sufficient parathyroid tissue is left to maintain a normal calcium and phosphorus level.

✓ for tetany Post Op

DISEASES OF CARBOHYDRATE METABOLISM

Introduction

When carbohydrates are taken into the body, they are converted into simple sugars which can readily be absorbed into the blood stream. Some of the sugar remains in the blood stream as glucose so that it is available when needed for energy. The excess sugar is carried to the liver, where it is stored as glycogen. When a demand for more energy arises, the liver reconverts the glycogen into glucose and releases it into the blood stream so that it can be carried to the muscles and other body tissues. In order for this process to take place, the hormone *insulin* is neces-

↑ insulin ↓ blood sugar
Hypo
↓ insulin diab mellitus

414 / NURSING CARE: DISORDERS OF THE ENDOCRINE SYSTEM

sary. Insulin is secreted by the *islets of Langerhans,* which are located on the surface of the pancreas.

An excess of insulin leads to a condition called *hypoglycemia* (low blood sugar). A deficiency in the supply of insulin or interference with the normal physiologic action of insulin results in a condition known as *diabetes mellitus.*

Special Diagnostic Tests and Examinations

Urinalysis. Sugar is not present in the urine of a normal person. When it is found in the urine, this is an indication of a high level of sugar in the blood, because excess blood sugar is spilled over into the urine.

Many unsuspected cases of diabetes mellitus have been discovered when a routine urinalysis was done as a part of a physical examination.

The testing of urine for sugar is now a relatively simple matter, and most diabetics check their own urine at home after they have been discharged from the hospital.

Blood Sugar. There is always a certain amount of sugar in the blood of a normal person (80 to 120 mg. of sugar per 100 ml. of blood). This sugar is constantly being used for the production of energy to carry on the daily activities of the body. However, an increase in the blood sugar level indicates a disorder of glucose metabolism. A high level of blood sugar is found in diabetes, in chronic liver disease and in overactivity of some of the endocrine glands.

Glucose Tolerance. All starches and sugars taken into the body must be eventually reduced to glucose before they can be absorbed into the blood stream and utilized by the body tissues for food and energy. When diabetes is suspected, the physician orders a glucose tolerance test to determine the patient's ability to utilize glucose.

In this test, a "fasting blood sugar"

and urinalysis are done first, and then the patient is given a solution of glucose to drink. Samples of urine and blood are taken later at regular intervals to determine their level of glucose. A normal patient's blood sugar will drop back to normal levels within 2 hours. A diabetic's blood sugar will remain high.

Diabetes Mellitus

also fats protein

Definition. Diabetes is a disease which results from an inability of the body to use and store carbohydrates in a normal manner. Even though insulin is necessary for the proper usage of carbohydrates, recent investigations have shown that other endocrine glands and their hormones may play some part in the development of the symptoms of diabetes.

The exact cause of diabetes is not known. However, there are at least four factors which may contribute to the development of this disease. These are:

1. There may be an inability to produce enough insulin because the pancreas is diseased or absent.

2. There may be an increase in the rate at which the body uses up insulin. This may be caused by overeating or by overactivity of the thyroid gland. Where this creates an insulin shortage, diabetes results.

3. There may be an increase in the rate at which insulin is destroyed in the body. It has been shown that the liver and other tissues contain an enzyme *insulinase* which can inactivate insulin.

4. There may be a drop in the efficiency of insulin due to liver disease or the introduction into the system of certain chemicals which impede insulin activity.[6]

Statistics indicate that from 20 to 50 per cent of all diabetic patients have a positive history of diabetes in the family. Authorities classify the trait as mendelian recessive. When a diabetic marries a nondiabetic who is not a carrier of the trait, none of their children will have diabetes, but all will be carriers. If two diabetics marry, all of their children will become diabetic eventually.

In older persons, heredity may be a predisposing factor rather than a direct cause of diabetes. In these persons, there seems to be a condition resulting from "using up" all the insulin the islets of Langerhans can produce, and the cells seem no longer capable of secreting sufficient insulin. Elderly diabetics usually have a less severe form of the disease than do younger persons, and they are less likely to develop ketoacidosis (diabetic coma). The vascular problems due to atherosclerosis are a common problem in the older diabetic.

Until the discovery of insulin, many diabetics who developed the disease in early childhood did not live to reach child-bearing age. Now that the disease can be controlled and diabetics are able to marry and have children, we can expect the incidence of diabetes to increase. At present, it is believed that there are more than one and a half million people in the United States who are known to have diabetes and probably as many more who have not yet been diagnosed as having the disease.[15]

There are four groups of people who are most susceptible to diabetes: those who are over 40 years of age, those who are overweight, women and those who have had diabetes in their family. Anyone fitting into any of these four categories should be tested for early signs of diabetes at least once a year.

Symptoms. The elevation of the blood sugar level and the presence of sugar in the urine are the two most outstanding symptoms of diabetes. These are found only by special laboratory work, however, and are not apparent to the person who has not yet sought medical attention. Other warning signals which a person may recognize as symptoms of illness are also present in diabetes. These symptoms are known as the three "polys": *polyuria* (increased urinary output), *polydipsia* (excessive thirst) and *polyphagia* (an increase in appetite).

Fatigue and muscular weakness, pruritus and numbness and tingling of the hands and feet are also symptoms of diabetes.

Treatment and Nursing Care. The treatment of diabetes must continue as long as the patient lives and demands his complete cooperation with the physician. For this reason, education of the patient is a very important aspect of the treatment.

Diabetes is never cured in the true sense of the word, but it may be controlled by diet and the administration of insulin according to the needs of each patient. There are also several systemic complications which may result from an excessive amount of sugar in the blood, and these must be diligently guarded against throughout the life of the patient.

According to the American Diabetes Association, a person's diabetes is well controlled when:

1. The person feels well.
2. He maintains normal weight on a well-balanced diet.
3. His urine tests are usually negative.
4. His blood sugar tests are usually normal.

As long as a diabetic can meet these four requirements and follows his doctor's orders faithfully, he need not worry about the progress of his disease or the development of complications.

DIET. The diet of each diabetic patient is calculated on an individual basis. There is no such thing as a "typical" diabetic and, since diabetes is an unstable and changing process, each patient's needs will change from time to time. Unfortunately, most nurses do not have sufficient background in nutrition to comprehend completely the many factors related to diet and the control of diabetes. Such a statement is not meant to point out a deficiency in the nurse's educational background, but rather serves to emphasize the need for a team approach to meeting the dietary needs of the diabetic patient.

In general, the diabetic diet is concerned with providing adequate nutrition with sufficient calories to maintain normal body weight and to adjust the intake of food so that the blood sugar is kept within safe limits. In recent years, less emphasis has been placed on caloric intake and restriction of carbohydrates and more attention paid to the regulation of body weight and blood sugar levels in each patient. It seems likely that the next few years will see a revision of the prescribed diets for diabetic patients. This trend suggests that the nurse who expects to give effective care to a diabetic patient must continue to read and to learn about the latest developments in patient care. It also means that just as we caution all patients on special diets to be sure to read the labels on foods that they purchase, we must also caution nurses to note the dates on the material they read so that they can keep abreast of the most current information available.

The American Diabetes Association and the American Dietetic Association have worked together to devise a simplified method of calculating a diabetic diet and planning a diabetic's meals. The booklet in which this information is published is entitled "Meal Planning with Exchange Lists." The principal foods are divided into six groups: milk, vegetables, fruits, breads, meats and fat. Each group contains foods that are similar in kind and have equal nutritional value in regard to carbohydrate, protein and fat. For example, more than 20 fruits from which the diabetic can choose are listed, each providing 10 grams of carbohydrate, a negligible amount of protein and fat and 40 calories per serving. Other lists contain similar information for a great variety of foods. With this simple method of choosing a menu from the exchange lists, a diabetic or a member of his family can calculate the caloric value and nutritional value with ease.

It is important that the diabetic patient not develop a defeatist or negative attitude toward his diet. Emphasis should be placed on the positive aspects of his diet, the foods he is allowed rather than those which are forbidden. He should not be made to feel guilty about experiencing difficulty with staying on his diet or the times he deliberately "cheats" and helps himself to foods that are not allowed. Each of us has our moments when we are likely to yield to the temptation to do what we know is not in our best interest. One of the most effective means of helping the patient follow his diet is by teaching him about food values and how they affect diabetes so that he can understand how food elements affect his health and well-being. This suggestion implies, of course, that the patient has access to persons who know and can impart to him the information he needs.

In order to help the diabetic and his family learn which foods he should eat and those he should avoid, the physician, the dietitian and the nurse must all participate in the instruction. Fortunately, there are available many well-written and clearly illustrated booklets and pamphlets which are most helpful to the diabetic and his family. Such organizations as the American Diabetes Association* and the American Medical Association† will send instructive material on request. This material not only covers diets, but also warns the diabetic against misleading or fraudulent information in regard to quick "cures" or special diets which will cure diabetes.

ADMINISTRATION OF INSULIN. There are some patients who cannot control their diabetes with diet alone. This is especially true of children who have developed diabetes at an early age and older diabetics with a moderate or severe case of diabetes. In these cases, exogenous insulin prepared by a pharmaceutical firm must be administered

---

*Address: 18 E. 48 St., New York 10017.
†Address: 535 North Dearborn Street, Chicago, Ill. 60611.

TABLE 19-2. INSULIN ACTIVITY*

Name	Time and Route of Administration	Onset	Peak	Duration of Action	Most Likely Time for Insulin Reaction	Most Likely Time for Sugar in the Urine
Fast action						
Regular	15–20 minutes before meals, S.C. (I.V. in emergency)	Rapid, within 1 hour	2–4 hrs.	5–8 hrs.	10 A.M. to lunch	During night
Crystalline	Same	Same	Same	Same	Same	Same
Semilente	½–¾ hr. before breakfast, deep S.C. (never I.V.)	Same	6–10 hrs.	12–16 hrs.	Before lunch	Same
Intermediate action						
Globin	½–1 hr. before breakfast S.C.	Within 2–4 hrs. (rapidity increases with dose)	6–10 hrs.	18–24 hrs.	3 P.M. to dinner	Before breakfast and lunch
NPH	1 hr. before breakfast, S.C.	Within 2–4 hrs.	8–12 hrs.	28–30 hrs.	Same	Before lunch
Lente	Same	Same	Same	Same	Same	Same
Slow action						
Protamine Zinc	Same	Within 4–6 hrs.	16–24 hrs.	24–36 hrs. plus	2 A.M. to breakfast	Before lunch and bedtime
(PZI) Ultralente	1 hr. before breakfast, deep S.C. (never I.V.)	Very slow– 8 hrs.	Same	36 hrs. plus	During night and early morning	

*Reprinted from Thompson: Pediatrics for Practical Nurses. 2nd edition. Philadelphia, W. B. Saunders Company, 1970. Adapted from Bergersen and Krug: Pharmacology in Nursing. 11th edition. St. Louis, The C. V. Mosby Co., 1969.

parenterally at regular intervals so that the body's metabolic processes can function normally. Exogenous insulin is a liquid hormonal preparation obtained from the pancreas of animals. Insulin was first discovered in 1921 by Sir Frederick G. Banting and Dr. Charles H. Best. This was plain insulin and is known today as regular insulin. This type of insulin will last in the body only 6 to 8 hours (see Table 19-2).

In 1936, a Danish physician, Dr. Hagedorn, discovered that by adding a protein (protamine) to insulin, its action could be prolonged to a period of 12 hours. It was later found that by adding zinc to the protamine, insulin blood sugar levels could be controlled for as long as 24 hours with a single injection. This combination of protamine, zinc and insulin is known as protamine zinc insulin or PZI.

The discovery of this long-acting insulin eliminated the need for several daily injections of regular insulin, but it did not prove to be ideal for those who had moderately severe or severe diabetes. In these cases, it was still necessary for the patient to take regular insulin in order to augment the action of the PZI.

The development of an intermediate-acting insulin which would strike a happy medium and reach its peak of action at some time between that of the fast-acting regular insulin and the long-acting PZI came only after much research and study. The

Intermediate Action

first to be used was *globin* insulin, and later NPH insulin and *lente* insulin were finally developed.

PZI, NPH and lente insulin are all cloudy and milky in appearance and must be thoroughly mixed before they are administered, so that the proper proportions of the crystals are given. This is done by *gently rolling* the bottle between the palms of the hands. The bottle is *not* shaken, because this produces air bubbles in the solution, which may alter the dosage being given.

Insulin is always measured in units. U-40 means that there are 40 units of insulin per ml. U-80 means that there are 80 units per ml. A specially marked insulin syringe must be used when administering insulin so that there will be no error in the calculation of the dosage.

The diagnosis of diabetes is usually definitely established by laboratory tests requiring admission to the hospital. Thus, a person learns he is a diabetic while he is a patient in the hospital. When the physician feels that the patient is ready to accept the fact that he is a diabetic, he may ask the nurse in charge to instruct the patient in self-administration of insulin. It is natural that there will be some resistance from the patient at first, and some patients never can bring themselves to the point of actually sticking a needle in their own skins. The practical nurse and all other members of the nursing staff must appreciate the patient's feeling in this matter and offer sympathetic encouragement and understanding. If the patient flatly refuses to learn to give his own insulin or is physically unable to do so, a member of the family is taught to give the injections under supervision before the patient is discharged from the hospital. Rotation of sites for insulin injections is necessary to avoid irritation and assure absorption.

The diabetic or a member of his family must also learn to test the urine for sugar and acetone and to give insulin according to the amount of sugar present.

SYNTHETIC HYPOGLYCEMIC AGENTS. All types of insulin must be given by injection. There are, to date, no insulin pills, capsules or liquids that can be taken by mouth. In recent years, at least three new drugs have been developed which act to lower the blood sugar. These drugs are rather limited in their usefulness because they do not take the place of insulin in the body and are effective only in older patients who have a relatively stable, nonketotic type of diabetes. They are of no value in a patient with ketosis or in diabetic acidosis.

Tolbutamide (Orinase) is a sulfonamide derivative. It reaches its peak in 5 to 8 hours and is very rapidly excreted. *Chlorpropamide* (Diabinese) reaches its peak in about four hours and is less rapidly excreted. Both of these drugs require that the diabetic have at least a small amount of insulin production. *Phenformin* (DBI) is another hypoglycemic agent that sometimes is used in the treatment of juvenile diabetes, but it does not take the place of insulin.

All hypoglycemic agents are capable of producing gastric irritation with nausea, vomiting and diarrhea. There also may be liver damage with jaundice, bone marrow depression or an allergic reaction. All patients taking one of these drugs should be informed of the early symptoms of hypoglycemia (drowsiness, nausea and deep breathing) because these drugs can produce hypoglycemic shock very rapidly.

Prevention of Complications. The diabetic is subject to a variety of complications. These may be the result of an extreme elevation in blood sugar, too much insulin or gradual changes within the blood vessels and other tissues.

The proper balance of glucose and insulin in the body may be compared to a scale. As long as there are equal parts on either side of the scale, there will be an even balance. In normal persons, this balance is maintained, but in a diabetic, the balance may be easily upset by failing to follow his diet, administering himself too much insulin or an infection or other illness which may increase the need for insulin in the body.

Too much glucose may produce a condition known as *diabetic coma*, and too much insulin may produce *insulin shock*. Both of these conditions may be found as complications of diabetes.

Table 19-3 describes the symptoms of diabetic coma as opposed to insulin reaction. In studying these symptoms, the reader must remember that each person reacts differently in a given situation, and not all of the symptoms will be present in every case. Some of the symptoms may be entirely absent, and some may not be as obvious as others.

The patient with diabetic acidosis must have immediate treatment, or the condition can be fatal. He is given insulin, glucose and water intravenously in doses calculated according to his current blood sugar level and uri-

nalysis. The urinalysis is done on an hourly basis until the diabetic acidosis is brought under control.

A mild insulin reaction may be relieved by a glass of orange juice or some other source of simple sugars. Severe insulin shock requires intensive treatment to prevent circulatory collapse. Glucose is often administered intravenously. The amount of glucose given is also calculated according to the patient's current urinalysis for sugar and his blood sugar level.

Diabetic coma, also called ketoacidosis or diabetic acidosis, is the result of a complicated chemical derangement in the body due to metabolic disturbances. When the body is unable to utilize carbohydrate for energy, it resorts to the metabolism of fat for its energy source. In diabetes, the amount of insulin is insufficient for proper carbohydrate metabolism, and so large amounts of fatty acids are removed from the body's adipose tissue to supply energy. The liver then breaks down these fatty acids into acetoacetic acid, which accumulates in the blood and

TABLE 19-3. SYMPTOMS OF DIABETIC COMA AND INSULIN REACTION

Diabetic Coma	Insulin Reaction
Gradual onset, may be more rapid in active children	Sudden onset, begins abruptly
Skin hot and dry, face may be flushed.	Perspiration, skin pale, cold and clammy
Deep, labored breathing	Shallow breathing
Nausea	Hunger
Drowsiness and lethargy	Mental confusion, strange behavior, nervousness
Fruity odor to breath	Double vision
Loss of consciousness	Loss of consciousness, convulsions (rarely)
Urine contains much sugar	There may be sugar in the urine, depending on the type of insulin and when it was taken
Blood sugar high	Blood sugar low

body tissues because the cells cannot handle it as rapidly as the liver produces it. This acid and two other chemicals into which it is converted are called *ketone bodies*. One of these chemicals is acetone, a highly volatile substance that causes a sweet, fruit-like odor to the breath in patients with metabolic acidosis. As the ketone bodies (two of which are acid) collect in the body fluids, they upset the normal acid-base balance, and the patient is said to be in *acidosis*. The ketoacids are excreted by the kidneys, and that is why a diabetic's urine is tested for acetone when ketoacidosis is suspected or likely to develop.

The person who has diabetes cannot always control his mealtime or emotional crises in his life any more than anyone else. He may be delayed by traffic or miss his train home after work and wait an hour or two for the next one. Or a death or sudden financial loss may cause him to become emotionally upset. Missing a meal can easily result in insulin reaction if the diabetic is taking an intermediate or long-acting insulin, and a sudden emotional upset may use up all available glucose and result in a drastic lowering of the blood sugar.

If the diabetic is alone and away from home at the time he suffers from insulin reaction or diabetic acidosis, his condition may be mistaken for drunkenness or mental derangement. To avoid confusion and delay in obtaining medical attention, all diabetics should carry identification cards (see Fig. 19-3) or wear identification bracelets stating that they are diabetics. Several drug companies as well as the American Diabetes Association have these cards available and will mail them upon request.

Other complications of diabetes arise from the fact that diabetics have a tendency to develop *arteriosclerosis*. The arteries which may be affected are the peripheral blood vessels, the vessels serving the kidney and those serving the heart. In view of this, it is obvious that such complications may easily lead to serious illnesses and even death.

The lower extremities of the diabetic are particularly susceptible to disturbances arising from poor circulation. That is why amputations of the lower limbs are a relatively common occurrence in many diabetics, especially those who have difficulty keeping the diabetes under control and their blood sugar level low.

Exercises and special care of the feet and legs as discussed previously under diseases of the peripheral vessels are essential in the prevention of complications arising from poor circulation of the lower limbs of the diabetic (see Fig. 19-5).

In addition to poor circulation, the diabetic also has an impaired resistance to infection. This situation demands meticulous care of the skin and careful attention to breaks in the skin through which bacteria may enter and cause an infection. It is believed that the high level of sugar in the blood provides an excellent breeding ground for bacteria, and they multiply much more rapidly in a diabetic than in a normal individual.

A slight cold or minor infection will also increase the need for insulin as the body speeds up its metabolism to fight the infection. The diabetic should know and understand this so that he will be prepared for an elevation of blood sugar and an increased need for insulin while he has an infection. He should be advised to notify his physician at once should an infection develop so that plans can be made for increasing the dosage of insulin when necessary.

Every nurse should appreciate the value of good habits of personal hygiene and recognize them as essential to the health of everyone. High standards of personal hygiene are even more important to the diabetic because they may mean the difference between life and death for him. He cannot afford to be careless in matters of cleanli-

EMERGENCY MEDICAL IDENTIFICATION

prepared by the
AMERICAN
MEDICAL ASSOCIATION
535 N. Dearborn St.
Chicago 10, Illinois

ATTENTION

In an emergency where I am unconscious or unable to communicate, please read the other side to know the special care I must have.

PERSONAL IDENTIFICATION

Name_____
Address_____
_____
_____
Religion_____

NOTIFY IN EMERGENCY

Name_____
Address_____
_____
Phone_____

Name_____
Address_____
_____
Phone_____

My Doctor is_____
_____
Address_____
_____
Phone_____

MEDICAL INFORMATION
(with date of notation)

Present Medical Problems_____
_____
_____

Medicines Taken Regularly_____
_____
_____
_____
_____

Dangerous Allergies_____
_____
_____

Other Important Information_____
_____
_____

Last Immunization Date
Tetanus Toxoid_____   Polio-Salk_____
Smallpox_____   Sabin_____
Diphtheria_____   Others_____
Typhoid_____
REMEMBER: This is the minimum medical and personal information needed by those who help you in an emergency. It is not designed to be a complete medical record. Check its accuracy with your doctor.

Figure 19-3. Front and back of identification card. This type of identification is recommended for all persons who have diabetes or some other type of chronic disease, or a serious allergy to certain drugs.

ness or fail to avoid extremes in eating, physical activities and exposure to infections. Every person who takes insulin must establish a regular pattern for meals, rest, work and play so that the amount of insulin available in the body at a given time will be in balance with the amount of sugar present. Physical exhaustion, emotional upsets or worry and anxiety can use up the supply of glucose in the blood and decrease the need for insulin.

Changes in vision are often associated with diabetes. These changes may

retinitis – inflamation of retena

be caused by a *retinis* or by the formation of cataracts. Regular visits to an eye specialist are necessary so that early changes in vision may be discovered and treatment begun before there is a serious loss of sight. Many visual disturbances are relieved when the diabetes is brought under control and the blood sugar lowered.

Education of the Patient and Family. There is probably no other chronic disease in which patient teaching is more important than in diabetes mellitus. The ultimate goal for patient in-

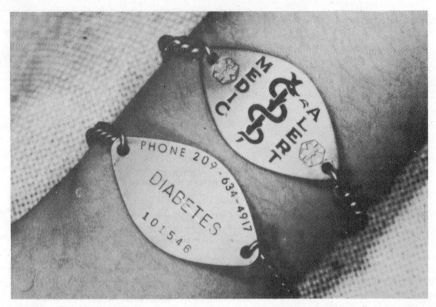

Figure 19–4. The Medic-Alert emblem may be worn as bracelet or necklace. Reverse side denotes specific medical problem of the wearer. (From Fish: Journal of Practical Nursing, March, 1970.)

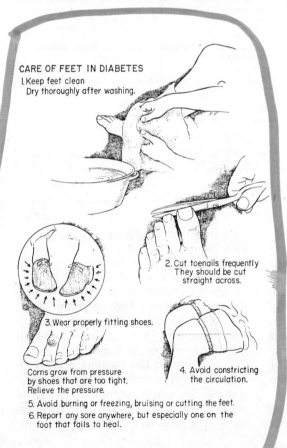

CARE OF FEET IN DIABETES
1. Keep feet clean
   Dry thoroughly after washing.

2. Cut toenails frequently
   They should be cut
   straight across.

3. Wear properly fitting shoes.

Corns grow from pressure
by shoes that are too tight.
Relieve the pressure.

4. Avoid constricting
   the circulation.

5. Avoid burning or freezing, bruising or cutting the feet.

6. Report any sore anywhere, but especially one on the
   foot that fails to heal.

Figure 19–5. The care of the feet in diabetes. (From Dowling and Jones: *That the Patient May Know,* W. B. Saunders Co., Philadelphia.)

struction is for the patient to be able to manage his illness insofar as he is physically and intellectually capable. His objectives are to <u>stay within the limits of his diet, check his urine routinely for sugar and acetone and administer his own medications</u> as they are prescribed for him.

Studies have shown that diabetic patients have many misconceptions about their illness and make serious errors in medication and diet. They become confused about the various types and strengths of insulin and the differences in insulin syringes. The exchange diet and its various serving portions create many difficulties for them when they first begin to follow directions for the diet. They often resort to old wives' tales and other cultural myths in desperation and many times do not mention these during instruction for fear of being ridiculed. Any student nurse who recalls her first introduction to diabetes can sympathize with the patient who becomes hopelessly lost in the details of diet, urinalysis and insulin administration.

It is not possible to teach self-care to a diabetic patient in a few short lessons. The amount of information the patient needs can be overwhelming if an attempt is made to teach him all at once the many things he will need to know. The nurse-instructor begins by <u>determining what the patient already knows about his illness and its management,</u> and then she proceeds in <u>small steps to build on that knowledge.</u> This progression, of course, implies that the nurse already knows the patient as a person. She is familiar with his background, his ability to learn and his attitude toward his illness.

It is especially important to <u>include the family</u> in the instruction whenever possible. The patient will need their support and encouragement as he strives for self-confidence in his ability to care for himself. If there are times during his illness that he cannot assume total responsibility for his diet and medications, he and his family will feel more secure if there is a family member who can assist him in his care. The patient, the family and those who teach them must have patience and a willingness to persevere in finding ways to manage an illness that demands continued surveillance and long-range planning as well as setting up immediate goals that can assure the patient some success and a sense of accomplishment.

Surveys of diabetic patients reveal that many of these patients have found the instruction they received woefully inadequate in helping them care for themselves when they leave the hospital and return home. They feel that most information about urine testing is incomplete, that they have many unanswered questions about self-administration of insulin and that they feel very insecure about dealing with insulin shock and acidosis. These findings suggest that instruction of the diabetic must be a continuing process that allows for frequent contact between the patient and the person giving instruction.

Hypoglycemia

Introduction. The term hypoglycemia refers to an <u>abnormally low level of glucose in the circulating blood.</u> The patient with this condition utilizes the available glucose in his blood at a very rapid rate, causing his <u>blood sugar to drop to a seriously low level within a few hours after he has eaten a meal or after exercise.</u>

In <u>most cases</u> of chronic hypoglycemia, there is <u>no known cause.</u> In others, the condition can be traced to a <u>tumor of the pancreas, liver disease</u> or a disorder of the <u>pituitary gland</u> or the <u>adrenal glands.</u>

Symptoms. The patient with hypoglycemia has a limited supply of glucose available for energy, so he feels <u>weak and faint, appears pale and may have slight tremors.</u> These symptoms are familiar to all of us who have, for some reason, gone too long without an adequate intake of food. If hypoglycemia becomes severe, there may be excessive perspiration, convulsions and coma. Many times the symptoms can be relieved temporarily by eating a carbohydrate food such as candy or by drinking a sweetened fruit juice.

Treatment. There is no cure for hypoglycemia when the basic cause is unknown. It can be controlled by diet and limiting of strenuous physical exercise to periods when glucose is readily available. The patient should eat regularly spaced meals that are high in protein. The body converts carbohydrates to glucose quite readily, but proteins are utilized more gradually, and a high protein diet is more likely to supply a more constant source of energy. Most physicians instruct hypoglycemic patients to carry candy or sugar with them at all times so that they can have a source of quick energy available in case they experience weakness and faintness.

DISORDERS OF THE ADRENAL GLANDS

Introduction

The adrenal glands are composed of two distinct parts, neither of which apparently has any direct functional relationship with the other. The adrenal medulla (middle portion) secretes two hormones, epinephrine and norepinephrine. These substances are secreted in response to stimulation from the sympathetic nervous system, and their effects are, in turn, almost the same as direct stimulation of the sympathetic nerves. Epinephrine prepares the body to meet stress or emergency situations and prevents hypoglycemia. Norepinephrine functions as a pressor hormone to maintain blood pressure.

The adrenal cortex (outer covering) secretes two major types of hormones, the mineralocorticoids and the glucocorticoids. It also secretes small amounts of androgenic hormones, which have effects similar to the male and female sex hormones. Normally the androgenic hormones have very little effect in comparison to the sex hormones secreted by the gonads, but in some abnormalities of the adrenal cortex, such large amounts of androgenic hormones are poured into the blood stream that they can present symptoms of sexual changes in the patient.

The mineralocorticoids and glucocorticoids are so named because of the effects they have on the body. The mineralocorticoids affect the electrolytes, particularly sodium, potassium and chloride. Without the mineralocorticoids, a person would die within three to seven days, because these hormones directly control fluid balance, blood volume, cardiac output, exchange of nutrients and wastes in each cell and, in effect, all chemical processes and glandular functions within the body. Little wonder that they are said to be "life-saving hormones." The glucocorticoids are almost equally important because they are essential to the metabolic systems for proper utilization of carbohydrates, proteins and fats.

Addison's Disease (Hypoadrenalism)

Definition. This disease is a result of underactivity of the adrenal cortex. It can be caused by an inflammation, infection or tumor of the adrenal gland which interferes with the production of secretions from the gland.

Symptoms. The symptoms in the early stages of Addison's disease are so vague they often are considered to be annoying but not serious enough to consult a physician. These symptoms include malaise, chronic fatigue, irritability and loss of weight. Pigmentation of the skin and mucous membranes develops later and gives the skin a brownish, "tanned" appearance.

Nausea and vomiting appear and become increasingly persistent, and the patient may eventually collapse with dehydration and circulatory failure.

Treatment and Nursing Care. Treatment of Addison's disease consists of replacement of the adrenal hormones lacking in the body. *Cortisone* is given in regular doses to maintain a proper level. Cortisone may be given as often as two to three times daily. Hydrocortisone, prednisone or prednisolone also may be used.

Infections are likely to increase the need for adrenal hormones just as they increase the need for insulin in a diabetic. Moderation in all activities and habits of good personal hygiene are as essential for the person with Addison's disease as they are for those suffering from diabetes.

Those who have Addison's disease should carry an identification card or wear an identification bracelet in the event they become ill from an acute episode while away from home. Such acute flare-ups may occur from failure to take the hormones regularly as ordered or from some physical or mental stress. During this acute stage, the patient may die from circulatory collapse and shock if treatment is not begun immediately.

Cushing's Syndrome (Hyperadrenalism) *cortex*

Definition. This disease is a result of an *increased* production of hormones from the adrenal cortex. It may be caused by a tumor or other disease of the adrenal gland, or it may result from overstimulation of the adrenal glands by the pituitary gland.

Symptoms. The person with Cushing's syndrome has a wide variety of symptoms too numerous to mention here. Briefly, it may be stated that the condition is characterized by a typical "moon" face, muscular weakness, abnormal sexual development and some mental disturbances.

buffalo hump

Treatment and Nursing Care. Treatment is usually based on the primary condition causing the increase in production of the hormones. But this is not always a simple matter, and in some cases, the cause cannot be found. Supportive treatment consists of administration of potassium chloride by mouth and measures which will improve the patient's general physical health and mental stability.

While potassium is being given, the nurse must keep an accurate record of the patient's intake and output. A low-sodium, high-potassium diet may be ordered as a means of maintaining the proper balance of these salts in the body.

Severe mental depression is often present, and the nursing staff must be alert for indications that the patient is contemplating suicide.

Surgical removal of the adrenal gland (adrenalectomy) may be carried out if other measures fail to relieve the symptoms of the disease. The surgeon leaves only an appropriate amount of adrenal cortical tissue so that normal function can be maintained.

Pheochromocytoma *medulla*

Definition. This is a relatively rare tumor that usually is located in the adrenal medulla but occasionally occurs in other chromaffin tissues of the sympathoadrenal system. It causes an increased secretion of epinephrine and norepinephrine, which in turn produces hypertension, severe headache, visual disturbances and tachycardia.

There is a test, called the Regitine test, that is specifically used for diagnosis of pheochromocytoma. The drug Regitine neutralizes the effect of epinephrine. If the blood pressure drops when the drug is administered, the presence of the tumor is strongly suspected.

In recent years, the Regitine test has been replaced for the most part by a determination of *catecholamines* (specifically, epinephrine and norepinephrine) in the urine. In pheochromocytoma, the level of these hormones is elevated. The normal range is 14 micrograms per 100 ml. of urine. Since these hormones are unstable, the test should be performed as soon as possible after the specimen has been collected. A special preservative may be added to the specimen if delay cannot be avoided.

Treatment of pheochromocytoma involves surgical removal of the tumor. During the postoperative period, the patient must be watched closely for extreme fluctuations in blood pressure. Although pheochromocytoma can be fatal, surgical treatment is usually successful, and the patient can be cured if there has been no damage to the cardiovascular system.

DISORDERS OF THE PITUITARY GLAND

Introduction

The pituitary gland (*hypophysis*) lies at the base of the brain and is connected with the hypothalamus by the hypophyseal stalk. It is only 1 cm. in diameter but is a key organ because it influences all systems and organs of the body. The hypophysis is divided into two distinct portions: the anterior pituitary, known as the *adenohypophysis*, and the posterior pituitary gland, known as the *neurohypophysis*. The adenohypophyseal hormones and their functions are presented in Table 19-1. One can readily see that hypofunction or hyperfunction of the gland can produce a variety of symptoms, depending on the particular organs involved.

Adenohypophysis

Gigantism. This condition results when hyperplasia or tumors of the adenohypophysis occur during the rapid growth before adolescence. Because there is overproduction of the growth hormone (somatropin) at a time when the epiphyses of the long bones have not become fused with the shafts, the bones lengthen very rapidly, and gigantism develops. The patient also may have diabetes mellitus as a result of overstimulation and eventual degeneration of the islets of Langerhans on the pancreas. Treatment involves irradiation of the hypophysis to reduce hormonal secretion. This is accomplished by insertion of a radioactive needle directly into the tumor or excessive glandular tissue.

Acromegaly. When there is an excessive secretion of the growth hormone after adolescence, the soft tissues continue to grow, and the bones grow thicker but not longer. In this situation, the disorder is called acromegaly. Enlargement is especially marked in the bones of the cranium, lower jaw, hands and feet. It also involves soft tissue such as that of the tongue and liver, which become greatly enlarged. Treatment usually is irradiation of the hypophysis in a manner similar to that used for gigantism. This reduces the secretion of hormones, but nothing can be done about the enlargement that has already taken place in the bones and soft tissues.

Dwarfism. Some types of dwarfism occur when there is undersecretion of the adenohypophyseal hormones. In one type, called the Lorain type, the condition is present at birth and, though the features of the body develop in proportion to one another, the rate of growth is much slower than normal. There is no mental retardation in the Lorain type of dwarfism. In other types, there may be thyroid deficiency and poor sexual development as well as retarded physical growth.

Panhypopituitarism in the Adult. This condition, also called Simmonds' disease, is very rare. It occurs as a result of tumors, surgical trauma or thrombosis of the hypophyseal blood vessels. There are three general effects of panhypopituitarism: thyroid deficiency, depressed secretion of adrenal glucocorticoids and loss of sexual function due to decreased production of hormones from the gonads, which depend on the pituitary gland for stimulation. The patient becomes emaciated, ages prematurely and loses sexual function. Treatment is by administration of hormones of the glands that depended on the adenohypophysis for stimulation.

Neurohypophysis

Diabetes Insipidus. This condition is characterized by the production of copious amounts of dilute urine, often as much as 15 to 20 liters in every 24-hour period. Diabetes insipidus occurs as a result of decreased production of the antidiuretic hormone (ADH). This hormone regulates reabsorption of water in the kidney tubules. When it is not present in sufficient amounts, the water remains in the tubules and is excreted as urine. Restriction of fluid intake does not control the excessive flow of urine, and the only satisfactory treatment is administration of posterior pituitary extract (pituitrin) on a regular basis for the rest of the patient's life.

CLINICAL CASE PROBLEMS

1. You are assigned to the evening care of Mrs. Tate, age 33, who had a thyroidectomy early that morning. Mrs. Tate has completely recovered from the anesthesia and has made a good recovery so far.

What precautions must you take in turning and positioning Mrs. Tate?

What special observations would you be expected to make while caring for this patient?

2. Mrs. Loomis is 62 years of age and has been a known diabetic for 20 years. She was admitted to the hospital with an infection of the great toe, re-sulting from improper care of an ingrown toenail. Before admission to the hospital, Mrs. Loomis had been taking Orinase and staying within the limits of her diet. With the development of the infection, she began have a 3+ and 4+ sugar with each urinalysis and finally informed her physician of her difficulties only after the infection was well under way.

What complications may develop from Mrs. Loomis' infection?

Why are these complications likely to develop, and how could Mrs. Loomis have avoided them?

What type of insulin would you expect her to receive while in the hospital?

REFERENCES

1. Beland, I. L.: *Clinical Nursing: Pathophysiological and Psychosocial Approaches,* 2nd edition. New York, The Macmillan Co., 1970.
2. Brunner, L. S., et al. *Textbook of Medical-Surgical Nursing,* 2nd edition. Philadelphia, J. B. Lippincott Co., 1970.
3. Burke, E. L.: "Insulin Injection." Am. Journ. Nurs., Dec., 1972, p. 2194.
4. Chellas, M.: "Insulin Reactions in a Brittle Diabetic." Nursing '72, May, 1972, p. 6.
5. DiPalma, J. R.: "Drugs for Diabetes." RN, Oct., 1967, p. 71.
6. Delger, H., and Seeman, B.: *How to Live with Diabetes.* New York, N. W. Horton Co., 1960.
7. French, R. M.: *The Nurse's Guide to Diagnostic Procedures,* 3rd edition. New York, McGraw-Hill Book Co., 1971.
8. Hornback, M.: "Diabetes Mellitus—The Nurse's Role." Nurs. Clin. N. Amer., Vol. 5, No. 1, 1970, p. 3.
9. Jacob, S. W., and Francone, C. A.: *Structure and Function in Man,* 2nd edition. Philadelphia, W. B. Saunders Co., 1965.
10. Krensnick, A.: "Diabetic Neuropathy." Am. Journ. Nurs., July, 1964, p. 106.
11. Martin, M. M.: "Insulin Reaction." Am. Journ. Nurs., Jan., 1967, p. 328.
12. Moore, M. L.: "Diabetes in Children." Am. Journ. Nurs., Jan., 1967, p. 104.
13. Nickerson, D.: "Teaching the Hospitalized Diabetic." Am. Journ. Nurs., May, 1972, p. 935.
14. Nordyke, R. A.: "The Overactive and the Underactive Thyroid." Am. Journ. Nurs., May, 1963, p. 66.

15. Rosenthal, A., and Rosenthal, J.: *Diabetic Care in Pictures,* 3rd edition. Philadelphia, J. B. Lippincott Co., 1967.
16. Shafer, K. N., et al.: *Medical-Surgical Nursing,* 5th edition. St. Louis, The C. V. Mosby Co., 1971.
17. Smith, D. W., et al.: *Care of the Adult Patient,* 3rd edition. Philadelphia, J. B. Lippincott Co., 1971.
18. Watkins, J. D., and Moss, F. T.: "Confusion in the Management of Diabetes." Am. Journ. Nurs., March, 1972, p. 526.
19. Weller, J. C.: "Oral Hypoglycemic Agents." Am. Journ. Nurs., March, 1964, p. 90.

SUGGESTED STUDENT READING

1. Chellas, M.: "Insulin Reactions in a Brittle Diabetic." Nursing '72, May, 1972, p. 6.
2. Dario, E. L.: "Nursing Management of Patients with Thyroid Dysfunction." Journ. Pract. Nurs., Sept., 1969, p. 33.
3. "Diabetics Speak Out: What Patients Say They Aren't Taught about Self-Care." Nursing Update, May, 1973.
4. DiPalma, J. R.: "Drugs for Diabetes." RN, Oct., 1967, p. 71.
5. Ellis, A. J.: "Ketosis: Condition Critical." RN, August, 1969, p. 45.
6. Fish, S. A.: "Medic Alert." Journ. Pract. Nurs., March, 1970, p. 29.
7. "Hypoglycemia." Nursing Update, July, 1972.
8. Kula, J.: "Diet and the Diabetic Patient." Journ. Pract. Nurs., May, 1972, p. 18.
9. Martin, M. M.: "Foot Disorders in Diabetes." Journ. Pract. Nurs., April, 1967, p. 32.
10. Martin, M. M.: "Insulin, the Life-giving Hormone," Part I and Part II. Journ. Pract. Nurs., March and April, 1968, p. 42.
11. Neuberger, S. C., and Johnston, H.: "Continuing Education in Diabetes." Bedside Nurse, Dec., 1970, p. 14.
12. Nickerson, D.: "Teaching the Hospitalized Diabetic." Amer. Journ. Nurs., May, 1972, p. 935.
13. Stewart, S.: "Day-to-Day Living with Diabetes." Am. Journ. Nurs., Aug., 1971, p. 1548.
14. Watkins, J. D., and Moss, F. T.: "Confusion in the Management of Diabetes." Am. Journ. Nurs., March, 1972, p. 526.

OUTLINE FOR CHAPTER 19

I. Introduction

A. Endocrine system is composed of ductless glands that pour their secretions (hormones) directly into blood stream.

B. Hormones are chemical substances that speed up or slow down activities of the cells of the body.

C. Overactivity or underactivity of a gland may cause disease.

II. Diseases of the Thyroid Gland

A. Special diagnostic tests—basal metabolic rate, radioactive iodine uptake, protein-bound iodine and cholesterol level.

B. Simple goiter—thyroid enlarged but not oversecreting thyroxine. Caused by deficiency of iodine in the diet.
  1. Symptoms—enlargement of the neck, dysphagia and dyspnea.
  2. Treatment and nursing care— Medications with iodine. Surgical removal of the goiter may be necessary if it is greatly enlarged.

C. Hyperthyroidism—a systemic condition resulting from overactivity of the thyroid gland and overproduction of thyroxine. Also called Graves' disease, toxic goiter or thyrotoxicosis.
  1. Symptoms—result of increased metabolic rate. Patient extremely nervous, tense and overactive, increasingly fatigued and very hungry. May be very unstable emotionally.
  2. Treatment—rest and diet high in carbohydrates, calories and vitamins. Drugs—iodine preparations, thyroid blocking agents such as propylthiouracil and radioactive iodine. Surgery— thyroidectomy.
    a. Preoperative care—observation of the patient for signs of overactivity or other indications that his metabolic rate may be too high for safety during surgery.
    b. Postoperative care—patient placed in high Fowler's position. Vital signs checked frequently, and patient watched for signs of bleeding or swelling in the operative area. Two most dangerous complications are thyroid crisis and tetany.

D. Hypothyroidism—underactivity of the thyroid gland with a deficiency in the production of thyroxine.
  1. Symptoms vary. In children, the symptoms of *cretinism* are retarded physical and mental growth. In adults, the condition *(myxedema)* is characterized by slurred speech, reduced mental

activity, sluggishness, dry and scaly skin and increased sensitivity to cold.

    2. Treatment with thyroid extract usually successful. *cytomel* *synthroid*

III. Disorders of the Parathyroids

A. Parathyroids are located on the posterior aspect of the thyroid. Parathyroid hormone regulates calcium and phosphorus concentration in body fluids.

B. Hypoparathyroidism (tetany) is due to a deficiency of parathyroid hormone.

    1. Can occur following thyroidectomy in which parathyroid tissue has been removed accidentally or with idiopathic atrophy of the parathyroid glands.

    2. Chief symptom is extreme irritability of muscle tissue resulting from calcium deficiency. ↓ Ca

    3. Acute condition treated by administration of calcium salts. Chronic condition treated by injections of parathyroid extract, vitamin D in massive doses and calcium salts.

C. Hyperparathyroidism (von Recklinghausen's disease) is due to excessive secretion of parathyroid hormone.

    1. Symptoms brought about by removal of calcium from bones and its accumulation in the blood include fatigue, kidney stones and changes in the skeletal system.

    2. Treatment is surgical removal of the excess glandular tissue.

IV. Disorders of Carbohydrate Metabolism

A. The hormone insulin that is secreted by the islets of Langerhans on the pancreas is necessary for proper utilization of carbohydrates. An excess of insulin leads to hypoglycemia; a deficiency in insulin leads to diabetes mellitus.

B. Diagnostic tests include:

    1. Urinalysis for sugar.

    2. Blood sugar level (a high level is found in diabetes mellitus, chronic liver disease and overactivity of some of the endocrine glands).

    3. Glucose tolerance (measures the body's ability to utilize glucose).

C. Diabetes mellitus is a chronic disease resulting from inability of the body to use and store carbohydrates normally.

    1. Exact cause not known. Contributing factors may include inability to produce enough insulin, increase in the rate at which the body uses up insulin, increase in the rate at which insulin is destroyed in the body and drop in the efficiency of insulin.

    2. Symptoms are polyuria, polydipsia, polyphagia, fatigue, muscular weakness, pruritus and numbness and tingling of hands and feet.

    3. Treatment. No cure, but it can be controlled by diet, proper exercise and administration of insulin or a hypoglycemic drug.

        a. Diet is generally low in carbohydrate, high in protein and moderate in fat. The patient is given an exchange list from which his menus are planned.

        b. Insulin is administered by hypodermie.

        c. Hypoglycemic agents may be used for some diabetics who develop the disease in adult life.

    4. A serious deficiency of insulin can lead to diabetic acidosis, which can be fatal. Too much insulin can cause an insulin reaction.

    5. The uncontrolled diabetic is more likely to develop arteriosclerosis with accompanying circulatory disturbances, especially in the lower extremities, and is prone to infections and visual disturbances.

D. Hypoglycemia is an abnormally low level of glucose in the blood.

    1. Condition can be due to a tumor of the pancreas, liver disease or a disorder of the pituitary or adrenal glands.

    2. Symptoms are weakness, pallor, excessive perspiration, convulsions and coma.

    3. Treatment of the primary disorder (if one can be found) is first step. Patient should eat high-protein, regularly spaced meals and should carry candy or sugar as a quick source of energy.

V. Disorders of the Adrenal Glands

A. The adrenal medulla secretes epinephrine and norepinephrine; the adrenal cortex secretes the mineralocortocoids, the glucocorticoids and the androgenic hormones.

B. Addison's disease (hypoadrenalism).
1. Result of underactivity of the adrenal cortex.
2. Symptoms—malaise, chronic fatigue, pigmentation of skin, dehydration and circulatory collapse.
3. Treatment—replacement of the adrenal hormones lacking in the body.

C. Cushing's syndrome (hyperadrenalism).
1. Result of increased activity of adrenal cortex.
2. Presents a wide variety of symptoms, including muscular weakness, abnormal sexual development and some mental disturbances.
3. Treatment of primary condition when it is known. Also supportive measures, administration of potassium chloride and a low-sodium, high-potassium diet. Surgical treatment is removal of most of the adrenal gland, leaving enough to provide necessary hormones.

D. Pheochromocytoma—a tumor located in the adrenal medulla or in other chromaffin tissues of the sympathoadrenal system.
1. Causes an increased secretion of epinephrine and norepinephrine.
2. Symptoms—hypertension, severe headache, visual disturbances and tachycardia.
3. Treatment—surgical removal of the tumor.

VI. Disorders of the Pituitary Gland

A. Introduction. The hypophysis influences all systems and organs of the body.

B. Gigantism. The growth hormone is overproduced during childhood, causing rapid growth and lengthening of the long bones. Patient also may have diabetes mellitus. Treatment involves irradiation of the tumor or excessive glandular tissue.

C. Acromegaly. Overproduction of the growth hormones after adolescence, affecting growth of the soft tissues and the bones of the cranium, hands, feet and lower jaw. Treated by irradiation of the hypophysis.

D. Dwarfism. Some types may be due to undersecretion of the adenohypophyseal hormones. May be some thyroid deficiency and poor sexual development as well as retarded physical growth.

E. Panhypopituitarism in the adult (Simmond's disease). A very rare disorder of the pituitary gland, causing thyroid deficiency, loss of sexual function and depressed secretion of the adrenal glucocorticoids. Treated by administration of deficient hormones.

F. Diabetes insipidus. Result of decreased production of the antidiuretic hormone (ADH). Characterized by production of copious amounts of dilute urine. Treated by administration of posterior pituitary extract (pituitrin).

20

Nursing Care of Patients With Disorders of the Reproductive System

VOCABULARY

Ectopic
Gynecology
Menopause
Perineum
Spermatozoa

INTRODUCTION

The male and female reproductive systems have one basic function in common: *procreation* or *reproduction of the species.* Aside from this similarity in function, there are some basic similarities in the structure of the male and female organs of reproduction. Generally, these organs may be divided into glands, tubes or ducts and reservoirs.

The glands of the female reproductive system are the ovaries, which lie on either side of the pelvis and are attached to the uterus. The ovaries are both *endocrine* and *exocrine glands* because they secrete hormones directly into the blood stream (estrogen and progesterone) and they also have external secretions which contain an ovum, or egg.

The glands of the male reproductive system are called the testes, and they too have internal secretions of a hormone (testosterone) and external secre-

tions, which contain the spermatozoa. The testes, like the ovaries, are oval; however, they are located outside the abdominal cavity in the scrotal sac. The prostate gland, which is located just below the bladder and completely surrounds the urethra, is one of several auxiliary glands which secrete a lubricant for the urethra.

The second group of organs are the tubes. In the female, these tubes are the uterine tubes, which conduct the egg from the ovary to the uterus, and the vagina, or birth canal, which serves as a passageway for either the menstrual flow or the products of conception, depending on whether or not the ovum has been fertilized.

In the male, the system of tubes is much more complex. These tubes include the epididymis, the ductus deferens, the ejaculatory duct and the urethra, and they are all responsible for transporting the spermatozoa from the testes to the outside.

The third group of organs consists of

the reservoirs. In the female, the ovary contains and allows for maturation of the egg, or ovum; the uterus serves as a reservoir for the fertilized egg and assists in its maturation and development until the birth of the infant.

In the male, the epididymis stores the spermatozoa until ejaculation, at which time the sperm are transported in the seminal fluid through the ducts to the outside.

The normal development and proper functioning of the reproductive organs in both the male and female depend to a great extent on the proper functioning of hormones from the pituitary gland.

In spite of the basic similarities mentioned previously, there are many and diverse pathologic conditions affecting the male or female reproductive system. This chapter is divided into Part I, which covers the female reproductive system, and Part II, which is concerned with the male reproductive system.

Part One. The Female Reproductive System

SPECIAL DIAGNOSTIC TESTS AND EXAMINATIONS

ASK BEFORE

Pelvic Examination

The examination of the genital organs by palpation and visualization is one of the most commonly used methods of diagnosing diseases of these organs. There are several duties and responsibilities of the nurse in assisting with this examination.

Physical and mental preparation of the patient is of utmost importance. The success of the examination will depend to a great extent on the ability of the patient to relax and cooperate with the examining physician. Proper draping of the patient and providing privacy for such an examination are considered to be an essential part of the nursing procedure, and every practical nurse is expected to know this procedure and carry it out efficiently and quickly without giving the patient the impression of being rushed into the procedure. The necessary equipment, such as a vaginal speculum, gloves and lubricant, must be assembled and conveniently arranged before the physician is summoned to begin the examination. The nurse should remain with the patient during the examination and assist her in dressing after the examination is completed. She should avoid all signs of haste or lack in interest in the patient's feelings and attitudes toward the examination. A few moments should be taken to explain the procedure if the patient does not know what to expect and to relieve her anxieties and fears by answering her questions simply and honestly. We repeat, *the success of the examination depends to a great extent on the patient's ability to relax and cooperate.*

BEFORE

While preparing her patient for a gynecological examination, the nurse must be sure to have the patient empty her bladder completely. Otherwise, the distended bladder will interfere with the examination.

The best time for a pelvic examination is between menstrual periods. This is sometimes taken to mean that a pelvic examination is dangerous and undesirable if the patient is bleeding. Actually, the presence of persistent vaginal bleeding for several weeks or months may indicate a serious disease which should be investigated *immediately,* rather than delaying the examination in the hope that the bleeding will stop. Thus, there is no reason that a pelvic examination should not be done when the patient is bleeding.

Sometimes patients who have an abnormal amount of vaginal discharge will administer a vaginal douche to themselves before going to the doctor's office, unaware that this procedure washes away secretions which may help the physician in diagnosing the cause of the discharge. The nurse may need to explain this to her patients so that they will understand why douching is not advisable immediately before a gynecological examination.

Smears and Cultures

In both of these tests, samplings of material from the reproductive tract are taken and examined in the laboratory. As is true for all other smears and cultures, these tests are useful in determining specific diseases present or the microorganisms causing the disease.

A Papanicolaou smear is used specifically for diagnosing cancer of the cervix. For further details on this particular type of smear and also for a cervical biopsy, the reader is referred to Chapter 10.

Dilatation and Curettage

This is actually a minor surgical procedure done under general anesthesia and may be used to treat certain diseases of the reproductive system. However, the endometrial tissue removed during the operation is often sent to the laboratory for microscopic examination to aid in the diagnosis of the patient's condition. For this reason, we consider dilatation of the cervix and curettage (scraping of the uterus) as both a diagnostic and therapeutic procedure.

Mammography

This is an x-ray examination of the soft tissues of the breast without the injection of a contrast medium. It can be used in diagnosing lesions of the breast such as tumors and abscesses but requires a skilled and experienced radiologist to read the films properly. One of the most difficult tasks is distinguishing between benign and malignant lesions, and so mammography cannot take the place of biopsy, palpation and other examinations of the breast. It should be accepted as one more means of detecting breast disorders rather than as a specific examination that eliminates the need for further study. It has been suggested that mammography could be useful in screening the general population for breast lesions that require further examination.

DISORDERS OF MENSTRUATION

Amenorrhea

Definition. The word "amenorrhea" means absence of menstruation, and this term is used to cover the absence of regular monthly periods at any time between the onset of puberty and the menopause. Amenorrhea is usually classified as *primary amenorrhea*, in which the menses have never occurred, and *secondary amenorrhea*, in which there is an absence of menstrual periods in women who have formerly had normal menstrual cycles. (See Table 20-1 for an explanation of the normal menstrual cycle.)

Symptoms. The symptoms of amenorrhea are obvious—there is simply no evidence of the monthly menstrual flow. The causes of amenorrhea are many and complex and are most often associated with disturbances in the hormonal activities of one of the glands, such as the ovaries, thyroid or pituitary gland. Other causes include malformations of the vagina or uterus, acute or chronic disease or some emotional disturbance. Sometimes the cessation of menstruation indicates pregnancy.

Treatment. The treatment of amenorrhea must be directed toward the

TABLE 20-1. PERIODS OF THE MENSTRUAL CYCLE*

First to Fifth Day	Sixth to Fourteenth Day	Fifteenth to Twenty-eighth Day
Menstrual Period	*Period of Growth and Repair*	*Secretory Period*
1. Endometrium sloughs away as menstrual flow begins.	1. Follicle grows and egg matures.	1. Progesterone and estrogen are secreted.
2. Progesterone and estrogen are no longer secreted.	2. Endometrium returns to normal state and then begins to thicken because of action of estrogen.	2. Endometrium continues to thicken and becomes filled with blood in preparation for receiving the fertilized egg.
3. New follicle starts to mature.	3. Ovulation occurs about fourteenth day, when follicle ruptures and releases the egg.	

°NOTE: In order for menstruation to occur, two organs are essential: (1) the uterus, because menstruation is the sloughing away of the lining of the uterus; and (2) at least part of one ovary, because the ovary secretes the hormones which cause the endometrium to thicken.

cause of the condition. Most physicians advise a thorough check-up by a gynecologist if a girl has not menstruated by her fifteenth birthday. All mature women who have an unexplained cessation of menstruation should consult a gynecologist, since absence of the menstrual flow may be symptomatic of many different diseases of the genital tract.

Dysmenorrhea

Definition. Dysmenorrhea refers to the association of pain with the menstrual flow. It is estimated that at least 50 per cent of all menstruating women experience some degree of discomfort during their menstrual periods at some time or other. However, this percentage cannot be considered an accurate statistic, because individuals react differently to pain and discomfort and most women do not have difficulty with every menstrual period.

Symptoms. It should be emphasized that menstruation is a normal function and should not be accompanied by severe cramps or a steady aching type of pain. Dysmenorrhea refers to an *abnormal amount* of pain and discomfort. Therefore, severe or persistent dysmenorrhea should be reported to a gynecologist.

Treatment and Nursing Care. Dysmenorrhea is treated according to its cause. Surgery is rarely indicated and then usually when congenital malformations or tumors are the direct cause of the condition. Endocrine disorders causing dysmenorrhea may be treated by the administration of hormones in some cases.

A woman's general physical condition and mental attitude toward menstruation may have a direct effect on the success of treatment for dysmenorrhea. The nurse may be of great help to young girls first learning about and adjusting to monthly periods if she will help them understand that menstruation should not restrict most of their usual activities. The person who is busy and happily engaged in her normal activities is less likely to be bothered by the minor discomforts of menstruation than one who considers the monthly cycle as a great inconvenience and an excellent opportunity to lie in bed and receive attention. Adequate rest, warm, soothing baths, removal of tight clothing and a well-balanced, nonconstipating diet should be all that is necessary for relief of the minor discomforts of menstruation.

Menorrhagia

Definition Menorrhagia is an excessive loss of blood in the menstrual flow during the regular monthly period. It is frequently due to a disturbance in the function of the endocrine glands, in which case it is called *functional bleeding*. Other causes may include uterine tumors, pelvic inflammatory disease and an abnormal condition of pregnancy.

Curettage of the uterine cavity is sometimes done for treatment of the condition as well as for diagnosis of the cause of the excessive bleeding.

Metrorrhagia

Definition. Metrorrhagia is uterine bleeding or spotting which occurs at times other than the regular menstrual cycle. Even a slight spotting should be reported to a gynecologist, since it may be the only symptom of a serious pelvic disease, as for example, malignant diseases of the genital tract.

INFECTIONS OF THE GENITAL TRACT

Gonorrhea

Definition. Gonorrhea is a venereal disease caused by a specific organism

called the *gonococcus.* Venereal diseases are infections usually spread by sexual contact.

Of the many venereal diseases, gonorrhea is the most common and, in spite of intensive efforts to eradicate the disease, it is still a menace to public health.

Symptoms. The symptoms of gonorrhea usually appear within 48 hours after exposure and include burning on urination and itching in the vaginal region. Within a few days, a profuse and purulent vaginal discharge appears. The disease spreads upward from the vagina, involving the endometrium (lining of the uterus) and then spreading to the uterine tubes. The symptoms of the acute stage may then subside somewhat, and the disease becomes chronic if left untreated. A definite diagnosis may be made by discovering the *gonococcus* in a specimen of the vaginal discharge.

Treatment and Nursing Care. In caring for these patients, the nurse must remember that gonorrhea is a highly infectious disease that may easily be spread to the eyes (gonorrheal conjunctivitis). In procedures such as douches or assisting with a pelvic examination, the nurse's hands must be thoroughly washed and kept away from the face. It is best if the nurse wears rubber gloves while administering any treatment which involves contact with the genital area or discharge from the vagina.

The antibiotics such as penicillin or streptomycin are used in the treatment of gonorrhea. Early treatment may prevent spreading the disease to others or complications such as sterility.

Syphilis

Definition. Syphilis is also a venereal disease, but it is a more generalized disease affecting the entire body and not limited to the genital organs only. It is caused by a spirochete, *Treponema pallidum.* The causative organism of syphilis cannot survive without moisture, and it can be destroyed with plain soap. Since the spirochete must be wet and warm to survive, syphilis is nearly always transmitted by direct bodily contact; it is extremely rare for the disease to be transmitted by inanimate objects such as toilet seats or eating utensils.

It is possible for an infant to be born with an active case of syphilis because the spirochete can pass the placental barrier once the fetus has reached the fourth month of development. About one half of the expectant mothers who have an active case of syphilis that is not treated will bear an infant with congenital syphilis. The disease can be fatal to the infant, or it can lead to physical deformities and mental disorders.

Diagnosis. A positive diagnosis of syphilis is established by finding the treponema in a smear made from exudate taken from a chancre. Blood tests such as the Wasserman, Mazzini, Kahn and Kolmer can also detect syphilis once it has been established in the body. This is usually within three weeks of the initial infection. A serologic test for syphilis (S.T.S.) can be falsely positive, however, and newer tests such as the TPI (*Treponema pallidum* immobilization) test are considered more accurate.

Symptoms. Unfortunately, the symptoms of syphilis are not very severe in the earlier stage of the disease. Some have a way of subsiding and then reappearing, and the infected person may not be aware of the serious and permanent damage being done to vital organs of his body until it is too late. This is doubly tragic because the disease can be cured and serious complications avoided if it is treated in its earliest stages.

There are three stages of syphilis: *primary, secondary* and *tertiary*. In the primary stage, a chancre or hard sore appears on the mucous membrane of the mouth or genitalia. The chancre is teeming with spirochetes, and so the individual is highly infectious at this stage. Within three days after infection, the spirochetes enter the blood stream, where they begin to multiply rapidly. Other symptoms of the first stage may include headache and some enlargement of the lymph glands near the chancre, but generally, the infected person does not feel very sick. The chancre and other symptoms disappear within three to eight weeks, and if the patient has used some salve or patent medicine with the mistaken idea that the chancre was a minor infection, he may falsely conclude that the medicine had cured him. Nothing could be further from the truth, because the disease has now entered the second stage, and spirochetes have invaded his blood stream.

Symptoms of the secondary stage of syphilis vary in individuals. Some may feel fairly well with only slight malaise or headache. Others may develop a skin rash or sore throat, or they may lose patches of hair from the scalp. There also may be some arthritis, neuritis or retinitis. Eventually these symptoms subside (though they may reappear), and the disease enters a latent period.

The tertiary stage of syphilis can begin one year after infection, but more often it is four or five years before the serious effects of the infection are first noticed. In some persons, the disease may lie dormant for 20 years before symptoms of the third stage appear. Since the spirochetes have had free access to all tissues of the body, the damage they have caused can present a wide variety of symptoms. The nervous system, blood vessels and eyes are most often affected.

Treatment and Nursing Care. Penicillin is the drug of choice in treating syphilis in its primary stage. Other drugs that can be used as alternatives in case of sensitivity to penicillin include tetracycline and erythromycin. Usually the patient receives a single, massive dose of long-lasting penicillin, which destroys the spirochetes in his body. He is instructed to return for periodic check-ups to be sure he is rid of the disease. There is no immunity conferred by an attack of the disease, and a person can become infected with syphilis again and again.

One of the most important aspects of treating and controlling syphilis and other venereal diseases is proper education of the public so that their cooperation can be gained. One promiscuous person can be responsible for infecting several others, who in turn become sources of infection for still others, and the chain reaction can be almost endless. Locating those who have been in contact with an infected person can be a time-consuming and often thankless job because it necessarily involves asking personal questions and requires convincing the contacts that a simple treatment can prevent very serious complications in later life. The nurse should realize that many infected persons are teenagers who fear being found out by their families and friends and who do not fully understand the disease or appreciate its seriousness. She must use tact and understanding with these patients, avoid treating them with disgust or censuring them and encourage them to cooperate with Public Health officials and other members of the health team who are striving to locate and treat infected persons.

Pelvic Inflammatory Disease

Definition. This is a general term used to include any inflammation in the pelvis *outside the uterus.* If the inflammation is located in the uterine tubes, it is called a *salpingitis;* if the ovaries are affected, the term used is *oophoritis;* and involvement of the pelvic peritoneum is called *pelvic peritonitis.*

The organisms causing the infection are usually introduced from the outside and then spread upward through the uterus without affecting the endometrium. Sometimes, however, in an infection following delivery, the inflammatory process may extend outward from the uterus and involve adjoining connective tissues of the pelvis. When this happens, the patient has a *pelvic cellulitis.*

Many people are under the impression that pelvic inflammatory disease is caused only by the gonococcus, probably because it was once the most common causative organism before the discovery of penicillin and the sulfonamides. Now that gonorrhea may be cured in its early stages before it spreads upward through the genital tract, it is less common as a cause of pelvic inflammatory disease. Any organism capable of producing an infection can cause pelvic inflammatory disease.

Symptoms. The patient with acute pelvic inflammatory disease is very ill and appears to be in acute distress. She experiences severe abdominal and pelvic pain, elevated temperature, nausea and vomiting and frequently has a purulent, foul-smelling vaginal discharge.

If the disease progresses to the chronic stage, there are usually disturbances of menstruation, backache and a feeling of heaviness in the pelvis.

Treatment and Nursing Care. Ideally the condition should be treated in its earliest stages so that further spread of the infection and complications from scarring of the tissues may be avoided. Antibiotics are administered for control of the infection, and hygienic measures to improve the general health of the patient are also employed.

The patient is usually placed on bed rest and positioned in a semi-Fowler's position so that any abscess which may form will be low in the pelvis, where drainage is most easily established. Heat is usually applied to the lower abdomen, and hot vaginal douches are ordered to facilitate drainage of the exudate from the site of the inflammation. Any change in the amount, color or odor of the vaginal discharge should be reported immediately.

The most common complication of pelvic inflammatory disease is *sterility*. This is a result of the narrowing or complete closure of the uterine tubes, which prevents passage of the sperm through the tube. Sometimes, even if the sperm can pass through and fertilize the egg, there is not room for the enlarged fertilized egg to pass back through the tube into the uterus, and it becomes lodged in the tube, thus leading to a *tubal* or *ectopic* pregnancy.

VAGINAL INFECTIONS

Trichomonas Vaginitis

Definition. This is an inflammation of the vaginal mucosa. It is a very common condition and is caused by the protazoon *Trichomonas vaginalis*, a parasite which thrives in the vaginal canal. Since these organisms are found in the vaginal secretions of women who do not have any symptoms at all, it is believed that other factors, such as changes in the physiologic condition of the vagina, contribute to the growth of the parasite and the development of an infection.

Symptoms. The symptoms of a trichomonal infection of the vagina include a persistent *leukorrhea* (white vaginal discharge), which causes irritation of the vaginal mucosa, and a swelling and inflammation of the vulva and perineum.

Treatment and Nursing Care. Trichomonal infections are very difficult to control and in many cases the condition may persist for years in spite of treatment. There are several suppositories and powders which may be prescribed for local application, but their success depends on the individual case. Vinegar douches which change the chemical environment of the vagina are often beneficial. Scrupulous cleansing of the perineum with soap and water after each voiding or defecation may help in the control of the primary infection and prevent a secondary infection from other bacteria.

Monilial Vaginitis

Definition. This is an inflammation of the vagina caused by *Candida albicans*, a member of the yeast family that thrives in warm, moist places. The condition is often seen in uncontrolled diabetics because the sugar provides an excellent medium for the growth of the yeast.

Symptoms. The most outstanding symptom is a watery vaginal discharge, often containing white, cheeselike flakes and producing severe itching and inflammation of the vulva.

Treatment and Nursing Care. If the condition can be traced to uncontrolled diabetes, it is obvious that lowering the blood sugar will greatly facilitate elimination of the infection. In other cases, local treatment is used. This consists of frequent applications of gentian violet or one of the other drugs used specifically for treating yeast infections. Douches are not advisable as long as the local medication is being applied.
No longer

TUMORS OF THE UTERUS

Definition

Tumors within the uterus are very common in women between the ages of 25 and 40. Those tumors which are benign are commonly called *fibroids* and involve the uterine wall. Malignant tumors most often affect the cervix; in fact, 66 per cent of the malignant disease involving the genital tract in the female are located in the cervix.

Symptoms

Bleeding is the most common symptom of all uterine tumors in their early stages. Later, as the tumor becomes larger, it causes symptoms of pressure within the abdominopelvic cavity.

Treatment and Nursing Care

The treatment of a nonmalignant tumor of the uterus is entirely different from that of a malignant tumor. It is well known that a malignant disease requires immediate surgical removal of the affected part and possibly additional radiation therapy to destroy any remaining malignant cells. A benign uterine tumor, however, may subside spontaneously, especially at the time of menopause, because it is at this time that ovarian hormones which stimulate the growth of these tumors are no longer secreted.

The choice of treatment of a benign tumor of the uterus depends on the age of the patient and the symptoms brought about by the tumor. In younger women, the tumor is removed surgically, and an effort is made to preserve the functions of the ovaries. Patients near the age of menopause or older may be treated conservatively unless severe bleeding or pressure symptoms require radium therapy or surgery.

UTERINE DISPLACEMENTS

Definition

The uterus is normally suspended in the abdominopelvic cavity by ligaments and is attached to the floor of the pelvis. It is not in a *fixed position,* however, and can be moved about to some degree. An extreme tilting of the uterus away from its normal position is considered to be abnormal and does create some difficulty. This condition is referred to as a uterine displacement.

Types of Displacement. The uterus may be bent forward or tilted backward. It may also slip downward out of its normal position. Figure 20-1 shows the major displacements of the uterus in comparison to its normal position.

Anteflexion is a bending forward of the uterus.

Retroflexion is a bending backward of the uterus.

Retroversion is a tilting backward of the uterus without bending.

Retrocession is a backward displacement of the uterus without bending.

Prolapse of the uterus is a falling or lowering of the uterus into the vagina.

Symptoms

Not all uterine displacements produce symptoms. Those that are severe cause symptoms of backache, feeling of heaviness or "drag" in the pelvis, white vaginal discharge and fatigue.

Treatment and Nursing Care

Treatment is considered necessary only when symptoms are annoying or cause discomfort. In minor displacements, the uterus may be replaced manually during a pelvic examination and a *pessary* inserted to hold the uterus in place. This is considered to be a temporary measure and is used to find out whether displacement is the cause of the patient's difficulties. In young women, if the pessary does prove to relieve the symptoms, the physician may correct the displacement by surgery. In this procedure, the ligaments are shortened so that they hold the uterus more securely.

In older women who are poor surgical risks, the pessary may be used permanently. Vaginal douches daily and frequent visits to the physician are necessary because this device is a foreign body in the vagina and is therefore likely to be irritating to the vaginal mucosa.

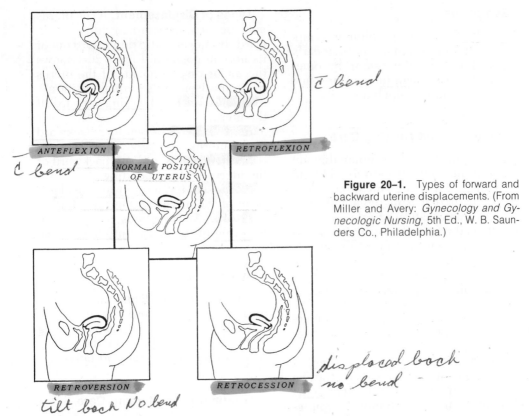

c̄ bend

c̄ bend

tilt back No bend

displaced back
no bend

Figure 20–1. Types of forward and backward uterine displacements. (From Miller and Avery: *Gynecology and Gynecologic Nursing*, 5th Ed., W. B. Saunders Co., Philadelphia.)

NURSING CARE OF THE PATIENT HAVING VAGINAL SURGERY

Introduction

Surgery of the female genital organs may be done by way of the abdomen or by way of the vagina. Surgical procedures such as those involving repair of the vaginal canal or pelvic floor, with restoration of these tissues and organs to their normal structure and function, will obviously involve vaginal surgery. Removal of part or all of the uterus, tubes and ovaries may be done by way of an abdominal incision or by way of the vagina. Table 29 gives a brief description of some of the more common types of gynecological surgery.

Preoperative Nursing Care

The physical preparation of the patient involves shaving of the pubic and perineal hair and a thorough cleansing of the area with a surgical detergent or pHisoHex. Care must be taken to clean between the folds of the labia and around the clitoris so that all secretions are removed. Vaginal douches may be ordered the evening and morning before surgery. Other physical aspects of the preoperative care are the same as for any patient having major surgery.

Postoperative Nursing Care

When the patient returns from surgery, she must be watched closely for signs of hemorrhage, because bleeding is a common complication of vaginal surgery. Some physicians do not allow patients with perineal stitches to wear perineal pads during the immediate postoperative period because they consider them to be a source of infection. The practical nurse should not apply any pads or dressings to the perineal area unless specifically ordered to do so.

TABLE 20–2. TYPES OF GYNECOLOGICAL SURGERY

Name of Surgical Procedure	Explanation
Dilatation and curettage	Widening the cervix and scraping away the inner lining of the uterus (endometrium).
Conization, or conical excision	Removal of a cone of inflamed tissues of the cervix. Conization is done with an electric cutting wire. Conical excision is done with a surgical knife.
Total hysterectomy	Removal of the entire uterus.
Radical panhysterectomy	Removal of the entire uterus, tubes, and ovaries.
Partial hysterectomy or surgical hysterectomy	Removal of part of the uterus, leaving a portion of the body of the uterus and endometrium.
Anterior and posterior colporrhaphy	Repair of the anterior and posterior wall of the vagina.
Salpingectomy	Removal of a uterine tube.
Oophorectomy	Removal of an ovary.

Some drainage containing blood may be expected following vaginal surgery, but any change in the amount or color of vaginal discharge should be reported immediately. A foul odor may indicate the presence of an infection. When caring for the patient with vaginal surgery, the nurse must always bear in mind the proximity of the rectum and recognize it as a source of infection. When cleansing the area or removing perineal pads, care must be taken to wipe from front to back and to avoid dragging the pad across the perineum from the rectum. Special irrigations of normal saline or a mild antiseptic may be ordered to keep the operative area clean, especially when there has been plastic surgery of the vagina or perineum. Heat lamps may be ordered once or twice daily to keep the area dry and to promote healing of the surgical wound. Aerosol sprays containing local anesthetics may be soothing and comforting when applied to the suture line.

Defecation may become a problem for the patient who has had a repair of the anterior and posterior walls of the vagina. To prevent straining at the stool and subsequent stress on the sutures, mineral oil is usually given each night at bedtime.

An indwelling catheter is usually inserted before or during surgery to insure proper drainage of the bladder. This catheter must be kept open so that distention of the bladder does not place an undue strain on the sutures of the repaired tissues. When the catheter is removed on the third or fourth postoperative day, the patient must be checked frequently for voiding so that the bladder is not allowed to become distended. If the patient cannot void, an order for catheterization must be obtained. The physician will also usually order that the patient's *residual urine* be checked.

Early ambulation and nursing measures to prevent pulmonary and circulatory complications are necessary, as for any patient having major surgery.

Mental depression and anxiety are commonly associated with surgical procedures involving removal of the female genital organs. The nurse must use much patience and tact in dealing with the patient who seems unreasonable or unduly worried about the changes brought about by the surgery. We cannot ignore the fact that such surgery may have altered the parts of her body which are closely associated with sexual activities and womanliness. In spite of a full explanation by the physician, the patient may continue to wonder about the effect the surgery may have on her femininity, her ability to have children or her fulfillment of her role as a wife. Even though such fears and anxieties are, in many cases, unfounded, the nurse must realize that the patient needs sympathetic care and understanding while she is going through this difficult period of adjustment.

ENDOMETRIOSIS

Definition

Endometriosis is a rather common disorder in which endometrial tissue (that of the inner lining of the uterus) is found outside the uterus, especially in the ovaries, recto-vaginal septum and other areas of the pelvis and abdomen. The misplaced tissue usually undergoes changes during the menstrual cycle in the same way normal endometrium does, and there may be some bleeding at the time of menstruation.

Symptoms

Because the aberrant endometrial tissue can cause bleeding into spaces that

have no outlet and are likely to be irritated by the blood, the patient experiences pain and often has adhesions in the area of bleeding. Other symptoms may include excessive menstrual flow, bleeding between menstrual periods and pain on defecation or during sexual intercourse. Some patients have dysmenorrhea that is so severe as to be almost incapacitating.

Treatment

The most efficient method for eradicating the symptoms of endometriosis is the removal of the ovaries, which are necessary for continued growth of endometrial tissue. This is not always a simple matter, however, because endometriosis is a disease of young women in their child-bearing years. If the patient is young and anxious for future pregnancies, the gynecologist usually tries more conservative treatment. This usually involves surgical removal of only one ovary or resection of an endometrial cyst of an ovary and fulguration of other areas of endometrial tissue in the pelvic or abdominal cavity. If the conservative treatment does not relieve the severe symptoms of endometriosis there may be no choice but to return the patient to surgery and remove both ovaries.

Although ectopic endometrial growths rarely become malignant, they can and often do lead to sterility. Most physicians advise their young patients with endometriosis to complete their families as quickly as possible before they become sterile.

OVARIAN TUMORS

Definition and Types

Tumors of the ovary are generally classified as benign or malignant. These new growths can arise from misplaced endometrial tissue (see the preceding discussion) or they can develop from tissues of the ovary itself. Some tumors are cystic, that is, sac-like structures, while others are solid. Dermoid cysts are neoplasms of the ovary that are believed to be the result of spontaneous growth of an unfertilized ovum.

Symptoms

Ovarian tumors do not, as a rule, present specific symptoms until they are fairly well advanced. For this reason, many malignant ovarian tumors are not detected until other organs have become involved. Some ovarian tumors such as the fibroma can become very large, weighing as much as fifteen pounds and interfering with normal motion of adjacent organs. Most ovarian tumors cause irregular bleeding, or there may be a palpable mass or a vague feeling of fullness in the abdomen. When an ovarian tumor is found in its very early stages, it is usually discovered during a routine examination.

Treatment and Nursing Care

If the tumor is benign, involves only one ovary and the patient is relatively young, the surgeon may treat it conservatively with surgical removal of the ovary and a section of the uterine tube, leaving the other tube and ovary intact. Patients with malignant tumors are treated more radically, usually with a panhysterectomy in which both ovaries, both uterine tubes and the uterus are removed. Radiation therapy is sometimes used to destroy the tumor and stop ovarian function when the patient is considered a poor surgical risk.

DISORDERS OF BREAST

Introduction

The most common disorder of the breast is cystic disease (dysplasia); the most serious is carcinoma or cancer of the breast. Cystic disease is not an inflammatory disease, even though it is sometimes called cystic mastitis. The condition usually presents only mild symptoms and requires no extensive treatment. If, however, there are multiple cysts and more severe symptoms of pain and tenderness, a simple mastectomy may be performed as treatment.

Carcinoma of the breast is the most common type of malignancy in females in the United States. It occurs most often during and after menopause and is more common in women who have a relative who has had the disease. For reasons not fully understood, the incidence of breast cancer is lower in women who have nursed babies. The cause of carcinoma of the breast is unknown. The belief that a blow to the breast can lead to cancer is unfounded and probably has arisen from occasions when, following a blow producing tenderness, a woman has sometimes been led to examine her breast and thus to discover an already present cancerous lump.

Signs and Symptoms of Breast Tumors

A lump in the breast is one of the prime symptoms of a breast tumor (see Fig. 20-2). Pain is symptomatic of cystic disease but is not usually associated with a malignant growth until it is in an advanced stage. Abnormal discharge from the nipple can be symptomatic of almost any breast disorder, but it should be considered significant and have prompt medical attention. Dimpling of the breast tissue and overlying skin and retraction of the nipple can occur when a tumor near the surface adheres to the underlying structures. Other symptoms include swelling or enlargement of one breast, a change in firmness or the appearance of a reddened area.

Treatment

The safest, most effective treatment for cancer of the breast is radical mastectomy, in which the entire breast, the pectoral muscles, the lymph nodes

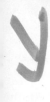

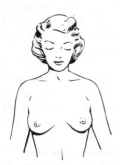

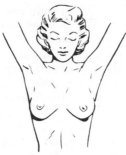

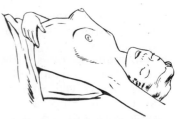

1. Careful examination of the breasts before a mirror for symmetry in size and shape, noting any puckering or dimpling of the skin or retraction of the nipple.

2. Arms raised over head, again studying the breasts in the mirror for the same signs.

3. Reclining on bed with flat pillow or folded bath towel under the shoulder on the same side as breast to be examined.

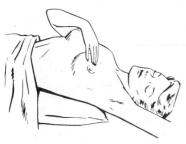

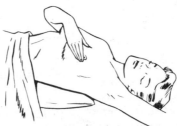

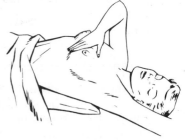

4. To examine the inner half of the breast the arm is raised over the head. Beginning at the breastbone and, in a series of steps, the inner half of the breast is palpated.

5. The area over the nipple is carefully palpated with flats of the fingers.

6. Examination of the lower inner half of the breast is completed.

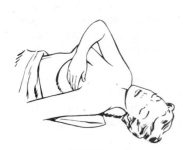

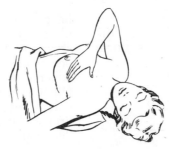

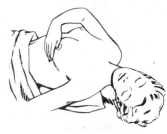

7. With arm down at side self examination of breasts continues by carefully feeling the tissues which extend to the armpit.

8. The upper outer quadrant of the breast is examined with the flat part of the fingers.

9. The lower outer quadrant of the breast is examined in successive stages with flat part of the fingers.

Figure 20–2. Self-examination of the breast. (From the American Cancer Society booklet "The Nurse and Breast Self-Examination," 1952.)

under the arm and all adjacent tissues are removed. A simple mastectomy may be performed for cystic mastitis, a well defined benign tumor or advanced malignant disease in which an ulcerated and draining carcinoma demands removal of the breast but cannot offer hope of a cure.

NURSING CARE OF THE PATIENT HAVING A MASTECTOMY

Preoperative Nursing Care

The physical preparation of the patient having a mastectomy differs very little from the routine preoperative care of any patient having major surgery. The emotional preparation, however, demands additional explanation of the type of surgery to be done and the formulation of plans for rehabilitation and prosthesis after surgery. These are the responsibility of the surgeon, but the nurse must be aware of the emotional upheaval that some patients experience when they realize that the breast must be removed. The same fears and anxieties associated with surgery of the genital organs are frequently seen in the mastectomy patient. Since the breasts are secondary sex organs, and as such are closely related to femininity and motherhood, it is only natural that removal of a breast will cause some emotional reaction. The nurse must try to understand her patient's problems in adjusting to this type of surgery and give her all the moral support and comfort she needs preoperatively as well as postoperatively.

Postoperative Nursing Care

A mastectomy is an extensive surgical procedure, one that may take 4 to 6 hours, and may involve the loss of more than a pint of blood. Transfusions are usually started during surgery and may be continued until several pints of blood have been given.

Since there is a loss of so much blood, the surgeon usually applies a pressure dressing over the wound to prevent further bleeding after surgery. This dressing must be watched carefully for signs of hemorrhage during the first few days postoperatively. In observing for bleeding, the nurse must remember to turn her patient and check the back of the chest as well as the front, because the blood may have seeped downward by gravity flow and collected on the bottom sheet. The pressure dressing may be reinforced but is never changed without specific orders to do so.

During the first 24 hours after surgery, there may be some swelling under the dressing, causing it to become tighter and constrict the blood vessels leading to the arm. When this happens, the patient will complain of numbness of the lower arm, inability to move the fingers or swelling of the lower arm. Such symptoms should be reported immediately.

In order to provide adequate drainage of serosanguineous fluid from the operative area, the surgeon may insert tubes that are connected to a spring-loaded portable suction apparatus (Hemovac). The drainage tubes are usually removed after the third or fourth postoperative day if the drainage has subsided. Directions for using the Hemovac are printed on the apparatus. The drainage obtained should be measured and recorded at least every eight hours. Large amounts of bright red blood may indicate hemorrhage and should be reported immediately. Deep breathing and coughing should be encouraged even though they will most certainly cause some discomfort in the operative area. The patient is usually allowed out of bed the first postoperative day. When getting the patient up, the nurse should be aware that the patient will have some difficulty in balancing herself as long as she cannot use one arm and will therefore be very likely to fall if she does not have adequate support from those helping her out of bed.

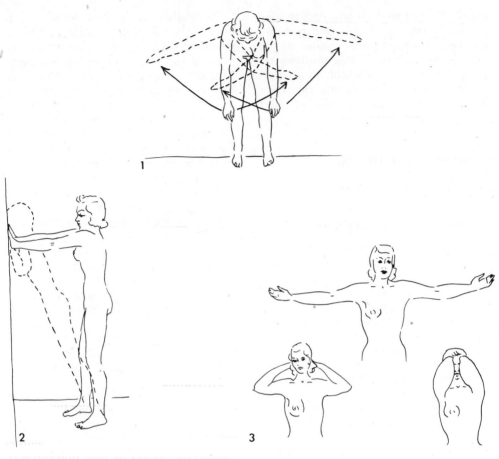

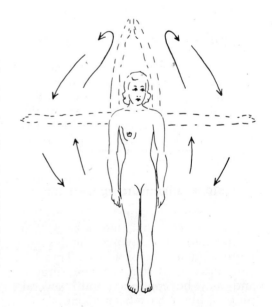

Figure 20–3. Arm exercise #1. Stand with feet 8″ apart. Bend forward from the waist, allowing arms to hang toward the floor by gravity. Swing both arms together, describing an arc from one shoulder to the other. Do not bend elbows. Stand and allow arms to fall to side. Arm exercise #2. Stand facing the wall at arm's length with feet 8″ apart. Place hands against the wall at shoulder level parallel to each other. Slowly flex the elbow, bending the trunk forward until forehead touches wall. Straighten elbows slowly until body is upright. Repeat. Note: Keep head, trunk and legs in straight line. Arm exercise #3. Stand with feet 8″ apart. Extend arms sideways to shoulder level. In rhythm: Flex elbows, clasping fingers at nape of neck. Rotate elbows forward until they touch. Rotate elbows sideways. Unclasp fingers and extend arms sideways at shoulder level. Repeat. Arm exercise #4. Lie on back with arms against the side of the body (use firm surface as floor with rug, pad or blanket, or firm mattress without a pillow). In rhythm: Raise arms to shoulder level (do not flex elbow). Extend arms above head. Return arms to shoulder level. Lower arms to side. Repeat. (From Wolf: Nursing Clinics of North America, December, 1967.)

Special exercises of the arm and shoulder on the affected side are begun as soon as the physician feels the patient may safely do them. Most patients are very cooperative and anxious to do these exercises regularly if they understand how these exercises will prevent deformities and disabilities. The most commonly used exercises are hand wall climbing, hair brushing exercises, elbow pull-in and paddle swinging.

These exercises are fully described and illustrated in the booklet, "Help Yourself to Recovery," published by the American Cancer Society and available at any local Cancer Society office. This booklet also contains some excellent information on the selection and fitting of breast forms and specially designed brassieres for the patient who has had a mastectomy. Other post-mastectomy exercises are shown in Fig. 20-3.

Part Two.   The Male Reproductive System

INFECTIONS OF THE MALE GENITAL TRACT

Introduction

A variety of pathogenic organisms may cause an infection anywhere within the male genital tract. The terminology used for each infection depends on the location of the infection. Urethritis, for example, is an inflammation of the urethra; prostatitis, an inflammation of the prostate; epididymitis, an inflammation of the epididymis; and balanitis, an inflammation of the glans penis.

Urethritis

Definition. This is simply an inflammation of the urethra. It may be caused by the staphylococcus, streptococcus, Escherichia coli (from the colon) or the gonococcus.

Symptoms. The patient with urethritis has symptoms of frequency and urgency and burning on urination. The urinary meatus is swollen and inflamed, and a discharge from the urethra may be present.

Treatment and Nursing Care. Medications used in the treatment of urethritis include the antibiotics and the local application of a mild antiseptic to control the infection. Hot sitz baths may relieve some of the discomfort associated with this condition. Fluids are forced to increase the flow of urine and aid in prevention of urinary complications.

Prostatitis

Definition. This is an inflammation of the prostate gland. It also may be caused by any pathogenic organism which has found its way into the male genital tract.

Symptoms. Because the prostate encircles the urethra just below the neck of the bladder, an inflammation of the prostate produces symptoms of urinary obstruction to some degree. There may be painful urination or difficulty in voiding. The patient also has tenderness and pain in the perineal area.

Treatment and Nursing Care. Prostatitis is treated by antibiotics and local applications of heat in the form of hot sitz baths or low rectal irrigations. Fluids are forced, and the patient is encouraged to rest in bed until the infection is under control.

Epididymitis

Definition. Inflammation of the epididymis may be caused by any pathogenic organism and is one of the most common infections of the male genital tract. It is a common complication of gonorrhea.

Symptoms. In epididymitis there is local pain and tenderness in the scrotal area. Walking may cause pain, and in order to protect the scrotum, the patient assumes an unnatural, stiff-legged gait. A high fever and extreme fatigue usually accompany epididymitis.

Treatment and Nursing Care. In the treatment of epididymitis, cold applications are applied rather than hot because extremely high temperatures may destroy the sperm cells. The scrotum should be elevated and an ice bag placed under it. Later, when the patient is allowed out of bed, an athletic support must be worn.

Balanitis

Definition. This is an inflammation of the glans penis. It is most often the result of *phimosis,* a condition in which the foreskin of the penis cannot be pulled back over the glans penis, thus preventing proper cleansing of the area.

Symptoms. The symptoms of balanitis are swelling of the penis with visible signs of a local inflammation.

Treatment. The first step in the treatment of balanitis is removal of the cause. The surgical procedure for correction of phimosis is *circumcision.* Antibiotics may be given for control of the infection.

Orchitis

Definition. This is an inflammation of the testicle. It is frequently found to be a complication of mumps in adult males. In many cases, this condition leads to sterility.

Symptoms. The symptoms of orchitis are very similar to those of epi-

didymitis. The patient experiences local pain and tenderness in the scrotal area and frequently has an elevated temperature.

Treatment. Because orchitis is a common complication of mumps in adult males, gamma globulin should be given routinely to all individuals past puberty who have been exposed to the disease and have not had mumps before. The orchitis is treated in the same manner as epididymitis.

TUMORS OF THE PROSTATE GLAND

Definition

Neoplasms, or the growth of new cells, within the prostate gland commonly occur in men over the age of 55. These tumors may be benign *(benign prostatic hypertrophy)* or malignant *(cancer of the prostate).*

Symptoms

Benign prostatic hypertrophy produces no symptoms until the growth becomes large enough to press against the urethra. Then the patient begins to experience difficulty in urinating, and in the later stages, there is complete obstruction of the urinary flow.

Carcinoma of the prostate is usually not discovered until the later stages of development, when it begins to cause symptoms of obstruction of the urinary flow. This is unfortuantely true of most malignant diseases and is all the more reason why persons past the age of 40 should have a complete physical checkup every 6 months, even though they may feel perfectly well.

Treatment and Nursing Care

Surgical removal of all or part of the prostate gland is the treatment of choice for tumors of the prostate.

Whenever a biopsy shows the tumor to be malignant, the entire prostate and its capsule must be removed.

The location of the incision and the amount of tissue to be removed will depend on the individual patient, his general physical condition and the type of tumor present.

Radical prostatectomy is the removal of the entire prostate gland and its capsule. The incision is made through the perineum.

Suprapubic prostatectomy is surgical removal of the prostate through an incision directly over the bladder. The bladder is opened, and the urethral mucosa is incised. The tumorous tissue is removed through this incision.

Retropubic prostatectomy involves a low abdominal incision, but the bladder is not opened.

Transurethral prostatic resection is removal of part of the prostate gland by way of the urethra. There is no surgical incision in this procedure, and the postoperative period is much shorter.

Preoperative Nursing Care. The patient who is admitted to the hospital for a prostatectomy will inevitably have some difficulty in voiding. The retention of urine may be so severe that an indwelling catheter is necessary to drain the bladder. In less severe cases, the patient may be able to void but probably cannot completely empty his bladder. In either case, the physician usually wishes to have an accurate record of the patient's intake and urinary output during the preoperative period.

Since most of the patients requiring a prostatectomy are older men beyond the age of 60, the nurse may need to give these patients the special attention required by all geriatric patients. Side rails should be applied to the bed, especially if a sedative has been given. Adequate explanation of the purpose of the indwelling catheter may help the patient accept this inconvenience more readily.

Preoperative medications are given according to the age and general physi-

cal condition of the patient, since elderly people cannot tolerate heavy sedation.

Postoperative Nursing Care. The postoperative nursing care of the patient will vary according to the type of surgery used in removing the prostate gland (see types of surgery described in the preceding material). The general principles of postoperative nursing care which apply to all patients having major surgery are necessary for the patient having a prostatectomy. In addition, the nurse must pay special attention to drainage through the catheter leading from the bladder. This is of primary importance because occlusion of the catheter may lead to more bleeding, cystitis or an upper urinary tract infection.

The patient who has had a transurethral resection will not have a surgical incision; however, this is still a major surgical procedure, and postoperative hemorrhage is always a possibility to be considered. In order to check the amount of drainage and loss of blood through the urethral catheter, the drainage bottle may be marked with adhesive tape. An excessive increase of bright red drainage in a given period of time should be reported.

The catheter and tubing should be checked frequently to make sure that they are not obstructed in any way. Clots or bits of tissue within the catheter may lead to severe spasms of the bladder, which are extremely painful. Before administering any analgesic medication, the nurse should first note whether or not the catheter is draining properly. If the catheter is obstructed, irrigations may be ordered by the surgeon. These irrigations should not be done without a written order and then only under sterile conditions, because infection is a very real danger after prostatectomy. If the patient continues to complain of severe pain even though the bladder is empty, the physician should be notified at once, because unusually severe pain and abdominal rigidity may indicate a perforated bladder.

When a suprapubic prostatectomy has been done, the surgical incision will lie directly over the bladder. The cavity left by the removal of the prostate may be packed with gauze or Gelfoam to prevent hemorrhage, or a large Foley catheter may be inserted into the cavity and traction applied so that the balloon of the catheter presses against the blood vessels. This traction is usually applied for as long as 6 to 8 hours and must not be disturbed while administering care to the patient.

Dressings over the wound must be changed frequently because they collect urinary drainage from the bladder. The skin around the surgical wound must be washed frequently to remove urine, which is very irritating to the skin.

The patient with a perineal incision usually returns from surgery with a small cigarette drain extending through the incision. There may be urinary drainage through this drain as well as through the urethral catheter in the bladder. The principles of cleanliness recommended for the patient having vaginal surgery are equally important in the care of the male patient with a perineal incision. Dressings over the incision must be changed as often as necessary to keep the patient dry and comfortable.

VASECTOMY

Within the past few years, there has been increased interest in birth control methods and family planning. Sterilization of the male through vasectomy has become more popular as an alternative method. An estimated 700,000 vasectomies were performed in the United States in 1971, and the number is expected to increase yearly.

The term "vasectomy" refers to a surgical procedure performed on the vas deferens for the purpose of interrupting the continuity of this duct, which conveys the sperm of the male at the time of ejaculation. The procedure varies according to the preference and training of the surgeon. In some instances, the vas deferens may be clamped bilaterally and a segment excised from each vas (see Fig. 20-4). This procedure is not reversible, and reestablishment of fertility at a later

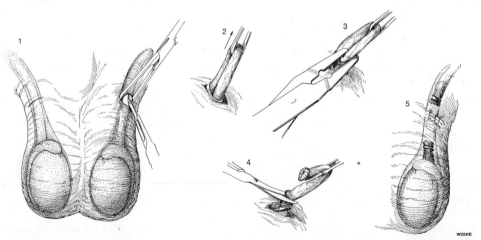

Figure 20–4. Vasectomy surgery: 1. Incision exposes the sheath which is then opened. Bilateral incisions are illustrated, but a midline incision may be used. 2, 3. Vas is exposed and occluded with two clips. Other occluding techniques can be used. 4. Segment of about half an inch is excised. 5. Vas is replaced in sheath and skin is sutured. (From Davis: American Journal of Nursing, March, 1972.)

date cannot be guaranteed. Most surgeons explain the outcome of the procedure to the patient and his wife and request that they sign a statement affirming their knowledge and understanding of the expected outcome.

Another type of so-called vasectomy does not involve removal of a section of the vas deferens but a simple ligation with sutures or clamps. This procedure usually does not provide permanent occlusion of the vas, and therefore does not eliminate the possibility of impregnation in the future. It is possible for the suture to disintegrate or to cut through the vas and allow for restoration of the patency of the tube.

There is no evidence that vasectomy affects the male sex hormone level in any way, since the vas is not an endocrine gland. There is also no physical reason for a vasectomy to affect the male's sexuality. If a man is contemplating surgery of this type, he should discuss it thoroughly with the surgeon and gain a full understanding of what to expect as a reasonable outcome.

The only immediate postoperative complication that usually occurs is pain. Other complications are extremely rare, even though infection and hematoma may develop because of the abundant blood supply to the scrotal area. The procedure is usually performed under local anesthesia in the physician's office or an out-patient clinic. The patient is given specific instructions in his responsibility for physical preparation preoperatively, such as cleaning and shaving the operative site.

CLINICAL CASE PROBLEMS

1. Your brother, whose wife is dead, has asked you to explain menstruation to his daughter, who is reaching the age of puberty. You know that the child has some idea of what to expect but most of her information has come from her friends who are no better informed than she. Her mother has been dead for two years, and even though you have tried, you have never been able to gain the child's confidence completely.

How would you go about explaining menstruation to her?

2. Miss Lawrence is a 40-year-old school teacher who has just had a radical mastectomy for treatment of cancer of the breast. She is a very well-adjusted person and does not seem to be seriously disturbed by her operation. She wishes to have some information on procuring a prosthesis and the exercises she should take to regain use of her arm and shoulder.

How can you help this person?

3. Mr. Williams, age 67, has been admitted to the hospital for a transurethral resection of the prostate. He is assigned to your care his second postoperative day. Mr. Williams seems disoriented and restless, and when you begin to give him his bath, he tells you that his bladder is full and he needs to urinate. You check the catheter and find that it apparently is not draining as it should.

What would you tell Mr. Williams about his need to void?

What would you do about the catheter that seems obstructed?

What observations should you make while caring for this patient?

What special precautions should be taken for his safety?

REFERENCES

1. Alford, D. A.: "Nursing Care of the Patient with Endometriosis." Nurs. Clin. N. Amer., Vol. 3, No. 2, 1968, p. 217.
2. Beland, I. L.: Clinical Nursing: Pathophysiological and Psychosocial Approaches, 2nd edition. New York, The Macmillan Co., 1970.

3. Brunner, L. S., et al.: *Textbook of Medical-Surgical Nursing,* 2nd edition. Philadelphia, J. B. Lippincott Co., 1970.
4. Celano, P., and Sawyer, J. R.: "Vaginal Fistulas." Am. Journ. Nurs., Oct., 1970, p. 2131.
5. Davis, J. E.: "Vasectomy." Am. Journ. Nurs., March, 1972, p. 509.
6. Egan, R. L.: "Mammography." Am. Journ. Nurs., Jan., 1966, p. 108.
7. Funnell, J. W., and Roof, B.: "Before and After Vaginal Hysterectomy." Am. Journ. Nurs., Oct., 1964, p. 124.
8. Gribbons, C. A., and Aliapoulios, M. A.: "Early Carcinoma of the Breast." Am. Journ. Nurs., Sept., 1969, p. 1945.
9. Gribbons, C. A., and Aliapoulios, M. S.: "Treatment for Advanced Breast Carcinoma." Am. Journ. Nurs., April, 1972, p. 678.
10. Iorio, J.: *Principles of Obstetrics and Gynecology for Nurses,* 2nd edition. St. Louis, The C. V. Mosby Co., 1971.
11. Kasselman, M. J.: "Nursing Care of the Patient with Benign Prostatic Hypertrophy." Am. Journ. Nurs., May, 1966, p. 1026.
12. Larsen, G. I.: "What Every Nurse Should Know about Congenital Syphilis." Nurs. Outlook, March, 1965, p. 52.
13. Mayo, P., and Wilkey, N. L.: "Prevention of Cancer of the Breast and Cervix." *Nurs. Clin. N. Amer.,* Vol. 3, No. 2, 1968, p. 229.
14. McGowan, L.: "Before and After Vaginal Surgery." Am. Journ. Nurs., Feb., 1964, p. 73.
15. Shafer, K. N., et al.: *Medical-Surgical Nursing,* 5th edition. St. Louis, The C. V. Mosby Co., 1971.
16. "V.D.: The Unconquered Menace." RN, March, 1970, p. 38.
17. Wolf, E. S.: "Nursing Care of Patients with Breast Cancer." *Nurs. Clin. N. Amer.,* Vol. 2, No. 4, 1967, p. 587.

SUGGESTED STUDENT READING

1. American Cancer Society (pamphlets): "Reach to Recovery" and "A Letter to Husbands."
2. Branson, H. K.: "The Nurse and Mutilation Reaction." Bedside Nurse, Sept., 1970, p. 26.
3. "Breast Cancer—Detection, Management, Rehabilitation." Journ. Pract. Nurs., May, 1971, p. 20.
4. Felton, C.: "The Long Road Home." Journ. Pract. Nurs., July-Aug., 1965, p. 34.
5. Fitzpatrick, G.: "Care of the Patient with Cancer of the Cervix." Bedside Nurse, Jan. and Feb., 1971, p. 11.
6. Harrell, H. C.: "To Lose a Breast." Am. Journ. Nurs., April, 1972, p. 676.
7. McGowan, L.: "Before and After Vaginal Surgery." Am. Journ. Nurs., Feb., 1964, p. 73.
8. Warren, J. C.: "Hormone Therapy in the Post-Reproductive Years." Bedside Nurse, May, 1970, p. 21.

OUTLINE FOR CHAPTER 20

I. Introduction

A. Reproductive system handles procreation or reproduction of the species.

B. Male and female organs of reproduction are glands, tubes or ducts and reservoirs.

1. Female glands (ovaries) secrete estrogen and progesterone and excrete ova. Male glands (testes) secrete testosterone and excrete spermatozoa.
2. Uterine tubes of female conduct ova from ovary to uterus. Vagina conducts menstrual flow or baby. Complex system of tubes in male serves as passageway for spermatozoa.
3. Reservoirs in female are the ovary and the uterus. In the male, the epididymis stores spermatozoa until ejaculation.

Part One   Diseases of the Female Reproductive System

I. Special Diagnostic Tests and Examinations

A. Pelvic examination.

B. Smears and cultures—sampling of material from the reproductive tract is taken and examined in the laboratory.

C. Dilatation and curettage—dilation of the cervix and curettage (scraping) of the endometrial lining of the uterus.

D. Mammography—x-ray examination of the soft tissues of the breast without injection of a contrast medium.

II. Disorders of Menstruation

A. Amenorrhea—absence of menstruation.

1. Causes—hormonal imbalance, malformation of the reproductive tract, chronic disease or emotional disturbance.
2. Treatment directed toward primary cause.

B. Dysmenorrhea—painful menstruation.

1. Severe pain, but not minor discomfort that usually accompa-

nies menstruation, should be reported to gynecologist.
2. Treatment concerned with primary cause.

C. Menorrhagia—an excessive loss of blood during menstruation.
1. Frequently due to an endocrine disturbance, uterine tumors or an abnormal condition of pregnancy.
2. Curettage of the uterine cavity sometimes done to relieve bleeding and to aid in diagnosis.

D. Metrorrhagia—bleeding at times other than menstrual cycle.
1. May be a symptom of serious pelvic disease and should be investigated.

III. Infections of the Genital Tract

A. Gonorrhea—a venereal disease caused by the gonococcus and spread by sexual contact.
1. Symptoms—purulent vaginal discharge, dysuria and itching. Can cause sterility.
2. Treatment—penicillin and streptomycin.

B. Syphilis—a venereal disease caused by a spirochete called *Treponema pallidum.*
1. Spread by direct bodily contact. Can be transmitted by a mother to her unborn child.
2. Diagnosis—presence of treponema in smear taken from chancre or by blood test.
3. Symptoms.
  a. Primary stage—chancre, headache and enlarged lymph glands.
  b. Secondary stage—no symptoms or patient may have rash, loss of hair in patches, sore throat or arthritis and neuritis.
  c. Tertiary stage—symptoms depend on organs affected; do not appear until damage has been done. Organs most often affected are the blood vessels and heart, nerves and eyes.
4. Treatment—penicillin or some other antibiotic in primary stage will cure and prevent complications. Disease in the tertiary stage beyond treatment.

C. Pelvic inflammatory disease—any inflammation in the pelvis outside the uterus.
1. Caused by microorganism that spread upward through the uterus and uterine tubes.
2. Symptoms—severe abdominal and pelvic pain, nausea and vomiting, foul-smelling, purulent vaginal discharge.
3. Treatment—antibiotics and measures to localize infection and prevent complications.

IV. Vaginal Infections

A. Trichomonas vaginitis—inflammation of the vaginal mucosa, caused by *Trichomonas vaginalis.*
1. Symptoms—persistent white vaginal discharge that irritates the vaginal mucosa and swelling and inflammation of the vulva and perineum.
2. Treatment—various suppositories, powders or other local applications may be used but infection difficult to control.

B. Monilial vaginitis—inflammation of the vagina caused by *Candida albicans.*
1. Symptoms—watery vaginal discharge containing cheese-like flakes and intense itching and inflammation of the vulva.
2. Treatment—local applications of drugs.

V. Tumors of the Uterus

A. Most common benign tumors (fibroids) involve the uterine wall. Malignant tumors most often affect the cervix.

B. Abnormal bleeding first symptom. If tumor grows it can cause symptoms of pressure.

C. Treatment. Benign tumors may subside at menopause or may require a simple hysterectomy. Malignant tumors demand prompt removal and possibly irradiation to eliminate the danger of metastasis.

VI. Uterine Displacements

A. An extreme tilting of the uterus away from its normal position in the pelvis.

B. Symptoms (may be none)—backache, feeling of heaviness in the pelvis, vaginal discharge and fatigue.

C. Treatment—insertion of pessary for milder cases; surgical fixation for more severe ones.

VII. Nursing Care of the Patient Having Vaginal Surgery

A. Preoperative perparation varies. Usually the patient is given a vaginal douche, the vulva and perineal area are shaved and cleansed with a surgical detergent and the intestines are emptied.

B. After surgery, patient is watched closely for signs of unusual bleeding. If there is no catheter, the patient must be checked for ability to void. Early ambulation or sitting up help prevent circulatory complications, such as thrombophlebitis and pulmonary complications.

VIII. Endometriosis (Endometrial Tissue Outside the Uterus)

A. Symptoms—severe pain in lower abdomen or pelvis, excessive menstrual flow, metrorrhagia and pain on defecation or during sexual intercourse.

B. Treatment—varies with location of misplaced tissue, age of patient and her desire to have children and severity of symptoms. Surgical removal of one or both ovaries or a panhysterectomy most often done.

IX. Ovarian Tumors

A. Symptoms very slow to develop. Irregular bleeding, palpable mass in abdomen and vague feeling of fullness in abdomen.

B. Treatment depending on type and size of tumor, age of patient and severity of symptoms. Surgery or radiation therapy common.

X. Disorders of the Breast

A. Cystic disease, also called dysplasia or cystic mastitis, is most common disorder of breast. Symptoms are mild and treatment (simple mastectomy) necessary for very few cases.

B. Carcinoma of the breast.
 1. Cause unknown.
 2. Symptoms are a lump in the breast, dimpling, retraction of nipple, abnormal discharge from nipple, swelling, change in firmness or appearance of redness.
 3. Treatment is radical mastectomy.

XI. Nursing Care of the Patient Having a Mastectomy

A. Simple mastectomy—removal of a breast. Radical mastectomy—removal of entire breast, underlying pectoral muscles and axillary lymph nodes.

B. Preoperative care—shaving and cleaning operative area and emotional support.

C. Postoperative care—pressure dressing watched closely for sign of hemorrhage, checked for being too tight and reinforced as necessary (changed only on specific orders). Deep breathing and coughing encouraged. Special exercises of arm and shoulder necessary to prevent deformities and disabilities.

Part Two   The Male Reproductive System

A. Urethritis—an inflammation of the urethra.
 1. Symptoms—frequent urge to void and burning on urination.
 2. Treatment—antibiotics and local applications of a mild antiseptic.

B. Prostatitis—an inflammation of the prostate gland.
 1. Symptoms—painful urination, difficulty in voiding and pain and tenderness in perineal area.
 2. Treatment—antibiotics, local applications of heat and bed rest.

C. Epididymitis—inflammation of the epididymis. A common complication of gonorrhea.
 1. Symptoms—local pain and tenderness in scrotal region, high fever and severe fatigue.
 2. Treatment—cold applications to scrotum, antibiotics and wearing an athletic support.

D. Balanitis—an inflammation of the glans penis often caused by phimosis.
 1. Symptoms—swelling and signs of local inflammation.
 2. Treatment—circumcision and antibiotics.

E. Orchitis—an inflammation of the testes. Can be a complication of mumps.
 1. Symptoms—pain and local tenderness in scrotal area and fever.
 2. Treatment—bed rest, elevation of scrotum and application of ice bags.

II   Tumors of the Prostate Gland

A. Classified as benign or malignant. Occur most often in men over 55 years of age.

B. Symptoms—tumors usually cause no symptoms until they have grown large enough to obstruct the flow of urine from the bladder.

C. Treatment is surgical removal of all or part of the prostate gland.

    1. Radical prostatectomy—entire prostate gland and its capsule removed.

    2. Suprapubic prostatectomy—removed by incision into the bladder.

    3. Retropubic prostatectomy—removed by low abdominal incision.

    4. Transurethral prostatic resection—removed by way of the urethra.

    5. Preoperative care—maintenance of urinary flow, protection of the patient from self-injury and adequate explanation of necessary procedures.

    6. Postoperative care—postoperative hemorrhage guarded against, urinary flow maintained and dressing changed to keep patient dry and comfortable.

III. Vasectomy—Removal of a Section from Each Vas Deferens for the Purpose of Preventing Impregnation

21

Nursing Care of Patients With Disorders of the Nervous System

VOCABULARY

Aneurysm
Cerebrospinal
Hematoma
Occiput
Palliative

INTRODUCTION

The nervous system is the communication system of our bodies. It acts as coordinator for all sensory and motor activities, receiving, interpreting and relaying messages which are vital to the proper performance of all the body's activities. The nervous system is composed of nerve cells and their branches, which interlace with one another to form a dense network of nerve tissue. There are a number of different types of nerve cells, but they all have two physiologic properties in common, *excitability* and *conductivity*.

Nerve cells are excited, or spurred into action, by a stimulus. This stimulus sets up an impulse which is conducted along the nerve pathways until it reaches the tissues of the organ which are controlled by the nerve cells. Should anything happen to impair the ability of certain nerve cells to receive and conduct impulses, the tissues which these cells control cease to function normally. An example of this would be trauma to the spinal cord. All parts of the body below the point of injury would be paralyzed and have no sensation of heat, cold, pressure or pain if the spinal cord had been severed and the flow of impulses interrupted.

Neurology is the branch of medicine concerned with the study of the nervous system and its diseases. It is a highly specialized branch of medical practice. Neurologic nursing also requires special training and scientific knowledge above the level of basic nursing. The practical nurse should become familiar with some of the more common neurologic terms and basic principles of neurologic nursing, but she should realize that most patients with serious neurologic disorders should be cared for by nurses who have had formal training as well as additional experience in the field of neurologic nursing.

Common Neurologic Terms

Paraplegia: paralysis of the lower extremities or lower part of the body.

Commonly associated with spinal injury.

Hemiplegia: paralysis of one side of the body. Commonly associated with cerebral damage.

Quadriplegia: paralysis of all four extremities.

Flaccid paralysis: paralysis in which the muscles are limp and flabby.

Spastic paralysis: paralysis in which the muscles are tense and rigid.

Amnesia: loss of memory.

Aphasia: loss of the ability to speak. In total aphasia, the individual cannot comprehend language in any form, written or spoken.

SPECIAL EXAMINATIONS AND DIAGNOSTIC TESTS

Neurologic Examination

The complete neurologic examination measures the ability of the body to perform certain motor and sensory functions. It is a very intensive and prolonged procedure, sometimes requiring several days to complete if the examination is done in its entirety. It is not within the scope of this text to cover the neurologic examination in detail, but some general aspects of the examination may help the practical nurse understand the purpose of the examination.

The *cranial nerves* control both sensory and motor activities within various parts of the body. The patient will be tested for his sense of taste, smell, sight and hearing. His facial expressions, gag reflex and ability to move his eyes are also included in the testing of the cranial nerves.

Groups of large muscles are tested for strength and coordination during a neurologic examination. The physician will evaluate the patient's gait while walking and running, his posture while standing and the strength of his hand grip.

Involuntary muscular contractions in response to a stimulus are called reflexes. These reflexes are impaired or entirely absent in some types of neurologic disorders. The knee jerk in response to tapping below the kneecap with a percussion hammer is a well known example of a reflex.

• When the physician suspects an inflammation or traumatic injury to the protective coverings of the brain and spinal cord, he will perform certain tests for signs and symptoms of meningeal irritation. Stiffness of the neck, unusual sensitivity of the skin and an involuntary flexion of the hip and knee joints when the head is flexed are all indications of an irritation of the meninges.

One of the primary symptoms of brain disorder is a change in the size of the pupils and their ability to react to light. Normally the pupils of the eye are of equal size and will constrict when exposed to light. It should be noted, however, that for some patients, a slight inequality in the size of the pupils can be normal. When checking the pupils for reaction to light, it is best to darken the room, allowing for dilation of the pupils, and then to shine a light into each eye from the side. It is also helpful to notice whether the pupil constricts quickly or slowly when the light is directed into the eye.

Pupils which remain dilated and fixed are indicative of brain damage. One pupil remaining fixed and dilated indicates increasing intracranial pressure. If both pupils remain constricted, there is probably damage to the pons.

The nurse who observes a patient for pupillary changes must be alert to minute changes and report her findings accurately. She should have some knowledge of the size of the pupils immediately after the accident or injury or at least know whether they have been equal in size. This information can give her a basis for comparison should change occur while she is observing the patient.

Lumbar Puncture

The meninges covering the brain and spinal cord are composed of three layers; the second, or middle, layer is called the *arachnoid* because it resembles a cobweb. The spaces within the arachnoid layer are filled with cerebrospinal fluid which bathes and protects the spinal cord and brain. To obtain a sampling of this fluid for examination in the laboratory, the physician inserts a hollow needle into the arachnoid space between the third and fourth lumbar vertebrae. The spinal cord does not extend this far down the vertebral column, so there is no danger of puncturing the cord with the needle. The specimen of spinal fluid obtained through a lumbar puncture is collected in a sterile test tube and sent to the laboratory for microscopic examination and chemical analysis.

The lumbar puncture (or spinal tap, as it is sometimes called) may also be done for any of the following reasons:

1. To measure the pressure within the cerebrospinal cavities.

2. To determine whether there is a blockage of the flow of spinal fluid.

3. To remove blood or pus from the arachnoid space.

4. To reduce intracranial pressure.

5. For spinal anesthesia.

6. To inject air for x-ray examination of the skull (pneumoencephalogram).

To reduce headache, the patient is usually kept flat in bed for at least 8 hours after a lumbar puncture.

Cisternal Puncture

In this type of spinal tap, the needle is inserted just below the occipital bone into the cisterna magna (see Fig. 21-1). Some authorities feel that this procedure is less likely to cause headache than a lumbar puncture. Cisternal puncture is often done in out-patient clinics and on children and other patients who are unable to cooperate during a lumbar puncture. Complications seldom occur, but the patient should be observed immediately after the procedure for signs of respiratory difficulty or the appearance of cyanosis.

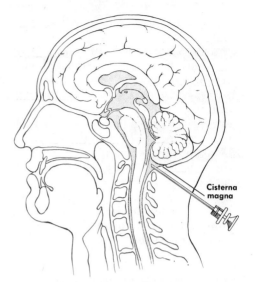

Figure 21-1. The position of the needle when a cisternal puncture is done. Note the needle length and the short bevel. (From Shafer et al.: *Medical-Surgical Nursing*, 4th Ed., The C. V. Mosby Co., St. Louis.)

Electroencephalogram

This test is similar in principle to the electrocardiogram, in that it magnifies electric impulses and records them on special graph paper, the difference being that in an electroencephalogram (EEG), the electrical impulses are generated by the activity of the brain cells. The electrodes for transmission of the impulses are placed at various sites on the head.

Preparation of the patient for the EEG is extremely important and can greatly affect the accuracy of the test. Stimulants and depressants can alter the brain's activity and are therefore restricted prior to the test. Medications are usually withheld unless they are specifically ordered by the physician. The nurse who is not familiar with the proper procedure for preparing a patient for an EEG should seek specific instruction in order to assure as much accuracy as possible.

X-ray Contrast Studies

There are three types of x-ray examinations commonly done in the diagnosis of intracranial disorders. These tests help determine the presence or absence of "space-taking" lesions such as tumors and other conditions such as atrophy of cerebral tissue and vascular disorders and malformations.

Angiography involves injection of a radiopaque liquid into the common carotid or vertebral arteries and taking a series of x-ray films as the solution fills the cerebral vessels. If a tumor is present in the brain, the blood vessels will appear dislocated or pushed aside at the tumor site. Other abnormalities such as aneurysms, thromboses or hematomas can also be diagnosed by angiography.

Pneumoencephalography utilizes a gas, usually air or oxygen, as a contrast medium. The gas is injected during a lumbar puncture, and then routine x-rays from varied angles are taken of the patient's head. Abnormalities of the brain structure will show up on the x-ray film. This procedure is not done if the patient shows signs of increased intracranial pressure, because the injected gas may serve to increase the pressure and damage the brain tissue.

Ventriculography involves the boring of two holes in the skull for the purpose of injecting air into the ventricles of the brain. This procedure must be done in an operating room. After air is injected, the wounds are closed and x-rays are taken of the skull. This type of test is most helpful in diagnosing and locating brain tumors.

Radioisotopes

Because some brain tumors accumulate more than a normal amount of radioactive isotopes, a substance such as radioactive iodine combined with serum albumin can be injected intravenously and then traced to the brain. Figure 21-2A shows the distribution of radioactive iodine in a normal brain scan. Figure 21-2B shows a dense area of radioactivity in the temporal area, suggesting a tumor that has accumulated the radioactive iodine.

GENERAL NURSING CARE OF THE PATIENT WITH A NEUROLOGIC DISORDER

The patient with a neurologic disorder has some *organic* disease of the nervous system. His condition should not be confused with mental derangements or emotional illness, which are psychiatric problems resulting from difficulties in adjusting to one's environment. Even though neurologic diseases do affect an individual mentally and emotionally, these effects are a direct result of physical changes and loss of function, or degeneration of nerve tissues.

There are many diseases that can cause disturbances in the functions of the nervous system. These include infectious diseases, tumors, trauma, disorders of the cerebral blood vessels and congenital malformations. The symptoms produced by these diseases are many and complex, and the nursing care required by each patient will depend on the type and location of the lesion and the effect the pathologic changes have on his ability to help himself. In serious neurologic disorders, the patient may have complete loss of function and control of many of his bodily activities. He will then be totally dependent upon those who care for him. In less serious neurologic diseases, there may be varying degrees of helplessness and dependency on others.

Problems of Nursing Care

Hygiene. Proper care of the skin to prevent pressure sores and breaks in the skin are especially important in neurologic nursing. We must remember that with a loss of motion of the various parts of the body, there is also a loss of feeling. The patient does not complain of discomfort from pressure or lying in one position too long because he does not *feel* any discomfort. He has been robbed of one of nature's ways of warning that something is wrong. This places an added respon-

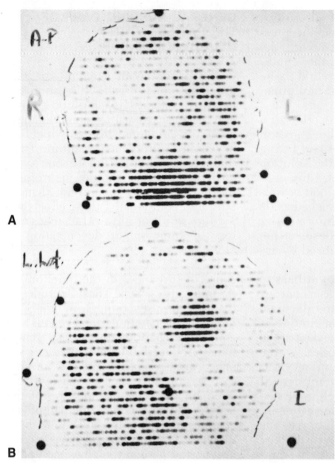

Figure 21–2. *A,* Normal brain scan. Note normal increased uptake in areas such as venous sinuses, nasopharyngeal mucosa, and scalp. *B,* Abnormal brain scan. Note large density seen in the left temporal area resulting from increased uptake by abnormal tissue. (Both courtesy of the Department of Nuclear Medicine, St. Mary's Hospital, St. Louis, Mo. From French: *Nurse's Guide to Diagnostic Procedures,* 2nd Ed., McGraw-Hill Book Co., New York.)

sibility on the nursing staff, since they cannot depend on the patient to remind them when he needs his position changed.

A regularly scheduled routine must be established for skin care, turning the patient and proper positioning so that the body is in good alignment.

Prevention of Complications. Prolonged bed rest and immobility create problems and allow for complications involving every major system of the body. These hazards of immobility are discussed in detail in Chapter 8 of this text. The patient with a neurologic disorder that produces paralysis or temporary loss of motion is subject to any and all of these complications arising from inactivity.

There are several types of beds and other devices that can be used to facilitate turning and positioning the patient so that the effects of immobility can be minimized. The CircOlectric bed described in Chapter 8 is especially helpful in the care of neurologic patients because it allows positioning the patient in a variety of ways and can be used for the patient who is also in traction. The tilt-table is a type of stretcher that can be adjusted so that the patient can assume an erect standing position. It allows for a gradual retraining of the patient in the ability to tolerate weight-bearing and a standing position. Both of these factors are important in preventing orthopedic, circulatory and respiratory complications.

This type of therapy is begun as soon as possible after neurologic injury, so that normal body function can be maintained whenever possible. It is a delicate and precise type of therapy that should be done only under the direction of a person who is familiar with its many advantages and few disadvantages.

Providing for Self-care

The nurse should not assume that all patients with neurologic disorders are totally helpless. She should take every opportunity to help the patient help himself as long as there are no contraindications for his doing so. If the physician grants permission for the patient to move about as much as he is physically able, the nurse may feel free to encourage her patient and provide him with the means to care for himself as much as possible. Doing too much for the patient may be as harmful to him as not doing enough.

The furniture in the patient's room should be arranged so that he can conveniently reach his bedside table and drawer if he wishes to get something for himself. Side rails should be applied to prevent falling out of bed and also to provide the patient with something to grasp so he can assist the nurses in turning him. A trapeze bar may be installed over the bed and the patient instructed in the way he might use this to lift himself up in bed or onto a bedpan.

Feeding himself may be slow or clumsy for the patient, but it is best if he manages this for himself as much as he is able. There are many things we do in the process of eating that require the use of both hands. For hemiplegics, such maneuvers as cutting up food, spreading butter or jelly on bread and opening milk cartons are extremely difficult if not impossible.

The patient should not be rushed through a meal nor made to feel that it would be best if he did not feed himself because he is so awkward. Accidental spilling of food or liquids should be treated as a matter of course and no comment made on the mess such accidents may make.

While encouraging the patient to help himself, the nurse should avoid pushing him into activities beyond his physical limitations. If the patient seems easily discouraged and unwilling to try to help himself, the practical nurse should consult the physician or nurse in charge and determine how much activity can be expected from the patient.

Emotional Aspects

In view of the fact that impairment of motion and sensory perception are so often the result of neurologic disorders, it is not surprising that emotional disturbances and personality changes should accompany these disorders. It is never easy for a formerly active person to adjust to a loss of his physical independence. Such a situation is extremely frustrating, and the patient may express his resentment in a number of ways. Emotional outbursts of anger or depression are not uncommon, and in some cases, the patient may show a loss of the will to live. The nurses who care for patients with neurologic disorders must be prepared for such emotional storms and crises and do their best to help these patients adjust to their illness and their handicaps and the problems they bring.

Perhaps the following quotation from a person whose muscles have been rendered all but useless by *myasthenia gravis* will help the reader gain some insight into the problems these patients must face.

If nurses and others would look past the body which is weak, and the face which probably looks expressionless, with its drooping lids or mouth half open because the patient is unable to close it, they would find a perfectly sane, reasonable human being. These patients are like a competent driver sitting in a faulty vehicle. No matter how hard he tries, he cannot make the car behave as he knows he could with a perfect machine which would respond to his control. However, it is not pity alone which is needed; in fact, that is usually not wanted. There are, however, some small things which mean much and can be done. The myasthenic is always a frustrated person because he usually has a strong will, and the greater his will, the greater the frustration when his muscles will not obey.*

Rehabilitation

The success of rehabilitation and preparation of the patient for his return to home, family and community will depend on the type of disorder affecting the nervous system. In some degenerative diseases such as multiple sclerosis, Parkinson's disease or myasthenia gravis, there is a gradual deterioration of the nerve cells and progressive loss of function. In these cases, rehabilitation is limited to keeping the patient happily occupied, if not gainfully employed, as the disease progresses.

When traumatic injury, cerebrovascular accidents (strokes) or tumors have brought about loss of function in specific areas of the body rather than a generalized paralysis, rehabilitation must be planned so that the individual is eventually able to function as an active member of the family and community in spite of his handicap. For further information on rehabilitation, the reader is referred to Chapter 8.

INFECTIOUS DISEASES OF THE BRAIN AND SPINAL CORD

Meningitis

Definition. Meningitis is an inflammation of the membranous linings of the brain and spinal cord. The infection may be carried to the meninges by way of the blood stream or by direct extension from neighboring tissues, such as from a severe infection of the

*Quoted from *Medical and Surgical Nursing II* by Amy Frances Brown. Philadelphia, W. B. Saunders Co., 1959, p. 568.

sinuses. Many different bacteria and viruses can cause meningitis, but when the disease occurs in epidemic form, it is usually caused by a specific organism called *meningococcus*. The disease is then spread by healthy meningococcal carriers.

Symptoms. The most outstanding symptom of meningitis is a severe and persistent headache that is greatly aggravated by shaking the head. There are also other signs of meningeal irritation; for example, pain and stiffness of the neck, irritability, photophobia and hypersensitivity of the skin. Nausea and vomiting and signs of an upper respiratory infection are usually present.

When meningitis is suspected, a spinal tap is done and the cerebrospinal fluid examined for the number and types of cells and organisms in it. In meningitis, the spinal fluid will often appear milky due to the increase of white cells suspended in the fluid.

In the late stages of severe meningitis, the back may be bowed so that the head is extended back toward the heels, and the trunk and legs are rigid.

Treatment and Nursing Care. Successful treatment of meningitis and prevention of permanent disability depend on early recognition and diagnosis of the disease. Once the causative organism has been determined, specific antibiotics are given in large doses. The drugs may be administered by mouth or intramuscularly, and penicillin is sometimes given directly into the spinal fluid circulation (intrathecally). Anticonvulsive drugs are given to control seizures. As long as the disease is in the acute stage, the patient is placed in strict isolation to prevent contamination of others. Meningococcal infection is spread by droplet infection, which means that all secretions from the respiratory tract are sources of infection.

Nursing care is primarily concerned with supportive measures to conserve the strength of the patient and close observation of the patient for signs of chills, elevation of body temperature and convulsions.

The patient's room should be quiet and dimly lighted. Sudden noises or a bright flash of light, such as occurs when an overhead light is switched on, may easily precipitate a convulsion. Every detail of the patient's environment must be considered and all stimuli which may excite the patient removed. It is obvious from his outward appearance that the patient with meningitis is acutely ill. He resents any disturbance because motion of the head or extremities increases pain and adds to his discomfort. He must be turned very gently and disturbed as little as possible for necessary treatments. Meningitis often produces mental confusion and delirium as well as the possibility of convulsions. Padded side rails and other safety measures should be used to prevent self-injury. Cool compresses on the forehead or an ice bag on the head often help relieve delirium.

Herpes simplex (fever blisters) frequently accompany meningitis. The presence of these sores, plus drying of the lips and mouth due to high temperatures and dehydration, demand special mouth care. The lips and mouth should be cleansed and lubricated at least every two hours during the acute stage of the disease.

Dehydration is often a problem, and most physicians wish to have a record kept of the patient's intake and output. Excessive vomiting or outward signs of early dehydration should be reported so that fluids may be given intravenously when necessary.

A decrease in peristaltic action of the intestines often occurs in meningitis, and thus leads to an accumulation of flatus and fecal material with severe abdominal distention. Rectal tubes, suppositories or small low enemas may be ordered for relief of this condition. Large amounts of water should not be given rectally because they may increase intracranial pressure and lead to convulsions or severe headache.

Once the acute stage of the disease is over, the patient is allowed to gradually resume his former activities. Residual effects of the disease, such as paralysis, deafness or visual defects, sometimes occur, but these sequelae of meningitis do not usually occur if the disease is diagnosed and treated in the early stages before permanent damage is done.

Encephalitis

Definition. Encephalitis is an inflammation of the brain tissues. The disease is most often caused by a virus or from toxins produced by the organisms which cause chickenpox, measles or mumps. Some chemicals such as lead and arsenic can also cause encephalitis.

Symptoms. The onset of encephalitis may be sudden or insidious and is characterized by headache, fever, extreme restlessness or lethargy and muscular weakness. The lethargy may progress to coma. Mental confusion, visual disturbances and disorientation may also be present.

Treatment and Nursing Care. The treatment of encephalitis is mainly symptomatic with general supportive measures to maintain the strength of the patient. Isolation of the patient may be necessary if the encephalitis is of the infectious type.

Side rails and constant attendance to prevent the patient from injuring himself are necessary during the period of disorientation. Mechanical restraints should be used only when absolutely necessary, for example, when the patient is receiving intravenous fluids and may dislodge the needle. The head of the bed and the side rails are padded, and a tongue blade wrapped with gauze is kept at the bedside in case the patient has convulsions.

The vital signs are carefully checked at frequent intervals so that any change may be reported immediately. If the body temperature becomes excessively high, measures are taken to bring it down to within normal limits. The environment of the patient is kept quiet and restful, and sedatives are sometimes given to control restlessness and induce sleep. Should the patient become extremely restless or display any signs of respiratory difficulty, his condition should be reported immediately.

The convalescent period for the patient with encephalitis is essentially the same as that for a patient with meningitis.

Poliomyelitis

Definition. Poliomyelitis is an acute inflammation of the anterior horn of the spinal cord. The disease may be caused by three different strains of viruses, all of which have a special affinity for nerve tissue. Since the discovery of the exact cause of poliomyelitis, it is now possible to immunize persons against this disease. The Salk vaccine and Sabin vaccine are used and have greatly reduced the incidence of poliomyelitis in this country.

Symptoms. Poliomyelitis may present such mild symptoms that the disease often goes unrecognized and leaves no residual paralysis. In fact, some authorities state that as high as 80 per cent of the people in this country have had poliomyelitis at some time without realizing they had the disease.

The symptoms of severe poliomyelitis are very similar to those of other neurologic infections. Signs of an upper respiratory infection, fever, severe headache and soreness and stiffness of the neck, back and hamstring muscles are usually present. As the disease progresses, paralysis may occur.

Treatment and Nursing Care. There is no cure for poliomyelitis and no specific treatment. It is a tragic disease in its more serious form, and the adage, "an ounce of prevention is worth a pound of cure," could not be more aptly applied than in this instance. In spite of the fact that im-

munization is possible, recent statistics show that almost half the schoolchildren in this country still have not been immunized against poliomyelitis. The nurse should take every opportunity to encourage parents to have their children protected against this crippling disease.

During the actue febrile stage of the disease, the patient is kept on complete rest. No specific positioning is necessary beyond maintenance of good posture and frequent turning. All muscular strain and rough handling should be avoided in moving the patient. The nurse should place the palms of her hands under the joints rather than on the muscular part of the extremities, because the skeletal muscles are subject to painful spasms when stimulated by pressure (see Fig. 21-3).

Urinary retention and fecal impaction are common problems, especially in patients with paralysis of the lower extremities. The urinary output is measured and recorded, and a careful checking of bowel movements is necessary. The nurse should not mistake a "dribbling" of overflow from a distended bladder as emptying of the bladder. She can determine bladder distention by gently pressing her hand over the bladder region. If the bladder is full, it is plainly felt under the palm of the hand.

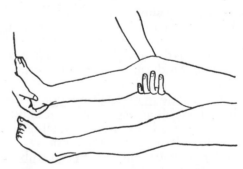

Figure 21-3. Proper method of handling a limb when muscle spasm is likely to result from stimulation. Note that the palms of the hands are used and the joints above and below the affected muscles are supported. (From Wiebe: *Orthopedics in Nursing,* W. B. Saunders Co., Philadelphia.)

The application of heat to the muscles for the relief of painful contractions has been found to be very helpful. The form of heat to be applied will depend on the wishes of the physician. Most patients with poliomyelitis are under the care of a physiotherapist who supervises the administration of hot packs and passive exercise of the extremities.

Patients with poliomyelitis frequently have difficulty swallowing and may also have respiratory problems requiring the use of an artificial respirator. These patients require expert nursing care from persons trained and experienced in this specialized area of nursing.

HEAD INJURIES

Definition and Types

A blow to the head may cause *open* injuries, with lacerations of the skin and scalp, and fracture of the skull; or *closed* injuries in which the scalp and skull remain intact but the underlying brain tissue is damaged. The term *"concussion"* is used to describe a closed head injury in which the brain is compressed by a portion of the skull at the time of the blow and temporary anemia of the brain tissue results. In a *contusion*, the brain tissue is bruised and swelling occurs, pressing the brain tissues against the skull.

Symptoms

The severity of brain damage from a head injury is best judged by the symptoms presented by the patient, the history of the type of blow received and whether or not the victim lost consciousness. No head injury should be considered completely harmless. They are all potentially dangerous because there may be a delayed reaction in which there is hemorrhage into the brain tissues or the formation of a blood clot (hematoma). These conditions build up over a period of time and result from weakening and rupture of the small blood vessels in the brain. Sometimes the bleeding is so slow that it takes weeks or even months for the symptoms of pressure within the skull to appear.

Aside from the obvious lacerations of the scalp or fractures of the skull which may be seen on x-ray, intracranial hemorrhage or the formation of a blood clot must always be considered a possibility in a head injury. The observations of the nurse in regard to the patient's behavior and the symptoms he manifests may be of great help to the physician in determining the extent of damage to the brain.

Treatment and Nursing Care

The patient with a head injury is treated conservatively at first unless a compound fracture of the skull demands surgical debridement of the wound and removal of splintered bone from the brain tissues. Other surgical procedures to relieve pressure from intracranial bleeding may be necessary if the pressure in the skull builds up to a dangerous level. (See the discussion that follows for nursing care of the patient having brain surgery.)

As we have stated previously, the nurse's observations are extremely important in the diagnosis and treatment of head injuries. Any one of the symptoms listed below should be reported immediately should they occur.

1. Changes in the patient's blood pressure, pulse or respiration.
2. Extreme restlessness or excitability following a period of apparent calm.
3. Deepening stupor or loss of consciousness.
4. Headache which increases in intensity.
5. Vomiting, especially persistent, projectile vomiting.
6. Unequal size of pupils.
7. Leakage of cerebrospinal fluid (clear yellow or tinged with pink) from the nose or ear.

8. Inability to move one or more extremities.

These observations are continued until the physician feels that the patient has passed the critical stage of his illness.

Most patients with head injuries are placed on bed rest and kept absolutely quiet until the doctor orders otherwise. Narcotics and other pain-relieving drugs may be prohibited by the physician if he thinks these will mask any of the symptoms the patient may exhibit. Positioning of the patient will also depend on the wishes of the physician. In some cases, he may order the patient flat in bed without a pillow, or, if there are signs of increased intracranial pressure and cerebral compression, he may order the head of the bed slightly elevated.

Patients who are unconscious must be watched closely for respiratory difficulties or inability to swallow. If the patient cannot swallow, his head must be turned to the side and his mouth and trachea suctioned as necessary to prevent aspiration of mucus into the lungs. A tracheostomy set and/or respirator may be required in severe head injuries in which there is severe respiratory embarrassment.

When delirium or disorientation is present and convulsions are anticipated, the patient must be protected from self-injury.

Sometimes the patient remains unconscious for weeks or months, and a stomach tube must be passed and tube feedings given regularly to maintain adequate nutrition. Intake and output records are kept, and the patient is observed for signs of urinary retention, incontinence, abdominal distention or bowel complications.

BRAIN TUMORS

Definition

Tumors of the brain are abnormal growths of cells within the brain tissue or the coverings of the brain. As with other tumors, the cause is not known.

Symptoms

There may be as many symptoms of brain tumors as there are functions of the brain. Symptoms may be produced by actual destruction of portions of brain tissue, or they may result from increased pressure within the skull and compression of the brain as the tumor grows inward.

The symptoms may appear gradually, or, if the tumor is a highly malignant, fast-growing type, they may appear suddenly. In a slow-growing type of tumor, the patient first shows personality changes, disturbances in judgment and memory, loss of strength or difficulties in speaking clearly. Headache and vomiting usually do not appear early in the disease because they are a result of increased intracranial pressure which occurs only after the tumor has grown to considerable size.

Treatment and Nursing Care

Brain tumors are treated by surgical removal of the tumorous mass and removal of adjacent tissues which may contain cancer cells. Radiation therapy may also be used in some types of tumors. Localization of the tumor is sometimes very difficult and is determined by observation of the patient's symptoms and by x-ray studies. If the tumor is located in the *cerebrum*, an operation called a *craniotomy* is done. In this procedure, a flap of scalp and bone is cut and pulled down, the dura (first meningeal layer) is opened, and the tumor is removed. Tumors in or near the *cerebellum* are removed through an incision under the occipital bone. This is called a *suboccipital craniectomy*, and part of the skull is permanently removed, leaving a defect in the skull.

If the tumor cannot be removed, a portion of the skull (usually in the temporal region) may be removed to relieve compression of the brain against the skull. The tumorous mass then bulges through the opening. This procedure is only a temporary measure to relieve the patient's symptoms.

NURSING CARE OF THE PATIENT HAVING BRAIN SURGERY

Preoperative Care

During the preoperative period in which diagnostic tests and x-ray examinations will be done to determine the location of the tumor, the nurse should familiarize herself with the patient's symptoms. She later uses these observations as a basis for comparison of the patient's condition postoperatively.

Physical preparation of the patient includes shaving of the scalp, which is a painful procedure physically, as well as an emotional shock for the patient. In most hospitals, the shaving of the scalp is done in the operating room after the patient has been anesthetized. The hair removed from female patients is saved so that a wig or other type of hairpiece may be made to cover parts of the head while the hair is growing back.

Postoperative Care

The patient's unit is prepared as soon as he is taken to the operating room. This includes the making of a postoperative bed as for other surgical patients, except that the linen is arranged so that the patient's head will be at the foot of the bed. This arrangement makes changing of the dressings and observation of the drainage from the surgical wound easier for the nurses and doctors and less disturbing to the patient. Side rails are applied to the bed.

Equipment assembled at the bedside should include: (1) a suction machine and two rubber catheters, (2) blood pressure apparatus, pencil and pad to record vital signs, (3) an emergency medicine tray containing stimulants and sedatives, (4) a tourniquet, needles and syringes, (5) a padded tongue blade, (6) a rubber airway, (7) a tracheostomy set (usually necessary only when surgery is done in the area of the cerebellum).

As soon as the patient returns from the operating room, he is placed on his side to facilitate drainage of mucus from the mouth and pharynx. Whether or not the head is elevated will depend on the wishes of the surgeon. The vital signs are taken and recorded at frequent intervals, and any change is to be reported without delay.

The dressings must be checked often for signs of drainage. If the dressings become soaked with drainage, they must be covered with a *sterile* towel to prevent contamination of the wound and possible meningitis.

A thin, watery, yellowish or pink-tinged discharge from the nose or ear may indicate a leakage of cerebrospinal fluid. This drainage is collected in a sterile gauze square loosely applied to the orifice from which the fluid is leaking. No attempt should be made to plug the orifice and stop the flow of fluid.

All of the preceding observations listed for patients with head injuries will apply to the patient having brain surgery.

Elevation of the body temperature may occur as a result of a disturbance of the temperature control center in the brain. Most surgeons wish to have the patient's temperature taken rectally every 2 hours for 24 hours after cranial surgery. Nursing measures to reduce the body temperature are used in the event that the temperature becomes excessively high.

As the patient recovers from the surgical procedure, his nursing care is planned according to his individual needs. Adequate nutrition and a normal fluid and electrolyte balance must be maintained, either through oral feedings or intravenous therapy, depending on the patient's ability to chew and swallow. Records of intake and output are kept, and the patient is observed for urinary retention or incontinence.

Plans for rehabilitation are made according to the residual effects of the surgery. Every attempt is made to salvage the patient's remaining abilities and use them to the greatest advantage. The prevention of complications by proper positioning, frequent turning and passive exercises during the postoperative period is one of the most important aspects of rehabilitation.

INJURIES OF THE SPINAL CORD

Definition

A person may suffer from injury to the spinal cord in a number of ways. When we speak of injury, our first thought is a violent, traumatic type of injury in which the spinal cord is severed or partially severed by a direct blow. Automobile accidents, gunshot wounds and other forms of violence do often inflict severe damage to the spinal cord, but tumors, degenerative diseases and infections can also impair the functions of the spinal cord and its branches.

Generally speaking, spinal cord injuries are classified according to their anatomical location; that is, *cervical, thoracic* or *lumbosacral.*

Symptoms

Whatever the cause of the damage to the spinal cord, the symptoms of the patient are essentially the same. A complete severance of the cord results in a total loss of function and control in the parts of the body below the point of injury. If the cord is severed in the cervical region, the paralysis and loss of sensory perception will include both arms and both legs. Severe injury to the cord above the level of the fifth cervical vertebra is often fatal because the *phrenic* nerves have their origin in the third, fourth and fifth cervical segments. Branches of these nerves play a major role in the control of respiration. Table 2-1 presents activities possible at varying levels of cord injury.

Injury to the spinal cord that does not involve complete severance of the cord may result in a temporary paralysis which will subside as the spinal cord recovers from the initial shock of the injury.

Treatment and Nursing Care

There are four main objectives in the treatment and nursing care of the patient with an injury of the spinal cord: (1) to save the victim's life, (2) to repair as much of the damage to the cord as possible, (3) to prevent further injury to the cord by careful handling of the patient and (4) to establish a routine of care which will maintain and improve

TABLE 21-1. ACTIVITIES POSSIBLE AT VARYING LEVELS
OF SPINAL CORD INJURY*

	Spinal Cord Level						
Activities	Cervical-5	Cervical-6	Cervical-7	Thoracic-1	Thoracic-6	Thoracic-12	Lumbar-4
Self-Care: Eating	−	+	+	+	+	+	+
Dressing	−	−	+ −	+	+	+	+
Toileting	−	−	+ −	+	+	+	+
Bed Independence	−	+ −	+ −	+	+	+	+
Wheel Chair Independence	−	+ −	+ −	+	+	+	+
Ambulation: Functional	−	−	−	−	+ −	+	+
Vocation: Homebound	−	−	+	+	+	+	+
Outside	−	−	−	+ −	+ −	+	+

*From Martin GraBois, Journ. Pract. Nurs., April, 1971, p. 23.
+ = capacity to accomplish task
+ − = questionable capacity to accomplish task
− = will not be able to accomplish task

the patient's physical condition, prevent complications and make his eventual physical, mental and social rehabilitation possible.

Immediate Care. As soon as a person suffers a sudden injury to the spinal cord, he must be handled with extreme care. Even though the nurse or doctor may not be at the scene of the accident to supervise the moving of the victim, he can teach others the proper emergency care of such injuries. If the injured person complains of neck pain, cannot move his legs and has no feeling in them, he should be treated as though he had a spinal cord injury.

Transfer of the patient to the hospital should be done only by trained ambulance attendants or other persons qualified to administer first aid. The victim is moved on a stretcher or board and taken directly to the hospital. His back is kept straight. *No pillow should be placed under the head;* however, rolled towels may be placed under the neck and small of the back so as to maintain the normal curvature of the spine.

In the emergency room of the hospital, the patient is treated for shock, and an examination is made to determine the extent of his injuries. His hospital room is fully prepared *before* he leaves the emergency room.

The type of bed to be used will be decided by the physician. In many cases, a Stryker frame or Foster frame is preferred. In other cases, a regular bed with cotton mattress and bed boards may be used, and the bed is made up so that the head of the patient is at the foot of the bed.

The physician may also apply traction to the neck through the use of a head halter or Crutchfield tongs (see Fig. 21-4).

Once the patient is in bed or on the orthopedic frame, the true test of nursing care begins. All the principles and practices of urologic, orthopedic and neurologic nursing must be used. The nursing staff must wage a continuous battle with three formidable enemies: *decubitus ulcers, urinary complications* and *orthopedic deformities.*

Skin Care. Frequent turning of the patient is made easier when the patient is on a frame, but it should be remembered that simple changing of position does not guarantee protection against decubiti. All points of pressure, especially the shoulder blades and sacral region, must be checked frequently, cleansed and dried often and gently massaged to increase circulation to the area.

One factor that contributes to the formation of decubitus ulcers is the poor circulation of blood to any part of the body which has been deprived of its nerve supply. This is because limited muscular activity makes the flow of blood sluggish and inadequate. In view of this, one must also realize that intramuscular injections *should not be given* in the areas of the body which have no "feeling," even though this may appear to be an advantage since the patient cannot feel the injection. The tissues at the site of the injection tend to become inflamed, and an abscess may develop because the medication is not properly absorbed into the blood stream.

Elimination. Kidney disorders are likely to develop because bladder function is partly controlled by the autonomic nervous system. A Foley catheter is usually inserted and irrigations of the bladder begun. In some cases, there is a return of bladder control after the initial "spinal shock" has subsided.

Liquids by mouth are pushed to 3000 ml. daily to insure adequate flow of urine and elimination of wastes. The juices of citrus fruits are not allowed because these tend to make the urine alkaline. It has been definitely established that an alkaline urine supports the growth of bacteria and the formation of renal stones. Apple, cranberry, grape and cherry juices are excellent substitutes for citrus juices.

Bowel function is also partially controlled by the autonomic nervous sys-

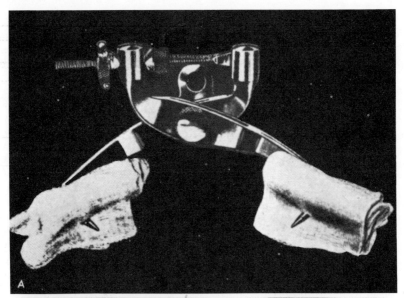

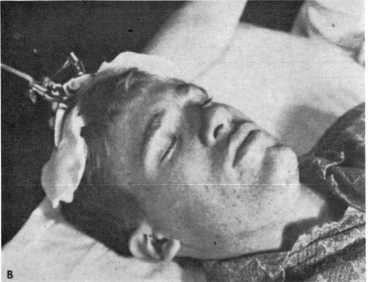

Figure 21–4. *A,* Crutchfield tongs. They are inserted through two holes drilled half way into the inner plate of the patient's skull. *B,* Direct alignment of patient's head with his cervical spine is always maintained; three persons are required to turn him on his side. (From Hunkele and Lozier: American Journal of Nursing, September, 1965.)

tem. When injury to the spinal cord impairs the flow of nerve impulses, there is a decrease in peristalsis. Thus, gas-forming foods and those that are high in residue are eliminated from the diet.

During the period immediately following injury to the spinal cord, the patient may be incontinent of feces because he does not feel the impulse to defecate. To avoid embarrassment and inconvenience, he should be offered the bedpan at frequent intervals. Later, a routine may be set up by the physician and nursing staff. This includes the use of suppositories, mild cathartics or low enemas to stimulate defecation at a given time each day until the patient is able to establish his own schedule for regularity of bowel movements. Establishing this routine takes some time and much patience, and the patient should understand that only with determination and a willingness to try again and again can this obstacle to his return to society be overcome.

Muscle Spasms. Immediately after a cord injury, the patient will usually have a flaccid type of paralysis. Later, as the cord adjusts to the injury, the paralysis will become *spastic*, and there will be strong, involuntary contractions of the skeletal muscles.

These muscle spasms may be violent enough to throw the patient from his bed or wheel chair and must be anticipated so that such accidents can be avoided. If the patient is on a frame, a protective strap is placed across the thighs. If the upper extremities are involved, he is likely to tip over glasses, water pitchers or anything within reach of his arms when he is seized with uncontrollable muscle spasms.

The patient and his family may interpret these spasms as a return of voluntary function of the limbs and will thus have false hopes of complete recovery. It is best if the nurse in charge or the physician explains to them that such is not the case.

Positioning of the Patient. Every nurse should be fully aware of the complications resulting from poor posture, in or out of bed. The principles and practices of good positioning of the patient who is bedridden have been described in detail in Chapter 14 of this text and in Chapter 15 under nursing care of a patient who has had a stroke. The only point to be emphasized here is a reminder that these principles and practices are of extreme importance in the care of a patient with an injury of the spinal cord. The success of his rehabilitation will depend to a great extent on the preservation of the remaining functions of his body.

Through the use of footboards, hand rolls, trochanter rolls, sandbags and other devices, the joints and muscles of the unaffected parts of his body can be kept intact (see Fig. 21-5). To allow the loss of these remaining assets through negligence on the part of the nursing staff is unforgivable. The partially paralyzed patient has so little to work with in his efforts to adjust to a new way of life, it seems incredible that anyone would willingly or knowingly deny him the little he has.

RUPTURE OF INTERVERTEBRAL DISC

Definition

The bodies of the vertebrae lie flat upon one another like a stack of coins. Between each of the vertebral bodies there is a disc of fibrous cartilage which acts as a cushion to absorb shocks to the spinal column (see Fig. 21-6). This disc may be ruptured by some type of injury such as lifting a heavy object or wrenching or falling on the back. When the disc ruptures, part of it squeezes out from between the vertebrae and pinches the adjacent nerve root by pressing it against the bone. Thus, the person suffers from what is sometimes called a "slipped disc." Another name for this condition is *hernia of the nucleus pulposus.*

Symptoms

Most ruptured or slipped discs occur in the lower lumbar and lumbosacral region. The patient experiences pain in the lower back, radiating down the back of one leg to the foot. Walking is extremely painful, and the discomfort is aggravated by coughing, sneezing or straining.

Treatment and Nursing Care

In most instances, the physician will treat the condition with conservative

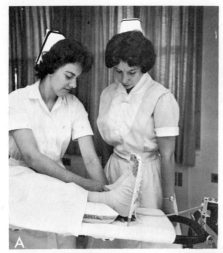

Figure 21–5. *A,* The patient's heels should be suspended above the frame, with the feet at a 90-degree angle against the foot support. Elastic bandages have been applied to improve circulation. Drainage tubing from the Foley catheter rests between the patient's legs and feet. *B,* This patient, being cared for on a frame and with Crutchfield tongs used for traction, illustrates several important points in care: arm pillows placed at shoulder height, hand rolls used to prevent contractures and a protective strap at midthigh to prevent injury or a fall from bed during a muscle spasm. (From Martin: American Journal of Nursing, March, 1963.)

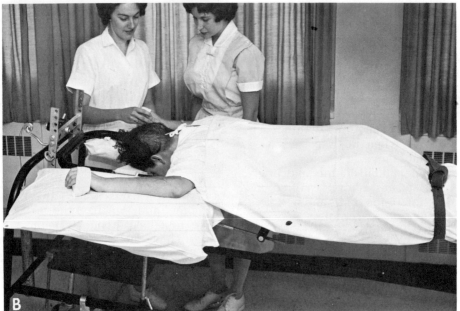

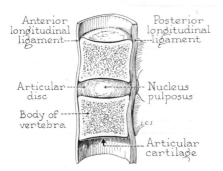

Figure 21–6. The articular disc, made of fibrous cartilage, is pictured here showing the manner in which it separates the body of each vertebra. When back strain or injury causes a slipping of the disc from between the vertebrae, there is a pinching of the spinal nerves located in that area. (From King and Showers: *Human Anatomy and Physiology,* 6th Ed., W. B. Saunders Co., Philadelphia.)

measures in the hope that surgical correction will not be necessary.

The patient is placed on a firm cotton mattress with bed boards under it. The bed is kept flat, and the patient is placed on bed rest. When he is turned off his back he is "log-rolled"; that is, he is turned without bending his back. In order to accomplish this, the patient folds his arms over his chest, flexes the knee opposite the side on which he is to turn and then is rolled over, just as a log would be rolled.

Hydrocollator packs or some other form of local heat is applied to reduce muscle spasm in the back. Pelvic traction may be applied and mild exercises ordered by the physician (see Fig. 21-7). These treatments are usually done under the guidance of a physiotherapist. Specially designed corsets or back braces are sometimes used to maintain proper alignment of the spine when the patient is allowed out of bed.

If these measures do not eventually relieve the symptoms, surgery is performed to relieve the damaged disc. The surgical procedure is called a laminectomy. The affected vertebrae may be fused together (spinal fusion).

The postoperative care is very much the same as for any patient with major surgery. The positioning of the patient following laminectomy is the same as before surgery: flat in bed and log-rolled to prevent bending the spinal column (see Fig. 21-8).

MYASTHENIA GRAVIS

Definition

The words "myasthenia gravis" literally mean *grave muscle weakness.* This disease is fairly uncommon, occurring most frequently in females in their early twenties and thirties.

Symptoms

Severe muscle weakness is the outstanding symptom. Any of the skeletal muscles may be involved, while the muscles of the intestine, bladder and heart are not affected.

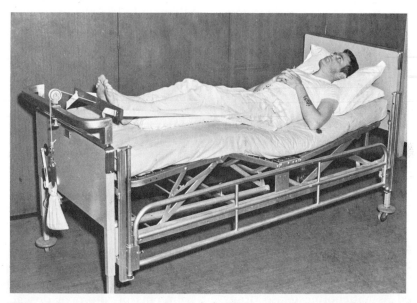

Figure 21-7. Patient in pelvic traction for relief of muscle spasm due to ruptured intervertebral disc. Note that knee rest is slightly elevated and pillow is used to support leg and prevent pressure against heels. (From Pasternak: American Journal of Nursing, February, 1962.)

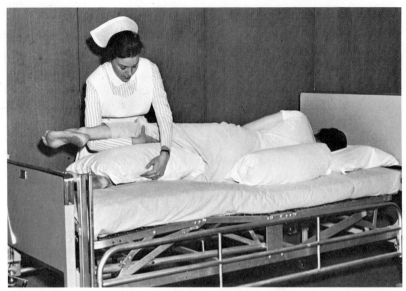

Figure 21–8. Proper alignment of back and support with pillows when patient is "log-rolled" following surgery. This method of turning and support is used for patient who has had laminectomy or a spinal fusion. (From Pasternak: American Journal of Nursing, February, 1962.)

The onset is gradual, usually beginning with double vision, ptosis (drooping) of the eyelids and progressive weakness in the arms and legs. The fatigue is relieved by rest but soon returns and is more severe than is to be expected from the amount of activity the person performs.

Diagnosis is established by administering an injection of *neostigmine.* If there is a dramatic return of strength within 15 to 20 minutes after the injection, the diagnosis of myasthenia gravis is confirmed. Another test using edrophonium (Tensilon) produces similar results, and the marked increase in muscular strength occurs within one minute of injection.

Treatment and Nursing Care

Neostigmine (Prostigmin) and *pyridostigmine* (Mestinon) are the two drugs most commonly used in treating myasthenia gravis. These medicines are classified as anticholinesterase drugs. They are used because they inactivate acetylcholinesterase, a substance that prevents accumulation of acetylcholine at the neuromuscular junction (point at which nerve impulses are transmitted to the muscle) (see Fig. 21-9). Since acetylcholine improves muscle strength in persons with myasthenia gravis (but not in normal persons), those drugs which remove the barrier to its accumulation indirectly prevent muscle weakness.

The correct dosage of anticholinesterase drugs is precisely calculated on an individual basis, with the aim of achieving a delicate balance between too much and too little acetylcholine at the neuromuscular junction. Stress in the life of the patient can quickly alter his need for the drug, and overmedication or undermedication can occur rather suddenly. Unfortunately, the symptoms of either too much or too little medication are quite similar. The patient, as well as members of his family and the nurse who is caring for him in the hospital, should be aware of the symptoms of improper dosage. These include dyspnea; poor tongue control which produces difficulty in swallow-

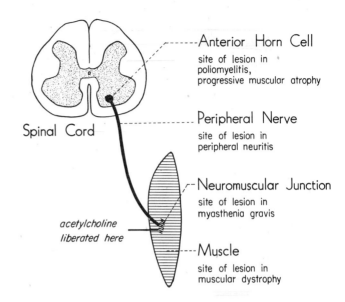

Figure 21-9. A cross section of the spinal cord showing sites of lesions in four nervous system disorders. Special attention is directed to the neuromuscular junction, site of the chemical abnormality present in myasthenia gravis. This lesion is the basis for present forms of treating the disease. (From Magee: Journal of Practical Nursing, November, 1965.)

ing, speaking and chewing; generalized muscular weakness; and psychic symptoms such as restlessness, anxiety and irritability. Should any of these symptoms occur, they should be reported to the physician immediately.

In addition to the problems arising from the anticholinesterase drugs, the myasthenic patient can also suffer from exaggerated and bizarre effects from a variety of drugs. These are presented in Fig. 21-10.

Before discharge from the hospital, the patient and one or more members of his family should be thoroughly instructed in the signs and symptoms of myasthenic and cholinergic states so that immediate medical help can be obtained should they occur at home. They should also be aware of the effects of emotional upsets and respiratory infections, which can bring on severe symptoms and a critical situation. The patient should obtain and wear at all times a Medic Alert emblem that identifies him as having myasthenia gravis.

The physician and nursing staff should give the myasthenic patient a thorough explanation of his disease and encourage him to learn all he can about his illness. The Myasthenia Gravis Foundation, with headquarters at the New York Academy of Medicine, 2 East 103rd St., New York City, 10029, promotes research for discovery of the cause and cure for the disease and disseminates information about the disease through its local chapters.

There are some myasthenic patients who become rapidly worse despite treatment by rest and medication. This severe weakness is called "myasthenic crisis," and may result in death from weakness of the throat muscles and respiratory failure. The patient with this condition is admitted to the hospital, and a tracheostomy and artificial respirator may be necessary to maintain life.

During the myasthenic crisis, a nurse should be in constant attendance, assisting the patient in maintaining a clear airway by suctioning the mouth and throat to remove mucus which cannot be swallowed and reassuring the patient by her calm and competent manner.

It is understandable that these patients are extremely apprehensive when left alone because they are too weak to summon help when needed.

Medications to be administered only after double checking with a physician who knows the patient has myasthenia gravis:

1. ACTH
2. STEROIDS
3. THYROID COMPOUNDS
4. RESPIRATORY DEPRESSANTS
5. SEDATIVES
6. PHENOTHIAZINES: Compazine, Thorazine, Sparine
7. MYCIN ANTIBIOTICS: Neomycin, Streptomycin, Kanomycin, Polymyxin B, Colistin, etc.
8. VASODILATING AGENTS
9. MORPHINE

Triple check before giving:

1. CURARE
2. QUININE
3. QUINIDINE
4. SUCCINYLCHOLINE

Many drugs are potentially dangerous to a patient with myasthenia gravis; many "harmless" drugs when administered to a myasthenic may precipitate an exacerbation. Dangerous oversights may be avoided if the front of the patient's chart is tagged with his diagnosis and a list of potentially hazardous drugs. A nurse asked to give any of the above drugs to a patient with myasthenia gravis would be wise to double check the order before giving the drug. (This is not meant to imply that these drugs are not used in treating patients with myasthenia gravis—only that they should be used with caution.)

(Based on chart tagging form: University of Virginia Hospital Department of Neurology)

Figure 21–10. List of drugs dangerous to the myasthenia gravis patient. (Based on a chart tagging form: University of Virginia Department of Nursing. From Blount, Mary, and Anna Belle Kinney, "Myasthenia Gravis: Nursing Essentials," Journal of Practical Nursing, June, 1972, p. 29.)

Emotional excitement uses up their limited amount of energy just as physical activity does. A quiet atmosphere and anticipation of the patient's every need will do much to conserve the patient's energy until he has recovered from the crisis. In some cases, there will be a spontaneous remission of symptoms in which the severe weakness subsides almost as rapidly as it appeared. The reason for this abatement of symptoms is not known.

PARKINSON'S DISEASE

Definition

Parkinson's disease is a chronic neurologic disease that is considered one of the major health problems of today because of its disabling effects and chronic nature. There are three major types of parkinsonism based on the causative factor. The first two types, arteriosclerotic and postencephalitic, are considered to be extremely rare. The third type, idiopathic (cause unknown), is by far the most common. The disease affects more males than females and occurs between the ages of 45 and 80 years.

Symptoms

There are two groups of symptoms which are characteristic of parkinsonism. The first, tremor, occurs when the body is at rest, decreases when there is voluntary movement and is absent when the patient is asleep. If the patient suffers stress and emotional tension, the tremor becomes more pronounced. The second symptom, rigidity, affects the skeletal muscles and produces poor body balance, a characteristic gait, loss of motion and body restlessness.

Treatment

Treatment of parkinsonism usually includes drug therapy, physical therapy and sometimes surgery. The most recent discovery that offers much hope to the victims of this disease is a drug called L-dioxyphenylalanine (L-DOPA). The drug is given in increasing doses until there is control of the symptoms. It is not without side effects, but these are relatively minor. Other drugs used may include antispasmodics and anticholinergic drugs. Surgery, once thought to be the best treatment, is successful only for patients who have minor symptoms, and the tremor and rigidity reappear as the disease progresses.

MULTIPLE SCLEROSIS

Definition

Multiple sclerosis is a chronic and progressive disease of the central nervous system. It is characterized by a sclerosing (scarring) of the myelin sheath which covers the nerve fibers and may occur anywhere along the nerve pathways. In a normal person, the myelin sheath functions in the same way as insulation on an electric wire. If the protective covering is worn away and replaced by scar tissue, nerve impulses cannot travel along the nerve pathways. Thus, the muscles do not receive these impulses and cease to perform in a well-coordinated and useful manner.

The cause of multiple sclerosis is not known. It tends to run in families, and most often affects persons between the ages of 20 and 40.

Symptoms

Multiple sclerosis has a very slow and insidious onset, with disturbances in vision, muscular weakness and gradual loss of coordination in muscular activities. The symptoms may completely subside for a while and then return with greater severity than before.

Treatment and Nursing Care

There is no cure for multiple sclerosis. Treatment is aimed at relief of symptoms and avoidance of infection, fatigue, poor nutrition or emotional upsets, all of which may precipitate an attack and increase the severity of the symptoms.

EPILEPSY

Definition

Epilepsy is a term used to describe sudden and uncontrollable seizures or "fits" in which the patient has muscular twitching and a temporary loss of consciousness. Epilepsy may be either a symptom or a disease in itself. When the seizures are due to a tumor, infection or injury to the brain, it is considered to be a symptom. When the cause is not known and no demonstrable pathology is found, the condition is called idiopathic epilepsy.

Although epilepsy has sometimes been considered to be an inherited disease it does not follow the laws of inheritance, and there are no dependable statistical studies to justify the importance some authorities have attached to heredity as a cause of the disease.

Symptoms

The signs and symptoms of epilepsy may vary from minor (petit mal) to major (grand mal). In a minor seizure, the attack may pass unnoticed by a casual observer because it often consists of only a very brief loss of consciousness and a "vacant stare" which lasts for a second or two.

The grand mal seizure is often preceded by an *aura.* This is a specific warning (varying in individual patients) which enables the epileptic to sense that an attack is coming on and prepare himself by lying down so that he will not be injured during the seizure. An epileptic may describe the aura as a flash of light, a dimming of vision, a peculiar odor, or any number of sensory changes of which he is aware just before the attack.

Treatment and Nursing Care

The care of a patient during a seizure is the same as for any person who is in convulsion (see Chapter 3).

The most useful and effective drugs for control of epileptic sezures are the barbiturates, diphenylhydantoin sodium (Dilantin Sodium) and trimethadione (Tridione). There are quite a few other anticonvulsant drugs that can be used when a patient cannot tolerate one of those listed above or when one specific drug loses its effectiveness for a patient. Toxic effects of anticonvulsants include drowsiness, rash, fatigue and sometimes blood disturbances. Patients taking these drugs regularly should remain under close medical supervision.

Through the efforts of the Epilepsy Association of America (111 W. 57 St., New York, 10019), the general public has become increasingly aware of the true nature of epilepsy. Research continues in an effort to find the cause and successful cure for this disease. In the meantime, we all have a responsibility to help these people gain steady employment and lead useful, active lives. Most epileptics are perfectly normal between seizures; they are not mentally retarded and are quire capable of becoming contributing members of our society if only they are given the chance to prove their worth.

CEREBRAL PALSY

Introduction

Cerebral palsy is a type of paralysis with lack of muscle coordination that is due to cerebral damage generally thought to occur at or near the time of birth. The exact cause is not known, but the condition is believed to be associated with oxygen lack, premature birth, blood type incompatibility, trauma during birth or infection involving the brain or meninges.

Symptoms

Although there may be a wide variety of muscular disorders and some disturbances of sensory perception, most cerebral palsy victims have one of three types: *Spastic paralysis,* in which there are exaggerated reflexes, increased deep tendon reflexes and muscle spasms; *athetoid type,* in which there are random and purposeless movements and a high degree of muscle tension; and *ataxic type,* in which there is a disturbance of coordination with poor balance and a staggering gait. The patient also may suffer from defects of hearing, vision or speech.

Treatment

There is no cure for cerebral palsy, but early muscle training and special exercises can be of benefit if they are started before a child develops faulty habits of movement and incorrect muscle patterns. In some cases, orthopedic surgery and the use of devices such as braces and casts can be used to correct orthopedic deformities and disabilities.

Attitude of the nurse. Most victims of cerebral palsy, be they men, women or children, long to be treated as normal, sane persons. For some reason, many people conclude that the speech difficulties and uncoordinated movements characteristic of cerebral palsy indicate mental retardation or total disability. Although the cerebral palsy victim may be somewhat slower and clumsier in accomplishing relatively simple tasks or more difficult to understand when he is talking, he can be

[handwritten in top margin: can understand adult language — Do Not treat as a child]

fairly independent if one is patient with him and willing to make the effort to communicate with him. What can happen to a person with this disorder when he enters a general hospital for a physical illness? We have presented below the memories of one cerebral palsy victim who was hospitalized for appendicitis. It is hoped that those who read her story will strive to have a better understanding of the problems such a person may encounter and avoid the common misconceptions about a cerebral palsy victim.

* * *

A Patient's Humiliation*

To the palsied patient, who cannot communicate clearly, any kind of operation can be terrifying. Terrified is how I felt when I entered a hospital for an appendectomy, recently. No member of my family could stay with me to interpret my needs, as I attended a boarding school 250 miles from home. Although the school is for the handicapped, I couldn't expect any of the nurses to be released from their regular duties at the school to stay at my side.

My first problem in the hospital arose when several nurses' aides came in to take a specimen of my urine. One of the problems of a cerebral palsy victim is that the harder he tries to do something, the tenser his muscles become, making the simplest commands almost impossible to obey. The aides tried everything to make me cooperate, but my tense muscles refused, no matter how hard I kept trying.

As they stood around my bed watching me, they began discussing my handicap. They discussed what a tragedy it was that I was so disabled and how sorry they felt for my parents. They must have thought me retarded, which frequently happens, as they ignored my presence. Several times, they spoke to me in language meant only for children. "Please try to go potty," was an example.

To anyone with normal intelligence, this would be very humiliating. In all my 19 years, I had detested self-pity, but now I wanted to turn my face to the wall and cry.

However, I knew crying wouldn't solve anything and would even make me seem more retarded. After about an hour the aides gave up and left. I knew they were exasperated.

In a little while, a familiar face appeared at my door. She was one of the student nurses who had been affiliated with our school for two weeks. As she was accustomed to cerebral palsied speech, we were able to begin a friendly conversation. I mentioned my problem with the aides and told her that if she would leave me alone for a few minutes I knew I would have success. Later, when she returned, my specimen was ready for the laboratory.

The pain in my side increased through the night robbing me of sleep. Two or three times I put on my signal light, but the nurse who came couldn't understand me either. She thought I was just restless. Finally, streaks of dawn appeared and I could hear breakfast trays rattling. I could hear the aides discussing me outside my door. "Do I have to feed her?" one asked.

"Yes, I did it last night and it's a slow and tedious job. She can't swallow too well and her head moves so much that she spills most of it."

"Well I guess I have to do it, but I dread it."

Knowing the nurses' aide dreaded feeding me made me all the more unsteady. I wanted to tell her that when I was in my wheelchair sitting at a table, I wasn't shaky at all; but I knew that to try talking to her was useless. It would not help.

The morning passed slowly. My pain subsided and I felt rather chipper by noon. As the afternoon wore on, my pain became worse again, and blood tests revealed that my white blood count was up and other symptoms of appendicitis were appearing.

The only thing I remember about my operation is being wheeled into the operating room and given an injection. When I came out of the anesthetic, I was terribly nauseated. Two of the school nurses and the principal were beside me when I awoke, but I was too sick to care. Later, after they left, I longed for their return because a tube had been placed in my nose, and the foot of my bed was raised on blocks. I knew no one would understand if I asked why these things were needed, so I didn't even try. Finally, after about three hours of misery, the tube was removed from my nose and I was able to drift into a peaceful sleep.

---

*Kay Stoll, in the American Journal of Nursing, October, 1965, p. 95. Reproduced by permission.

Shortly after I awoke in the morning, mom came. Words cannot express my happiness in seeing her. I was alone no longer; someone was there who could understand what I said and needed. For the next five days mom was beside me doing most of my personal nursing herself. On the following Sunday, I was released from the hospital and driven back to school. There were many depressing moments during my hospital stay. Some could not have been avoided; others might have been if personnel had known that what I needed most was to be treated as any patient would be—and as the 19-year-old adult I am.

* * *

CLINICAL CASE PROBLEMS

1. John Powers, age 16, is admitted to the hospital with a diagnosis of meningitis. He had been ill several days before admission and complained of having a head cold and aching all over. The morning of admission he began to experience severe headache and stiffness of the neck and was taken to the doctor's office by his parents.

Two days after his admission to the hospital, John is assigned to your care. He is beginning to feel better but has still not completely recovered from the acute stage of his illness. John is a very popular teenager, and his friends and classmates are anxious to visit him and keep him company and they cannot understand the doctor's order restricting visitors.

What special precautions should you take while caring for this patient?

How can you keep him quiet yet help pass the time for him?

What special observations should you make while caring for John?

How can you help his friends understand his need for rest?

2. Mrs. Lewis has been in the hospital for five days following an automobile accident in which she received a severe blow to the head, but there was no open wound and no fracture of the skull. She regained consciousness the day after the accident but is still somewhat disoriented and confused. You are assigned to the care of Mrs. Lewis the fifth day after the accident.

What special observations must you make in caring for this patient?

What equipment would you need at the bedside?

What problems in nursing care would you expect this patient to present and how would you go about solving them?

3. Mr. Connors is admitted to the hospital with a diagnosis of rupture of an intervertebral disc. The physician has chosen to treat the condition conservatively and orders the patient placed on a cotton mattress with bed boards under it.

How would you give the patient a bed bath and back care?

What special treatment would you anticipate his receiving which might require alteration in the scheduling of his A.M. care?

How would you serve his meals if his head cannot be elevated?

Will he need any help with his tray?

REFERENCES

1. Blount, M., and Kinney, A. B.: "Myasthenia Gravis: Nursing Essentials." Journ. Pract. Nurs., June, 1972, p. 26.
2. Carozza, V. J.: "Understanding the Patient with Epilepsy." Nurs. Clin. N. Amer., Vol. 5, No. 1, 1970, p. 13.
3. Fowler, R. S., and Fordyce, W.: "Adapting Care for the Brain-Damaged Patient." Am. Journ. Nurs., Oct. and Nov., 1972, p. 2056.
4. French, R. M.: The Nurse's Guide to Diagnostic Procedures, 3rd edition New York, The McGraw-Hill Book Co., 1971.
5. Gardner, A. M.: "Responsiveness as a Measure of Consciousness." Am. Journ. Nurs., May, 1968, p. 1035.

6. GraBois, M.: "Nursing Guidelines for the Rehabilitation of the Quadriplegic and Paraplegic Patient." Journ. Pract. Nurs., April, 1971, p. 24.
7. Haber, M. E.: "Parkinson's Disease—Challenge to the Professions." Nurs. Clin. N. Amer., Vol. 4, No. 2, 1969, p. 263.
8. Henderson, G. M.: "Teaching-Learning for the Rehabilitation of the Spinal-Cord Disabled Individual." Nurs. Clin. N. Amer., Vol. 6, No. 4, 1971, p. 655.
9. Hilkmeyer, R., et al.: "Nursing Care of Patients with Brain Tumors," Am. Journ. Nurs., March, 1964, p. 81.
10. Hunkele, E., and Lodzier, R.: "A Patient with Fractured Cervical Vertebrae." Am. Journ. Nurs., Sept., 1965, p. 82.
11. Miller, B. E.: "Assisting Aphasic Patients with Speech Rehabilitation," Am. Journ. Nurs., May, 1969, p, 983.
12. Parsons, L. C.: "Respiratory Changes in Head Injury." Am. Journ. Nurs., Nov., 1971, p. 2187.
13. Plummer, E. M.: "The MS Patient." Am. Journ. Nurs., Oct., 1968, p. 2161.
14. "Quadriplegic Adolescent." Issues in Rehabilitation, moderated by M. Levine. Nursing '72, June, 1972, p. 28.
15. Queensbury, M. M., and Lembright, P.: "Observation & Care for Patients with Head Injuries." Nurs. Clin. N. Amer. Vol. 4, No. 2, 1969, p. 237.
16. Trigiano, L. L.: "Independence Is Possible in Quadriplegia." Am. Journ. Nurs., Dec., 1970, p. 2610.
17. Welch, Sr. R.: "Tilt-Table Therapy in Rehabilitation of the Trauma Patient with Brain-Damage and Spinal Cord Injury." Nurs. Clin. N. Amer., Vol. 5, No. 4, 1970, p. 621.
18. Wershow, H. J.: "Muscular Dystrophy: A Positive Approach to Care." Nursing Outlook, Jan., 1966, p. 49.
19. Young, J. F.: "Recognition, Significance and Recording of the Signs of Increased Intracranial Pressure." Nurs. Clin. No. Amer., Vol. 4, No. 2, 1969, p. 223.

SUGGESTED STUDENT READING

1. Blount, M., and Kinney, A. B.: "Myasthenia Gravis: Nursing Essentials." Journ. Pract. Nurs., June, 1971, p. 26.
2. Cooper, U. S.: "Cryogenic Neurosurgery." Journ. Pract. Nurs., Sept., 1968, p. 21.
3. "Epilepsy—Today's Outlook." Journ. Pract. Nurs., Nov., 1966, p. 37.
4. Golub, S.: "Parkinson's Disease Today." RB, Oct., 1967, p. 59.
5. GraBois, M.: "Nursing Guidelines for the Rehabilitation of the Quadriplegic and Paraplegic Patient." Journ. Pract. Nurs., April, 1971, p. 24.
6. Magee, K. R.: "Myasthenia Gravis." Journ. Pract. Nurs., Nov., 1965, p. 23.

7. Miller, B. E.: "Assisting Aphasic Patients with Speech Rehabilitation." Am. Journ. Nurs., May, 1969, p. 983.
8. Neuberger, G. J.: "Epilepsy—What Is It?" Bedside Nurse, Oct., 1970, p. 21.
9. Schneider, K.: "Care of a Young Patient with Paraplegia." RN, Nov., 1969, p. 48.
10. Sudduth, A. L.: "Comprehensive Care of the Traumatic Paraplegic." RN, May, 1970, p. 59.
11. TeWinkle, M. B.: "Observation and Care of the Patient with a Head Injury," Parts I and II. Journ. Pract. Nurs., Nov., 1971, p. 23.

OUTLINE FOR CHAPTER 21

I. Introduction

A. Nervous system is body's communication system.

B. All nerve cells are excitable and conductive.

C. Impairment of nerve cells' ability to receive and conduct impulses affects normal function of tissues controlled by those nerves.

II. Special Examinations and Diagnostic Tests

A. Complete neurologic examination is a very intensive and prolonged procedure in which physician may test normal functioning of cranial nerves, strength and coordination of groups of large muscles and involuntary muscular contractions.

B. Tests done for signs of irritation of the meninges.

C. Lumbar puncture—needle inserted into spinal cavity to measure pressure or to obtain specimen of spinal fluid.

D. Cisternal puncture—spinal tap needle is inserted just below the occipital bone into cisterna magna.

E. Electroencephalogram records the activity of brain tissues.

F. X-ray studies of the skull are done after injection of a contrast medium.

    1. Angiography involves injection of a radiopaque solution.

    2. Pneumoencephalography utilizes a gas as contrast medium.

    3. Ventriculography uses air injected via two holes bored in the skull.

G. Radioisotopes used to locate tumors of the brain.

III. General Nursing Care of the Patient with a Neurologic Disorder

A. Patient suffers from some organic

disease of the nervous system rather than from mental illness or personality disorder.

B. Patient may not be able to move or to recognize dangers of immobility.

C. Nurse should guide patient to help himself.

D. A neurological disorder can cause severe emotional upset. Patient will need help in adjusting to his illness.

E. Patient is rehabilitated to live a full life within the physical limitations imposed by his illness.

IV. Infectious Diseases

A. Meningitis is an inflammation of the membranous linings of the brain and spinal cord.

1. May be caused by a variety of organisms (meningococcus causes epidemics).
2. Symptoms are severe headache, stiff neck, nausea, vomiting and signs of upper respiratory infection. Spinal fluid contains increased number of white cells and causative organisms.
3. Treatment and nursing care. Specific antibiotics and anticonvulsants may be given. Provide rest and fluids.
   a. Patient may be isolated, as all secretions from nose and mouth are highly infectious.
   b. Protect patient from injury during delirium and convulsions.
   c. Small, low enemas prevent abdominal distention.

B. Encephalitis is an inflammation of the brain tissues.

1. Caused by a virus or toxins from organisms and some chemicals.
2. Symptoms are fever, headache and extreme restlessness or lethargy and muscular weakness.
3. Treatment and nursing care is like that of the meningitis patient. Check vital signs frequently.

C. Poliomyelitis is an acute inflammation of the anterior horn of the spinal cord caused by three different strains of viruses. Vaccine is now available.

1. Symptoms may be so slight as to cause no great discomfort. Severe infection produces signs of upper respiratory infection, fever, severe headache, stiff neck and sore back and hamstring muscles. Paralysis may occur as disease progresses.
2. Treatment and nursing care. There is no cure. Give patient complete bed rest and apply heat to muscles. Watch for urinary retention and fecal impaction, respiratory failure and difficulty in swallowing.

V. Head Injuries

A. Concussion is a closed injury in which a portion of the brain tissue suffers from a temporary anemia. Contusion is bruising and swelling of brain tissues.

B. There may be a delayed reaction to any head injury.

C. Extent of damage to the brain is determined by patient's behavior and symptoms.

D. Treatment is conservative unless fracture or increased intracranial pressure is present. Patient placed on bed rest and kept quiet until physician decides danger has passed. May need help in swallowing or breathing.

VI. Brain Tumors (Abnormal Growths of Cells Within the Brain or Its Coverings)

A. Symptoms are quite varied. There may be personality changes, disturbances in judgment and memory, loss of strength, speech and visual disturbances, headache and vomiting.

B. Treatment: tumors must be removed surgically or destroyed by radiation.

VII. Nursing Care of a Patient Having Brain Surgery

A. Preoperative observations are used as a basis for comparison after surgery.

B. Postoperative care. Vital signs are taken frequently. Dressings are checked and reinforced when necessary.

VIII. Injuries of the Spinal Cord

A. Are classified as cervical, thoracic or lumbosacral.

B. Symptoms depend on location of nerve damage and severity of damage.

C. Treatment: repair damage to cord, prevent further injury to spinal cord by careful handling and immobilization, improve patient's physical condition, prevent complications (decubitus ulcers, urinary complications and orthopedic deformities) and make rehabilitation possible.

D. Nursing care is concerned with proper care of skin, attention to proper elimination, prevention of muscle spasms and proper positioning of patient.

IX. Rupture of Intervertebral Disc

A. Symptom is pain in lower back and one leg.

B. Treatment and nursing care. Patient given bed rest with firm spinal support and heat to relieve muscle spasm. Pelvic traction sometimes used. Surgical treatment (laminectomy and spinal fusion fuses the affected vertebrae together.

X. Myasthenia Gravis (Grave Muscular Weakness)

A. Symptoms—severe muscle weakness and fatigue.

B. Treatment—drugs (usually neostigmine and pyridostigmine).

XI. Parkinson's Disease

A. A degenerative disease of the nerve cells in the brain. Cause unknown.

B. Symptoms—tremor and rigidity of the skeletal muscles.

C. Treatment—drugs to produce mild relaxation and sedation. Surgical treatment successful in some cases.

XII. Multiple Sclerosis

A. A chronic and progressive disease of the central nervous system. Cause unknown.

B. Symptoms—slow onset with disturbance in vision, muscular weakness and gradual loss of coordination. There may be remissions of symptoms after which they are more severe.

C. Treatment—symptomatic. No cure.

XIII. Epilepsy (Sudden and Uncontrollable Seizures)

A. May be symptom of a disorder of the brain or idiopathic (in which there is no pathology).

B. Symptoms. Grand mal—severe convulsive movements and loss of consciousness. Often preceded by some sensory change. Petit mal—seizure very mild with only momentary loss of consciousness.

C. Treatment—protection from injury during convulsion and anticonvulsants.

XIV. Cerebral Palsy

A. A type of paralysis with lack of muscle coordination. Due to cerebral damage possibly stemming from oxygen lack at birth, traumatic birth, premature delivery or infection.

B. Symptoms—exaggerated reflexes, poor coordination of voluntary muscles, high muscle tension and sometimes a defect of hearing, speech, or vision.

C. Treatment—early muscle training and special exercises. Orthopedic surgery, braces or casts can correct some orthopedic deformities and disabilities. Patient to be as independent as possible.

22

Nursing Care of Patients With Disorders of the Eyes, Ears and Throat

VOCABULARY

Equilibrium
Intraocular
Labyrinth
Malaise
Ossicle
Prosthesis

Part One.   Disorders of the Eyes

INTRODUCTION

According to statistics, there are two million persons in the United States who have inadequate vision even with glasses and another million who are blind. In fact, probably a little over half the people in this country have defective vision to some degree. The emotional, physical and financial burdens brought about by such visual defects would be impossible to estimate.

The sense of sight is such a priceless possession it would seem that everyone would exercise extreme care in taking care of his eyes, yet many of the persons included in the preceding statistics could have prevented their loss of vision if they had known and applied the fundamental principles of good eye care. Some of them may have been ignorant of these principles, others may have deliberately neglected their eyes and still others may have been hopelessly confused by misinformation and superstitious beliefs. Whatever the reason for improper eye care, all members of the health team have the responsibility of health education in prevention of injuries and diseases of the eyes.

In her work or at home among friends and relatives, the practical nurse will have many opportunities to correct mistaken ideas and give factual information about the eyes and their care. Some of the basic facts of eye care are listed below.

1. The term "eyestrain" has been greatly abused and overused. It has often been a catchall to explain various and sundry visual defects and diseases of the eye. It is actually very difficult to

strain the eye. Inadequate light or excessive use of the eyes for close work can cause the eye muscles to become overly tired, just as any other muscle of our bodies becomes tired from overuse, but such use will not damage the eyes any more than straining to hear a distant sound can damage the ears. The eye muscles should be rested periodically while the person watches television, reads, sews or performs other activities which require constant use of the eyes. If the eyes seem to tire easily, or if there is headache, burning, itching and redness of the eyes, this is not eyestrain. These are symptoms of a visual defect and are an indication that the person's eyes should be examined by a physician.

2. Adequate diet and good nutrition play an important role in the conservation of sight, but eating large amounts of carrots and other yellow vegetables will *not improve eyesight.* A lack of vitamin A in the diet often results in an inflammation of the lids and conjunctiva and an increased sensitivity to light. A deficiency of vitamin B in the diet can cause irreparable damage to the retina and permanent visual defects.

3. Normal eyes do not require irrigations or periodic "washing out" with boric acid solutions or other commercial preparations. The normal secretions of the conjunctiva and tear glands are sufficient to lubricate the eye and remove small particles of dust which may collect in the eye. Accumulation of purulent material or itching and burning of the eyelids may indicate diseases and should be reported to a physician.

4. Children do not outgrow crossed eyes. Until a baby reaches the age of 6 or 9 months, he may have some difficulty focusing his eyes, but this condition should not persist past that age. Neglect of crossed eyes *(strabismus)* can cause a serious loss of vision. It is generally agreed by ophthalmologists that the sooner treatment is begun, the better the chance of correcting the con-dition and preserving the child's eyesight. A child who has only one crossed eye will not use the affected eye and will eventually become blind in that eye if the condition is not corrected.

5. Every person over the age of 40 should have a periodic examination of the eyes. It is particularly important that a test for glaucoma be made at the time of the examination, since this disease usually does not present symptoms of pain or discomfort until it reaches the advanced stages. It is also believed that this disease runs in families, and any person who has a relative with glaucoma should be especially alert for the development of the disease in himself.

6. Every year there are at least 100,000 schoolchildren who suffer from some serious accidental injury to the eye. Many of these accidents could be avoided if parents, teachers and the children themselves were made aware of the danger of sharp pencils, paper wads, small stones or other objects children may be tempted to hurl at one another while playing.

7. Visual defects cannot always be corrected by the purchase of a pair of glasses or the changing of the lenses in glasses. Many people who otherwise demand the best medical care for their physical ailments will not hesitate to purchase "reading glasses" from a dime store counter in an effort to improve their vision, or consult an optometrist for treatment of a serious eye disease. Both practices are foolish. The dime store clerk is only trained to collect the price of the glasses and make the correct change. A reputable optometrist will usually refer the person to a physician when he recognizes the need for medical treatment of the eyes, but he is not qualified to diagnose diseases of the eye, and much precious time may be lost while he futilely attempts to correct the condition by changing the lenses of the patient's glasses.

8. One of the reasons for improper care of the eyes stems from the layman's confusion about the terminology

used to designate the various persons concerned with the prescribing and fitting of eye glasses. The nurse should know and understand the various functions and qualifications of such persons so that she can offer intelligent advice to those who seek her help on disorders of the eye.

An *ophthalmologist* or *oculist* is a medical doctor who specializes in the diagnosis and treatment of visual defects and diseases of the eye.

An *optometrist* is one who is trained only in scientific examination of the eyes for the purpose of prescribing glasses. He is not a physician and cannot treat diseases of the eye.

An *optician* is one who is trained to make glasses and optical instruments. He grinds the lenses and fits glasses according to a prescription from the ophthalmologist or optometrist.

DIAGNOSTIC TESTS AND EXAMINATIONS

Snellen Chart

This chart is quite familiar to most of us, even though we may not have known it by name. The chart is usually designed so that there is one large letter at the top and subsequent rows of letters under it, each row in smaller print than the one above it. The Snellen chart is read from a distance of exactly 20 feet, and the letters are scaled according to normal vision. A person with normal visual acuity can read the top letter from a distance of 100 feet, the second row of letters from 70 feet, the third at 50 feet and so on down to 10 feet for the last row of letters.

The visual acuity of the person being tested is expressed as a fraction. The numerator indicates the distance between the patient and the chart (20 feet), and the denominator indicates the distance at which a person with normal vision can read the letters. For example, 20/50 vision means that the person being tested can only read the letters of the third row at a distance of 20 feet, while a person with normal visual acuity could easily read these letters from a distance of 50 feet. If the vision is 20/20, it is considered to be normal distance vision. A vision of 20/200 is used in defining blindness.

Near Vision

In order to test an individual's ability to see objects close at hand, the physician uses a test known as *Jaeger's Test Types.* The patient is given a card which is printed with different sizes of ordinary printer's types. The smallest and finest type is used for line one and each successive line is printed with larger types. A piece of cardboard is placed over one eye and each eye is tested separately.

Refraction

When light rays enter the eye, they are "refracted" or bent so that they focus on the retina. The lens, aqueous humor and vitreous humor are responsible for bending these light rays. Disorders of the lens which prevent the proper focusing of light rays upon the retina are diagnosed by a *refraction.* This eye examination makes use of various glass lenses of different shapes through which the patient reads the Snellen chart. When he chooses the lens through which he can best read the chart, the ophthalmologist prescribes the same kind of lenses to be ground by the optician and fitted as glasses for the patient.

Intraocular Pressure

The chambers of the eyeballs in front of the lenses are filled with a watery substance called the *aqueous humor.* This fluid is constantly being produced and drained off in equal proportions so that there is a normal amount of pressure within the chambers. An increase or decrease in the amount of pressure being exerted by the aqueous humor within the chambers of the eye can be measured with an instrument called a tonometer. The testing of intraocular pressure is extremely important in the diagnosis of glaucoma, in which intraocular pressure is increased.

COMMON VISUAL DEFECTS

The most common visual defects are those of refraction. This means that light rays entering the eye are not "refracted," or bent, at the correct angle and therefore do not focus on the retina. Errors of refraction may be caused by a number of structural defects within the eyeball itself. For example, if the eyeball is constructed so that the distance between the lens and retina is too short, the light rays focus behind the retina. This causes difficulty in seeing objects close at hand and is called farsightedness (hyperopia) (see Fig. 22-1).

If the opposite is true, and the lens is situated too far from the retina, the light rays will converge and focus in front of the retina. The individual then has difficulty in seeing objects at a distance and is referred to as nearsighted. Nearsightedness is called myopia.

Light rays from distant objects do not enter the eye at the same angle as light rays from near objects. When we look off into the distance and then quickly look down at a book in our hands, our eyes must make an adjustment to the difference in the light rays entering the eye. This adjustment is called accommodation and is accomplished by ciliary muscles and ligaments which change the shape of the lens, making it more rounded or flatter (see Fig. 22-2).

As we grow older, our ciliary muscles become less elastic and cannot readily accommodate to the needs of distant and near vision. This hardening of the ciliary muscles occurs in many persons over 40 years of age and is known as presbyopia. Bifocal glasses are usually prescribed for this condition because they allow for two sets of lenses in one pair of glasses, one set for viewing distant objects and one for seeing close objects.

Astigmatism is a visual defect resulting from a warped lens or irregular curvature of the cornea, either of which will prevent the horizontal and vertical rays from focusing at the same point on the retina. Actually, there are very few people who have perfectly shaped eyeballs, and so there are very few who do not have some degree of astigmatism. If the astigmatism is very slight, the eye can accommodate for its imperfec-

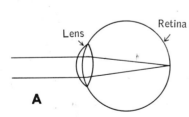

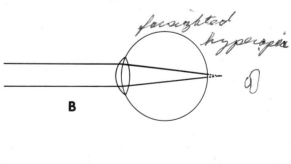

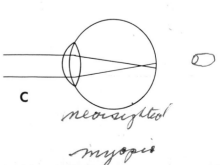

Figure 22–1. *A,* Normal vision. Lens bends light rays so that they focus directly on the retina. *B,* Hyperopia. Lens is too close to retina. Thus light rays converge at point beyond the retina. *C,* Myopia. Lens is too far away from retina, causing light rays to converge before they reach the retina. (Modified from Sackheim: *Practical Physics for Nurses,* 2nd Ed., W. B. Saunders Co., Philadelphia.)

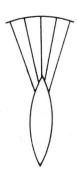
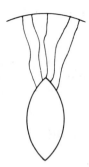

Ligaments tight—lens flattened   Ligaments relaxed—lens more rounded

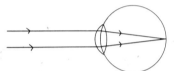
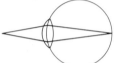

Rays from a distant object are focused   Rays from a nearby object are properly
on the retina by a flattened lens   focused on the retina by a more
                                                rounded lens

Figure 22–2. Defects of the eye. (From Sackheim: *Practical Physics for Nurses,* 2nd Ed., W. B. Saunders Co., Philadelphia.)

tion by changing the shape of the lens. If there is a serious error of refraction, the eyes will tire very easily or the person will have defective vision because the eyes cannot change the shape of the lens enough to compensate for the abnormality. The treatment for serious errors of refraction is the prescription of artificial lenses and the fitting of glasses so that the light rays are brought into proper focus on the retina.

INJURIES AND INFECTIONS OF THE EYE

Foreign Bodies

The human eye is situated within the eye socket of the skull so that it is partially protected from direct blows. The quick-acting lids, the eyelashes and the eyebrows also serve to protect the eye from injury. But in spite of nature's attempts to protect the eye, there are still many instances in which foreign bodies become lodged in the eye (see Fig. 22-3).

If the foreign body is not deeply embedded in the tissues of the eye, it can easily be removed by touching it with the corner of a clean handkerchief. Should the object remain lodged in spite of this effort to remove it, a physician should be consulted at once. Many eyes have been damaged and vision permanently impaired by a layman's well-meaning attempts to remove foreign objects from the eyes.

Conjunctivitis

Definition. The term "conjunctivitis" is used to describe any inflammation of the mucous membrane lining the upper and lower lids and covering the front part of the eyeball. This condition may be caused by a number of organisms, including the staphylococcus, streptococcus and gonococcus. "Pinkeye" is a conjunctivitis caused by a specific organism called the Koch-Weeks bacillus.

Symptoms. Objective symptoms of conjunctivitis include redness and

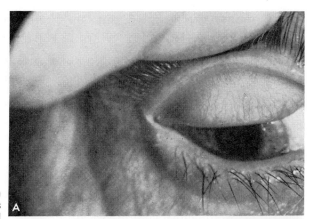

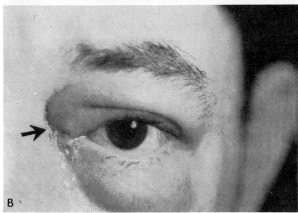

Figure 22-3. *A,* Foreign body often can be seen only if the upper lid is everted. *B,* Acute meibomitis (internal sty) may require surgical treatment. (From Gordon:American Journal of Nursing, November, 1964.)

swelling of the conjunctiva and the production of a watery secretion in the eyes. Later this secretion may become purulent and, if not properly treated, the eyes may be partially closed and covered with crusts of dried exudate. In addition to these outward signs, the patient may also complain of local itching and burning.

Treatment and Nursing Care. Conjunctivitis should be treated as quickly as possible and all precautions taken to prevent its spread to other persons. "Pinkeye" is highly infectious and is quite common in schoolchildren.

The treatment of conjunctivitis will depend on the organism causing the infection. Some types of conjunctivitis may resist local treatment of antibiotic ointments and eye drops and require the administration of antibiotics systemically. Gonorrheal conjunctivitis

demands immediate attention because of the danger of blindness as a result of the infection. In this type of conjunctivitis, the exudate from the eyes must be handled with extreme care and isolation precautions taken to prevent spread of the disease to the eyes of others.

In addition to the administration of ointments or eyedrops ordered by the physician, nursing care is also concerned with hot or cold moist compresses and irrigations of the eye to remove the exudate and relieve the local itching and burning.

Sty (Hordeolum)

Definition. The sty is one of the most common infections of the eye. It is usually a staphylococcus infection of a follicle of an eyelash.

Symptoms. Redness, burning, and itching of the eyelids are usually the first symptoms of a sty. Very soon after these symptoms develop, a small pustule forms on the lid, and the lid becomes red and swollen. Even though a sty is not especially painful, it may be very annoying and uncomfortable. A general state of poor health or a need for glasses may predispose a person to repeated development of stys.

Treatment and Nursing Care. Most stys will rupture and drain without incision if warm, moist compresses are applied regularly to the affected eye. Those which do not respond to this treatment must be surgically incised by a physician.

Infections of the meibomian glands (small lubricating glands around the edge of the eyelids) are often mistaken for sties. These infections cause considerably more pain than the more common sty and usually do not respond to hot wet compresses alone. If antibiotic ointments do not eliminate the infection, surgical treatment is necessary. Frequent infections of the eyelids can be symptomatic of diabetes mellitus.

Cataract

Definition. The word "cataract" literally means a waterfall. The term is used to designate an opacity of the lens of the eye because the vision of the person with this condition is impaired as if he were trying to see through falling water. His vision is blurred because the lens of the eye is cloudy and opaque, thus preventing proper entrance and focusing of light rays on the retina.

Cataracts are sometimes present at birth (congenital cataracts). But they most often occur as a result of the aging process and are found in persons in their seventies or eighties (senile cataracts).

Treatment. The only effective method of treating cataracts is surgical removal of the affected lens. This procedure is called a cataract extraction. It should be understood that while this procedure does improve vision, it does not restore the eye to a perfectly normal condition. The patient must have glasses prescribed, and they must be worn at all times. The reason this is necessary is that the process of accommodation (see the preceding discussion) is no longer possible once the lens has been removed. The glasses prescribed are usually bifocals. The practice of waiting until a cataract has grown to full maturity (ripened) is no longer practiced, and the present trend is toward removal of the lens as soon as the cataract is noticed.

Nursing Care of the Patient Having a Cataract Extraction

PREOPERATIVE CARE. Since the great majority of these patients are elderly and therefore most likely to be suffering from some additional chronic disease, the nurse must remember the need for applying the principles of geriatric nursing in administering nursing care to a patient with a cataract. Fear, anxiety over the surgery and confusion about the expected results of the surgery are all factors to be considered in the preparation of the patient for the operation.

When the patient is admitted to the hospital, he should be given adequate instruction in the physical layout of his room and the ways in which he can call for the nurse should he need her. Side rails are usually necessary to prevent falls, and the patient should be cautioned against getting out of bed without assistance.

Preoperative medications include the local application of an antibiotic ointment to reduce the chances of a postoperative infection, and the administration of mydriatic eyedrops to dilate the pupil. The drugs must be given with extreme care and accuracy, especially if only one eye is affected. If the symbols "o.d." and "o.s." are used to designate the right eye and the left eye, the nurse must be sure that the medication is applied to the correct eye.

POSTOPERATIVE CARE. The patient may receive a general anesthetic for this surgical procedure, or the physician may prefer to use a local anesthetic. There are several advantages to a local anesthetic, but his choice will depend on the general health of the patient and his ability to cooperate with the surgeon.

In either case, the nurse must help the patient understand the importance of avoiding stress on the suture line within the eye. Coughing, sneezing, squeezing the eyelids or sudden movements of the head should be avoided. Policies regarding the amount of bodily activity allowed the patient vary in different institutions, and some doctors permit their patients more freedom than others. In recent years, there has been a trend toward allowing the patient more activity, and many patients begin ambulation the day after surgery. The surgeon is usually very clear and explicit in his instructions to the patient and the nursing staff, so there should be no excuse for failure to follow his orders precisely. *ambulate per Dr orders*

As long as the patient has dressings and eyeshields over both eyes, he will need the same considerations as one who is blind. If he is allowed out of bed, he must have assistance (see Fig. 22-4).

Compresses and saline irrigations of the eye are usually ordered to remove drainage and exudate from the eyes. It should be remembered that the eyeball itself is never touched during this procedure. Only the lids are cleansed, using gentle vertical strokes and working from the inner corner of the eye outward. If some bits of exudate cannot be removed with this gentle cleansing, they should be left for the surgeon to remove.

Occupational therapy and some diversional activities should be planned

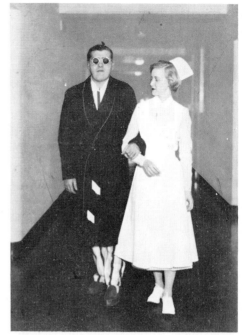

Figure 22–4. When a patient is allowed up to walk after eye surgery, the nurse must realize that attempting to walk with both eyes covered is a frightening experience. The nurse who assists the patient must give adequate guidance and a feeling of safety, yet not make the patient feel that he is being pushed forward. This is accomplished by having the patient hold the guide's arm and by giving precise verbal directions, including an estimate of the distance to be covered. (Courtesy of Cora L. Shaw, Institute of Ophthalmology; and the American Journal of Nursing.)

to prevent boredom and help the patient pass the long hours of waiting. Before the patient goes home, he will receive instructions from the physician about the amount of activity he may be allowed. Usually he is told that lifting, bending or otherwise straining his muscles should be avoided. He will also be told when he must return to the doctor's office for checkups and the prescribing of glasses.

Adjusting to cataract glasses can be very frustrating and even frightening for the patient and will require much patience and understanding from those trying to help him during this difficult period. The lenses of cataract glasses are very thick, and the edges tend to curve straight lines. This produces a kind of rounded tunnel vision in which everything in the peripheral vision curves around the center, depth perception becomes greatly distorted and the patient has great difficulty judging distances. If he turns his head suddenly, the curved lines are set in motion, and his only clear vision is directly through the center of the glasses. Another problem is a blind area, between 11 and 20 feet away, in which the patient cannot see objects. Thus, he has the unnerving experience of seeing someone approach him, disappear from his sight and then reappear much closer to him. In time, the patient will adjust to this, and he will barely notice the blind spot, but at first, such a difficulty can be very frightening and discouraging.

The nurse can help the patient in his adjustment by reassuring him that such difficulties are to be expected at first, and that eventually he can become accustomed to his glasses. He should be instructed to move slowly at first, feeling his way through doorways and other close quarters through which he feels unable to move about. He should make a special effort to get into the habit of moving his head from side to side rather than shifting his eyes, and he must always try to look directly through the center of his glasses. The adjustment can be more rapid if the patient is able to use his hands and eyes for fine work such as knitting, carving, whittling or sewing. This type of precision work trains the eyes to focus through the cataract glasses properly and also serves as a form of occupational therapy that can do wonders for the morale of a person who could barely distinguish between light and dark shadows before surgery.

Glaucoma

Introduction. The aqueous humor (watery fluid) which flows within the eyeball in front of the lens is normally constant in volume and exerts a well-balanced pressure within the chambers of the eye. When there is an increase in production of the aqueous humor, or when there is a hindrance to its outflow, the pressure within the eyeball increases. This increase of intraocular pressure can damage the optic nerve and produce varying degrees of visual impairment. Glaucoma is the condition in which increased intraocular pressure is present. It usually results from an obstruction to the outflow of the aqueous humor in the anterior chamber of the eye.

Symptoms. "Glaucoma must be considered a very serious condition because (1) it is frequently not diagnosed, (2) it often leads to irreversible loss of vision and (3) the disease process may be extremely difficult to slow down."

The disease is particularly treacherous because symptoms during the early stages are very mild, and many patients are not aware that anything is wrong until vision has been completely lost in one eye or until headache and pain in the eye during an acute attack bring about a visit to the physician.

The National Society for the Prevention of Blindness lists the following symptoms as danger signals of glaucoma:

1. Glasses, even new ones, don't seem to help.
2. Blurred or hazy vision which clears up after a while.
3. Trouble in getting used to darkened rooms, such as at the movies.
4. Seeing rainbow-colored rings around lights.
5. Narrowing of vision at the sides of one or both eyes.

The society also recommends a regular eye examination at least two years after the age of 40. Since one of the earliest indications of developing glaucoma is an elevation of eye pressure, use of a tonometer to test the degree of intraocular pressure is an important part of the eye examination (see Fig. 22-5).

Treatment and Nursing Care. Glaucoma is primarily treated medically. If the medications are not effective

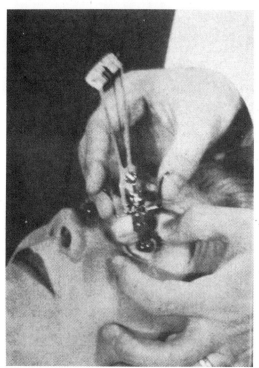

Figure 22–5. The tonometer is used to measure pressure within the eye. The eyes are anesthetized with a local anesthetic and the tonometer is touched to each eye and a measurement taken. (From Weinstock: American Journal of Nursing, April, 1973.)

and the disease continues to progress, a surgical procedure involving removal of a section of the iris (iridectomy) may be performed so that outflow of the aqueous humor is established.

The first drugs used in the treatment of glaucoma are usually those which constrict the pupil (miotics). Pilocarpine, which acts on the sphincter muscle of the pupil, and eserine and neostigmine, which inhibit the nerve impulses to the pupil and prevent dilatation, are the drugs most often used. Other drugs, such as Diamox and other carbonic anhydrase inhibitors, which decrease the production of aqueous humor, are often used in conjunction with the miotic drugs.

Glaucoma is essentially a chronic disease. It develops slowly, and if left untreated, will relentlessly progress to total blindness in the affected eye. Both eyes are usually involved, although one may show evidence of the disease before the other will. This disease is the main cause of blindness in adults in this country and as such must be considered of primary importance in education of the public about the disease.

The patient with glaucoma is usually not hospitalized unless he suffers an acute glaucomatous attack. In this instance, he will experience a severe pain which may be localized in the eye or may involve the entire head. The pain is so excruciating that nausea and vomiting will often occur. During this episode, the patient should be kept very quiet and disturbed as little as possible, and sedatives and analgesics for relief of pain are given until the attack subsides. If the condition is not treated, the attack may persist for several days or weeks, and complete blindness will result.

There is evidence that emotional upsets, worry or poor general health further aggravate glaucoma and precipitate attacks of acute symptoms. The patient and his family will need help in understanding the disease and avoiding situations which increase intraocular pressure. These include family arguments, quarrels and other situations which produce mental anxiety and tension. Physical exertion, heavy lifting or tight-fitting clothing may also increase the pressure. Use of the eyes should be limited, and watching television, sewing or reading should be interspersed with periods of rest for the eyes.

Detached Retina

Introduction. The retina is the innermost layer of the eye. It is composed of two layers: a pigmented layer that is in close contact with the choroid (vascular wall) of the eye and that supplies nutrients for both layers, and a sensory layer that receives visual stimuli and therefore is essential to normal vision. In detached retina, there is a hole or tear in the two layers, and vitreous fluid leaks under the retina, separating it from the vascular wall and depriving it of its blood supply. Once the retina is detached from the wall of the eye, it no longer receives a clear image, and vision is greatly impaired.

There are many possible causes of detached retina. The condition can result from a sudden blow or a penetrating injury to the eye or following surgery of the eye. Predisposing factors include myopia and diabetic changes in the retina.

Symptoms. There may be a gradual or sudden onset, depending on the cause and size and location of the area involved. The patient may see flashes of light and then, days or weeks later, notice cloudy vision or loss of central vision. Another common symptom is the sensation of spots or moving particles in the field of vision. In severe cases, there may be complete loss of vision.

Diagnosis of detached retina can be done with a direct ophthalmoscope, but it is greatly simplified by a newer instrument called a stereoscopic indirect ophthalmoscope. This instrument permits visualization of the entire retina and produces an image of the retina with less magnification and distortion.

Treatment and Nursing Care. The only treatment for retinal detachment is surgery. During the preoperative period, the patient is usually extremely apprehensive because of his fear of blindness and will need reassurance that newer techniques of surgery promise success in more than 85 per cent of all cases of retinal detachment. Physical preparation of the patient includes instillation of eye drops that dilate the pupil. These eye drops are extremely important and must be given precisely as ordered by the surgeon. Prior to surgery, the upper and lower eyelashes of the affected eye are clipped close to the lid margin using scissors whose blades are covered with petroleum jelly so that the eyelashes adhere to the blades and do not fall into the

eye. The patient's face is usually washed several times with a surgical soap. Male patients must be clean-shaven so that adhesive dressings can be applied without difficulty.

There are several new surgical procedures used for the repair of detached retina. Almost all of them utilize diathermy to seal the retinal break firmly so that vitreous fluid cannot leak between the retina and the choroid and thereby produce recurrence of retinal detachment. Another aim of surgery is to drain off fluid that has accumulated so that the retina can be returned to its normal position.

The amount of activity allowed during the postoperative period will depend on the type of surgery done and the specific directions of the surgeon. Patients having the newer types of surgery are usually allowed out of bed the day after surgery, though they must use care not to move their heads too vigorously. Others who have had sutures applied to hold the retina in place may be confined to bed for two weeks postoperatively, and they must keep their heads as still as possible during that time.

NURSING CARE OF THE PATIENT HAVING EYE SURGERY
Determine how much a pt sees
Preoperative Care

During the preoperative period, the individual needs of each patient anticipating surgery of the eye must be determined and his nursing care planned accordingly. Some patients will have nearly normal vision, while others may be almost totally blind. At the time of admission the nurse should make a special effort to orient the patient to his environment. This is true for every patient having eye surgery, for even though he may be able to see fairly well before surgery, he may have his eyes bandaged after the operation. The physician or nurse should explain times, she must know whether the patient can feed himself and whether there are restrictions on food or fluid intake. If the patient is allowed out of bed, he must take care not to jar his head or move too suddenly; all straining and lifting must be avoided. The patient and his family should be encouraged to follow the physician's directions faithfully during the convalescent period at home so that nothing will be done to jeopardize the success of the surgery.

GENERAL PRINCIPLES IN THE CARE OF THE BLIND

Emotional Aspects of Blindness

Those of us who are fortunate enough to have adequate vision cannot fully realize the tremendous adjustments to be made by those who are deprived of their sight. If we were to put on a blindfold and stumble through one day of our usual activities, we might have some slight comprehension of the obstacles to be overcome, but we still would not experience the same sense of hoplessness and despair which besets those who have lost their sight. We would have the satisfaction of knowing that we could regain our sight by simply removing the blindfold. The permanently blind person has no such promise in the future.

These feelings of depression and despair in the person who has lost his sight are to be expected and are considered by some psychologists to be a necessary step in the direction of adjustment to blindness. The following quotation from an article in the January 1956 edition of the American Journal Nursing may emphasize and clarify this very important point in the care of those who have lost their sight.

The important lesson for all who work with the blind—friends, nurses, and ophthalmologists—is to realize that the various stages through which the newly blinded

person passes are fundamental to his rehabilitation. Unfortunately, we are told there seems to be a "concerted effort of society to prevent the patient from accepting his blindness." Everyone—frequently even the doctor who is treating the patient—tries to "cheer him up," to prevent him from grieving; many even offer hope that his sight may yet return. Rarely is any hope offered that the patient may yet have a full life as a blind man, and that it is only a *different kind of life* he must learn to live.

The patient must, in fact, "die as a sighted person in order to be reborn as a blind man," and he usually experiences a very welcome relief from struggle once he accepts his condition. Once he realizes that he is a new person, he can begin to investigate both his limitations and his capacities, and actually learn a new way of life.

Special Rules to Follow in Helping a Blind Person

1. Remember that the person is blind, not deaf. There is no reason to shout at him or address him as though he were either deaf or a child. Speak normally, and do not try to avoid using the words "I see." Blind people use this phrase themselves without hesitation.

2. Speak to the blind person as you enter the room, and do not touch him until after you have spoken to him. This prevents startling or frightening him when he may not have heard you enter the room.

3. The prevention of accidents is an important part of the care of the blind. Aside from the physical effects of bumping into objects or falling over them, the blind person also suffers from a loss of self-confidence and security if he cannot move about safely and independently. Doors should be kept closed or completely open. They must never be left ajar. If it is necessary to move a piece of furniture in the patient's room, tell him about its new location.

4. When you leave the room, tell the blind person that you are going. He will not then resume the conversation

the reason for postoperative bandaging of both eyes, if this is expected, so that the patient will not be upset by the bandages when he recovers from anesthesia. In most instances, especially following cataract extraction, the unaffected eye is covered so that the patient will not be tempted to move his eyes during the immediate postoperative period.

Preoperative medications such as ophthalmic ointments and eye drops must be given exactly on time because they are important to the success of the surgery. When these medications are instilled, the eye is held open by resting the fingers on the bones of the face. Never press against the eyeball. The hand administering the drops should be firmly pressed against the patient's forehead so that any sudden movement of the head will not cause the container to injure the eye. After the eyelids are separated, the patient is asked to look up, and the medication is administered along the lower lid. The patient is then instructed to close his eye slowly so that the medication will not be squeezed out of the eye.

Physical preparation for surgery may include an enema or suppository to evacuate the lower bowel. This is done to prevent straining at stool during the immediate postoperative period. If the eyelashes are to be clipped, they should be cut with small curved scissors with blunt points. Petroleum jelly is applied to the blades of the scissors so that the eyelashes will adhere to the blade and will not fall into the eye. Some physicians direct the patient to wash his face with surgical soap several times during the evening before surgery, and a sterile eye pad may be placed over the eye.

If the nurse notices any symptoms of a respiratory infection or allergy that will bring about coughing and sneezing during the postoperative period, she should notify the surgeon. Since such violent motions can bring about hemorrhage within the eye or rupture the surgical incision, the physician may postpone surgery until a later date.

Postoperative Care

In all types of eye surgery, word is gentleness. The patien must be firmly supported wh transferred from the operating stretcher to his bed, and all m by those moving him should deliberate and gentle. While fined to his bed, small pillow used on either side of his hea support it in the proper pos member that you should alw softly before touching a patie blind or wearing bandages eyes. If he did not hear you room or was napping at the entered, he may be fright move suddenly and violentl feels someone touch him. O older patients who are unab erate may need someone i attendance to prevent their the bandages. Nausea and vomiting can wreak havoc cate suture lines in the patient becomes nauseate and liquids should be withh physician notified so tha emetic drug can be ordered pain in the eye may indic rhage and should be bro attention of the physician i

Irrigations of the eye ar presses sometimes are ore move exudate and reduce the eyelids and surround These procedures must b the utmost care, cleansing and avoiding any contact ball.

Because there can be difference in the amount activity allowed a patient tioning preferred by the practical nurse must be th miliar with the individua patient who has had surge She should know wheth patient can be turned on sides or whether he must his back, whether pillow under the head and how of the bed may be rai later and find that he is talking to someone who is not there.

5. Pity is neither expected nor appreciated by the blind. They only want to be treated as normal people and would prefer to ask for your help when they need it rather than have you do everything for them. It is also important to remember that there are no such things as "extra senses of blindness" which many people mistakenly believe blind people are given to compensate for their loss of sight. Whatever the blind person has learned about living with his blindness he has accomplished through hard work and determination.

6. If you are assigned to the care of a blind person admitted to a general hospital, determine the amount of assistance the patient desires and needs. Do not embarrass him by assuming that he is helpless, but avoid neglecting him when he needs your help. When serving a meal to the blind patient, tell him what foods are in his plate and their location (see Fig. 22–6). Do not use a straw or drinking tube unless requested by the patient, because it may be awkward for him to use. If you must feed him all of the meal, work slowly and calmly. Inform him of hot

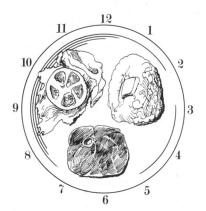

Figure 22–6. Telling the patient that his meat is at 6 o'clock, potato at 2 o'clock and vegetable at 10 o'clock helps him to locate them on his plate.

and cold foods, and alternate dishes rather than feed him all of one thing and then another. Avoid talking too much and forcing the patient either to stop eating or to answer you with a mouth full of food. Whenever possible, allow the patient to feed himself finger foods such as bread and raw vegetables or fruit. Bear in mind that your goal is to help the patient maintain his dignity and self-respect while meeting his personal needs.

Part Two. Disorders of the Ears

INTRODUCTION

It is estimated that one out of every ten persons in this country suffers from hearing loss to some degree. Deafness, like blindness, burdens its victims with emotional problems as well as physical, financial and social handicaps. Communication with others is of primary importance in daily living; to be deprived of the essentials of social intercourse leaves most individuals completely out of the group. Because this is true, the person who hears only distorted sounds or no sounds at all tends to withdraw from others and live within a world of his own.

Children who have hearing difficulties may be considered disobedient, stupid or even seriously mentally retarded. A baby who is deaf at birth has great difficulty learning to speak because he cannot hear the words of the language and therefore is unable to repeat them. The adult who has a hearing deficiency may lose his job and alienate his friends because of his handicap in communicating with others.

Normal hearing depends on the conduction of sound waves through the ear to the auditory nerve and the transmission of impulses along this nerve to the brain. Sound is described as occurring in waves because the vibrations of sound are similar to the ripples in a pond produced by throwing a pebble into the water. The length of the waves determines its *frequency;* the height of the waves determines the sound's *intensity.* Both of these are important in the detection of sound by the human ear.

A loss of hearing may be *sensorineural or conductive.* A sensorineural loss of hearing is brought about by a disorder of the eighth cranial nerve (the auditory nerve) and is sometimes called nerve deafness. Conductive loss of hearing occurs when there is a barrier in the canal, drum or middle ear which prevents the progress of sound waves from the environment to the auditory nerve. Obstruction of the movement of the tiny ossicles within the middle ear will also produce a conductive loss of hearing.

SPECIAL DIAGNOSTIC TESTS AND EXAMINATIONS

Tuning Fork Tests

The tuning fork is a simple, inexpensive instrument which may be used to test hearing. The fork is struck with a rubber reflex hammer, and its vibrations produce sound waves which can be heard by a person with normal hearing.

The *Weber test* is done by striking the tuning fork and then placing the handle of the tuning fork on the patient's forehead. If the patient has normal hearing or is equally hard of hearing in both ears, he will hear the sound in the middle of his head. A comparison of hearing acumen in both ears can be made with this test.

The *Rinne test* is done by striking the tuning fork and then placing the handle against the mastoid bone. The fork is removed and struck again; this time it is held beside the ear. The patient is then asked in which position he heard the sound better or longer. The Rinne test is used to determine whether a hearing loss is sensorineural or conductive.

Audiometry

The audiometer is a special machine used in the measurement of sound perception. It is especially useful in the testing of speech perception, because it is in this area that loss of hearing creates the most problems. The administration of tests using the audiometer requires special training and experience and must be done by an audiologist. A list of all the hearing centers where these tests are available may be obtained by writing to the American Hearing Society, 919 Eighteenth Street, N.W., Washington, D.C., 20006. Address

INFECTIONS OF THE EAR

Otitis Media, Tympanitis

Definition. Otitis media is an abscess or inflammation of the middle ear (tympanum). It is the most common of all ear infections and usually is a complication of an acute infection of the throat or sinuses. Otitis media may also occur as a result of the collection of fluid within the middle ear due to an allergy.

Symptoms. Pain in the ear, fever and drainage from the ear are the common symptoms of this condition. In some cases of chronic otitis media, these symptoms may be controlled by the administration of antibiotics, and the only indication of an inflammation will be a loss of hearing.

Treatment and Nursing Care. General treatment of otitis media is rest and the relief of pain through the use of analgesics and the application of heat

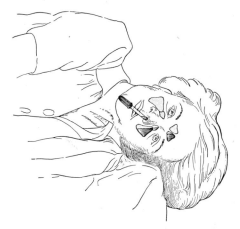

Figure 22–7. Recommended position for administering nose drops to patient who has otitis media and needs to have the eustachian tube kept open and draining. (From Boies et al.: *Fundamentals of Otolaryngology,* 4th Ed., W. B. Saunders Co., Philadelphia.)

to the ear. Antibiotics are given to inhibit the growth and development of the causative organisms. Because of the danger of eliminating the symptoms without curing the disease, most physicians also administer hearing tests during and after treatment, to be sure that the infection has completely subsided and there is no remaining fluid left containing pathogenic organisms.

Incision and drainage of the eardrum to allow for removal of the inflammatory exudate from the middle ear is called a *myringotomy.* This procedure may also be done as a diagnostic test to determine the presence of specific types of pathogenic organisms in the fluid.

Nosedrops may be given at regular intervals during the day so that the eustachian tube is kept open and drainage encouraged. These drops are given with the head inclined toward the affected ear (see Fig. 22–7).

Mastoiditis

Definition. Mastoiditis is a bacterial infection of the cells of the mastoid bone. The infection is usually streptococcal and spreads to the mastoid from the middle ear.

Symptoms. Earache with tenderness in the area of the mastoid bone and elevation of the body temperature are the outstanding symptoms of mastoiditis. Upon visual examination, the eardrum appears congested and is bulging. Incision of the eardrum brings about the flow of a large amount of purulent, foul-smelling drainage. The drum may rupture spontaneously if the pressure behind it becomes too great.

Treatment and Nursing Care. When antibiotics were first used in the treatment of the middle ear infections, it was hoped that the spread of infection to the mastoid cells would be prevented, thereby eliminating mastoiditis as a complication of otitis media. Unfortunately, this has not happened. Instead, the antibiotics often mask the symptoms, giving the impression that complete recovery has taken place, when in reality the infection smolders and spreads from the middle ear to the mastoid cells.

When mastoiditis is diagnosed, it is treated surgically and with medication. The first step is usually myringotomy to drain off the purulent matter and the administration of antibiotics and sulfonamides to destroy the causative organism. If x-ray examinations of the mastoid bone show that there is necrosis of the bone cells, the surgical removal of the cells becomes necessary. The operation is called a *mastoidectomy* and may be simple or radical, depending on the amount of dead bone tissue which must be removed.

Nursing Care of the Patient Having a Mastoidectomy

PREOPERATIVE CARE. Physical preparation of the patient is basically the same as for other types of major surgery. The hair should be washed before the day of surgery and the area around the affected ear shaved (see Fig. 22–8).

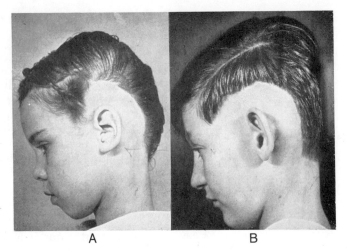

A   B

Figure 22–8. Area to be shaved for mastoid operation *(A)* on female patient and *(B)* on male patient. Note that hair of male patient has been parted very low on side of head where surgery is to be performed. (From Manhattan Eye, Ear and Throat Hospital: *Nursing in Diseases of the Eye, Ear, Nose and Throat,* 10th Ed.)

Many of these patients are children, and the nurse must recognize the need for eliminating safety hazards and providing emotional support for the child during the preoperative period. If possible, the same nurses should be assigned to the care of the child during the preoperative and immediate postoperative periods. This gives the child a sense of security and reduces the anxiety produced by únfamiliar surroundings and the child's natural fear of pain and discomfort.

POSTOPERATIVE CARE. When the patient returns from the recovery room, he must be watched closely until fully conscious so that he will not disturb the surgical dressings or any drains which may have been inserted during the operation. Very small children may require tongue-blade restraints on their arms to keep their hands away from the operative site. Bleeding, elevation of temperature or changes in the vital signs should be reported immediately.

The patient is usually placed on a semisoft diet of foods which require a minimum of chewing until the soreness in the operative area has subsided.

DISORDERS OF THE INNER EAR

Introduction

The inner ear is a very complex structure located deep in the temporal bone. It consists of bony and membranous labyrinths filled with fluid, and its functions are hearing and maintaining equilibrium. Because of the location and complexity of structure of the inner ear, its disorders are difficult to treat and tend to become chronic, producing loss of hearing that can be permanent.

Labyrinthitis

This is an inflammation involving the labyrinths of the inner ear, usually occurring as a complication of chronic otitis media. The symptoms of labyrinthitis include loss of hearing in the affected ear, dizziness with nausea and vomiting and abnormal jerking movements of the eyes *(nystagmus).*

Treatment is aimed at removal of the source of infection and relief of symptoms. Antibiotics may be given in massive doses to control the infection, which often is quite persistent and difficult to clear up completely. The patient is kept in bed to minimize vertigo and to avoid injury from falls. Side rails must be applied to the bed, and the patient should be told the reason for this and why he should not try to get out of bed without assistance. Dimenhydrinate (Dramamine) or other drugs to control motion sickness may be given. If the source of infection is a chronic mastoiditis that does not respond to medical treatment, a mastoidectomy may be done.

Meniere's Syndrome

This is a group of symptoms in which there is an increase in fluid within the spaces of the labyrinths with swelling and congestion of the mucous membranes of the cochlea. The symptoms include attacks of dizziness, ringing in the ear (tinnitus), headache, poor coordination that makes walking difficult or impossible and loss of hearing. Any sudden movement of the head or eyes during an attack usually produces severe nausea and vomiting. The condition occurs most often in persons who have had chronic ear disorders and allergic symptoms involving the upper respiratory tract. The exact cause is unknown.

Diagnosis of Meniere's syndrome usually is not difficult, but since these symptoms could indicate a tumor of the auditory mechanism, a special test may be done to confirm the diagnosis. This test, called the caloric test, involves instilling very warm or cold fluid into the auditory canal. A patient with Meniere's syndrome will experience a severe attack, while a normal person will complain of only slight dizziness. A person with a tumor of the auditory mechanism will have no reaction at all.

Treatment of Meniere's syndrome is primarily concerned with relief of symptoms; there is no cure for the

condition, although it does disappear spontaneously in some cases. In order to control edema and reduce pressure in the inner ear, the patient may be placed on a low-sodium diet, his fluid intake restricted and his urinary output increased by means of a diuretic drug. Drugs such as Dramamine and Bonamine may be given to control nausea and vomiting. The patient is kept quiet in bed to avoid aggravating his symptoms. He may be very irritable and withdrawn and refuse to eat or drink because of fear of vomiting. One should be very careful to avoid increasing his irritation by jarring his bed, turning on bright overhead lights or making loud noises.

These measures help control the severe symptoms during an attack, but the patient's hearing is not improved. If the attacks continue and are very severe in spite of medical treatment, surgical destruction of the eighth nerve may be necessary. Although this produces permanent deafness in the affected ear, the severe attacks are eliminated and in most persistent cases of Meniere's syndrome, the patient will have experienced a serious or even total loss of hearing eventually, no matter what treatment was used.

Otosclerosis

Definition. Much of our hearing depends on the proper vibration of the small bones of the inner ear. The stapes, or stirrup, is particularly important because it transmits the sound waves to the fluid in the semicircular canals. In otosclerosis, the stapes becomes fixed and cannot move because of destruction of normal bone and the laying down of sclerotic bone cells. When the stapes is locked in a fixed position, it cannot vibrate and therefore is no longer able to transmit sound waves.

Symptoms. The patient who has otosclerosis has a peculiar type of hearing disability. He has difficulty hearing the voices of others, yet his own voice sounds unusually loud to him. In response to this, he lowers his voice to the point that he can scarcely be understood by others. His reaction is characteristically one of criticism in which he complains that everyone is mumbling and they do not pronounce their words distinctly. His attitude can be understood when we realize that because of cranial bone conduction of sound waves, he does not have an overall loss of hearing and can hear fairly well over a telephone or in a noisy atmosphere in which other people are speaking loudly above the surrounding noise.

Treatment and Nursing Care. Otosclerosis may be treated by a properly fitted hearing aid or by surgical means. Newer methods of surgery, using a microscope because the ossicles of the middle ear are so small, have greatly increased the success of surgical treatment of this condition.

The operative procedure is called a *stapedectomy*, in which the stapes is removed and is replaced with a prosthetic device. This device may be a steel wire and fat implant, a wire and a segment of vein or a vein graft with polyethylene tubing. In any case, the prosthesis is attached to one end of the incus (anvil of the middle ear) so that sound can be transmitted to the inner ear (see Fig. 22-9).

The surgical procedure is extremely delicate and would not be possible without the fairly recently developed dissecting binocular microscope and

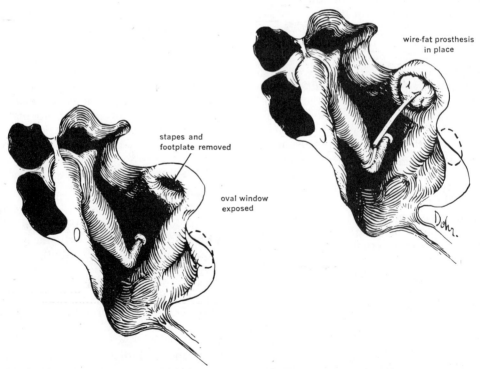

Figure 22–9. In otosclerosis, spongy, vascular bone invades and fixes the footplate of the stapes, normally movable on its annular ligament. A stapedectomy restores air-conductive hearing by providing a new movable pathway from middle ear to inner ear. A prosthesis, which may be made of earlobe fat and stainless steel wire, of wire-Gelfoam, of a Teflon-wire piston or of polyethylene #90 tubing, can replace the stapes and footplate. At left, the middle ear tissue is removed, and at right, the wire-fat prosthesis is shown in place. (From De Laney: American Journal of Nursing, November, 1969.)

other modern surgical instruments that allow visualization and manipulation of the very small structures of the middle ear.

Postoperative nursing care is concerned with keeping the patient quiet and flat in bed for forty-eight hours. The head is turned so that the operative ear is uppermost. When the patient is allowed to move about, he must be warned that dizziness is likely to occur, especially if he turns his head suddenly. Side rails are applied to the bed, and the patient must have assistance when getting out of bed and walking. Coughing, sneezing and other violent movement of the head should be avoided, and the patient must be warned not to blow his nose, as this may introduce organisms into the middle ear via the eustachian tube. The physician will instruct the patient in which activities are allowed and which are to be avoided during his convalescence at home.

NURSING CARE OF THE PATIENT HAVING SURGERY OF THE EAR

Preoperative Care

The nursing care of the patient during the preoperative period usually is rather routine except for administration of ear drops or other special medications and treatments. The physical preparation may or may not involve removal of some of the hair from the scalp. Most patients having a mastoidectomy do have some hair removed on the affected side. Male patients should be clean-shaven the morning of surgery. The external ear and surrounding skin should be thoroughly cleaned, preferably with a surgical soap. Female patients with long hair should have it braided or pinned back securely so that it will not become soiled by drainage from the ear or serve as a source of infection at the operative site.

Postoperative Care

Positioning of the patient after surgery will depend on specific instructions from the physician. Usually the patient is placed flat in bed, and his head is supported so that he does not turn it from side to side. In addition to noting the vital signs, the nurse should watch for signs of injury to the facial nerve. These would include inability of the patient to close his eyes, wrinkle his forehead or pucker his lips. Such symptoms should be reported to the surgeon. If they appear later than 12 hours after surgery, they may be due to edema, and the physician may order a loosening of the dressings.

Precautions such as side rails to the bed should be taken to avoid injury due to dizziness and loss of balance, which can occur temporarily as a result of disturbance to the equilibrium mechanism. When the patient is allowed up and about, he should have someone in attendance to prevent falls.

Because the ear is so near the brain, a special effort must be made to avoid contamination of the operative area. Dressings may be reinforced to keep them dry, but excessive drainage must be reported to the surgeon. The patient must keep his hands away from the bandages, and if he is unable to do so, he should be restrained.

Sneezing, coughing and nose-blowing are all ways in which the operative site may be disturbed to the detriment of the patient's welfare. If sneezing cannot be controlled, the patient should be told to keep his mouth open while sneezing so that the force of the sneeze will exit through the mouth rather than the eustachian tube. Sneezing and blowing the nose also may force bacteria and other infectious material into the operative area.

The nurse should know beforehand exactly what outcome is to be expected from the surgery. If the patient's hearing is slightly impaired immediately after surgery because of edema or bandages but is expected to improve in time, she should know this so that she can sincerely reassure the patient that it will improve. She should be able to give encouragement to her patient but must avoid giving false hopes or telling him that he has nothing to worry about when he will indeed have to make an adjustment to a disability.

GENERAL PRINCIPLES IN THE CARE OF THE DEAF

Terminology

The terms "deaf" and "hard of hearing" are sometimes taken to mean the same thing, when, actually, they represent two separate conditions.

The *deaf* are those in whom the sense of hearing is entirely absent. The *congenitally deaf* are those who are born without the sense of hearing, the *adventitiously deaf* are those who are born with the sense of hearing but, by illness or accident, have lost their hearing.

The *hard of hearing* are those in whom hearing is defective but not totally absent.

Signs of Hearing Loss

Many cases of deafness could have been prevented if the condition had been detected in the early stages and treatment begun. The value of public health education in the early signs of hearing loss cannot be estimated. Nurses must be familiar with the following signs and accept some of the responsibility for educating parents and teachers in the health of the ears and preservation of the sense of hearing:

1. A listless or weary expression.
2. Frequent requests for repetition.
3. Mispronunciation of words.
4. Habitually turning one ear toward the speaker.
5. Inattention or failure to respond when questioned.

6. Voice or speech peculiarities.
7. Continued failure in school.
8. Earache, head noises, discharging ears.
9. Tendency to avoid people.

THE NURSE AND THE DEAF AND HARD OF HEARING

We have discussed earlier the emotional aspects of hearing loss (see introduction to Part II of this chapter). When a person who is deaf or hard of hearing enters a hospital, he brings with him some of the emotional scars resulting from his struggle to live with his handicap. Like the blind patient, he does not want pity. He *does* appreciate understanding and consideration from those who must care for him while he is ill. The following rules are given in the hope that they will help the nurse when she is assigned to the care of patients who suffer from a loss of hearing.

1. Do not shout at the person who is hard of hearing. Speaking slowly and distinctly is more help than raising the voice.

2. Face the person when you speak to him. Your facial expressions are helpful in understanding what you are saying, even if the person cannot read your lips.

3. Keep questions to a minimum, but when you must ask a question, phrase it so that his answer will require more than a yes or no. For example, "What is your name?" is better than "Are you Mr. Lowe?" In this way you avoid getting an incorrect answer from the patient who does not wish to ask you to repeat the question and will just say "Yes" because he thought you had asked if he was Mr. Long.

4. Because the patient either cannot hear or often misinterprets the sounds he does hear in the unfamiliar surroundings of the hospital, he is more likely to be upset and frightened his first few days in the hospital. He will

appreciate frequent visits from the nurse to reassure him that she is genuinely interested and close at hand should he need her.

The Hearing Aid

Many hearing aids are bought, worn for a few days and then relegated to the depths of a dresser drawer. This unfortunate situation is often the result of improper fitting of the hearing aid and inadequate instruction in its use.

The hearing aid should do more than amplify sound. Less expensive aids do make sounds louder, but they often distort the sounds. The patient who has a conductive hearing loss but normal sensory function is usually satisfied with amplification alone because he has no problem with sound perception. The patient who has sensorineural hearing loss may actually have poorer hearing with the hearing aid than without it if the appliance distorts sounds as it amplifies them.

It is obvious, then, that the choice of a hearing aid and the preparation and instruction of the patient are very important factors in the successful use of such an appliance. Just as the proper fitting of glasses for correction of visual defects demands more than a trip to the local dime store for a pair of reading glasses, the fitting of a hearing aid requires more than purchasing an amplifier and applying it to the ear. The person who wishes to improve his hearing through the use of a hearing aid must have persistence, determination and adaptability. He must be willing to cooperate with the audiologist who prescribes the aid, learn to use the aid intelligently and care for it properly.

Part Three. Disorders of the Throat

PHARYNGITIS

Definition

The throat has been described as the "crossroads of the human body." It has openings leading from the nose and ears and also serves as a passageway for food and air. It is little wonder, therefore, that inflammation of the throat (pharyngitis) is such a common condition. Considering the exposure of the throat to the hordes of bacteria present in our environment, it is remarkable that more infections do not occur there.

Symptoms

Most of us are quite familiar with the symptoms of pharyngitis—the dry, "scratchy" feeling in the back of the throat, slight fever, chills and malaise. These symptoms are usually accompanied by a sinusitis or an inflammation of the nasal mucosa.

Treatment and Nursing Care

Local treatment consists of hot saline throat irrigations and, if the discomfort is severe, the application of an ice collar to the throat. Aspirin gargles (5 grains of aspirin and ½ tsp. of baking soda dissolved in a glass of warm water) are also helpful in the relief of local symptoms. Antibiotics or sulfonamides are sometimes given to prevent secondary infection if the patient has a chronic illness or is physically weak and debilitated.

TONSILLITIS

Definition

An inflammation of the tonsils is usually caused by streptococci or staphylococci and is completely different from pharyngitis even though the symptoms may be somewhat alike. Acute tonsillitis may occur repeatedly, especially in those who have a low resistance to infection. Chronic tonsillitis usually produces enlargement of tonsillar tissue and adjacent adenoidal tissue as well.

Symptoms

Acute tonsillitis occurs most often in young children. There is an elevation of the temperature, sore throat, general malaise and chills. Inspection of the throat reveals redness and swelling of the tonsils and surrounding tissues.

Chronic infection of the tonsils produces symptoms which may not be as dramatic but most certainly are capable of making the person uncomfortable. The child with chronic tonsillitis and enlarged adenoids has frequent colds and appears to be in poor health. He gives the impression of being dull or mentally retarded because he constantly holds his mouth open to breathe, and he often has difficulty in hearing. These children also are mouth breathers when they sleep and are very likely to snore.

Treatment and Nursing Care

Acute tonsillitis is treated with hot saline throat irrigations and the administration of specific antibiotics for the destruction of the causative organism. Bed rest, nursing measures to reduce the fever and liquid diet to minimize trauma to the tonsils are also included in the treatment.

Chronic tonsillitis is treated surgically when accompanied by enlargement of the tonsils and adenoids. The practice of indiscriminately removing

tonsils "just in case tonsillitis may develop" has been discontinued. Most physicians usually will not remove the tonsils unless the child fails to respond to medical treatment and has symptoms of enlarged tonsils and adenoids.

Nursing Care of the Patient Having a Tonsillectomy and Adenoidectomy

Preoperative Care. Most tonsillectomies are performed on young children who have had no previous admissions to a hospital and are not yet old enough to fully understand the need for the surgical procedure. Every nurse who expects to care for a child in a hospital should have a thorough understanding of the essentials of child psychology. Even those nurses who have had training and experience in pediatric nursing are sometimes surprised to find that they are not able to gain the confidence and cooperation of a child and allay his fears and anxieties while he is in the hospital. It is to be expected, therefore, that those who do not understand children are even less likely to have any success in this area of nursing. The reader is referred to texts on pediatric nursing and child psychology for the essential principles of child care.

Physical preparation of the patient having a tonsillectomy involves administration of preoperative medications as ordered and restriction of the patient's diet for 6 to 8 hours prior to surgery. It is especially important that the child's temperature be taken for signs of fever, so that an elevation of temperature or any signs of an upper respiratory infection may be reported. Surgery is usually postponed if these signs are present.

Postoperative Care. Following tonsillectomy or adenoidectomy, the nurse's chief concern is observation for hemorrhage. Even though about one million tonsillectomies are performed in the United States each year, and nurses may tend to become somewhat complacent about the routine care of these patients, it must be remembered that *a tonsillectomy or adenoidectomy should never be considered a minor operation.*

Since hemorrhage is always a possibility following a tonsillectomy, the vital signs are checked quite frequently. If the patient appears to be swallowing often, seems unusually restless or has a change in pulse rate and blood pressure, excessive bleeding should be suspected even though there are no outward signs of bleeding. An ice collar may be placed around the neck to reduce swelling and prevent the oozing of blood from the operative site.

Even though it is difficult to keep a child in one position for very long, he should be kept on his side or abdomen as long as there is drainage from the surgical wound. If the child is thrashing about in the bed when recovering from the anesthesia, it is best to collect secretions from the mouth in a large towel rather than use a metal emesis basin which may injure him. Older children may sit up in semi-Fowler's position after they have recovered from the anesthesia and are often more comfortable this way. A younger child usually can be kept calm and quiet if someone holds him and rocks him. This is not spoiling the child; he needs to keep as quiet as possible to prevent hemorrhage from the operative site, and he needs love and affection to reassure him at a time when he is frightened and uncomfortable. It should be emphasized that every child is an individual. He has his own likes and dislikes, his own preferences. The nurse who bears this in mind is more likely to keep her patient calm and cooperative than the one who insists on following the rules to the letter.

The postoperative diet usually consists of ice-cold liquids, ice cream, jello, custards and other semisolid foods for the first 24 hours. Citrus fruits, hot fluids and rough foods should be avoided until the throat has completely healed.

CANCER OF THE LARYNX

Introduction

Cancer of the larynx occurs most often in men of middle age or older, but it can strike anyone, especially those over the age of 18. It is one of the most easily cured of all malignancies because of its location and adjacent tissues, and about 80 per cent of all cases treated by early surgery are cured. The cause of cancer of the larynx is not known, but there is some evidence that predisposing factors are cigarette smoking, chronic laryngitis, abuse of the vocal cords and a familial tendency toward cancer.

Symptoms and Diagnosis

Since the larynx, sometimes called the voice box, is directly concerned with the production of vocal sounds, a tumor of the larynx will quickly produce persistent hoarseness that does not respond to usual methods of treatment. After the cancer has spread beyond the vocal cords (and is much more difficult to treat), the symptoms may include difficulty in swallowing or breathing, a sensation of having a lump in the throat, cough, enlarged lymph nodes in the neck and pain in the region of the Adam's apple.

Diagnosis is established by visualization of the larynx via a laryngoscope and microscopic examination of the sample of tissues taken from the tumor.

Treatment

There are two types of surgical procedures that may be done for treatment of laryngeal malignant disease. If the tumor is restricted to the vocal cords, the surgeon may perform a partial lar-

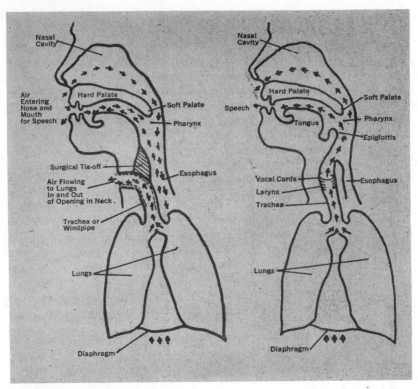

Figure 22–10. Airflow after laryngectomy *(left)* and in a normal person. (From Adler: American Journal of Nursing, October, 1969.)

yngectomy in which the thryroid carti-lage is split and only the tumor and involved portion of the vocal cords are removed. In more advanced cases, me-tastasis may demand a total laryngecto-my, in which the surgeon excises the entire larynx, epiglottis, thyroid carti-lage, hyoid bone, cricoid cartilage and two or more rings of the trachea.

A partial laryngectomy does not per-manently eliminate voice sounds. A tracheostomy may be done for tempo-rary facilitation of breathing, but this eventually is closed, and the patient may resume talking after the operative area is healed completely.

In a total laryngectomy, the trachea is diverted to a surgically constructed opening (stoma) in the neck. The pa-tient then has a permanent tracheosto-my with no connection between the nose and mouth and the lower respira-tory system and must depend on the

stoma for breathing. The laryngectomy tube is inserted in the stoma and re-sembles a tracheostomy tube except that it is somewhat shorter and wider. Usually the laryngectomy tube can be removed within six weeks after sur-gery.

Nursing Care. The patient who has had a laryngectomy will require ade-quate instruction in the care of his stoma and laryngectomy tube. He will need help and guidance in facing a future in which he will not be able to speak until he learns esophageal speech or uses an artificial "voice box." He also may have difficulty eating and swallowing until he gets accustomed to the sensations of choking and gagging that frequently occur with a laryngec-tomy.

Feedings through a nasogastric tube may be prescribed by the physician if the patient has great difficulty swallowing or if the surgeon feels that there is danger of contaminating the operative area. Tube feeding is then given at regular intervals, and the nasogastric tube is inserted before each feeding and removed when the feeding is completed. Some patients can be taught to pass their own tubes and give their own feedings because this gives them a feeling of independence. Others will refuse to take any active part in the procedure.

Protection of the tracheal opening from dust and lint can be accomplished by a simple gauze covering or high-necked clothing. The patient also should be told to avoid swimming and to use care when taking a shower or tub bath so that water is not aspirated through the opening. In order to protect the patient from inhalation of extremely cold air (he no longer breathes through his nose and mouth, which normally warm inspired air) the patient may wear a small scarf over the opening during the winter weather.

Proper rehabilitation of the patient plays a very important part in his acceptance of surgery and its consequences. Many persons are able to learn esophageal speech in which they first master the art of swallowing air and then moving it forcibly back up through the esophagus. They then learn to coordinate lip and tongue movements with the sound produced by the air passing over vibrating folds of the esophagus. The sounds may be somewhat hoarse, but they can be understood as speech and are more natural than the sounds produced by an artificial larynx.

In various parts of the United States, there are several groups organized for laryngectomy patients who wish to get together for social and rehabilitation purposes. These clubs have names like Lost Cord, New Speech, New Voice and Esophageal Speech. Information regarding these clubs and other aspects of post-laryngectomy rehabilitation can be obtained by writing to the American Speech and Hearing Association, 1001 Connecticut Ave., Washington, D.C. 20036.

ADDRESS

CLINICAL CASE PROBLEMS

1. Mr. Wilson, aged 72, is admitted to the hospital for surgical treatment of cataracts of both eyes. His poor eyesight has prevented his earning a living for quite a few years, and he has been totally dependent on his son. He did not consult a doctor until recently because he has always heard that cataracts had to be "ripe" before they could be treated, and he felt that he could not afford frequent trips to the doctor when nothing could be done for his eyes.

When you take Mr. Wilson to his room after admission to the hospital, he tells you that he is used to being "almost blind" and can take care of himself. He does not want side rails on his bed and insists he can get up to the bathroom without any help. From your observations of the patient, you can see that Mr. Wilson does need help but is apparently too proud to ask for it.

The day after his operation Mr. Wilson is again assigned to your care. He seems more cooperative and somewhat frightened by his experience in the hospital. He is very anxious to walk down the hall and the doctor has stated that he can be ambulatory for a very brief period of time.

What nursing problems are presented by Mr. Wilson's attitude of independence when he is admitted to the hospital?

What precautions must be taken for his safety?

What special nursing care will he require postoperatively?

How will you accompany Mr. Wilson as he takes a walk down the hall?

2. A neighbor tells you that her 4-year-old son seems to have more than his share of colds and sore throats. She feels that these could be eliminated by having the child's tonsils removed, but her physician advises against surgery. The neighbor asks your advice about changing doctors, because she is convinced that a tonsillectomy is the only solution to the frequent colds and sore throats.

How would you advise this person?

3. Janice is a 7-year-old who has been admitted to the hospital for a tonsillectomy and adenoidectomy. She has been emotionally prepared for the stay in the hospital and seems happy and satisfied before surgery.

Following the surgical procedure, Janice is taken to the recovery room and then is brought to her room after she has recovered sufficiently from the anesthesia. When she is placed in the crib bed, she begins to thrash about, screaming for her mother. All this activity causes an attack of vomiting and increases the flow of blood from the operative site. The mother of the child becomes very upset and cannot stay with her. The nurse in charge gives Janice a sedative and then asks you to stay with her and keep her quiet.

How will you handle the secretions from the operative site?

How would you keep the child quiet?

4. Mr. Lavant, age 52, and his wife, age 50, have heard about a glaucoma screening clinic being held in their community. They are interested in attending the clinic but very apprehensive about the kind of tests that will be done. They ask your advice and whether you think they should spend time going when they have no symptoms of glaucoma or any other eye disease.

How would you explain the tests that might be done?

Could you explain glaucoma in terms they would understand?

What do you think might be the purpose of the screening clinic?

REFERENCES

1. Adler, S.: "Speech after Laryngectomy." Am. Journ. Nurs., Oct., 1969, p. 2138.
2. Bender, R. E.: "Communicating with Deaf Adults." Am. Journ. Nurs., April, 1966, p. 757.
3. Brockhurst, R. J., and O'Donnell, C. T.: "Detachment of the Retina." Am. Journ. Nurs., April, 1964, p. 96.
4. Bruegger, S. L.: "Contact Lenses." Am. Journ. Nurs., Sept., 1965, p. 92.
5. Chodil, J., and Williams, B.: "The Concept of Sensory Deprivation." Nurs. Clin. N. Amer., Vol. 5, No. 3, 1970, p. 453.
6. Condl, E. D.: "Ophthalmic Nursing: The Gentle Touch." Nurs. Clin. N. Amer., Vol. 5, No. 3, 1970, p. 467.
7. Conover, M., and Cober, J.: "Understanding and Caring for the Hearing Impaired." Nurs. Clin. N. Amer., Vol. 5, No. 3, 1970, p. 497.
8. DeLaney, R. E.: "Stapedectomy." Am. Journ. Nurs., Nov., 1969, p. 2406.
9. Flowers, A. M.: "Eelctronic Mechanical Aids for the Laryngectomized Patient." Nurs. Clin. N. Amer., Vol. 3, No. 3, 1968, p. 529.
10. Gordon, D. M.: "The Inflamed Eye." Am. Journ. Nurs., Nov., 1964, p. 113.
11. Haddad, H. M.: "Drugs for Ophthalmologic Use." Am. Journ. Nurs., Feb., 1968, p. 325.
12. Jackson, G. D.: "How Blind Are Nurses to the Needs of the Visually Handicapped?" Nurs. Outlook, Sept., 1965, p. 34.
13. Moore, M. V.: "Diagnosis: Deafness." Am. Journ. Nurs., Feb., 1969, p. 297.
14. Nilo, E. R.: "Needs of the Hearing Impaired." Am. Journ. Nurs., Jan., 1969, p. 114.
15. Nordstrom, W.: "Adjusting to Cataract Glasses." Am. Journ. Nurs., July, 1966, p. 1578.
16. Pitorak, E. F.: "Laryngectomy." Am. Journ. Nurs., April, 1968, p. 780.
17. Ronnei, E. C.: "Hearing Aids." Am. Journ. Nurs., May, 1963, p. 90.
18. Seaman, F. W.: "Nursing Care of Glaucoma Patients." Nurs. Clin. N. Amer., Vol. 5, No. 3, 1970, p. 489.
19. Smith, D. W., et al.: *Care of the Adult Patient,* 3rd edition. Philadelphia, J. B. Lippincott, 1971.
20. Weinstock, F. J.: "Emergency Treatment of Eye Injuries." Am. Journ. Nurs., Oct., 1971, p. 1928.
21. Weinstock, F. J.: "Tonometry Screening." Am. Journ. Nurs., April, 1973, p. 656.

SUGGESTED STUDENT READING

1. Bender, R. E.: "Communicating with Deaf Adults." Am. Journ. Nurs., April, 1966, p. 757.
2. Carbary, L.: "When Your Patient Wears an Artificial Eye." Practical Nursing, July-August, 1962, p. 20.
3. Davis, R. W.: "Care of the Patient with Laryngectomy." Bedside Nurse, Nov., 1970, p. 13.
4. Olson, N.: "A Mother's View of Tonsillectomy." Am. Journ. Nurs., May, 1969, p. 1024.
5. Pamphlets from American Foundation for the Blind, 15 West 16th St., Washington, D.C.

OUTLINE FOR CHAPTER 22

Part One Disorders of the Eyes

I. Introduction

A. Fundamentals of good eye care:
  1. Headache, burning, itching and redness of the eyes are symptoms of a visual defect.
  2. Adequate nutrition conserves but does not improve eyesight.
  3. Normal eyes do not require irrigations.
  4. Children do not outgrow crossed eyes.
  5. Every person over the age of 40 should have periodic eye examinations.
  6. Teaching eye safety to children in school could prevent many accidental injuries.
  7. Visual defects cannot always be corrected by eye glasses.

II. Diagnostic Tests and Examinations

A. Snellen chart—composed of increasingly smaller rows of type. Visual acuity expressed as a fraction comparing subject's distance (20 feet) with distance at which a person with normal vision can read the row. 20/20 is normal.

B. Near vision tested by a card with different sizes of types (Jaeger's Test Types).

C. Refraction—patient reads the Snellen chart through differently shaped lenses.

D. Intraocular pressure—tonometer measures amount of pressure being exerted by the aqueous humor within the chambers of the eye.

III. Common Visual Defects

A. Errors of refraction—light rays bent so that they do not focus properly on the retina.
  1. Myopia (nearsightedness)—light rays converge and focus in front of the retina. Individual has difficulty seeing distant objects.
  2. Hyperopia (farsightedness)—light rays focus behind the retina. Person has difficulty seeing objects close at hand.
  3. Presbyopia is improper accommodation of the ciliary muscles and ligaments in switching between distant and near vision.
  4. Astigmatism results from a warped lens or irregular curvature of the cornea.

IV. Injuries and Infections of the Eye

A. Foreign bodies—patient should be referred to physician if body is not easily removed.

B. Conjunctivitis is an inflammation of the mucuous membrane lining the upper and lower lids and covering the front part of the eyeball.
  1. Symptoms are redness, swelling of conjunctiva, watery secretion, burning and itching.
  2. Treatment depends on organism causing infection. Antibiotic ointments, steroids and hot or cold moist compresses may help.

C. Sty (hordeolum) is an infection of a follicle of an eyelash.
  1. Symptoms are redness, burning and itching of the eyelids. Pustule develops on the eyelid.
  2. Warm, moist compresses usually cause rupture and draining of the pustule, or surgical incision may be made.

D. Cataract—an opacity of the lens of the eye.
  1. Symptoms—blurring of vision.
  2. Treatment—surgical removal of the affected lens and prescription of eyeglasses.
  3. Nursing care
    a. Preoperative care—ophthalmic ointments and eye drops.
    b. Postoperative care—no stress on sutures by coughing, sneezing or suddenly turning head. Physical activity depending on orders of surgeon.

c. Adjustment to cataract glasses which is frustrating and discouraging.

E. Glaucoma—a condition in which increased intraocular pressure produces varying degrees of visual impairment.

1. Cause is an obstruction to the outflow of aqueous humor in the anterior chamber of the eye.
2. Symptoms: in an acute attack, the patient has severe headache or pain in affected eye, nausea and vomiting. Chronic glaucoma is characterized by vision that is blurred or hazy and then clears up after a while, trouble adjusting to dark, narrowing of vision and seeing halos around objects and lights.
3. Treatment with myotics and drugs that decrease production of aqueous humor may help; otherwise, removal of a section of the iris (iridectomy) may be necessary.

F. Detached retina—separation of the retina from the vascular wall of the eye.

1. Possible causes are sudden blow or penetrating injury, diabetic changes in the retina, myopia.
2. Symptoms: patient sees flashes of light and spots or moving particles and has cloudy vision or loss of central vision.
3. Treatment and nursing care— only treatment is surgical repair of tears or holes in retina, removing accumulated fluid and securing the retina in its normal position. Physical activity determined by directions of surgeon.

V. Nursing Care of the Patient Having Eye Surgery

A. Preoperative period: orient patient to his surroundings, explain procedures, watch for allergies or respiratory infection and cleanse intestinal tract. Ophthalmic drops or ointments exactly as ordered.

B. Postoperative period:

1. Position patient according to specific orders of surgeon, keep patient quiet and undisturbed and limit patient's activity.
2. Sudden pain in eye may indicate hemorrhage in operative area.
3. Instruct patient to avoid sudden, violent movements of the head.

VI. General Principles in the Care of the Blind

A. Emotional impact of blindness can be quite severe. Patient must be allowed to express his fears and gradually to adjust to his new way of life.

B. Special rules in helping blind person:

1. Do not shout.
2. Always speak as you enter his room, and notify him when you are leaving.
3. Blind persons want to be treated as normal persons, not pitied.
4. Remember that whatever independence a blind person has acquired is the result of hard work and determination.

Part Two   Disorders of the Ears

I. Introduction

A. One with hearing difficulties tends to withdraw and live in a world of his own owing to difficulty in communicating with others.

B. Loss of hearing can be due to a nerve defect (sensorineural) or to a barrier to the conduction of sound waves through the ear.

II. Special Diagnostic Tests and Examinations

A. Tuning fork tests:

1. Weber test compares hearing acumen in each ear.
2. Rinne test determines whether hearing loss is sensorineural or conductive.

B. Audiometry—audiometer measures sound perception.

III. Infections of the Ear

A. Otitis media, or tympanitis, is an inflammation of the middle ear; often a result of acute infection of the throat or sinuses.

1. Symptoms are pain, fever and drainage from ear.
2. Treatment includes rest, analgesics and antibiotics and possibly myringotomy (incision and drainage).

B. Mastoiditis is inflammation of the mastoid bone. Infection is usually streptococcal.

1. Symptoms are earache with tenderness in the area of the mastoid bone, fever and congestion of ear drum.
2. Treatment involves myringotomy and antibiotics and possibly mastoidectomy (surgical removal of infected mastoid cells.).
3. Nursing care of the patient having a mastoidectomy:
   a. Preoperative care—wash hair and share area around ear. Become acquainted with children and make them feel secure after surgery.
   b. Postoperative care—prevent disturbance of drains or bandages, watch for bleeding, elevation of temperature or change in vital signs and give soft diet requiring little chewing.

IV. Disorders of the Inner Ear

A. Introduction. Inner ear is concerned with hearing and maintenance of equilibrium. Inaccessibility makes disorders difficult to treat.

B. Labyrinthitis—inflammation involving the labyrinths of the inner ear.
   1. Symptoms—loss of hearing in affected ear, dizziness, nausea, vomiting and nystagmus.
   2. Treatment—antibiotics, bed rest and drugs to control nausea. Possibly mastoidectomy for patients with chronic mastoiditis.

C. Meniere's syndrome—group of symptoms occurring as a result of increased fluid in labyrinthine spaces with swelling and congestion of mucous membranes of the cochlea.
   1. Symptoms—tinnitus, headache, poor coordination, loss of hearing and nausea and vomiting when head is moved.
   2. Treatment—bed rest, antiemetics, restruction of fluid intake and sometimes surgical destruction of eighth nerve.

D. Otosclerosis—a fixation of the stapes due to destruction of normal bone and the laying down of sclerotic bone cells.
   1. Peculiar type of hearing loss in which patient's own voice seems much louder than others'.

2. Treated surgically. Patient kept quiet after surgery and positioned so that operative ear is uppermost. Coughing, sneezing or sudden movements of head to be avoided.

V. Nursing Care of the Patient Having Surgery of the Ear

A. Preoperative care: shave operative area, clean ear and pin hair back securely.

B. Postoperative care: patient is usually kept flat in bed with head kept still. Put side rails on bed.
   1. Watch for signs of injury to facial nerve.
   2. Avoid postoperative infection; it could spread to brain or meninges.
   3. Patient should avoid sneezing, coughing or blowing his nose.

VI. General Principles in the Care of the Deaf

A. Deafness is total loss of hearing. Many people are "hard of hearing" but do have some sense of hearing.

B. Signs of hearing losss include listless or weary facial expression, inattention or inability to understand what is being said, voice or speech peculiarities, mispronunciation of words, continued failure in school and tendency to avoid others.

VII. The Nurse and the Deaf

A. Offer understanding and consideration, not pity.

B. Avoid shouting.

C. Face the person when you speak to him.

D. Keep questions to a minimum and phrase them so that more is required than yes or no answer.

E. Frequent visits to the patient while in the hospital will help him feel more secure and less isolated from others.

F. The hearing aid must be fitted properly and patient given adequate instruction in its use and care.

Part Three   Disorders of the Throat

I. Pharyngitis (Inflammation of the Throat)

A. Symptoms—dryness, irritation in back of throat, slight fever and malaise.

B. Treatment—hot saline gargles and aspirin, and antibiotics or sulfonamides for severe infection.

II. Tonsillitis

A. An inflammation of the tonsils, usually streptococcal or staphylococcal.

B. Symptoms—sore throat, fever, chills, general malaise. Chronic infection can lead to enlargement of tonsils and adenoids.

C. Treatment—acute: hot saline gargles, bed rest and antibiotics. Chronic tonsillitis with enlargement of adenoids may require tonsillectomy and adenoidectomy.

III. Nursing Care of Patient Having Tonsillectomy and Adenoidectomy

A. Preoperative—temperature checked.

B. Postoperative—vital signs checked frequently. Patient kept on his side or abdomen as long as there is drainage from the throat. Diet restricted to soft, nonirritating foods until throat is healed.

IV. Cancer of the Larynx

A. Most easily cured of all malignant diseases.

B. Predisposing factors—smoking, chronic laryngitis and abuse of vocal cords.

C. Symptoms—hoarseness at first. Later, pain in throat, difficulty in swallowing, lump in throat and pain in region of Adam's apple.

D. Treatment—partial or total laryngectomy.

1. Patient who has had partial laryngectomy retains function of speech.

2. Total laryngectomy patient has permanent opening in trachea and must learn new speech pattern.

23

Accident and Emergency Nursing, Disaster Nursing

PREVENTION OF ACCIDENTS

Home Safety

According to statistics compiled by the U.S. Department of Health, Education and Welfare, home accidents cause more than one fourth of all accidental deaths. The principal victims of accidental deaths occurring in the home are children under 5 years of age and elderly persons over 65. Since persons in these age groups spend a large percentage of their time in the house, it is imperative that safety hazards be removed from their environment if these accidental deaths are to be prevented.

Nurses, physicians and other persons concerned with the safety and welfare of others must take an active part in the education of the public in regard to home accidents and the ways in which they can be eliminated. The two most dangerous rooms in the house are the kitchen and the bathroom. Falls account for almost one half of the accidental injuries sustained in the home. Fig. 23-1 shows some of the most common hazards and how they can be avoided.

Highway Safety

Motor vehicle accidents are the leading cause of accidental death in the United States. The National Safety Council estimates that automobile accidents kill a person every 15 minutes and injure someone every 30 seconds. This means that every year there are over 38,000 Americans killed and over one million disabled by some type of injury sustained in a traffic accident.

The two major causes of motor vehicle accidents are human failure and mechanical failure. Of these two, human failure is by far the greater danger. Improper driving, which causes almost 90 percent of all accidents, may be due to drinking alcohol, taking drugs, lack of alertness and fatigue, excessive speed or emotional instability of the driver. Mechanical failure is often not detected as the cause of an accident; however, there has been much interest recently in the lack of built-in safety devices and inspection for safety hazards in new automobiles, and it is hoped that many instances of mechanical failure as the cause of accidents will soon be greatly reduced.

Water Safety

The advent of the 40-hour work week and extended vacations have provided more leisure time and more opportunity for Americans to enjoy water sports.

515

HOME SAFETY CHART

KITCHEN

For gas or coal stove, have vents or flues; keep windows open a crack

Never light stove with kerosene or gasoline

Turn off all flames after cooking

Repair any gas leakage

Use potholders, asbestos pads

Keep handles of pots and pans turned in

Keep knives, sharp instruments and poisons such as bleach out of children's reach

Wipe up spills on floor

Keep electric appliances in good working order

STORAGE AREAS

Always keep cellars, attics, garages neat

Throw out newspapers and oily rags at once: they can start fires

Clean and disinfect area where garbage is kept, and dispose of it frequently

Never place poisonous substances in drinking glasses, cold drink bottles or other containers that have been used for food or drink

Always label poisonous compounds; read labels of poisons you have purchased

LIVING ROOM

Be sure floors are not slippery

Replace frayed or torn carpets

Use rubber mats under rugs to prevent slipping

Cover electric sockets

Replace frayed electric cords

Keep electric cords off floor where people walk

Place heaters a safe distance from walls

Use screens around fireplace

Remove sharp edges from furniture

Check ashtrays for lit matches or cigarettes

FURNACE

Have it checked every year, especially for leaks in tank of oil-burning furnaces

Never light furnace with gasoline or kerosene

BATHROOM

Use rubber mat in tub

Keep soap in sturdy container

Store medicines out of children's reach

Keep all medicines capped and labeled

Throw out old medicines

Dispose of razor blades immediately after use

BEDROOMS

Do not smoke in bed

Use rubber mats under scatter rugs

STAIRWAYS

Cover with carpeting or rubber safety treads

Replace torn or frayed carpeting

Keep stairs cleared of toys and cleaning equipment

Install handrails, proper lighting

Use gates at top and bottom if there are young children

Figure 23–1.

With this increased participation in water-centered activities, there has been a proportionate increase in accidental deaths and injuries in or on the water. Many of these accidents could have been prevented if the simple rules of water safety had been observed. These rules include using good judgment about the choice of swimming area, proper supervision of children and adults who are not strong swimmers, diving only in areas where the water is sufficiently deep and is free of rocks or other obstacles and avoiding overexertion or swimming distances beyond one's ability. Above all, one should know how to handle an emergency should it arise. Panic and unthinking actions frequently cause the loss of life of the person in trouble as well as the would-be rescuer.

Rescue for a drowning person requires a cool head and deliberate action. First, the rescuer should call for help. If possible, he should try to reach the victim without going in water over his head. It is often possible to reach him by extending an arm, towel, rope or pole, or any long and sturdy object that is handly. When the victim has grasped the object, he can be pulled slowly to shore. If a boat is available, it should be used for rescue of the person who is beyond reach by other methods.

A swimming rescue is very difficult even for the most experienced swimmer, primarily because the victim is frightened and is abnormally strong in such a situation and is quite capable of drowning both himself and his rescuer. After the rescued person is brought out of the water, he must be given artificial respiration if he is not breathing. If he is breathing, he should be placed in a reclining position and covered with a blanket or coat. His head should be turned to one side so that if he vomits, he will not aspirate the vomitus into his lungs. If the person is conscious, he may be given plain water, tea or coffee to drink. He should not be given any alcoholic beverages. The ordeal of nearly drowning can place an added burden on the heart and circulatory system. For this reason, it is advisable to have the victim continue to lie down and rest even though he appears to be all right.

GENERAL PRINCIPLES OF FIRST AID

1. Try to keep calm and think before acting.

2. Concentrate on what should be done first and the manner in which to proceed step by step. Move slowly and deliberately so that you can gain time to think things through and at the same time instill confidence in those you are trying to help.

3. Identify yourself as a nurse. This will serve to reassure the victim and onlookers.

4. Summon help or have someone call the local police department or physician or ambulance if necessary.

5. Make a careful but quick examination and evaluation of the extent of injuries sustained by the victim or victims. Obviously the more serious condition such as stoppage of breathing or severe bleeding must have top priority in the order of treatment. The following list of actions shows their order of importance:

    a. Maintain a patent airway.

    b. Stop bleeding.

    c. Prevent or treat shock.

    d. Protect wounds with a dressing if a sterile or clean bandage is available.

    e. Keep the victim in a reclining position. If he is found in another position and damage to the spine is a possibility, do not attempt to force the person to lie straight.

    f. Keep the victim covered.

    g. Reassure the victim and make him as comfortable as possible.

    h. Observe the victim frequently and re-evaluate his condition at regular intervals until a physician or ambulance arrives.

CONTROL OF BLEEDING

The only emergency conditions that have priority over control of hemorrhage are cessation of breathing and a sucking wound of the chest. Severe bleeding can rapidly lead to irreversible shock resulting from reduced circulating blood volume and circulatory collapse.

Application of Pressure

Bleeding usually can be controlled by placing a sterile or clean cloth over the wound and applying firm, steady pressure with the palm of your hand.

Or the area may be wrapped snugly with a clean bandage over several layers of cloth placed over the wound. Do not wrap the area so tightly as to constrict circulation completely. This would, in effect, be the same as applying a tourniquet, a measure that is used only as a last resort (see the following section). The flow of blood to the wound can be decreased somewhat by elevating the injured part and immobilizing it in some way.

If the bleeding is copious and impossible to stop with a pressure bandage, the artery leading to the wounded area should be compressed. The six principal pressure points for control of arterial bleeding are pictured in Figure 23-2. These pressure points are extremely important because uncontrolled bleeding from an artery can be fatal in a very

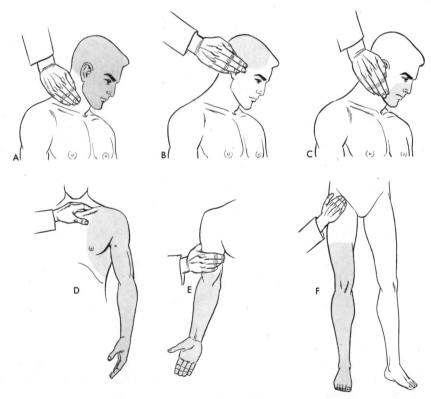

Figure 23–2. Location of the more commonly used digital pressure points. Shaded areas are those within which hemorrhage may be controlled by pressure on the specific artery. *A,* Carotid artery; *B,* temporal artery; *C,* external maxillary artery; *D,* subclavian artery; *E,* brachial artery; *F,* femoral artery. (From Crawford: Nursing Clinics of North America, June, 1967.)

short time. Blood issuing from an artery will be bright red in color and will gush forth in spurts at regular intervals; blood from a severed vein leaks slowly and steadily and is dark red in color.

Use of Tourniquets

Application of a tourniquet to prevent hemorrhage is recommended *only as a last resort* when other methods have failed and hemorrhage threatens the life of the victim or when an injured extremity has been amputated or severely crushed or mangled. The tourniquet has been used more often than it should have been, so if you are in doubt, do not apply one. The reason for this is obvious when we realize that a tourniquet can, by obstructing the flow of blood to a part, deprive its tissues of vital nutrients and permanently damage them, resulting in loss of the limb.

To apply a tourniquet, one needs several thicknesses of gauze or cloth to make a pad to be placed under the tourniquet, a wide strip of fabric long enough to go twice around the limb and a stick for tightening the tourniquet. Place the pad on the inside of the limb above the point of bleeding. Wrap the tourniquet around the limb over the pad and then tie the loose end with a half knot (overhand knot). Insert the stick and tie again with a full knot. The tourniquet is then tightened by twisting the stick until bleeding stops (see Fig. 23-3). Once the tourniquet has been applied, it should be released by a physician. Always leave the tourniquet uncovered so that it can be seen by others who may not be aware it has been applied. If this is not possible, write a note to the effect that a tourniquet has been applied, giving the location and the time of application of the tourniquet.

SHOCK

The term shock is extremely difficult, if not impossible, to define precisely. It has become something of a

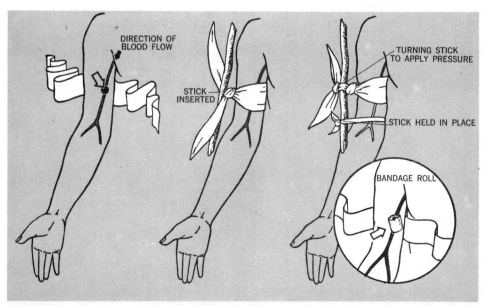

Figure 23–3. To apply a tourniquet for control of arterial bleeding of the arm: Wrap a gauze pad twice with a strip of cloth just below the armpit and tie with a half knot; tie a stick at the knot with a square knot. Slowly twist stick to tighten. Loosen tourniquet every ten minutes. (From *The Modern Medical Encyclopedia,* Western Publishing Company, Inc., New York.)

catchall word that is used to cover a multitude of clinical situations and a variety of symptoms. These situations may vary from simple fainting to total circulatory collapse and death. In emergency nursing, shock is usually *neurogenic* (caused by psychologic factors such as pain, fright or trauma) or *hematogenic* (caused by decreased blood volume, as in severe bleeding, or loss of plasma, as in burns). Shock also may be caused by a "heart attack" which greatly reduces cardiac output and results in collapse of the peripheral vascular system.

Symptoms

The symptoms indicative of shock are the result of complex pathologic and psychologic mechanisms. These involve inadequate blood volume, reduction of the cardiac output, loss of tone in and collapse of the blood vessels near the surface of the body, increased permeability of the capillaries with a shift of the body fluids from one compartment to another and alterations in the chemical characteristics of the blood.

Not all of the signs and symptoms of shock need be present in every patient; they can occur in varying combinations and in different degrees of severity, depending on the cause of shock and the patient's response to it. The classic symptoms and signs of shock include cold, moist skin, especially of the extremities; pallor, especially of the lips and fingers; and rapid and weak pulse, decreased blood pressure, listlessness, thirst and oliguria.

Management of Shock

Whenever possible in an emergency situation, the nurse must do what she can to prevent shock or at least to lessen its severity. She can do this by acting quickly to control bleeding, relieving pain through proper splinting or positioning and treating the wound. There are several defense mechanisms of the body which are automatically called into action as soon as injury occurs. By supporting these mechanisms through simple nursing measures, the nurse can reduce the severity of shock and diminish its effects upon an accident victim.

Since most emergency cases are accompanied by some degree of psychogenic shock, it is extremely important to reassure and comfort the victim. This will help to keep him calm and reduce physical tension and activity so that his energies can be fully utilized by the natural defense mechanisms of the body. Maintaining normal body heat helps to ensure adequate circulation. To do this, one must protect the patient from cold and dampness, but remember that applications of extreme heat to the surfaces of the body only serve to aggravate circulatory collapse and tend to increase loss of vital body fluids through perspiration. The "shock position" (with the head slightly lower than the feet) will improve circulation to the brain and heart. This position is contraindicated in head injuries.

As soon as the patient arrives at a hospital or clinic where equipment is available, other measures are taken to control shock. These may include administration of whole blood or plasma to restore the circulating blood volume, oxygen to relieve respiratory embarrassment and narcotics for the control of pain.

BURNS

The two hazards to be guarded against in the emergency treatment of burns are infection and shock. All burns must be considered potentially dangerous because the skin is one of the body's first lines of defense against the invasion of pathogenic organisms. It also plays an important role in the maintenance of fluid balance and body temperature. The destruction of relatively large areas of skin can cause loss of vital body fluids and electrolytes, produce profound changes in the blood vessels and alter the chemical activities of the cells and tissues of the internal organs.

The severity of complications of a burn will depend on the amount of body surface destroyed by the burn and the depth of the burn. The degrees of burn (first, second and third) and the means by which the extent of a burn are determined are discussed in Chapter 13 of this text.

Minor Burns

If the burned area is small and appears to be a first degree burn, the affected area should be immersed in cold water immediately. An alternative to this is applications of cold compresses, using ice cubes and a sterile gauze pad or clean cloth. By applying cold, it is possible to reduce somewhat the pain of the burn. A minor burn should be covered with sterile petroleum jelly or a paste of baking soda and water and then loosely bandaged.

Major Burns

The burned area should be covered with a clean, dry dressing. This can be a sheet, towel or other freshly laundered piece of linen. It should be made of tightly woven cotton so that air is kept from the wound and the possibility of infection is reduced. The victim should be transported to a hospital as soon as possible.

No attempt should be made to remove clothing from a burned area. Never apply absorbent cotton, oily substances or ointments to a major burn. Blisters should not be disturbed because they serve as a protective covering over the wound.

If there is an unavoidable delay in getting the patient to a hospital and he is conscious and able to swallow, he should be given fluids to drink. The ideal is a solution of a half teaspoonful each of salt and baking soda in one quart of water. The patient is encouraged to drink small amounts of the solution at 10 to 15 minute intervals unless nausea develops and vomiting seems likely. Intravenous fluid therapy and more extensive medical treatment of major burns are discussed in Chapter 13 of this text.

Chemical Burns

Strong chemicals capable of burning the skin and mucous membranes will continue to destroy tissue unless they are diluted and removed immediately. For this reason, one must act quickly to irrigate the area with large amounts of water until all traces of the chemical have been removed. Once this has been done, the burned area is covered with a dressing, and the patient is then transported to a hospital.

Chemical burns of the eye also require extensive irrigation followed by application of a clean dressing.

POISONING

The annual number of cases of poisoning in the United States is almost one half million. Of these, approximately two thousand are fatal, and a large majority are accidental. Prevention of accidental poisoning begins with a realization that there are literally hundreds of thousands of poisonous substances in our environment. Every home has a variety of poisons sitting on the shelves of the medicine cabinet, under the kitchen sink or in the laundry room, utility room and garage. Children are the most frequent victims of poisoning, and medicines account for one half of all accidental poisonings of children under the age of five years. Aspirin has consistently been the leading cause of death in accidental poisoning in children of this age. Other poisons frequently ingested by children include bleaches, soaps and detergents, insecticides and vitamin and iron preparations. Recently there has been an increase of poisoning in children who have ingested their mothers' birth control pills.

Prevention

As a member of the health team, the practical nurse must do all she can to educate the public in the ways in which accidental poisoning can be prevented. She should remember the simple rules given below and use every opportunity to teach them to her friends and neighbors.

1. Destroy all medicines that are no longer being used. An overdose can be fatal, especially to a child. In some instances, drugs undergo chemical changes with age and become toxic compounds.

2. Store poisons and inedible products separately from edible foods.

3. Do not transfer poisonous substances from their original container to an unmarked one. NEVER place a poison in a container (such as a soft drink bottle) that is normally used for edible solids or liquids.

4. Never tell a child that the medicine he is being given is candy. Tell him it is a drug to make him feel better and that is must be taken only as the doctor has directed.

5. Always read the labels of chemical products before using them.

Symptoms of Poisoning

The symptoms of poisoning vary according to the poison taken and the time that has elapsed since it first entered the body. Poisoning should be suspected if the victim becomes ill very suddenly and there is nearby an open container of a poison or a drug. In children, one should be alert to the possibility of poisoning when there is a peculiar odor to the breath or when there is evidence that the child has eaten leaves or wild berries. Always remember that children are naturally very curious and that a substance need not taste good for a child to place it in his mouth and swallow it.

Other symptoms of poisoning include pain or burning sensation in the mouth and throat, nausea, vomiting, disorientation, visual disturbances, loss of consciousness or a deep unnatural sleep.

General Principles of First Aid for Poisoning

All cases of poisoning demand immediate action. The longer the delay in treatment, the greater the chance of the poison being absorbed in the body and permanently damaging body tissues.

Always save the container and any of its contents that may help in identification of the poison. If the container cannot be found and the type of poison is not known, try to save a sample of vomitus for analysis and identification.

Swallowed Poisons. Generally, the first step is *dilution* of the poison, immediately followed by *removal* of the stomach contents. In the absence of a stomach pump, one must induce vomiting. A liquid such as water or milk will serve to dilute the poison. (Exceptions to this rule are listed below.) Vomiting is induced by placing a spoon or an index finger down the back of the throat to stimulate the gag reflex. An emetic such as 2 tablespoons of salt in a glass of warm water can be used. Be sure that during the vomiting episode, the victim is positioned so that the vomitus will not be aspirated into the lungs and cause damage there.

Antidotes to specific poisons are often printed on the label. The specific antidote should be administered as soon as the stomach has been emptied of the poison. If the poison cannot be identified, activated charcoal is recommended as an antidote because of its absorbent properties.

When a patient has swallowed a *corrosive poison*—for example, a strong acid or alkali—vomiting is contraindicated because there is the danger of further irritating and damaging the upper intestinal tract. There is also the possibility of aspiration of the corrosive substance into the respiratory tract during vomiting. Antidotes for corrosive compounds are as follows: for *strong acids,* use milk, water or milk of magnesia (1 to 2 cups for children, up to 1 quart for adults). For *strong alkalies,* use milk, water, any fruit juice or vinegar (1 to 2 cups for children, up to 1 quart for patients five years or older).

Other cases in which *vomiting should not be induced* include when the victim is in a coma or unconscious, is having a convulsion or has swallowed petroleum products, such as gasoline, kerosene, lighter fluid and some furniture polishes.

Inhaled Poisons. Transport the patient to fresh air immediately: do not let him walk. Loosen tight clothing. Apply artificial respiration as needed. Keep the patient warm and quiet. Do not give alcohol or any stimulant.

Barbiturate Poisoning. The barbiturate drugs are those most frequently used in suicide attempts. Approximately 50,000 cases of barbiturate poisoning are hospitalized every year in the United States. Symptoms include depression of respirations and reflexes, stupor or coma, dilated pupils and flushed face. The patient may be able to respond to questions, but his answers will be very slow. Without adequate treatment, the patient succumbs to respiratory failure and cerebral edema. Pneumonia is a common sequel to barbiturate poisoning that has not proved fatal.

Emergency treatment must be instituted quickly if the patient's life is to be saved. The drug should be removed from the stomach by inducing vomiting or using a stomach pump. Artificial respiration is administered if breathing has ceased or is irregular and shallow. In the hospital, drugs that stimulate circulation are given, and efforts are made to maintain a normal fluid and electrolyte balance. To counteract the depressing effect of barbiturates on the central nervous system, analeptic drugs (stimulants or restoratives) are given. Drugs of this type include picrotoxin,

strychnine and bemegride. If the barbiturate is a long-acting type, an artificial kidney may be used to remove the drug from the blood stream.

There is often a delayed reaction to barbiturate poisoning, and the patient must be watched closely for several days after ingestion for signs of depression of the central nervous system.

Poisoning by Morphine, Bromides and Other Sedatives. The patient who has taken or been given an overdose of a sedative drug will suffer from severe depression of the central nervous system, with resultant depression of respiration, involuntary reflexes and some voluntary actions. The symptoms are similar to those listed previously for barbiturate poisoning. Emergency measures include administration of strong coffee or tea to provide a stimulant (caffeine) and attempts to keep the patient awake; he should not, however, be forced to walk, as this will only tire him and deplete his energies. If the patient is unconscious, it will be necessary to keep the air passages open and artificial respiration should be administered if respiration has ceased.

Hospital treatment of narcotic poisoning includes administration of oxygen, use of a respirator as needed, frequent suctioning and administration of available specific antidotes. In recent years naloxone (Narcan) has been used as a narcotic antagonist that counteracts the depressant effects of morphine, codeine and other opiates. The drug shows promise as a means of reversing the depression of respiration, and some authorities suggest that it may be an effective means of treating some forms of drug addiction. It is used with caution, however, when drug overdose and respiratory depression are suspected in a narcotic addict, because naloxone quickly precipitates withdrawal symptoms in one who has been taking opiates over an extended period of time.

A tracheostomy is sometimes required when depression is severe. The patient's vital signs must be noted at frequent intervals and any changes reported to the physician in charge. To facilitate drainage of bronchial secretions, the patient is positioned so that the head is slightly lower than the feet. He must be turned frequently to prevent the development of pneumonia, which is always a hazard in cases of this type.

Poisoning by Carbon Monoxide and Other Lethal Gases. The inhalation of poisonous gases brings about an emergency situation in which death can occur in a matter of minutes. Carbon monoxide unites readily with hemoglobin, thereby replacing vital oxygen in the blood stream and rapidly producing a depletion of oxygen supply to body tissues. The first tissues to be affected are those of the nervous system, which cannot survive more than a few minutes once their supply of oxygen is gone. The patient first becomes drowsy, has a headache and experiences visual disturbances; he then sinks rapidly into a coma. The skin is a bright cherry red in color, owing to the presence of the carbon monoxide in the blood.

As soon as the victim of an inhaled poison is found, he must be carried to a source of fresh air, such as an open window or door, or outside and away from polluted air. The rescuer must be careful that he, too, is not overcome by inhaling the poisonous gas. Artificial respiration is begun immediately if the victim is not breathing. He should be kept warm and quiet and must not be allowed to walk about.

Hospital treatment includes administration of oxygen and supportive measures to prevent shock and maintain normal respiration. The patient must be observed carefully for signs of central nervous system damage and heart failure. Although he may appear to have recovered once oxygen has been administered, there can be residual effects of the poisoning that may be fatal.

Food Poisoning. This type of poisoning is produced by the toxins of bacteria present in contaminated food. The term "ptomaine poisoning," so frequently associated with food poisoning, is actually a misnomer. Ptomaines are substances formed by the decomposition or "spoilage" of protein foods. The digestive system is able to cope with these substances, and they do not necessarily cause illness. Decomposing food is not of itself necessarily harmful, but since foods in the process of decomposition frequently harbor pathogenic organisms and serve as excellent media for their growth, they should be avoided.

PREVENTION. Cleanliness, good personal hygiene and proper preparation and handling of foods are essential to the prevention of food poisoning. Fig. 23-4 presents the basic rules of prevention.

SYMPTOMS AND TREATMENT. Food poisoning should be suspected when more than one person in a group, family or community is affected by an acute febrile gastrointestinal disturbance. The onset is sudden, with nausea, vomiting, diarrhea and abdominal cramps. Emergency treatment generally consists of lavage or the induction of vomiting (if not already present) to remove the poisonous food from the stomach. Food is withheld, drugs are administered to control the diarrhea if it is present, and sedation and parenteral fluids are administered. If diarrhea is not a symptom, a saline cathartic may be given to remove the bacteria from the lower intestinal tract.

TYPES. Food poisoning may be bacterial or chemical; however, the chemical types are not true food poisonings but a toxic condition caused by poisonous mushrooms, toxic berries or foods that have not been cleansed of insecticides or other chemicals.

Botulism is the most dangerous type of food poisoning; about 65 percent of

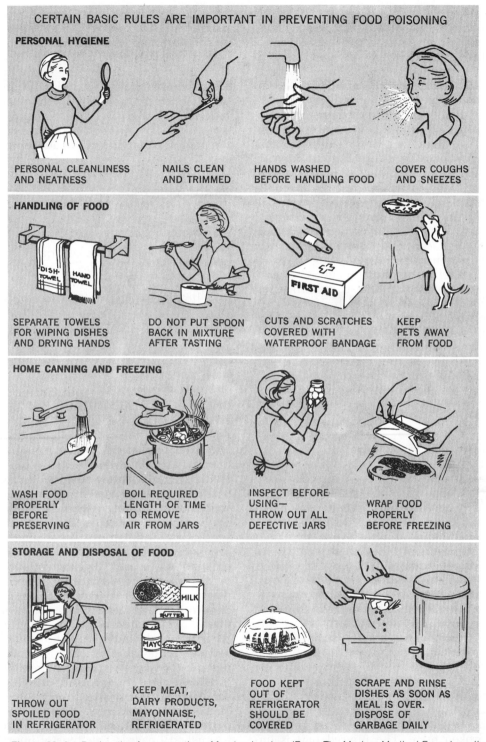

CERTAIN BASIC RULES ARE IMPORTANT IN PREVENTING FOOD POISONING

PERSONAL HYGIENE

PERSONAL CLEANLINESS AND NEATNESS

NAILS CLEAN AND TRIMMED

HANDS WASHED BEFORE HANDLING FOOD

COVER COUGHS AND SNEEZES

HANDLING OF FOOD

SEPARATE TOWELS FOR WIPING DISHES AND DRYING HANDS

DO NOT PUT SPOON BACK IN MIXTURE AFTER TASTING

CUTS AND SCRATCHES COVERED WITH WATERPROOF BANDAGE

KEEP PETS AWAY FROM FOOD

HOME CANNING AND FREEZING

WASH FOOD PROPERLY BEFORE PRESERVING

BOIL REQUIRED LENGTH OF TIME TO REMOVE AIR FROM JARS

INSPECT BEFORE USING— THROW OUT ALL DEFECTIVE JARS

WRAP FOOD PROPERLY BEFORE FREEZING

STORAGE AND DISPOSAL OF FOOD

THROW OUT SPOILED FOOD IN REFRIGERATOR

KEEP MEAT, DAIRY PRODUCTS, MAYONNAISE, REFRIGERATED

FOOD KEPT OUT OF REFRIGERATOR SHOULD BE COVERED

SCRAPE AND RINSE DISHES AS SOON AS MEAL IS OVER. DISPOSE OF GARBAGE DAILY

Figure 23–4. Basic rules for prevention of food poisoning. (From *The Modern Medical Encyclopedia*, Western Publishing Company, Inc., New York.)

the cases are fatal. It is caused by *Clostridium botulinum,* which most often grows in foods that have not been properly canned at home. A neurotoxin produced by the organism affects muscular coordination and causes an inability to swallow, talk or breathe. Early recognition and emergency treatment are necessary to prevent death. The patient is given an antitoxin that neutralizes the neurotoxin. Supportive measures include use of a respirator to facilitate breathing and intravenous fluids to maintain normal fluid and electrolyte balance.

A strain of staphylococcus known as *Staphylococcus aureus* frequently grows in creamed foods that have not been refrigerated adequately. Custards, cream pies, mayonnaise and processed foods of the type used for picnics are often the source of this type of food poisoning. The illness is rarely fatal, and symptoms are usually limited to nausea, vomiting, diarrhea and abdominal cramps. The patient should be kept quiet and given sedation and parenteral fluids as necessary.

FRACTURES

A fracture is a break in the continuity of a bone. The types of fracture and their specific treatments are discussed in Chapter 14 of this text.

Symptoms of a fracture include pain and swelling in the area, deformity and limited motion. One should always treat a suspected fracture as a real one, since proper first aid measures will be beneficial whether or not a true fracture is present.

Emergency treatment is aimed at immobilization of the affected part so that soft tissues in the areas adjacent to the bone will not be damaged further. The term "splint it as it lies" means exactly that. An inexperienced person should never attempt to straighten or set a broken bone. The injured part is immobilized in the position in which it is found at the time of injury and is supported firmly so that it will not be jarred when the victim is being moved to the hospital or doctor's office.

If the broken bone has pierced the skin and bleeding is severe, apply direct pressure over the wound (see Control of Bleeding, p. 518). Try to avoid introducing infectious agents into the wound, and remember also the need for the prevention and treatment of shock.

HEAD INJURY

The victim of a blow to the head may suffer a skull fracture or concussion. In either case, he should be kept quiet and no stimulants should be given. Since there can be a delayed reaction in injury to the brain, all head injuries should be considered serious and should have the attention of a physician. The symptoms, treatment and nursing care of head injuries are discussed in Chapter 21.

CHEST AND ABDOMINAL WOUNDS

Victims of automobile accidents frequently suffer from severe chest wounds as a result of violent contact with the steering wheel and column. Victims of stabbing can also have open chest wounds which create serious respiratory difficulties. An open or "sucking" chest wound is one in which pneumothorax results from penetration of the pleural cavity. This type of wound should be covered with an occlusive dressing, that is, one made of plastic wrap, aluminum foil or any other material which seals the wound and prohibits the flow of air into the pleural cavity. The occlusive dressing is held in place by a pressure dressing.

A "flail" chest results from fracture of three or more ribs, each in two places, so that a portion of the rib cage is crushed inward. This type of injury produces "paradoxical respirations," which means that upon inhalation, the affected portion moves inward rather than outward. The condition is treated by splinting the affected portion of the chest using a small pillow, folded sheet or other bulky material and taping it securely in place. The victim is given oxygen to help compensate for respiratory deficiency.

Impaled objects, whether protruding from the chest, the eye, the abdomen or any other part of the body, should never be removed at the scene of the accident if at all possible. The protruding object should be left in place until specifically ordered removed by a physician who is in attendance. First aid measures include stabilizing the object as much as possible to avoid its being moved around in the wound, controlling bleeding and applying a dressing over the wound and around the object.

Abdominal injuries resulting from improperly worn seat belts, penetrating objects, blunt instruments and sharp cutting edges are all potential sources of damage to internal organs and hemorrhage. If internal hemorrhage is suspected, the victim should be observed closely for symptoms of shock and handled very gently when being moved. Lacerations which cause evisceration or spilling of the abdominal contents are treated with warm, moist dressings which help preserve the viability of the intestines. No attempt should be made to replace the organs through the open wound. Medical treatment should be obtained as quickly as possible and the dressings kept moist until such treatment is available. [4]

ELECTRIC SHOCK

When an electric current passes through the body, it can cause severe shock to the entire body, cessation of breathing, circulatory failure and serious burns.

Emergency treatment involves artificial respiration if breathing has ceased, general measures to treat shock

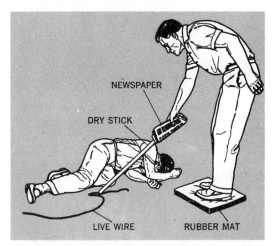

Figure 23–5. To separate a victim from live electric wire without suffering similar shock, stand on rubber mat or dry board in rubber-soled shoes. Move wire with dry stick held with dry paper or dry gloves. Don't touch until sure wire contact is broken. (From *The Modern Medical Encyclopedia*, Western Publishing Company, Inc., New York.)

and emergency treatment of a major burn when one is present. The proper procedure for separating a victim from a live conductor of electricity is described in Figure 23-5. Remember that water serves as a conductor of electricity and wet objects can transmit a fatal electric current to a person trying to rescue the victim of electric shock.

A person who is struck by lightning suffers from electric shock.

EMERGENCY CHILDBIRTH

It is often assumed that practical nurses should be able to assist a mother and infant in an emergency delivery outside the hospital environment. Such an assumption can be foolish if the nurse has not yet studied obstetrical nursing or has been allowed only to observe but never participate in the delivery of an infant in the hospital. The simple steps given here are presented only as emergency first aid measures to be undertaken when a physician or more experienced person is not available.

1. Place the mother on her back in a comfortable position.

2. Keep the vaginal area as clean and free from contamination as possible.

3. Do not attempt to pull or push the infant through the birth canal.

4. Wipe the infant's nose and mouth with a clean cloth to remove mucus from his air passages.

5. Leave the infant between the mother's knees and cover him with a blanket or clean cloth.

6. The cord does not require attention unless a physician cannot be available within an hour. After that length of time, the cord should be cut if the placenta (afterbirth) has been expelled. Tie the cord securely about two inches from the navel and again at about six inches. Cut the cord between the two places, using a knife or scissors that has been sterilized by boiling or soaking in a disinfectant.

7. Save the placenta for the physician's inspection.

8. If there is no medical help available after the placenta is expelled, gently massage the fundus of the uterus to stimulate contraction and reduce bleeding. The fundus can be felt as a fairly large lump in the mother's abdomen just below her navel.

ANIMAL BITES

Family pets, especially dogs and cats, are the most common source of animal bites. When a wild animal such as a squirrel or fox attacks and bites a human being without provocation, one should always suspect rabies as the cause of the animal's unusual behavior. All animal and human bites should be treated as potentially dangerous because of the presence of pathogenic microorganisms in the mouth, which can cause a serious infection.

Treatment

The wound should be washed immediately with soap and hot running water for 5 to 10 minutes. It is then covered with a clean bandage and a physician is consulted. If medical help is not readily available, it is best to make the wound bleed, probing it with a sharp, sterile instrument if necessary. Later the physician may decide to give tetanus toxin or toxoid to provide adequate immunity.

The possibility of rabies must always be considered in an animal bite. The animal must be confined and observed for signs of the disease. If he has been killed, his head should be sent to a laboratory for examination. If a diagnosis of rabies in the animal has been confirmed or if there is no proof that the animal has been immunized against rabies, the victim is given passive immunization through a series of injections known as the Pasteur treatment. This treatment has serious complications and can be fatal, but since rabies itself is always fatal, the Pasteur treatment is recommended by most authorities.

SNAKE BITE

Although bites from poisonous snakes are rare in the United States, one should be able to differentiate between venomous and nonvenomous bites and should initiate treatment immediately when a snake bite does occur. The poisonous snakes in the United States are the pit vipers (copperheads, rattlesnakes and cottonmouths or water moccasins) and the coral snake, a brightly colored snake found in the southern regions of this country.

A venomous snake bite is distinguished by two fang marks, the immediate sensation of pain in the area and swelling and discoloration at the site of injection of venom. Nonpoisonous snake bites appear as small scratches or lacerations.

Treatment

Nonpoisonous snake bites are treated as simple wounds and require washing with soap and water and the application of a mild antiseptic. Venomous snake bites, which can be fatal, demand immediate and vigorous treatment. The formula TISA is used to designate the steps of treatment; i.e., *tourniquet, incision, suction* and *antivenin.* Since bodily activity increases circulation and subsequent distribution of the venom throughout the body, the victim must be kept quiet and given no stimulants.

Tourniquet. The tourniquet (see the preceding discussion for details) is applied between the fang marks and the trunk of the body. It should be moderately tight so as to impede venous flow but not to stop arterial flow of blood. It must be loosened every ten minutes for one full minute and is left in place until a physician has administered antivenin or given further treatment.

Incision. A cut about 1/4 inch deep and 1/4 inch long is made directly over each fang mark.

Suction. Removal of the venom from the site of injection can be done by applying a suction cup from a snake bite kit or with the mouth. The latter is quite safe if there are no open sores or cuts on the lips or mouth through which the venom can enter the blood stream.

Antivenin. This is an immunizing agent made of horse serum, and as such, is capable of causing a serious allergic reaction in hypersensitive persons. For this reason, the antivenin should be administered only by a physician under conditions in which the allergic reaction can be controlled.

INSECT BITES OR STINGS

Insect attacks, especially multiple stings from bees or wasps, can be quite serious or even fatal in small children or in persons who are highly allergic to the venom. If signs of anaphylactic shock—extreme swelling, respiratory difficulty or loss of consciousness—develop, the patient must receive medical treatment immediately. Whenever a person has a systemic reaction to an insect sting, time is a crucial factor in whether he suffers severe or even fatal symptoms. A specially prepared emergency kit for treatment of venomous stings should be readily available to all persons known to have had a previous reaction, and a kit should also be a part of emergency equipment in all first aid stations. A kit of this type may contain a syringe of aqueous epinephrine, but since the medication can lose its potency over a period of time, it should be checked periodically for brownish discoloration and replaced as needed.

A kit that should be available to persons known to be hypersensitive usually contains an epinephrine inhaler rather than aqueous solution. It also contains Isuprel in 10 mg. tablets, a tourniquet, tweezers and antiseptic towelettes. The individual is instructed to dissolve one Isuprel tablet under his tongue and to repeat in 5 to 10 minutes if needed. The inhaler is used if the Isuprel does not relieve symptoms or if dyspnea develops. The tourniquet is applied loosely enough to allow for feeling a pulse in the wrist or ankle when applied to an extremity. The tweezers are used to remove the stinger *without* squeezing the venom sac. The sting is then wiped with an antiseptic towelette and a cold pack applied. Further medical attention should be obtained.

Less serious stings of bees, wasps, yellow jackets and hornets are treated by application of a paste of baking soda and water and cold compresses. Meat tenderizer has also been found effective in relieving the symptoms of minor insect sting reactions.

Bites from venomous spiders, scorpions and other poisonous insects are treated in the same manner as poisonous snake bites.

A tick, which can carry diseases such as Rocky Mountain spotted fever, is removed by placing a drop of turpentine or mineral oil on its body, and removing it with tweezers once its head has been withdrawn from the skin. If the tick is removed too quickly, its mouthpiece will be left in the skin and will serve as a source of irritation and infection. After the tick is removed, wash the area with soap and water and apply a mild disinfectant. If there is some question as to whether or not the tick may be carrying an infectious disease in a particular area of the country, a physician should be consulted.

INJURIES DUE TO EXTREME HEAT

Heatstroke

This rare condition, also called sunstroke, is the result of a serious disturbance of the heat-regulating center in the brain. Normally the body will respond to higher environmental temperatures by increased perspiration and other internal mechanisms which keep the body temperature within normal limits. In heat stroke, these mechanisms fail to function properly, and the patient's temperature rises, the skin becomes dry and hot, and there may be convulsions and collapse. Since the body temperature may go as high as 108 to 110° F. (42°C.), the patient is likely to die if his condition is not treated.

He should be placed in a shady, cool place and cooled immediately by sprinkling with water and fanning. As soon as possible, he should be immersed in cold water or have ice packs applied to lower his temperature. Care must be taken that his temperature is not lowered too quickly. The extremities are massaged so that adequate circulation is maintained.

The person with this disorder of the heat-regulating center may experience heatstroke any time he is exposed to extremely high temperature, and he may need to adjust his life so that he can avoid repeated episodes of heatstroke.

Heat Exhaustion (Heat Prostration)

This condition is caused by excessive sweating, which removes large quantities of salt and water from the body. The patient appears to be in shock with cool, damp skin, pallor, increased pulse and heart beat, dizziness or stupor. There may also be muscle cramps and poor coordination. Treatment is aimed at replacing the essential salts and fluids. He should be placed in a cool place and kept quiet. As much salt and water or tomato juice (one teaspoon of salt to a glass of liquid) as he can drink is administered. If he is unable to swallow the salt solution, replacement fluids are administered intravenously. Muscular cramps may be relieved by gently massaging the affected muscles.

Sunburn

Immediate treatment of a minor sunburn involves cool compresses using a solution of magnesium sulfate (Epsom salts) or sodium bicarbonate (baking soda) to relieve the discomfort. If chills, fever, swelling or gastrointestinal disturbances occur, the patient should receive medical attention.

INJURIES DUE TO EXTREME COLD

Prolonged exposure to cold can bring about a serious lowering of the body temperature *(hypothermia)* or a localized injury to tissues that is known as *frostbite.*

In hypothermia, the victim has suffered from a generalized reaction to the cold. The emergency treatment is aimed at returning the body temperature to normal limits as soon as possible. It is now believed that gradual rewarming is not necessary and may be more harmful than rapid rewarming. The patient is placed in a warm bath and then wrapped in warm blankets. Do not apply hot water bottles or electric heating pads directly to the skin. The use of hypothermia in certain surgical procedures is discussed in Chapter 6.

Frostbite produces a constriction of blood vessels, damages the vessel walls and tissue cells and leads to the formation of blood clots (thrombosis). It occurs most often on the fingers, toes, cheeks and nose, where exposure is usually greatest and blood supply is most easily restricted by cold. Symptoms include numbness and pallor in the area, a prickling sensation and eventually edema as fluid escapes from damaged vessel walls.

The affected area should be warmed by immersion for about ten minutes in water heated to a temperature of between 90 and 100° F. Handle the part gently and *never* rub or massage the area. The practice of rubbing with ice or snow is dangerous and completely ineffectual. Rubbing the area can cause further damage to the tissues. Wrap the area in sterile or clean bandages, being sure to separate skin surfaces, as between the fingers. Give the patient hot coffee or tea to drink. Hospital treatment may include surgical debridement of dead tissue and skin grafting if the deeper tissues are destroyed by gangrene due to inadequate circulation.

THE UNRULY PATIENT

The use of tranquilizing drugs has greatly reduced the occurrence of violent behavior in persons who are temporarily unable to control their emotions. This reduction does not mean, however, that psychiatric emergencies no longer occur or that the nurse will never need to know how to handle such

a patient. When a person becomes greatly agitated and experiences an uncontrollable urge to do violence to others, he is extremely frightened and usually welcomes help in regaining control if it is offered in the correct way.

It is recommended that success in dealing with an unruly patient is more likely to occur if help is offered on a one-to-one basis. Several persons trying to talk to him or subdue him may only add to his fright and disorientation. If, however, physical restraint becomes necessary, one should be sure that enough persons are at hand to control the patient.

When the nurse is talking to a person who is unruly, it is best that she use his name frequently, tell him who she is and what she is trying to do and express genuine concern about his feelings and the situation he is in. It may be necessary to help the patient by exerting some outside controls. These may be verbal or physical, but physical force should be used only after it is apparent that talking with him is not going to calm him. One may simply tell him to stop screaming or to sit down or to put down an object that he apparently intends to use as a weapon. If verbal control does not work, it may be necessary to restrain the patient who is overwrought. If restraints are used, the patient should not be left alone immediately after he has been restrained, since this action will give him the impression that he is being punished for wrongdoing rather than aided to control himself.

It is strongly suggested that any nurse who works regularly in an emergency room, psychiatric unit or other setting where she will have occasion to deal with violent patients obtain additional information and training in handling such situations. Lack of knowledge and experience in emergency psychiatric situations can be detrimental to the patient as well as to those who are trying to help him.

THE HOSPITAL EMERGENCY ROOM

In recent years, the hospital emergency room has become a combination doctor's office, outpatient clinic and facility for treatment of minor as well as major emergencies. Surveys show that there are an increasing number of patients going to emergency clinics with ailments that should be treated by a family doctor. There are various reasons for this trend, but the most common factor seems to be the certainty of medical help in an emergency room regardless of the hour of day or night.

This additional burden of nonemergency cases somewhat changes the roles of the various members of the emergency room staff. Since the main purpose of nursing is to help meet the needs of those who require medical attention, the nurse is in no position to be critical of those who come to the emergency room seeking such help. She must be able to screen patients rapidly, use good judgment in discerning their individual needs and handle each case with tact and diplomacy. When a true emergency arises, she must work quickly and effectively, remembering the basic principles and techniques she has learned in her classes. In some instances, the nurse may be expected to go beyond the limits of the traditional functions of a nurse in order to save a life. Certainly, therefore, the emergency room nurse must be a mature, thinking person, able to cope with a tremendous variety of situations.

The general procedures and policies in regard to keeping records, obtaining diagnostic x-rays and laboratory examinations and carrying out the final disposition of the patient will vary in each institution. The nurse must familiarize herself with these policies and procedures as soon as she is assigned to the emergency unit and certainly *before* attempting to assist in the care of an emergency in which time is precious and a few minutes can mean the difference between life and death. In addition to this orientation to policies, the nurse must know the location of each item of emergency equipment and exactly what her duties will be in operating such equipment. She should become familiar with the drugs most commonly used in emergency situations, and she must know where these drugs are stored, how they are administered and by whom. She should learn her responsibilities in assisting with various emergency procedures such as tracheostomy, thoracotomy, transfusions and suturing of wounds. And, above all else, she must maintain a calm, dignified attitude, deal with her distressed patients tactfully and, at the same time, work quickly and efficiently.

Conduct of the staff in the emergency unit is one of the most important and perhaps least understood aspects of emergency care. The patient and his family may be experiencing one or more of a variety of emotions—anger, guilt, anxiety, fright or depression— and cannot be expected to be in complete control of their emotions. The personnel in an emergency unit are, in effect, "living in a fish bowl." Their every movement, facial expression and attitude become magnified and are under close scrutiny by persons in a highly sensitive state of mind and mood. These distraught persons need moral support and reassurance that everything possible is being done for the injured person in the quickest and most efficient way possible. Relatives and friends of injured persons sometimes spend what seems to them endless hours sitting in corridors and waiting rooms. So do the non-emergency patients who are waiting to see a doctor. They naturally become resentful and upset if they observe emergency clinic personnel indulging in social conversation, reading or drinking coffee together in apparent oblivion of the distress of those around them. These practices, are, unfortunately, not uncommon, and each member of the

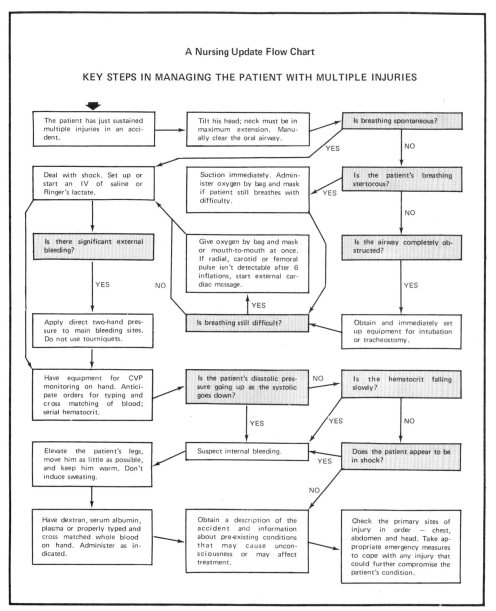

Figure 23–6. From Nursing Update, May, 1971.

staff should be aware of the need for professional conduct in the emergency room. The nurse must be careful of her choice of words and the tone of her voice when answering questions, and she must always try to convey the impression that she is indeed interested in each patient as a person and sincerely concerned about his welfare.

DISASTER NURSING

Introduction

A disaster may be defined as any catastrophe in which numbers of persons are plunged into helplessness and suffering. Natural disasters include epidemics, earthquakes, explosions, hurricanes, tornadoes, fires, floods and transportation accidents. War-caused disasters result from enemy attacks with chemical, biological, nuclear, psychological and conventional weapons.

Whether the disaster is a natural one or war-caused, it will involve physical injuries, loss of property and interruption of the normal activities of daily living. The victims often will be in need of food, clothing, shelter, medical and nursing or hospital care and other basic necessities of daily life. Nurses have traditionally accepted the responsibility for helping in times of disaster, and the practical nurse must realize that she has a definite role in helping to relieve the suffering inflicted by such tragedies. She should actively participate in community planning and civil defense programs so that in time of disaster she will be prepared to function effectively as a member of the health team.

Disaster Agencies

The governmental agencies in disaster planning on a national, state and local level are the Office of Civil Defense and the U.S. Public Health Ser-vice. The voluntary organization that traditionally provides nursing care and the basic essentials of shelter and food during a natural disaster is the American Red Cross. In most communities, the local civil defense agency and the Red Cross work together to formulate disaster plans so that their services are coordinated with each other and with other planning agencies for other essential services such as transportation, communication and welfare.

Special courses in civil defense and disaster nursing are usually offered by the Office of Civil Defense, Red Cross and professional organizations. These courses help the nurses and volunteer workers in the community understand the function of each agency in a particular type of disaster and serve to coordinate the planning for each kind of emergency nursing.

Responsibilities of the Nurse

In the following list are the responsibilities of nurses in regard to disaster planning and citizen and health care in a disaster. These are presented in a booklet published under the direction of the U.S. Department of Health, Education and Welfare Public Health Service.

All nurses should:

1. Be prepared for self-survival and for performing emergency nursing measures.
2. Know the community disaster plans and organized community health resources.
3. Know the meaning of warning signals and the action to be taken.
4. Know measures for protection from radioactive fallout.
5. Know measures for prevention and control of environmental health hazards.
6. Be prepared to interpret health laws and regulations.
7. Know and interpret community resources for citizen preparedness, such as first aid, and medical self-help courses.

The practical nurse will find that in many types of disaster, she may need to improvise because of lack of equipment. She must always bear in mind the basic principles of nursing that she has been taught and has practiced in the hospital environment. If there is a great disparity between need and availability of medical and nursing personnel, she may be called upon to exercise leadership and discerning judgment in determining the condition of each victim, use of supplies and equipment and detection of changes in the environment that might be hazardous to health.

Functions of the Nurse

Some of the functions of the licensed practical nurse are listed below. These functions are comparable to the ANA-NFLPN "Statement of Functions of the Licensed Practical Nurse" and are recommended by the U.S. Department of Health, Education and Welfare.

A. Participates in planning and providing nursing care for large groups of persons under extreme duress in various types of disaster situations by:

1. Providing for the emotional and physical comfort and safety of large numbers of disaster victims with limited supplies, equipment, utilities, and personnel through:
   a. Understanding the emotional stress caused by personal fear, problems of displacement of people and separation of families, increasing anxiety and continuing danger.
   b. Helping people with different cultural backgrounds and religious beliefs to accept and adapt to shelter and disrupted living conditions under crowded and often adverse situations.
   c. Recognizing and understanding the effect of disrupted social and economic patterns, such as personal and material losses, emotional trauma, and crowded living conditions.
   d. Encouraging patients to verbalize their concerns and fears and guiding them in performing certain tasks.
   e. Participating in the development, revision, and implementation of nursing procedures designed to insure the comfort and safety of patients and personnel under chaotic conditions.
   f. Providing for basic instruction to disaster victims in the aspects of appropriate self-care, encouraging them to further provide for their own needs and the needs of others.
2. Observing, recording, and reporting to appropriate persons (record and report forms may have to be improvised):
   a. General physical and mental condition of patients and signs and symptoms which may be indicative of change.
   b. Stresses in human relationships between patients and patients' families, visitors and personnel.
3. Performing nursing procedures within the framework of a disaster situation by utilizing skill and judgment for the good of the greatest number of people:
   a. Administering medications and treatments as directed and improvising supplies, equipment and techniques as necessary.
   b. Carrying out precautionary measures, including the maintenance of a safe and sanitary environment and the separation of patients with communicable diseases.
   c. Performing emergency first aid measures.
   d. Utilizing improvised supplies and observing aseptic

techniques such as sterilization.

4. Working toward restoration of community and family life according to available resources by:
   a. Encouraging individual self-help and work therapy.
   b. Encouraging activities of family living, with adaptations designed to attain and maintain a sanitary and healthy environment.
   c. Applying the principles of deformity prevention by using improvised equipment and available resources.
   d. Utilizing existing community facilities and resources, including family and neighbors, for continuing patient care.

B. Promoting the effectiveness of the health service agency in disaster preparedness through:
   1. Knowing and interpreting the disaster plan of the health agency.
   2. Understanding the relationship between the agency plan, the local government plan and the local Red Cross plan.
   3. Promoting maintenance and restoration of community health by participating in the control of environment health hazards.

CLINICAL CASE PROBLEMS

1. While driving home from work one afternoon, you come upon the scene of an accident. There are two victims inside the wrecked automobile and one lying on the side of the road. The two persons in the car are bleeding moderately from small lacerations. One is unconscious and has a large bruised and swollen area on his forehead. The other person is hysterical and cannot move his leg without great pain. The victim lying on the side of the road has no visible signs of injury, but he is not breathing.

Which victim is treated first? How is he treated?

If help is available, what should be done for the apparent fracture?

If help is not available, what would you say to the victim with the fracture?

How would you control moderate bleeding?

2. While you are working in the Emergency Unit late one evening, there is not much work to do, and you hear one member of the staff complaining in a loud voice about "people who don't seem to know what the word emergency means." She is referring to several persons who have come in with nonemergency ills and are waiting to see a physician.

What impressions are being given by the complaining nurse's comments?

What can you do to use your time productively while there is a lull in activity in the Emergency Room?

Have you or has a member of your family ever been a patient in a serious emergency situation?

3. A friend of yours who is a Red Cross volunteer driver tells you about a course being offered by the Civil Defense Office and asks you to join her in taking the course.

Do you think you could gain anything by taking a course in civil defense planning?

What do you know about disaster nursing plans in your community?

What would you do if a hurricane hit your community one night while you were asleep?

4. You have answered a call for help during a disaster following a tornado in your community. When you

arrive at the hospital you are asked to take care of a person with multiple injuries until a physician can see him.

Read the flow chart (Fig. 23-6) and explain what you would do to help this person.

REFERENCES

1. "Animal Bites: When and What to Worry About." Nursing Update, July, 1971.
2. Brunner, L. S., et al.: *Textbook of Medical-Surgical Nursing,* 2nd edition. Philadelphia, J. B. Lippincott Co., 1970.
3. Chandler, J. G.: "The Physiology and Treatment of Shock." RN, June, 1971, p. 42.
4. Committee on Trauma, American Academy of Orthopedic Surgeons: *Emergency Care and Transportation of the Sick and Injured.* Menasha, George Banta Co., 1971.
5. "Dealing Firmly with the Violent Patient." Nursing '72, July, 1972, p. 29.
6. Fink, M., et al.: "Narcotic Antagonists." Am. Journ. Nurs., July, 1971, p. 1359.
7. Francis, B. J.: "Current Concepts in Immunization." Am. Journ. Nurs., April, 1973, p. 646.
8. Kilpatrick, H. M.: "The Frightened Patient in the Emergency Room." Am. Journ. Nurs., May, 1966, p. 1031.
9. Magnussen, A.: "Who Does What in Defense, in Natural Disaster." Am. Journ. Nurs., March, 1965, p. 118.
10. Miller, R. R., and Johnson, S. R.: "Poison Control Now and in the Future." Am. Journ. Nurs., Sept., 1966, p. 1984.
11. *Modern Medical Encyclopedia.* New York, Golden Press, 1965.
12. "Naloxone." Nursing '72, May, 1972, p. 17.
13. Nott, L. M., and Petty, T. L.: "Acute Respiratory Failure." Am. Journ. Nurs., Sept., 1967, p. 1847.
14. O'Boyle, C.: "A New Era in Emergency Services." Am. Journ. Nurs., Aug., 1972, p. 1392.
15. "Priorities in Managing the Patient with Multiple Injuries." Nursing Update, May, 1971, p. 3.
16. Renshaw, D. C.: "Psychiatric First Aid in an Emergency." Am. Journ. Nurs., March, 1972, p. 497.
17. Rodman, M. J.: "Poisonings and Their Treatment." RN, Nov., 1972, p. 57.
18. Russel, F. E.: "Injuries by Venomous Animals." Am. Journ. Nurs., June, 1966, p. 1322.
19. Shafer, K. N., et al.: *Medical-Surgical Nursing,* 5th edition. St. Louis, The C. V. Mosby Co., 1971.
20. Sullivan, C. M.: "Preparedness May Mean Survival." Am. Journ. Nurs., Nov., 1965, p. 121.
21. "Water Sport Injuries." Nursing Update, June, 1972.
22. Weinstock, F. J.: "Emergency Treatment of Eye Injuries." Am. Journ. Nurs., Oct., 1971, p. 1928.

SUGGESTED STUDENT READING

1. "Animal Bites: When and What to Worry About." Nursing Update, July, 1971.
2. Beatty, C. J.: "Guess Who's Dying at Dinner?" RN, Nov., 1972, p. 52.
3. Chandler, J. G.: "The Physiology and Treatment of Shock." RN, June, 1971, p. 42.
4. Committee on Trauma, American Academy of Orthopedic Surgeons: *Emergency Care and Transportation of the Sick and Injured.* Menasha, George Banta Co., 1971.
5. "The Emergency Room Nurse." Journ. Pract. Nurs., March, 1966, p. 20.
6. Kerr, R. R.: "The LPN as ER Nurse." Journ. Pract. Nurs., Aug., 1969, p. 32.
7. Kretzger, M. P., and Engley, F. B.: "Preventing Food Poisoning." RN, June, 1970, p. 50.
8. Rodman, M. J.: "Poisonings and Their Treatment." RN, Nov., 1972, p. 57.
9. Tyler, M. L.: "Getting a Proper Fit with an Ambu Mask." Nursing '72, April, 1972, p. 25.
10. U.S. Department of Health, Education and Welfare, Public Health Service: "The Role of the Licensed Practical Nurse in National Disaster." 1967.
11. Weinstock, F. J.: "Emergency Treatment of Eye Injuries." Am. Journ. Nurs., Oct., 1971, p. 1928.

OUTLINE FOR CHAPTER 23

I. Prevention of Accidents

A. Home safety.
   1. More than one fourth of all accidental deaths occur in the home.
   2. Principal victims are children and the elderly.
   3. Education of the public will help prevent accidents.
B. Highway safety.
   1. Motor vehicle accidents are leading cause of death in this country.
   2. Two major causes of such accidents are human failure and mechanical failure.
C. Water safety.
   1. Observing the common-sense rules of water safety helps prevent accidents.
   2. Rescue methods vary. Attempt a

swimming rescue only if you are experienced.

3. Artificial respiration may be necessary.

4. Have victim lie down, and treat for shock.

II. General Principles of First Aid

A. Think before acting.

B. Move slowly and deliberately, and act with confidence.

C. Evaluate injuries and summon help.

D. Treat respiratory failure and hemorrhage first.

E. Prevent or treat shock.

F. Observe victim carefully and frequently for signs of change in his condition.

III. Control of Bleeding

A. Place clean or sterile dressing over wound, and apply firm, steady pressure with hand or wrapping. Do not wrap wound so tightly as to constrict circulation to distal parts.

B. Elevate and immobilize the injured part.

C. If pressure to wound does not decrease blood loss from wound, apply pressure to pressure point above the artery serving the wounded area.

D. Use of tourniquet must be last resort, as when other methods fail and victim's life is in danger or when limb is amputated, severely mangled or crushed.

1. Tourniquet should be removed only by physician.

2. Do not cover tourniquet.

IV. Shock

A. Types are neurogenic and hematogenic.

B. Symptoms due to inadequate blood volume, loss of tone and then collapse of peripheral vessels and shift of body fluids. They are pallor, weak pulse, clammy skin and thirst.

C. Management of shock:

1. Reassure and comfort the patient.

2. Maintain body heat.

3. Place head lower than feet.

4. Restore circulating blood volume, relieve respiratory embarrassment and control pain.

V. Burns

A. Two dangers are shock and infection.

B. Minor burns should be immersed in ice water or covered with cold compresses. Apply sterile petroleum jelly or a paste of baking soda and water and cover with loose bandage.

C. Major burns.

1. Cover with clean, dry dressing, and transport victim to hospital or clinic.

2. Give him fluids to drink.

3. Never apply ointments or disturb blisters.

D. Chemical burns.

1. Flush with water.

2. Cover with a dressing, and transport victim to hospital.

VI. Poisoning

A. Education can help prevent accidental poisoning.

B. Symptoms—poisoning should be suspected if victim becomes suddenly ill and if there is a peculiar odor to the breath and an open container nearby. Save container or vomitus for identification.

C. Swallowed poisons.

1. Induce vomiting, except for corrosive poisons or petroleum products.

2. Give specific antidote if it is known, or give universal antidote.

D. Inhaled poisons.

1. Transport victim to source of fresh air.

2. Give artificial respiration as necessary.

3. Keep victim warm and quiet; do not give alcohol or stimulants.

E. Barbiturate poisoning.

1. Most frequent in suicide attempts.

2. Induce vomiting.

3. Obtain medical help immediately, or patient may die of respiratory failure.

F. Poisoning by morphine and other sedatives which cause severe depression of the central nervous system.

1. Administer coffee or strong tea.

2. Give artificial respiration as needed.

3. Obtain medical help immediately.

G. Poisoning by carbon monoxide and other lethal gases.

1. Transport victim to source of fresh air.

2. Administer artificial respiration and oxygen.
3. Keep victim warm, and avoid stimulation.

H. Food poisoning due to toxins produced by bacteria in contaminated foods.

1. Prevented by proper preparation, storage and handling of food.
2. Onset is acute with severe gastrointestinal disturbances.
3. Treatment—remove from intestinal tract, and begin supportive measures.

VII. Fractures

VIII. Head Injury

A. Keep patient quiet.
B. Have a doctor see victim.

IX. Chest and Abdominal Wounds

A. Sucking chest wound treated with occlusive dressing.
B. Impaled objects protruding from a wound are *not* removed. The object is stabilized and dressings applied around it.
C. Flail chest is splinted with small pillow or other bulky material.
D. Open wound of abdomen with evisceration is covered with warm, moist dressing.

X. Electric Shock

A. Give artificial respiration, and treat burns as needed.
B. Use caution in separating victim from source of electric current.

XI. Emergency Childbirth

A. Avoid contamination as much as possible.
B. Do not pull infant through birth canal.
C. Cut cord if medical help is not available within an hour.
D. Save placenta for physician's inspection.
E. Massage the fundus after expulsion of the placenta.

XII. Animal Bites

A. Treat wound immediately.
B. Pasteur treatment may be necessary if examination of the animal reveals the possibility of rabies.

XIII. Snake Bite

A. Nonpoisonous snake bite is treated as minor wound.
B. Poisonous snake bite is treated by tourniquet, incision, suction and antivenin.

XIV. Insect Bites or Stings

A. Serious stings require immediate attention.
B. Apply paste of baking soda and water or meat tenderizer and cold compresses to less serious stings.
C. Apply a drop of turpentine or mineral oil to ticks, and remove. Wash the area with soap and water, and apply an antiseptic.

XV. Injuries Due to Extreme Heat

A. Heatstroke (sunstroke)—a disturbance in the heat-regulating mechanism in the brain allows patient's body temperature to become extremely high. Cool with cool water.
B. Heat exhaustion (heat prostration) is caused by excessive loss of salt and water through perspiration. Treated by replacement of these substances.
C. Sunburn—treat minor burn with solution of baking soda or Epsom salts and water. Major burns require medical attention as soon as possible.

XVI. Injuries Due to Extreme Cold

A. Hypothermia is a drastic lowering of body temperature. Patient is rewarmed by warm bath and blankets.
B. Frostbite is a local condition associated with constriction of blood vessels and damage to tissue and vessel walls.

1. Rewarm quickly by immersion in warm water.
2. Do not rub; handle very gently.

XVII. The Unruly Patient

A. Patient who is violent is terribly afraid.
B. Identify yourself, and speak to the patient, using his name frequently.
C. Try simple commands to help patient gain control of himself.
D. If physical restraint is used, be sure enough people are available to subdue the patient. Do not leave him alone immediately after he is restrained.

XVIII. The Hospital Emergency Room

A. Increasing number of nonemergency cases being treated in the hospital emergency units.

B. Become familiar with procedures, policies and equipment of the institution.

XIX. Disaster Nursing

A. A disaster involves loss of property, physical injuries and interruption in activities of daily living on a large scale.

B. Agencies involved in planning disaster nursing are Office of Civil Defense, Red Cross and other local voluntary organizations.

C. Nurse's responsibilities:
   1. Know community disaster plans.
   2. Provide leadership and nursing care.

D. Functions of the nurse:
   1. Provide for emotional and physical comfort and safety of victims.
   2. Work to increase effectiveness of local disaster planning agency.

GLOSSARY

Abduction—The withdrawal of a part away from the center of the body.

Absorption—The taking up of fluids or other substances.

Adduction—The act of drawing a part toward the center of the body.

Aerosols—Solutions of a drug or a bactericide that can be atomized into a fine mist.

Albumin—One of a group of simple proteins that yield only amino acids or their derivatives on hydrolysis.

Alkali—One of a group of compounds that form salts when united with acids and soaps when combined with fats. A base, or substance capable of neutralizing acids.

Alopecia—Loss of hair from a part of the body that is normally hairy.

Altruistic—Unselfishly thoughtful or working for the welfare of others.

Amino acids—A group of organic compounds that form the chief structure of proteins.

Anaerobic—Able to grow only in the absence of oxygen.

Analgesic—Relieving pain.

Aneurysm—A bulging outward of a portion of a blood vessel that has been damaged by disease or weakened by a congenital defect in the vessel wall.

Ankylosis—Abnormal fixation and immobility of a joint.

Antigen—A substance that stimulates the formation of a specific antibody and which reacts specifically with its antibody.

Anxiety—A feeling of extreme uncertainty and fear.

Aphasia—A defect in or the loss of the power of speech.

Apprehension—A mental state of fear in which danger or harm to oneself is anticipated.

Arteriography—X-ray filming of an artery following injection of a contrast medium.

Asepsis—Absence of infectious material; freedom from infection.

Aspiration—The act of breathing or drawing in.

Atelectasis—Incomplete expansion or collapse of the alveoli of a segment or entire lobe of the lung.

Atom—The smallest part of an element that can exist and still retain the chemical properties of the element.

Atrophy—A wasting away or reduction in size of a cell, organ or part of the body.

Audiology—The science concerned with the sense of hearing.

Autoclave—An apparatus used to apply steam under pressure for the purpose of sterilization.

Autoimmunity—The immune reaction of an organism to its own tissues.

Avitaminosis—A condition due to a lack of one or more vitamins in the diet.

Balanitis—Inflammation of the glans penis, usually associated with phymosis.

Benign—Not malignant; not having a tendency to recur; having a favorable outcome.

Bilirubin—A red bile pigment formed from the hemoglobin of red blood cells.

Biology—The science of physical life or living matter in all its forms and phenomena.

Blepharitis—Inflammation of the edges of the eyelids.

Bradycardia—Abnormal slowness of the heart beat and pulse.

Bronchioles—The smaller subdivisions of the bronchial tubes.

Bursa—A sac or sac-like structure filled with fluid that acts as a cushion and prevents friction between two moving parts.

Calorie—A unit of heat. In the study of metabolism, a calorie is the amount of heat required to raise the temperature of 1 kg. of water 1 degree centigrade.

Cannula—A tube for insertion into the body. It usually encases a trocar that is used during insertion and then removed.

Capillary—Any one of the minute, hair-like vessels that connect the smaller arteries with the smaller veins.

Carrier—An individual who harbors in his body the specific organisms of a disease but does not have the symptoms and thus can spread the infection undetected.

Catalyst—A substance that alters the speed of a reaction but does not form part of the final product.

Caustic—Burning or corrosive; capable of destroying living tissue.

Cauterize—Applying a caustic substance, hot iron or electric current as a means of killing tissue.

Cerebrospinal—Pertaining to the brain and spinal cord.

Cervix—Neck or neck-like part.

Coma—A state of unconsciousness in which the affected person is unresponsive to even the most powerful stimuli.

Concussion—A severe jar or shock, or the condition that results from such an injury.

Conduction—The transmission or transfer of sound waves, nerve impulses or electrical charges.

Contour—The outline or configuration of the body or one of its parts.

Contracture—A condition in which there is fixed resistance to the stretching of a muscle. It results from fibrosis of the tissues surrounding a joint or from disorders of the muscle fibers.

Curettage—Scraping the walls of a cavity such as the uterus.

Cyst—A sac or sac-like structure, usually abnormal, containing liquid or semi-solid matter and often caused by blockage of a passage.

Cytology—Study of cells.

Cytotoxic—An agent poisonous to cells.

Debilitated—Weak; lacking strength.

Debridement—The removal of all dead tissue and foreign matter in or near a wound.

Defibrillator—An apparatus used to counteract convulsive twitching of the heart muscle by application of electric impulses to the heart.

Dehydration—Removal of water from the body or a tissue; or the condition resulting from excessive loss of water.

Delusion—A false belief that cannot be changed by reason, argument or persuasion.

Dermatology—The branch of medicine concerned with diagnosis and treatment of skin disorders.

Deviation—A turning away from the center or from the normal course.

Diaphragm—1. The dome-shaped muscle separating the throacic and abdominal cavities and aiding in the function of respiration. 2. Thin partition.

Diastole—The period of dilation of the heart when the ventricles fill with blood.

Diathermy—The generation of heat produced by the resistance of body tissues to the passage of high frequency electric impulses.

Diffusion—The process of passing through or spreading widely through a tissue or structure.

Dilatation—The condition of being stretched beyond normal dimensions.

Disability—A condition in which one is deprived of power or crippled.

Disinfectant—An agent that destroys pathogenic organisms.

Distention—The state of being enlarged.

Duct—A tube, pipe or channel for conveying liquid, air or other matter.

Dysphagia—Difficulty in swallowing.

Dyspnea—Difficult or labored breathing.

Dysuria—Painful or difficult urination.

Ectopic—Located away from the normal position.

Electrolyte—A compound which, when in solution, will conduct an electrical current by means of its ions.

Element—Any one of the basic parts or constituents of a thing. In chemistry, a simple substance that cannot be broken down by ordinary chemical means.

Embolism—The obstruction of a blood vessel by a clot, plug of fat or other substances brought there by the blood.

Empathy—Entering through imagination into the feelings or motives of another.

Enzyme—A complex protein produced in living cells and able to act as a catalyst in chemical change, particularly in the changing of a substrate for which the enzyme is specific.

Epiphysis—The end of a long bone, usually wider than the shaft and resembling a knob. It is either made up of cartilage or separated from the shaft by a disc of cartilage.

Equilibrium—A state of balance.

Erythema—Redness of the skin produced by congestion of the capillaries.

Eschar—A hard crust or scab produced by a burn or corrosive agent.

Euphoria—An exaggerated feeling of well-being or bodily comfort.

Exacerbation—Increase in severity of a symptom or disease.

Excreted—Thrown off as waste matter in a normal discharge.

Exfoliate—To fall off in scales or layers.

Expiration—The act of exhaling air from the lungs.

Extension—A stretching out or prolonging in time, space or direction.

Exudate—Material that has escaped from blood vessels and has been deposited in or on tissues, usually as a result of inflammation.

Facade—A front or outward part of anything.

Facies—The appearance of or expression on a face.

Febrile—Pertaining to fever.

Fibrin—A whitish, insoluble protein that forms the essential protein of a blood clot.

Filtration—The passage of a liquid through a straining device.

Fissure—A cleft or groove.

Fistula—An abnormal passage.

Flaccid—Weak or limp.

Flatus—Gas in the intestinal tract.

Flexion—The bending of a limb of other part.

Fulguration—Destruction of tissues by the application of electric sparks that are controlled by a movable electrode.

Fundus—The base or part of a hollow organ that is farthest removed from its mouth.

Geriatrics—The branch of medicine concerned with problems peculiar to old age and aging.

Gerontology—The scientific study of all problems of aging.

Gingivitis—Inflammation of the gums.

Globulin—Any one of a class of proteins. Gamma globulins are plasma proteins that react with specific harmful agents such as bacteria, viruses or toxins that invade the body.

Glycosuria—The presence of abnormal amounts of glucose in the urine.

Gynecology—That branch of medicine concerned with the diagnosis and treatment of disorders of the female genital tract.

Hematinic—An agent that increases the hemoglobin level and the number of red blood cells.

Hematoma—A tumor containing blood that has escaped from an injured vessel.

Hematuria—Blood in the urine.

Hemiplegia—Paralysis of one side of the body.

Hemolysis—Destruction of red blood cells with the liberation of hemoglobin.

Hemoptysis—The spitting of blood or blood-stained sputum.

Hepatic—Pertaining to the liver.

Hormone—A chemical substance, formed in certain parts of the body, that has a specific effect on the activity of a certain "target" organ.

Hydrocele—A collection of fluid, especially in the scrotal sac.

Hydrolysis—The splitting of a compound into fragments by the addition of water.

Hypercalcemia—Excessive amount of calcium in the blood.

Hyperpnea—Abnormal increase in the rate and depth of respiration.

Hypersensitive—Having an abnormally increased sensitivity, especially in regard to a reaction to certain substances which are innocuous to a normal person.

Hypothalamus—That portion of the brain that forms the floor and part of the lateral wall of the third ventricle. It exerts control over visceral activities, water balance, body temperature and sleep.

Idiopathic—Without a known cause, self-originating.

Idiosyncrasy—1. A feeling, liking or aversion peculiar to a single person or group. 2. An abnormal sensitivity to some drug, protein or other agent that is peculiar to a person.

Immunity—Security against a particular disease or poison.

Impaction—The condition of being firmly lodged or wedged.

Incoherent—Confused, disconnected.

Inspiration—The act of drawing air into the lungs.

Intercostal—Situated between the ribs.

Interdependent—Mutually dependent.

Interstitial—Pertaining to or situated in the interstices or interspaces of a tissue.

Intracranial—Within the skull.

Intraocular—Within the eye.

Intussusception—A telescoping of one part of the intestine into the lumen of an immediately adjacent segment.

Isotope—Any of two or more forms of a chemical element having the same chemical properties and the same atomic number, but different weights or radioactive behavior.

Lacrimal—Pertaining to the tears.

Leiomyoma—A benign tumor arising from smooth muscle.

Lipoid—Resembling fat.

Lumen—The space within a tubular organ such as a blood vessel.

Lymphatic—Pertaining to or containing lymph.

Malignant—Tending to become progressively worse and to have a fatal outcome.

Mediastinum—1. Septum or partition. 2. A partition formed by the two pleurae between the lungs, including the enclosed space in which are all the viscera of the thorax except the lungs.

Menarche—The beginning of menstruation.

Menopause—Cessation of menstruation.

Meninges—The three membranes that cover the brain and spinal cord: the dura mater, pia mater and arachnoid.

Necrotic—Pertaining to the death of tissue.

Neoplasm—Any new or abnormal growth, such as tumor.

Nevus—A mole or birthmark.

Nodular—Pertaining to a swelling or protuberance.

Occiput—The back of the head.

Occlusion—The state of being closed or shut off.

Occult—Concealed from observation.

Ocular—Pertaining to the eye.

Oxidation—The act of combining or causing to combine with oxygen.

Palliative—Providing relief, but not a cure.

Palsy—Paralysis.

Paracentesis—Surgical puncture of a cavity for the aspiration of fluid.

Pathogenic—Producing disease.

Pectoral—Pertaining to the chest or breast.

Pedicle—A base or stem-like part.

Penetration—The act or power of going into or through.

Perineum—The area between the anus and the genital organs.

Phagocyte—Any cell that ingests microorganisms or other cells and foreign particles.

Phimosis—Restriction of the foreskin so that it cannot be drawn back over the glans penis.

Placebo—A pill or injection given to a person as medicine but actually containing no active ingredients.

Platelet—A circular disc that is one of the blood elements and concerned with coagulation of blood.

Poultice—A soft, hot, moist mass of mustard, herbs or other medicines applied to the body for therapy.

Prophylaxis—Prevention of disease; preventive treatments.

Radiopaque—Not transparent to x-rays or other radioactive substances.

Reaction—The response of a part to stimulation.

Reflex—An involuntary action in direct response to stimulation of a nerve.

Remission—An abatement or lessening of the symptoms of a disease; also, the period during which such an abatement occurs.

Residue—That which remains after the removal of other substances.

Resistance—The act of withstanding or opposing.

Resorption—The act of absorbing again.

Sclerosis—A hardening, especially hardening of a part from inflammation.

Secrete—To separate or elaborate cell products.

Sinus—1. A cavity or hollow space. 2. An abnormal channel or opening allowing the escape of pus.

Spermatozoon—The male germ cell produced by the testes.

Spore—A single cell which becomes free and is capable of reproduction. It can flourish without oxygen and can develop resistance to pasteurization.

Stasis—A stoppage of the flow of blood or other body fluids in any part.

Stoma—Any minute pore, orifice or opening on a free surface.

Supine—Lying with the face upward.

Susceptible—Readily affected or acted upon.

Synthesis—The artificial building up of a chemical compound by uniting its elements.

Systemic—Pertaining to or affecting the body as a whole.

Systole—The period of contraction of the heart, especially contraction of the ventricles.

Tachycardia—Excessively rapid action of the heart.

Therapeutic—Pertaining to the art of healing; curative.

Thoracentesis—Surgical puncture of the chest wall with drainage of fluid.

Thromboplastin—A factor essential to the production of thrombin and proper coagulation of blood.

Tinnitus—A noise or ringing in the ears.

Toxic—Poisonous.

Transmitted—Transferred; carried across.

Trauma—A wound or injury.

Tremor—An involuntary trembling or quivering.

Trocar—A sharp-pointed instrument used with a cannula for piercing a part of the body.

Vascular—Pertaining to or full or vessels.

Virulent—Exceedingly pathogenic, noxious or harmful.

Vital—Necessary to or pertaining to life.

Volvulus—A knotting or twisting of the bowel, producing intestinal obstruction.

INDEX

Page references to illustrations are printed in *italics;* page references to tables are followed by the letter t.